Scientific principles in nursing

SEVENTH EDITION

Scientific principles in nursing

Shirley Hawke Gragg, R.N., B.S.N., M.R.E.
Formerly Instructor in Nursing, East Tennessee State University School of Nursing,
Johnson City, Tennessee

Olive M. Rees, R.N., M.A.
Chairman, Health Science Division; Director, Associate Degree Program in Nursing,
Golden West College, Huntington Beach, California

With 257 illustrations

The C. V. Mosby Company
Saint Louis 1974

Seventh edition

Copyright © 1974 by The C. V. Mosby Company

All rights reserved. No part of this book may be reproduced
in any manner without written permission of the publisher.

Previous editions copyrighted 1950, 1953, 1958, 1962, 1966, 1970

Printed in the United States of America

Distributed in Great Britain by Henry Kimpton, London

Library of Congress Cataloging in Publication Data

Gragg, Shirley Hawke.
  Scientific principles in nursing.

  First-2d ed. by M. E. McClain; 3d-5th ed. by M. E.
McClain and S. H. Gragg.
  Includes bibliographies.
  1. Nurses and nursing. I. McClain, Mary Esther,
1900-   Scientific principles in nursing.
II. Rees, Olive M., joint author. II. Title.
[DNLM: 1. Nursing care. WY100 G737s 1974]
RT41.G8 1974   610.73   73-22272
ISBN 0-8016-1952-1

TS/CB/B 9 8 7 6 5 4 3

Preface

THE SEVENTH EDITION of *Scientific Principles in Nursing* suggests the use of a theoretical model for the process of nursing that should assist in guiding the student toward forming habits of patient care leading to a high probability of success.

The escalating demands upon nursing to assume its full share of responsibility toward attaining and maintaining the quality of health care delivery, in keeping with the changing times and human needs, causes attention to be focused on the public's expectation for better-prepared practitioners. The demand is for nurses equipped with the knowledge and behaviors essential to promoting the individual's wellness, preventing disease and injury, and facilitating the patient's progress from illness toward optimum health. Hence, a variety of selected physiologic, psychologic, and sociologic concepts are suggested that supply the nursing student and practitioner with a rational approach to planning patient care that meets the needs of the individual as he responds holistically to his environment.

It is intended that the ideas presented will provide fruitful ways of translating concepts into nursing behaviors as the student is led to apply scientific principles through problem-solving activities in utilizing the modified adaptation model described in Chapter 6.

Throughout the book the interdependent nature of health problems is recognized, and understanding of the concepts of stress and homeostasis is presented as a basic component in planning and implementing holistic patient care.

Though many persons have been inspirational in the preparation of this revision, we wish to express our appreciation for manuscript review to nursing instructors of Golden West College, Huntington Beach, California (Miss Jean Kirkpatrick, Mrs. Nancy English, Mrs. Shirley Matachak, and Mrs. Winifred Wilson). We are also grateful to Sister Callista Roy, who reviewed Chapter 6.

Recognition is also due to Bill Parsons and Tom Minter, for photographic work; to the Golden West College nursing students; and to Mrs. Lillimae Hester and other personnel of Hoag Memorial Hospital, Newport Beach, for their part in making the photography possible.

We are deeply indebted to the staff and faculty of the East Tennessee Baptist Hospital and School of Nursing, Knoxville, Tennessee, for the use of their clinical facilities, personnel, and library, and also for their assistance in photographic work and other illustrations.

Other special contributors to whom we express our appreciation are Mrs. Mary Ruffin Griffin, of East Tennessee State University, for her help on home care nursing plans and advice on community and public health nursing; Mrs. Lillian D. Riddick, formerly of Temple University, for her assistance in our research in terminal and long-term care; Chaplain Fred Linkenhoker, East Tennessee Baptist Hospital, for his advice in spiritual and religious areas; Mrs. Gay C. Warren, of East Tennessee Baptist Hospital, for our range of motion illustrations; and Mrs. Dolly Lorene Farris, of Jackson Memorial Hospital, Miami, Florida, for various suggestions throughout the book in relation to patient teaching.

We are grateful to student nurses Vicky Brock, Cheryl Bryant, Ronald Coker, and Steven Robinson, who so generously gave of their time to participate in our projects, and to Mrs. Betty Shelley, Mrs. Margaret Parsons, Rebecca Daugherty, Betty Roope, Charlotte Accuff, Norma Jean Miller, Cheryl Dothard, Peggy Orren, and Cecil Murphy, who helped in various ways during the final stages of the production of the manuscript, enabling us to make this revision a reality.

Shirley H. Gragg
Olive M. Rees

Contents

Scientific principles in nursing

UNIT ONE
Introduction

1 Nursing

AN INTERPRETATION

NURSING IN THE 1970's
The dilemma of health care delivery

Nursing, like every other profession in the 1970's, is in the midst of unparalleled change. The individual nurse may well inquire into the pressures forcing the fast-moving and challenging changes in the nursing profession and be concerned about the direction of these changes and their ultimate effect upon the practice of nursing and the future role of the profession in our society.

The social forces affecting nursing are closely related to the problems of keeping pace with increasing public pressure for a system of health care delivery that will make quality care readily available to all people when and where needed and at a cost society can afford. This growing philosophic belief in the worth and dignity of the individual is being felt with increasing impact by the health professions, including nursing. The stimulus is to find ways of providing quality health care that incorporate the modern advances in medical and scientific research and the increased understanding of man himself,

which wlll lead to improved patient care. Surely the knowledge, skills, and resources sufficient to accomplish this goal are accessible.

A major task of nursing in the 1970's may prove to be that of translating principles into responsible practice while keeping abreast of the phenomenal demands of modern society for improved health service. The nursing profession should play a large and indispensable role in improving the quality, effectiveness, and cost of the health care expected by the American people. The public demand now is that health care be considered from the viewpoint of the consumers of health services as well as of the providers of these services. A part of the total problem has been the gap between the ideal and reality in these viewpoints. Efforts are being directed toward closing this gap through providing the public with an opportunity for a voice in the design and operation of health systems development that will meet the changing demands.

Health care includes not only the diagnosis, treatment, and rehabilitation asso-

3

ciated with acute and chronic illness but also early case finding, prevention, health maintenance, and health education. In its entirety, health care is the sum of care provided by all health disciplines. Modern comprehensive health care involves the integration of the skills and services of many professions, often in a team approach, with each member seeking to achieve the common goals.

It is anticipated that nursing must assume an increasingly larger place and extended scope of practice within the community of health professions if the goal of ready availability of quality health care is to be achieved for all citizens.

What is nursing?

In modern society nursing is viewed as a desirable and necessary human service in that it is a way of assisting persons who are sick, aged, or otherwise incapacitated to cope with their needs in illness and, within their existing potential, to regain or attain responsibility for self-care. Self-care is the responsibility of the individual to care for himself in order to maintain his mental and physical health; if self-care is not maintained, illness or death is inevitable. The nurse may guide and instruct other persons to maintain wellness through self-care.

Nurses may manage and maintain the required self-care for incapacitated persons, guiding and instructing them as they move toward recovery and resumption of their own self-care (for others, to death with dignity), or they may instruct and supervise others who are assisting patients.

Among the essential elements of nursing practice, which is the provision of nursing services directly to patients, are those that are related to maintaining or restoring normal life functions (respiration, elimination, nutrition, circulation, rest and sleep, locomotion, and communication), observing and reporting signs of changes

in the patient's status, assessing his physical and emotional state, assessing environmental factors, formulating and implementing a plan for the provision of nursing care based on medical therapy and other factors affecting the patient and his family, and integrating the services of other health personnel.

In providing these services, the nurse functions as a responsible member of a health care team by interpreting and carrying out the instruction of the physician, by collaborating with professional colleagues in the planning and delivery of health services, and by acting independently when the needs of the patient and the principles of nursing practice so indicate.

Many attempts have been made to define nursing in specific and precise terms. While there are many statements in the literature that help to picture the nature, scope, dimensions, and concerns of nursing, as yet they do not seem to adequately describe how and why nursing is specifically unique and different from other human services.

Nursing and the total health services concept

It is helpful to view nursing in relation to the current overall concept of health care and to note that the focus of the nurse practitioner within this concept is on the individual patient and the process through which his individual needs may be met. While nursing literature reflects this philosophy, it is the practice of the individual nurse that must demonstrate that the true focus of the profession is on patient health care needs rather than on professional prerogatives.

The nursing process in today's complex society can be considered most realistically as a part of the changing pattern of total health services. In a recent report, the World Health Organization Expert Committee on Nursing suggests that any com-

4

plete health service will make provision for its operations within the following five broad categories.

1. The *health maintenance stage* is the most opportune time for applying and teaching all that we know about health (for example, principles of hygiene, nutrition, and mental health) to assist the individual in maintaining or attaining his highest potential for healthful living. During this stage the individual would, ideally, choose for himself courses of action most favorable to his own human functioning, referred to as self-care. A deep concern of nursing is the need of the individual for the power of self-care action on a continuous basis in order to maintain life, health, and well-being. Self-care is viewed as a requirement for every individual in order to avoid illness and death. It is a learned behavior and, therefore, is the content of health teaching of the nurse.

2. The *increased risk stage* is a predisease stage in which specific preventive measures can be applied most effectively to protect the individual who has an increased risk of a health problem or problems.

3. The *early detection stage* is the stage in which the focus is on identifying the individual who is in the early stages of an illness and, through early diagnosis and therapy, preventing unnecessary suffering, expense, and possible loss of life.

The second and third stages of complete health service afford a most fruitful area for extending the role of nursing. In the provision of health care, the nurse is a provider of personal health care services, working interdependently with the physician and other health professionals in the task of keeping people well through supporting self-care in the stages during which preventive measures and early detection and treatment are most successful in promoting health and well-being. In currently popular terminology, the level of nurse functioning in these first three stages of health services (level referring to type of preparation) is primarily *distributive.*

4. The *clinical stage* is the stage to which the individual too often progresses when his early symptoms were neither prevented nor diagnosed. The clinical stage still represents the area of greatest concentration of health care in the United States.

Again, in current terminology, the level of nurse functioning during the clinical stage is termed *episodic,* in accordance with the recommendations presented in *An Abstract for Action.*

5. The *rehabilitation stage* is the stage in which there is the most opportunity for preventing disability; it often overlaps with the preceding stages. The goal is to prevent disability, or when this is not possible, to assist the individual to achieve his maximum potential within his degree of disability, or when there is no possibility of rehabilitation and death is inevitable, to assist the patient in facing death with courage and dignity.

Elements of the nursing process

The essential elements of the nursing process in providing direct patient care may be derived from these various stages of health services. The nursing process forms the framework through which the nurse functions to meet specific responsibilities in the provision of patient care. These elements are presented in greater detail in Chapter 3, as phases of the problem-solving process. There are variations in outlining the nursing process and in the terminology appearing in the literature. However, the phases of the nursing process as here outlined are intended to be a beginning application of the problem-solving steps in working through the nursing process. These elements, which will be discussed in greater detail in Chapter 3, are the following:

1. Assessing the needs of patients who

5

have potential and/or actual health problems and identifying the related nursing problems

2. Collecting information about the patient's identified problems, which the nurse uses in stating the objectives to be achieved
3. Developing an appropriate nursing care plan in terms of the data collected and the relevant nursing principles
4. Exercising judgment in implementing the nursing care plan to provide optimum quality of nursing care
5. Evaluating the success of the nursing care plan in meeting the patient's individual needs, adjusting the plan accordingly to assist the patient in restoring and/or maintaining health, and achieving his potential for independence

This is a very brief introductory summary of the nursing process, which will be further described in later chapters. It is emphasized at this point that the nurse must be aware of the patient's medical problems and therapy when defining the nursing problems, formulating the objectives of nursing care, and evaluating the success of the plan of care. It is also important to remember that while for purposes of study the steps in the nursing process appear to be entirely separate and discrete actions, in reality they are interrelated and ongoing. Assessment and evaluation are constantly in progress in order that the plan of care may be promptly adjusted and improved according to changes occurring in the patient's status.

According to Orem in *Nursing: Concepts of Practice,* the need for nursing care exists when the individual is unable to engage in the amount and quality of self-care necessary to maintaining "life and health, in recovering from disease or injury, or in coping with their effects." An implication that may be inferred from this statement is that one of the major goals of patient care is to develop the patient's

fullest potential for independent functioning for self-care. The individual nurse contributes to this goal in conjunction with other members of the health care team. Today's nurse must be prepared to (1) assume responsibilities and functions concerned with health problems of individuals, sick or well, and (2) provide a range of service that the patient cannot provide for himself.

Current literature contains many descriptions and arguments about the expanded nursing role; primary care; extended practice; and pediatric, family, geriatric, and independent nurse practitioner. There is a great deal of divergence of opinion about nurses taking on these expanded roles with the intent of helping to meet the pressing health care needs of our society. Most of the prevailing differences of opinion about nursing can be related to the rapid change and uncertainty that seem to characterize modern society. When confusion exists, much of it can be viewed as stemming from the strain on the existing traditionalism that is still to be found in hospitals, medicine, and nursing and that is a reflection of the turbulence in a transitional society. In this formative period the student may find that concentration on the acquisition and application of scientific principles in approaching the study of nursing will be a means of keeping in step with the demands of contemporary society for better quality of nursing care.

A study of history reveals how world events and discoveries have influenced the development of nursing, its achievements through the years, what is being done now, and what may be done in the future. At any point in time, the history of nursing reflects the conditions and developments of the society within which it existed, and it can therefore be viewed as a product of growth and change throughout recorded history. Perhaps the changes occurring in society from one decade to the next and the resulting effect on the profession partially account for the continued delay in formulating a definition of nursing and a statement of its functions that is satisfying to all.

Some understanding of the important historical developments that have been influential in molding our present-day concepts of nursing will enable students to appreciate more fully the nature of the long struggle for professional advancement that has led to the current critical issues in the profession and that will assist them in recognizing the present as a vital and exciting period in which to be entering the field. Hopefully, it may also bring deeper appreciation of our heritage in nursing and inspire more thorough pursuit of learning and the achievement of excellence in the care of patients, based on the application of scientific principles. Perhaps the student will be stimulated to gain a more complete understanding of contemporary nursing through study of its colorful and often dramatic history as portrayed in the Suggested Readings that are listed at the end of the chapter and in other nursing literature.

EDUCATIONAL PREPARATION FOR NURSING

As changes occur in the health care delivery system and in nursing responsibilities, nursing education must also change to provide education for all levels of nursing practice in whatever setting they are located or by whatever title the nurse may function.

Currently the state laws recognize two types of nurses. Each type of nurse is eligible to take the specialized licensing examination on the basis of education, the requirement being completion of a state-approved program in nursing:

Registered nurse (RN). There are three recognized types of educational programs preparing graduates to qualify for licensure as a registered nurse. They are:

1. Programs in senior colleges or universities leading to the baccalaureate degree with a major in nursing, usually 4 years in length
2. Associate degree in nursing programs in community or junior colleges, 2 years in length
3. Diploma programs, usually sponsored by hospitals, approximately $2\frac{1}{2}$ to 3 years in length

Licensed practical (vocational) nurse (LPN, LVN). Approved programs are usually 1 year in length and may be sponsored by community colleges, hospitals, or other health agencies.

Some states have laws providing for licensure of applicants on the basis of experience rather than on their background of educational preparation for nursing.

Although there are many variations in nursing education programs, depending on the type of institution in which they are located and the length of the program, important common denominators can be recognized in qualified programs, regardless of the individual setting. Some identifiable commonalities in contemporary basic nursing education that seem to be emerging include the following:

1. Curricula emphasizing liberal education as essential for knowledgeable practice of nursing
2. Development of integrated core courses
3. Objectives developed in terms of desired student behavior that encourage the ability to weigh values, to form independent judgments about the care of patients, and to arrive at decisions on an intellectual level
4. Commitment of the nurse to the need for creative and therapeutic use of self in interacting with the patient
5. Learning experiences designed to develop understanding of fundamental principles and the application of theory in the practice of nursing
6. An atmosphere that stimulates students to think clearly and to be creative in their nursing performance and that encourages continuing edu-

cation for preparation beyond completion of the basic program in nursing

Nevertheless, a great deal of confusion has been created by the existence of these widely differing types of preparation for registered nurse licensure. There are many unresolved questions regarding the functioning of these variously educated nurses, and problems exist in the utilization of the registered nurse and the licensed practical (vocational) nurse in the provision of quality patient care. The problems of nursing service organization are further complicated by the addition of aides, orderlies, and other ancillary workers who usually receive only short-term, on-the-job instruction given by the employing health agency.

It is apparent that with the great variation in current systems of preparation for health care personnel, nursing service must be provided with guidelines for quality control of patient care in order that the variously prepared health care personnel may function in roles commensurate with preparation and experience.

The inadequacies of preparation received by health professionals, including nurses and physicians, are receiving a great deal of attention as momentum increases for developing extended roles in nursing. A possible remedial course of action is that health education centers would undertake curriculum development and innovative planning that would prepare practitioners for the physician-nurse team concept in optimum health care delivery systems. The opportunity for maximum levels of functioning in an interdependent relationship could then be provided for both professions. Planning for educational preparation and for specific professional roles would need to proceed concurrently so that the educational preparation would be designed to prepare the practitioner to function at the highest level of competence within the pattern of the health care delivery system. Continuing education,

structured for all health professionals, would encourage professional gains, improved quality of patient care, and personal rewards.

In the midst of the current pressures encouraging nursing to take on extended roles by incorporating some basic medical skills within a nursing and family-oriented context, there are insistent voices within the profession reminding us that nursing has its own body of knowledge, its own unique professional practice, and that it is this practice of nursing that should be developed and given operational independence (in the role of independent nurse practitioner), rather than creating expanded roles with specified medical care responsibilities, which, some believe, would still leave nursing with uncertain identity.

There is a great deal of concern in the nursing profession that sound guidelines for qualitative standards in nursing education and nursing practice be developed. Within the framework of the professional organizations, efforts are underway to define the nursing activities and responsibilities for nurses prepared at varying educational levels.

MAJOR NURSING ORGANIZATIONS

Much effort has been expended through the nursing organizations, and on the part of individual nursing leaders, to establish nursing as a profession. The two major national nursing organizations are the American Nurses' Association and the National League for Nursing. In addition, there are several special interest organizations—for example, the Association of Operating Room Nurses—that exert considerable strength in the upgrading of professional responsibilities in the specialty area.

American Nurses' Association. The American Nurses' Association (ANA) has a long history of service to nurses and to the public. It was developed originally out of the need felt by nurses before the turn of the century for working together in concerted action to resolve the issues confronting them. The primary concern of the Association has always been the welfare of the individual nurse and the protection of the public served by the profession. During the early, formative years of the developing profession, ANA worked diligently for improved standards of nursing education, for registration and licensure of all nurses educated according to these standards, and for improved employment standards. Through the efforts of ANA leadership the public has been protected from unsafe nursing care by unprepared individuals calling themselves nurses.

In recent years the structure of the organization has been revised to provide for many more functions and services. For example, its Economic Security Program has been centered on the welfare of the individual nurse, recognizing that the quality of patient care improves when the nurse finds working conditions satisfying rather than frustrating.

Among the current activities pertinent to present-day issues are efforts to establish functions, standards, and qualifications for nursing practice; to establish standards of nursing education and foster implementation through appropriate channels; to develop standards of nursing service; to establish a code of ethical conduct for practitioners; to promote research designed to advance nursing knowledge; and a number of other points.

Membership in ANA begins with the local district association. Registered nurses are eligible to apply for membership in the district association, usually in the area of residence or employment. Membership in the district association automatically confers membership in the state association, in ANA, and in the International Council of Nurses. Since licensure in good standing as a registered nurse in at least one state is a membership requirement, only registered nurses can become members. Therefore, ANA is the official, professional organization representing American nurses. It is the organization through which nurses themselves establish functions, activities, and goals of their profession. It serves as a spokesman for nursing in accordance with the wishes of its membership.

National League for Nursing. The central purpose of the National League for Nursing (NLN) is conveyed by the much publicized phrase from its Certificate of Incorporation: "... that the nursing needs of the people will be met."

While it is true that NLN and ANA have similar goals, each organization has its own programs, activities, responsibilities, and functions. NLN's membership includes not only nurses but any other interested persons, whether lay people or other members of the health team, who are concerned with nursing education or service and community health agencies. Both organizations are concerned with improved nursing care, but ANA accomplishes its work primarily through nurses themselves and within the nursing profession, while NLN works within the community and in association with individuals and groups outside of nursing but who are interested in nursing and better nursing care.

The League maintains a variety of services, including the accreditation service for schools of nursing, the evaluation and testing service, and the consultation service. All of the League's programs are intended to benefit both nursing and the public.

ANA's official publication is the *American Journal of Nursing,* while that of NLN is *Nursing Outlook.*

National Student Nurses' Association. The National Student Nurses' Association (NSNA) was established in 1953 for the purpose of aiding in the preparation of nursing students for the assumption of professional responsibilities that will eventually be theirs as registered nurses. To accomplish this purpose, NSNA has established an organizational pattern similar to ANA. The policies and programs of

9

NSNA are approved through its House of Delegates, whose membership consists of elected representatives from the state associations.

Activities of NSNA include preparation for membership and participation in ANA, stimulation of interest in and understanding of the programs and services of NLN, and assistance in the development and growth of the individual student by fostering good citizenship. Ongoing projects and services of the organization vary with changing circumstances and needs.

The official publication is the *American Journal of Nursing.* However, the quarterly *NSNA News Letter* is a valuable publication for keeping the membership aware of activities and issues, within both NSNA and the profession.

THE NURSE AND THE LAW

Some knowledge of the law is essential, for as a member of a health service occupation, any nurse may be involved in situations that can lead to litigation. Therefore, the nurse needs to be aware of the extent of personal responsibilities and privileges assumed in the nursing role. A brief introduction to the legal aspects of nursing is included here to aid the nursing student to begin understanding both the nurse's legal responsibilities and privileges and the patient's rights.

The nursing student

The relationship of the student and the school of nursing is, in effect, that of a contract, even though it may not be in writing, which continues while the student is enrolled. Both the student and the school have responsibilities in this relationship.

The school of nursing must meet the criteria for approval by the state board of nursing in the individual state. One of the universal state board minimum requirements is that the school must maintain a faculty competent to instruct the student in both the theory and the practice of nursing. The faculty is expected to be competent to guide the student in practicing nursing skills safely for the patient, himself, and others.

The legal right for the student to practice those nursing skills that are the legal prerogative of the registered nurse is conferred by the Nursing Practice Act in most of the states, and it is also usually included in the state board of nursing's rules and regulations. In most states, the provision is so stated that the student has the legal right to practice when the assignment is a part of the approved program of the school of nursing. This implies that the student does not have this legal right of performance in any other situation.

Written contractual agreements between the nursing school and the health agency provide the basis for determining the responsibilities of both the school faculty and the agency's nursing service personnel for the guidance of the student and for the welfare and safety of the patient. Most agency contracts specify that the student is under the direct assignment, supervision, and evaluation of the school's instructor. However, it is well to note that the student's legal right to practice the skills and techniques of the licensed nurse does not rest primarily upon the fact that the nursing instructor is licensed as a registered nurse but rather on the legal provision in the Nursing Practice Act, in most states.

It is assumed that the intention of the student entering a school of nursing is to be an ethical, courteous, and cooperative person who is conscientious in abiding by the law and who will, therefore, assume the responsibility for taking seriously the instruction and guidance offered while enrolled in the nursing school.

Instructions regarding the care of patients should be followed meticulously, but with the exercise of judgment on the student's part, remembering that every individual is legally responsible for his own acts. Furthermore, in actual patient care, the nursing student has been held by the courts to the higher standard of care of the registered nurse. The reason for holding the nursing student to this higher standard is that the patient has the right to assume that all services of the hospital, including nursing care, will be provided by competent persons with professional training and skill.

A vital point for the student's awareness is the need to recognize one's own limitations of ability, training, and experience. In the event of being assigned to a task that calls for skills not possessed, the student's responsibility would be to seek the assistance of the instructor or the immediate supervisor. In all situations the courts hold the nursing student responsible for exercising reasonableness of conduct in carrying out nursing responsibilities as measured against that of other reasonably prudent nurses in professional performance under the same or similar circumstances.

Legal relationships with physicians and the practice of medicine also are areas of concern for the student. The medical staff should be able to expect competent performance of the nurse consistent with education, experience, and legal limitations and no more. It is important for the nurse to have a clear understanding of these matters and of acceptable ways of handling irregularities that may arise.

The patient's rights

The patient is an individual with the legal rights of any other person, plus additional rights that are his by virtue of being a patient. Among the patient's legal rights to be observed by the nurse are the following:

Right of privacy. Any information about the patient, whether appearing on the chart or otherwise, is by law confidential; the patient must give permission in writing for release of medical information. For example, a young unmarried woman was admitted for an abortion. One of the nurses who was a neighbor of the patient's family told another neighbor about the nature of the patient's problem. Later the patient brought suit against the nurse for *defamation of character.* A patient may sue if he can prove malicious gossip about himself on the part of hospital personnel. The patient, or legal guardian, must also give permission for the taking or release of photographs. The instructor and/or student using a patient's record for study purposes must not identify the patient in any way without his permission.

Freedom from injury. Any patient has the right of safe care. However, if he is very ill, either mentally or physically, the law gives him further consideration because he must depend upon the care administered by others at a time when his mental acuity is diminished and he is least responsible for himself. The patient should not be fearful for his safety from injury.

Protection of belongings. The hospital is obliged to give safe care to the personal belongings that the patient brings with him. This includes clothing, valuables, and such items as his dentures, prosthesis, and the like, and it also extends to diagnostic specimens removed from the patient.

Competent professional care. This right of the patient has already been discussed in relation to the responsibility of the nursing student to exercise reasonable conduct in the performance of nursing.

This information has been presented as a brief introduction to the legal aspects of nursing. For further study the references on the Suggested Readings list at the end of the chapter will be found helpful.

SUMMARY

The unparalleled changes occurring in nursing during the 1970's are viewed in relation to the phenomenal demand on modern society for improved health care delivery services. The challenge for nursing is to play a large and indispensable role in improving the quality, effectiveness, and cost of health care that is expected by the American people.

Nursing in modern society is considered to be a desirable and necessary human service in that it is a way of assisting individuals toward attaining or maintaining self-care, leading to mental and physical health.

In providing the essential elements of nursing practice, the nurse functions as a responsible member of a health care team or may act independently when the needs of the patient and the principles of nursing practice so indicate. As yet there is no one definition that adequately describes how and why nursing is specifically unique and different from other human services. However, today's nurse must be prepared to assume responsibilities and functions concerned with health problems of individuals, sick or well, and provide a range of services that the patient cannot provide for himself.

The stages of complete health services are used as a framework for studying the nursing process through which the individual patient's needs may be met. The phases of the nursing process are presented as a beginning application of the problem-solving steps that are used in working through the nursing process.

Current confusion regarding nursing has been increased by the existence of widely differing types of preparation for registered nurse licensure and other levels of health care personnel; the problems are further complicated by the need for quality control guidelines in patient care.

As changes occur in the health care delivery system and in nursing responsibilities, nursing education must also change to provide appropriate education for all levels of nursing practice in whatever setting they are located or by whatever titles nurses may function.

The major national nursing organizations have through the years accomplished much toward protection of the public and toward bettering the welfare of the individual nurse, recognizing that the quality of patient care improves with better working conditions.

A brief introduction to the legal aspects of nursing has been included for aiding the nursing student to begin understanding both the nurse's legal responsibilities and privileges and the patient's rights.

SUGGESTED READINGS

Auld, Margaret E., and Birum, Linda H.: The challenge of nursing, St. Louis, 1973, The C. V. Mosby Co.

Bernzweig, Eli P.: Nurse's liability for malpractice, New York, 1969, McGraw-Hill Book Co.

Brown, Elta: Nursing: a health care specialty, Nursing Clinics of North America 6:353, June, 1971.

Cherescavich, Gertrude: Florence, where are you? Nursing Clinics of North America 6:217, June, 1971.

Freeman, Ruth B.: NLN at twenty: challenge and change, Nursing Outlook 72:376, June, 1972.

Greenidge, Jocelyn: Community nurse practitioners—a partnership, Nursing Outlook 73:228, April, 1973.

Hazzard, Mary E.: An overview of systems theory, Nursing Clinics of North America 6:385, September, 1971.

Keller, Nancy S.: The nurse's role: is it expanding or shrinking? Nursing Outlook 73:236, April, 1973.

MacArthur, M. Christine: New challenges for visiting nursing, Nursing Clinics of North America 6:467, September, 1971.

National Commission for the Study of Nursing and Nursing Education: An abstract for action, Jerome Lysaught, Director, New York, 1970, McGraw-Hill Book Co.

Orem, Dorothea E.: Nursing: concepts of practice, ed. 1, New York, 1971, McGraw-Hill Book Co.

Rockefeller, Mary C.: Why I believe in the League, Nursing Outlook 72:380, June, 1972.

Spalding, Eugenia K., and Notter, Lucille E.: Professional nursing, ed. 8, Philadelphia, 1970, J. B. Lippincott Co., pp. 422-543.

Three challenges to the nursing profession, selected papers from the American Nurses' Association Convention, 1972.

Thurston, Hester I.: Education for episodic and distributive care, Nursing Outlook 72:519, August, 1972.

Walker, A. Elizabeth: Primex—the family nurse practitioner program, Nursing Outlook 20:28, January, 1972.

2 Orientation to health care

NURSING AND HEALTH CARE

The nurse plays an important role in the field of health care not only when disease is present but also in health teaching that may aid in the prevention of disease. To fulfill this role, the nurse must know what community facilities are available and how they can be used in providing continuity of patient care.

Knowledge of the health picture of the community gives the nurse understanding of how effective previous methods of care have been and serves as a guidepost in plotting future nursing activities in the provision of health care and health education. A concept of health that leads the nurse to the study of the whole man in relation to physiologic and socioeconomic factors—that is, the totality of man in his environment—is basic to functioning as a nurse in the contemporary field of health care. This approach to the study of nursing will assist the student to select and apply major scientific principles from the areas of psychology, anatomy, physiology, chemistry, physics, microbiology, sociology, and other related disciplines.

This chapter will briefly present the general framework in which health care is being practiced in the current transition period as it moves from an era in which acute illness was the rule to the contemporary period in which coping with chronic diseases is a greater need and the wide application of positive health practices is essential. The coordinated efforts of many different kinds of health personnel are now required to develop health education

13

for all and to provide early detection, diagnosis, and effectve treatment of diseases. Within this multidisciplinary framework of health provision, the nurse contributes significantly to the comprehensive and continuous care provided for patients in many different settings in and out of institutions.

In the past, nursing was primarily care of the sick. In today's evolving health care system the role of the nurse is extending into the area of preventive medicine. Legislative changes are expected that will permit the nurse to assume greater responsibilities in the area of primary care. In fact, one is hearing that "nursing is health care."

NEED FOR HEALTH CARE
Changing concepts of health care

Need for the provision of health care has been recognized in the United States since the early colonial period, when high mortality rates were a reflection of epidemic diseases (cholera, smallpox, yellow fever, diphtheria, malaria, typhoid, and tuberculosis) and the lack of proper medical and nursing care. Physicians were inadequately prepared and few in number, and the therapeutic agents available to them were generally ineffective for treating health problems with which they were confronted. Scientific knowledge regarding the causes, modes of transmission, and treatment of prevalent diseases was lacking.

With limited knowledge of the etiology of disease, the major preventive controls were mostly sanitary measures that included quarantine, paving streets, draining marshes, and building waterworks. These measures were of some effect in lowering mortality rates from diseases such as cholera, typhoid, malaria, and typhus. However, symptomatic care of the sick and wounded, provisions for the indigent, and burial of the dead seem to have been the major extent of accomplishment in health care during those eras when health was considered to be merely the absence of illness and disease.

For centuries there had been conflicting theories regarding the cause of the devastating epidemics that seriously threatened the public health. By the late nineteenth century sufficient knowledge had been accumulated to resolve the age-old conflict over the miasmatic theory of disease (the idea that disease was spontaneously generated in filth, decaying organic material, swamps, cesspools, and the like) versus the theory that a particular disease was caused by a living particle that could be transferred from one person to another.

One of the scientific advances most significant to ushering in a new and modern epoch of health care was the development of bacteriology, which brought proof that infectious diseases are caused by microorganisms. The developing concept of disease prevention was furthered through the identification of sources and modes of transmission of disease, the introduction of immunology and innoculation against specific disease, and other discoveries in the physical, biologic, social, and medical sciences. These advances led to the establishment of modern diagnostic and therapeutic measures demonstrating effectiveness in the solution of many health problems.

Striking results were achieved through application of new scientific knowledge in the control of infectious disease. Epidemics were greatly suppressed, but it became apparent in the early twentieth century that new social phenomena were developing and bringing with them new health hazards. Industrialization and rapid urban growth were being accompanied by a host of social problems related to health and well-being. Public attention focused on poverty, malnutrition, and congested slum areas with high maternal and infant mortality rates. Beginning efforts were direct-

14

ed toward alleviating the health problems attending these social conditions.

Social responsibility for health matters

Out of the pressures of increasing social awareness and the new scientific knowledge being applied to the problems of health there emerged an ideology that eventually led to the establishment of an expanded public health service to provide for the rapidly increasing and pressing health needs of the population.

The task of organized public health came to be viewed as that of applying the knowledge and practices that contribute to maintaining the health of the individual and of the aggregate population through use of both preventive and curative measures in the detection, diagnosis, and treatment of disease and through rehabilitation. Society's attitude toward health and disease had evolved into a basic concern for the conservation of life and health, with activities directed toward promoting the health and well-being of all segments of society.

This view of the role of society in the responsibility for health promotion and maintenance represented a marked change from the past. Formerly these matters were thought to be largely the responsibility of the individual. With the increasing complexity of our contemporary society has come recognition that health is many faceted and its promotion and maintenance must be approached on a variety of fronts, that it encompasses many activities beyond the control of one individual, that health is not only a public and therefore national responsibility but also a global concern requiring the scientific and technologic resources of all nations.

Socioeconomic factors affecting health

The relationship between health problems and socioeconomic factors is sometimes obvious, as in the illness of a person suffering from malnutrition resulting from insufficient food supply. Other effects of modern social change and one's economic status in society may be less apparent. However, it is generally assumed that one's health is affected by the society in which he lives and that the health of an economic group is often directly related to economic status. In general, the higher the economic status, the better is one's opportunity to provide factors contributing to health, such as optimum nutrition, favorable living conditions, education and medical care, and the practice of good personal hygiene. However, it does not always follow that the individual will make wise use of the opportunity for positive health maintenance.

Much information is beginning to appear about the effects of social change and the resulting stress on the individual. Stress, usually thought of as a physical, chemical, or emotional factor in bodily or mental tension, is being considered as a possible causative factor in disease.

Within the last decade the problems of environmental health have come under the careful scrutiny of a great many citizens, including health professionals, scientists, and legislators. Various authorities in the field of environmental health are now pointing out that it has become clear to this generation that the capacity of man to improve conditions of living are achieved in proportion to the understanding of evolving and interacting environmental forces. This idea seems valid and challenging, as reflected in the frequency of news items describing pollution of air, water, and land; contamination of food by chemicals jeopardizing health; and the threat of radiation hazards.

It seems ironic that the past successes in the application of scientific principles in sanitation and communicable disease control, though lowering the death rate caused by some of the biologic hazards in the environment, have contributed to the current world population crisis that is

15

compounding the socioeconomic health problems now facing society. It is common knowledge that the present world population of over $3^1/_2$ billion is expected to nearly double by the end of this century and that the present growth of world resources may be insufficient to support mankind's needs for living harmoniously in peace, prosperity, and dignity. Behind the conflicts of ideologies in the world today are the problems of increasing hunger, poverty, and overcrowding.

Unless the expansion of food production can keep pace with the staggering population growth, the majority of the world's people will be increasingly faced with the vicious cycle of poverty, ignorance, malnutrition, disease, and early death. Food, and its relation to health, continues to be a primary concern of man because it affects to a high degree his ability to keep well, to work, to be happy, and to live long. Although the people of the United States are probably better fed than any other people in the world, it is evident that there are still nutritional problems of major health importance to be solved in this country as well as in other countries of the world.

COMMUNITY AND PERSONAL HEALTH
Definition of health

Ideally everyone should be in a state of health, a condition that is now generally accepted to mean *complete mental, physical, and social well-being, which maximizes the individual's ability to function in a normal manner.* Obviously this is an affirmative definition that acknowledges that health is more than the mere absence of disease or infirmity. Health is a positive, dynamic state that can be thought of as giving rise to physical and mental efficiency as well as to satisfaction with life.

Implied in the definition of health is acceptance of the physiologic concept of homeostasis, which, simply stated, is the maintenance within the body of a constant internal environment necessary for cellular survival. For normal functioning of the cell, its components and conditions of cell fluids are held in a state of balance through the cooperation of the different body systems.

Disease is a state of imbalance of one or more cell components or conditions of cell fluids. (Similar imbalance may also accompany trauma.) According to this theory of disease, the disequilibrium involves cellular components—water, salt, nutrients, gases, or hormones—or the constancy of the fluid surrounding the cell when disturbed by foreign substance, such as bacterial toxins or mechanical obstacles. When the imbalance is too great for the protective and restorative mechanisms of the body, the state of health is adversely affected, a situation often necessitating medical or surgical intervention.

The concept of homeostasis has gradually expanded beyond the relatively narrow application just described to include mental and social aspects as well as physiologic ones. Homeostasis is now generally thought of as including the maintenance of (1) body balance, (2) psychologic and emotional balance, (3) cultural, social, and political balance, and (4) spiritual and philosophic balance. With this broad view of health and homeostasis, health care has become a tremendous task, requiring effort toward maintaining and, when needed, restoring balance within the individual and within his environment.

In contrast with the definition of health, *disease may be defined as any condition that actually or potentially hinders individual function.*

Health and illness (disease) are at opposite ends of the health-illness continuum. This does not necessarily mean that health and illness are absolute terms or that they are exact opposites. Rather, they are relative terms in that the individual may have a potentially illness-producing

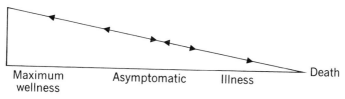

Fig. 2-1. Health-illness continuum. Health and illness tend to merge but may represent patterns of adaptive change along the continuum. The direction of change may be reversible, depending upon the quality of the individual's adaptive efforts.

condition, yet it does not hinder his ability to function in a normal manner. He is asymptomatic, but signs and symptoms may develop and he will then move further toward the illness end of the continuum (Fig. 2-1). For example, an asymptomatic polyp may be present but the individual would be healthy according to the definition of health, unless malignant changes were to occur, in which case he would become ill if untreated. The goal in preventive health care is to maintain equilibrium between health and illness, with the balance in favor of maximum wellness for the individual. Thus it can be inferred that the interaction among many constantly changing factors is responsible for producing a particular condition along the health-illness continuum.

Adaptation

In accordance with the health-illness continuum concept, man is seen as a *biopsychosocial* being constantly interacting with his changing environment. In order to maintain equilibrium on the health-illness continuum in this changing environment, he must successfully cope with the constantly changing factors or succumb to illness. The coping mechanisms man uses for adapting adequately to life situations are biologic, psychologic, and social in origin—for example, such responses include the bodily reactions of homeostasis, inflammation, the clotting mechanism, and the like and psychologic mechanisms for warding off anxiety

(adaptive or defense mechanisms). The sum of the mechanisms that maintain relative constancy of the body's internal environment constitutes *homeostasis.*

Stress, which may be thought of in terms of a multiplicity of changes that take place in the body as a result of a stress agent (or stressor), is always a threat to homeostasis. The stressor causes disruption of homeostasis. When the disruption is so serious that the body is not capable of regaining homeostasis by itself, damage or disease occurs and medical therapy may be necessary to correct it. Stress agents are derived from the internal or external environment and may be mechanical, microbial, chemical, physiologic, or psychologic. Whatever the nature of the stressor, it tends to be disruptive to homeostasis.

Adaptation is a term used to describe the work expended by the body in attempting to maintain homeostasis and to ward off the effect of the stressor. In other words, through adaptive mechanisms stress is counteracted. Hans Selye first stated this theory of stress which, in his words, "embraces all of the various mechanisms through which the body responds to the 'stress of life.'"* Through his research, Selye was able to produce experimentally and consistently a set of symptoms that he named the *stress syndrome.* He noted that no matter what stressor was

*Selye, Hans: The stress of life, New York, 1956, McGraw-Hill Book Co., p. 101.

17

used, these certain changes always occurred, which were atrophy of the thymus gland and lymphatics, enlargement of the adrenal cortex, gastrointestinal ulcers, and weight loss.

From these findings Selye developed the "general adaptation syndrome," a term used to indicate the chain of event in the three stages of physiologic changes in response to stress. The reasons for all of these changes are not entirely clear but may be summarized as follows (Fig. 2-2):

Alarm stage (or reaction). In the initial response to the stressor, sodium and chloride levels in extracellular fluids fall while potassium rises. Blood glucose falls first but rises later. There is loss of body weight. The stress situation calls out ACTH (adrenocorticotropic hormone, secreted by the pituitary gland). The response is increased production of adrenocortical hormones: *cortisone*, which inhibits inflammation, acting on carbohydrate metabolism, and *aldosterone* and *desoxycorticosterone,* which stimulate inflammation, exerting influence on mineral metabolism.

Stage of resistance (adaptation). In re-

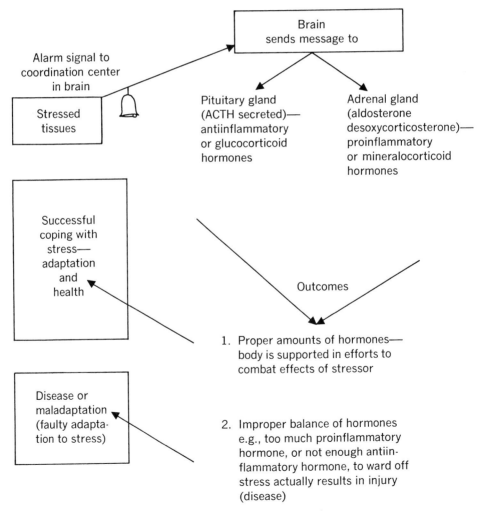

Fig. 2-2. General adaptation syndrome.

sponse to the alarm the body fights back. A proper balance of hormones supports the body's effort to combat the effects of the stressor (that is, adjusts to the stress). Body weight tends to stabilize.

Stage of exhaustion. When exposure to stress is prolonged and severe enough, the acquired adaptation is lost and exhaustion follows because there is a limit to the adaptation energy of the individual.

When the body is unable to adapt, *maladaptation diseases* may follow from faulty adjustments to stress. Selye's research showed that certain cardiovascular and rheumatic diseases can be produced experimentally in animals by administering overdoses of desoxycorticosterone or aldosterone, resulting in the assumption that stress can give rise to conditions that stimulate excessive secretion of these hormones.

Diseases thought to be those of maladaptation include inflammatory diseases of the skin and eyes, diseases of the joints, a type of hypertension, eclampsia, and nephrosis. Also, it appears that the general adaptation syndrome (GAS) has some relationship to other disturbances, including allergies, digestive diseases, metabolic diseases, and a number of others. Since not every individual reacts to a stressor in the same way or to the same degree, it is apparent that there are other factors influencing the results, such as age, sex, genetic factors, or external factors such as faulty diet or drugs. It follows, then, that health and disease may represent patterns of adaptive change along the health-illness continuum and that life depends upon the quality of that adaptation.

Adaptation and the nursing process

Through assessment of the patient's situation, the nurse is able to gain awareness of the responses that indicate the sufficiency (or failure) of the body's effort to combat the effects of the stressor. Accurate observation of both local and general signs and symptoms will give the nurse a fund of knowledge about the patient upon which to begin a plan of care best suited to meeting the needs for comfort and safety of the individual patient and for supporting his adaptation efforts in the illness situation. Through assessment indicating the nature of the adaptation in progress, the nurse learns to pick up the cues that provide a rational basis for wise decision-making by the nurse in the patient's behalf and through which nursing intervention may be designed so that it fosters adaptation to the greatest extent possible for the patient. The Suggested Readings at the end of the chapter develop the nursing application more fully.

Personal health

The subject of individual physical fitness has received much publicity through a wide variety of publications that usually stress the importance of achieving and maintaining an optimum personal health level. Fundamental health habits, which are the simple routine practices developed for the purpose of giving greater freedom and more efficient use of body and mind, are commonly stressed throughout school systems. At this point the student should, therefore, have the basic information and experience needed to keep feeling and looking well in usual circumstances and be able to adjust adequately to the changing activities of life.

The ability to maintain a favorable personal health situation is of utmost importance to the individual nurse for a variety of reasons. Obviously, the nurse may be subjected to many health hazards in performing professional responsibilities and needs a high degree of physical and emotional stamina in order to withstand illness and incapacity. It should also become apparent to the student that the nurse whose actions and appearance imply personal knowledge and understanding of the values of good health will

19

have a greater advantage as a missioner of health than will the one who gives the impression of having neglected personal health and appearance.

Although the student may assume that he has sufficient information and experience for maintaining his own health, it is well to keep in mind that education of individuals in personal and community hygiene is a slow process, complicated by the oft-repeated experience that knowledge of health alone does not guarantee that one will be healthy.

Community health

Community health is a broad term generally accepted as referring to the organized efforts of all agencies in the community that are directed toward promoting health, including both private and governmental agencies. Distinction between public and community health efforts may be made on the basis of financial support. *Public* refers to being "tax supported." In this sense public health agencies may be thought of as those that are tax supported and therefore governmental. *Private,* voluntary organizations are not tax supported.

In the past few years, advances in the total field of community health have been enormous, largely as the result of combined legislative controls and application of the science of public health. Public health efforts have been instrumental in preventing disease, prolonging life, and promoting health through organized community measures for the sanitation of the environment, the control of community infections, the education of the individual in principles of personal hygiene, the organization of medical and nursing service for the early diagnosis and prevention of disease, and the development of social machinery in the attempt to ensure to every individual in the community a standard of living adequate for the maintenance of health.

The average modern community's local resources for health include the private physician, the hospital, the health department, and private health agencies. The health of each individual is dependent not only on his own knowledge of disease but also on the medical facilities available in the community.

Knowledge of community organizations for health and social problems is a necessity for every nurse to function effectively as a member of the health team in the care and instruction of patients. Every nurse must be cognizant of the social needs of patients, conversant with agencies that can show the patient or his family how he can be helped, and able to guide patients to appropriate sources of aid or advice. Health education is a special function of nurses employed by public and voluntary health agencies that participate in supplying home nursing, preventing the spread of communicable diseases, and giving health instruction in clinics, in homes, and in schools.

AGENCIES FOR HEALTH CARE
Classification of health agencies

The mid–twentieth century has been a period of unprecedented development in the organization of services for health care devoted to improving the physical and mental well-being of specific population groups. Although health organizations vary considerably among the different nations and from one state to another within the United States, existing agencies have been classified into three basic groups:

1. Official agencies, which are operated by the federal, state, or local governments and are tax supported.

2. Voluntary agencies, which are private organizations supported by endowments, donations, campaign subscriptions, patient fees, membership dues, or contracts. They are operated as nongovernmental agencies under an independent board.

3. International agencies, which include organizations that function cooperatively through the efforts of several nations, though usually initiated by one of the more advanced countries. These agencies are concerned with the broad scope of world-wide health problems.

Official agencies of the United States

The powers of the federal government in health activities have been inferred from the United States Constitution through interpretation of such phrases as "to promote the general welfare." These powers, strengthened over the years through Supreme Court decisions and socially accepted practices, permit opportunity for leadership by the United States government in developing and establishing policies and health organizations to meet changing community needs.

In 1939 the Federal Security Agency was established to bring together the federal programs that promoted social and economic security, educational opportunity, and the health of the nation's citizens. Health activities were regrouped and consolidated in 1946 by changes made possible under the Reorganization Act, passed by the United States Congress in 1945. In 1953 the Federal Security Agency became the United States Department of Health, Education, and Welfare. This department is the main channel through which the United States government contributes to nationwide services for health, education, and social security. A few of its activities are direct federal operations, but most are on a cooperative basis, with the states operating the services and the federal government setting basic standards and sharing the cost. Activities include community, family, and individual services.

The United States Public Health Service is the oldest organization included in the United States Department of Health, Education, and Welfare. Its important functions may be stated in terms of its eight main divisions: (1) marine hospitals and relief, (2) foreign and insular quarantine and immigration, (3) sanitary reports and statistics, (4) domestic quarantine, (5) scientific research, (6) venereal disease control, (7) mental hygiene, and (8) personnel and accounts. The National Institutes of Health in Bethesda, Maryland, research center for the United States Public Health Service, conduct research into causes of illness and methods of preventing and treating specific diseases. They also aid nonfederal institutions and investigators engaged in research by means of grants.

The Children's Bureau in the Social Security Administration, under the Department of Health, Education, and Welfare, has an extensive program. Its functions are the investigation and reporting of matters pertaining to the welfare of children among all classes of people and administration of federal grants to states under the Social Security Act for maternal and child health, crippled children, and child welfare service.

The Office of Vocational Rehabilitation is engaged in helping handicapped workers return to active employment. Rehabilitation is a three-part process: (1) medical and surgical care to repair disabilities as far as possible, (2) necessary education and training to fit the worker for employment in which he can make the most of his capacities and in which his disability will not stand in the way, and (3) helping the worker in getting suitable work and giving him on-the-job guidance until he is reestablished as a wage earner.

Through the federal health agencies, the states are given consultant services, with freedom to plan programs to meet their respective needs, and matching funds are given for buildings, education, and other projects.

The activities of the state health departments are threefold: (1) to advise, and in some degree supervise, local health

21

departments, (2) to provide direct services to local communities, such as laboratory service, vital statistics, and hospitalization of certain kinds, and (3) to cooperate with other states and with the federal government in interstate health affairs. The state renders advisory service with some degree of supervision and may actually take charge of a situation in an emergency.

The functions of state health organizations may be put under five broad headings: (1) sanitation, (2) control of communicable diseases, (3) public health education, (4) individual health protection and promotion, and (5) research in disease prevention (Fig. 2-3).

Most communities include in their activities the organization, through community effort, of a medical and nursing service for the early diagnosis of disease in the individual and for the prevention of permanent defects. Many health departments arrange for suitable care, by clinics or otherwise, for those individuals in the community who cannot pay for essential preventive services.

Some portion of the time and attention of each of the major divisions of a health department is devoted to research and inquiry. It is the obligation of the health department to demonstrate effective methods and to stimulate public interest in such medical, dental, and nursing services as may be necessary for the promotion of the health of the individual.

Local health organizations may be county or city sponsored. City departments of health find their form and functions in the city charter. Protection of the public health is one of the functions of the

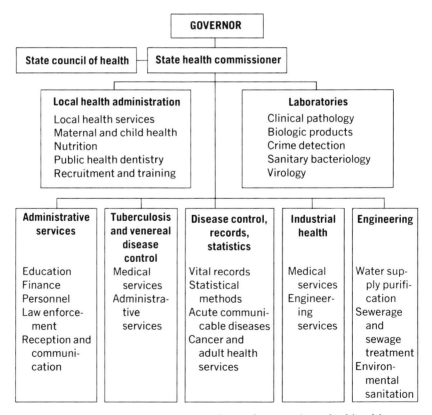

Fig. 2-3. Typical organization chart of a state board of health.

city government. Certain functions are centralized, such as sanitation of water, sewage disposal, milk inspection, and industrial health services, whereas direct services to the people are decentralized. Direct services include well-baby clinics, tuberculosis clinics, school health, and dental hygiene. The health department may be charged with the duty of caring for the medically indigent in their homes or in institutions. A few health departments have been empowered to administer public clinics and hospitals for all ages and all groups of the population. A typical organization chart of a city health department is given in Fig. 2-4.

Voluntary agencies in the United States

Public health was just becoming a function of government at the beginning of the twentieth century. Official agencies developed gradually, and for certain health problems in some localities they were slow in taking any action. As a result, physicians and laymen voluntarily organized national, state, and local health agencies to combat a specific disease or condition.

The voluntary (nonofficial, private, non–tax-supported) agencies were designed to arouse public interest and to secure public support for additional facilities for diagnosis and treatment.

Some of the nonofficial agencies are the American Cancer Society, the National Tuberculosis Association, the American Heart Association, the National Committee for Mental Hygiene, the National Society for the Prevention of Blindness, the National Society for the Hard of Hearing, the American Child Health Association, and the Visiting Nurse Association. Many

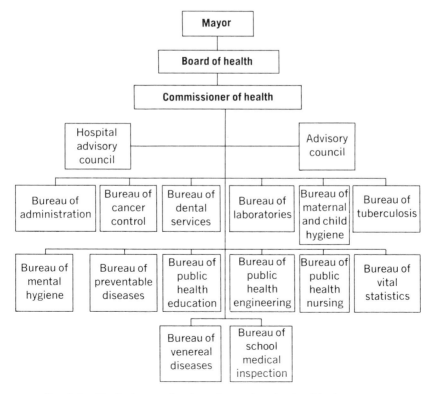

Fig. 2-4. Typical organization chart of a city health department.

national nonofficial agencies, however, are found in every city. There may be a local agency with a different name but with the same functions as an established national organization, yet in no way affiliated with it.

An example of service supplied by a voluntary agency is the home nursing provided through the Visiting Nurse Association, whose purpose is to give care to the sick at a price that the patient can pay. The price ranges from the full cost of the visit to free service. With actual bedside nursing, the visiting nurse teaches health and care during illness. It is a generally accepted idea that every nurse who enters a home should be prepared to give definite and suitable health instruction.

The Red Cross, one of the earliest voluntary health agencies and the only one that has a quasi-official status, offers courses in home nursing and first aid as one of its services. The home courses are for homemakers and others interested in learning proper and safe methods of caring for the sick at home, whereas the first-aid courses teach emergency care and preventive measures.

International agencies

The international official governmental agency in public health is the World Health Organization (WHO), a part of the United Nations, which held its first meeting in 1948 (Fig. 2-5). There are now more than 120 member countries in all parts of the world. Its headquarters are at Geneva, Switzerland, with regional offices to serve the areas of Southeast Asia, the Eastern Mediterranean, the Americas, Europe, Africa, and the Western Pacific. It is a collective instrument to prevent and control disease, promote physical and mental health, expand scientific knowledge, and contribute to the harmony of human relations on a world scale. Its emphasis is laid not only upon quarantine, control of epidemics, and other defensive measures but also upon positive aggressive action

toward health in its broadest sense. The first objective of this organization is disease prevention; the second is the positive improvement of physical and mental fitness.

The World Health Organization emphasizes certain fields of activity because these fields have high rates of world attack. Its interest is centering about infant and maternal hygiene, malaria, tuberculosis, veneral disease, and nutrition. The present top priorities in its promotion of world health, briefly stated, appear to be (1) expanding health research, (2) training health workers and developing training programs, and (3) promoting long-term national health planning.

TRENDS IN ORGANIZED HEALTH EFFORTS

Relatively recent federal legislation is an indication of the increasing role and influence of the federal government in health care. The intent of contemporary health legislation has been to initiate integrated, federal-state-local programs that will stimulate the development of better community health services by establishing regional jurisdictions in the management of health and social problems. The objective of this approach is to develop concerted regional and local efforts in solving the more pressing health and social problems confronting American communities during the remainder of the twentieth century, thus improving the health and welfare of the entire nation.

This trend in health-related legislation, sometimes referred to as "creative federalism," is evident in several of the laws passed by the Eighty-Ninth United States Congress in the 1965-1966 session. The following brief summary of legislation cites a few such laws as examples.

Federal legislation

Public Law 89-239 created the Regional Medical Program for Heart Disease, Cancer, Stroke, and Related Diseases.

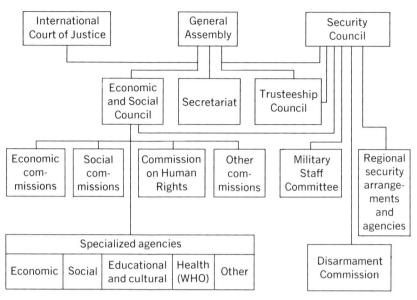

Fig. 2-5. Organization chart of the United Nations to show the place of the World Health Organization.

One of its goals was to reduce the gap between the potentialities of medical science and actual medical practice. An Administration on Aging was created by the Older American's Act (P. L. 87-73), which established joint federal, state, and local government responsibility for the health and welfare of older people.

Most significant in federal legislation is the Comprehensive Health Planning and Public Health Services Act (P. L. 89-749) passed by Congress on November 3, 1966, in "an effort to remove some of the barriers to optimal health care for every person in the country." It provides comprehensive planning for efficient use of all health resources at local and regional levels to assure the highest level of health attainable for every individual. This goal is to be accomplished through partnership of all levels of governmental and voluntary agencies, organizations, and individuals, with federal grants being made available to the states for comprehensive health planning and community health service. New approaches to disease control and new sources of health manpower are emphasized in the act. It provides that each

state be divided into regions to bring comprehensive health planning closer to the people served. It also provides a local center for receiving information on all of the multifaceted health problems in the local region that will exercise priority determination in the planning, analysis, solution, and implementation of these activities.

Despite the apparently improved situation in health care, there has been for some time an awareness of growing discontent in regard to the high cost and availability of quality professional health services for various segments of the population. It appears that probably 80% of the American public receives little or inadequate medical care for one reason or another.

The urgency of doing something, especially for elderly persons, who are most apt to have inadequate incomes and may therefore be unable to meet the rising cost of medical care, has long been recognized. After much controversy, the 1965 Congress passed an amendment to the Social Security Act (Title XVIII), which is commonly known as *Medicare.* Under this

25

legislation a federal program of health insurance providing funds for hospitalization and other specified services has been established for persons 65 years of age or older. Although this insurance coverage is not complete, the benefits available to most of the aged are more advanced than they were prior to Medicare.

Title XIX, known as *Medicaid,* was also passed as an amendment to the Social Security Act in 1965. The purpose of Medicaid was to establish a consolidated medical care program for all those identified as eligible for public assistance by the individual states. It provides a formula for financing the program by matching federal and state funds.

Among other discernible trends affecting the current crisis in health care there are at least the following factors that are of particular interest to the individual nurse.

Trends affecting health and health care

The amount of national expenditures for health purposes has been increasing at an enormous rate. The effects of technologic and scientific advancements related to health have been dramatic, producing major changes that have altered price standards and expectations of patients.

The vast array of complicated diagnostic and laboratory equipment and other aids now widely available for the physician and other health personnel in the prevention, diagnosis, treatment, and rehabilitation of patients have made better health care possible. The computer can be cited as an example of the type of equipment that is necessary for modern medical technology. These advances in science and technology have not only expanded medical ability to help the patient but have greatly increased its complexity, with the result that more and more effort needs to be given to the organization and delivery of health care. Some of the resulting changes and their effects include the following:

1. Medicine has changed from an individualized general practitioner type profession to a very complex, highly specialized, interdependent system that can almost be called an industry. In 1931 general practitioners comprised about four fifths of the active practicing physicians, while at present more than one half of the actively practicing physicians are specialists.

2. The development of new health careers with increasing specialization of all health manpower levels has added to the complexity.

3. Significant alteration in the relationships between different types of health care personnel has been a consequence of the growing complexity of the health field.

4. Fragmentation in patient care is becoming a consequence of specialization and accounts for the increasingly crowded emergency rooms and clinics.

5. With the trend toward fragmented and uncoordinated health service, the care given tends to become chiefly episodic.

6. The foregoing problems have combined to produce increasingly serious inefficiencies in the delivery of health care and rising cost of health care, which is reflected in increased charges to patients.

Since about 1960 private consumer expenditures for health care have reportedly increased about $20 billion annually. It is quite unlikely that the cost of health care to the consumer will decrease, since the trends appear to be moving toward further development of scientific and technologic advances and for some continuing degree of inflation. Hence, there seems to be a growing demand for seeking ways of ensuring economy in the delivery of health services.

Among socioeconomic and demographic factors significantly related to health care utilization are:

1. Population increases resulting in mounting demand for health services. The Bureau of the Census predicts an increase in the population of the United States

from approximately 205 million to about 361 million by the year 2000.

2. Shifts in proportion of age groups in the total population are occurring; according to projections, by 1990 over half of the population will be under 20 years or over 65 years of age, which certainly will affect both the economy and the kinds of health problems that are most prevalent.

3. Personal consumption expenditures for health care are being affected by other factors such as increasing mobility of the population and educational and income levels.

THE HOSPITAL AS A HEALTH AGENCY

The evolution of the American hospital as a community health agency has kept pace with the dramatic advances that have characterized medical technology and the entire health care field from about 1900 to the present. The hospital has progressed from a custodial institution where sick people went only as a last resort to emerging, modern, comprehensive medical care centers in which the patient expects to be treated successfully. In fact, many hospitals now have follow-up care plans that extend the patient's care beyond the hospital into the community and link the hospital staff and resources to the patient and his family in the home situation.

The word "hospital" is derived from the Latin word *hospes*, which means "a guest." When hospitals were first established in centuries past, they were intended as places of shelter and entertainment. This meaning still holds true in the sense that the patient is a guest of the institution. The hospital is composed of patients, doctors, nurses, and other members of the health team who function in meeting the needs of sick and injured persons.

The advancement of the hospital is important to the nurse, because the greater portion of nurses spend years of employment in this complex, ever-changing insti-

tution. The nursing student should develop a thorough understanding of the true meaning of a hospital as an institution and view it not only as a physical plant but also as a group of people with a common objective.

Classifications

Hospitals are usually classified in two major ways: (1) according to the type of patient or service offered and (2) according to ownership or control. Under the type of service offered, there are two groups of hospitals—general and special. A general hospital cares for patients with many kinds of conditions, including those receiving medical, surgical, pediatric, and obstetric care. Many general hospitals also have facilities for patients with psychiatric and communicable diseases. A special hospital limits its service to a particular condition, sex, or age—for example, tuberculosis, maternity, and pediatrics.

Under ownership, hospitals are separated into either (1) governmental and nongovernmental or (2) public and private. Public or government hospitals are divided into federal, state, county, and city. The army, navy, Veterans Administration, and United States Public Health Service hospitals are owned and controlled by the federal government. State hospitals may be either general or special. Many state hospitals are for psychiatric patients. County and city hospitals may also be general or special, depending on the needs of the community. The majority of hospital beds are owned and operated by the government at the federal, state, or local level.

Nongovernment, or private, hospitals may be owned or controlled by a church, a fraternal order, an industry, or a private group of doctors or citizens. Private hospitals are for the care of those who can afford to pay in part or in full for hospitalization. Many private hospitals also have provisions for giving free care. Financial support for these hospitals may be derived from

27

trust funds, endowments, stocks, donations, earnings, and other types of income.

Accreditation

Hospitals may be evaluated according to quality of service rendered. Certain professional organizations such as the American Hospital Association, the American Medical Association, the American College of Physicians, and the American College of Surgeons have set standards for the quality of care delivered. Hospitals meeting the minimum standards are accredited through the *Joint Commission on Accreditation of Hospitals,* which was established by these professional organizations as the means of conducting the accreditation process.

Functions

All hospitals, regardless of their control, perform somewhat similar functions within a community. Although the major purpose of the hospital is the care of the sick, many modern hospitals are now educational centers for the teaching of nursing, medicine, nutrition, social work, and other specialties, and the students in all of these fields obtain much of their professional experience within the hospital walls. Many institutions also make some effort to prevent disease and to promote health among families of the community by planning with the family for care at home. Specific functions of the hospital may include (1) diagnosis, (2) medical treatment, (3) surgical treatment, (4) prevention of disease, (5) education, and (6) research.

Health care has become a leading industry in the United States, and the financial aid provided by federal, state, and local government has given great impetus to health work. A larger number of people are currently using hospital facilities because of improved economic conditions and health hospitalization insurance plans in which more than 80% of the population is enrolled. Hospital insurance may be thought of as prepaid medical care, whether it be through individual or group insurance plans.

There is urgent need to effect a more even distribution of hospital facilities between urban and rural areas. A solution to the problem has been attempted by federal legislation that encourages doctors to set up practice in rural areas, thus opening the way for other allied fields to follow.

Organization

The governing body of a hospital, usually called the board of trustees, is responsible for the policies of the institution. Directly at the head of the hospital is the administrator, to whom authority and responsibility for management is delegated by the governing board. He directs the two divisions of hospital work—the business management and the professional care of patients. The business management includes accounting, utilities, maintenance, engineering, housekeeping, and purchasing. Under the professional care of patients are found the medical department —including diagnostic and treatment facilities—social service department, dietary department, nursing department, and other special areas.

The medical department has within it various clinical services: medical, surgical, obstetric, pediatric, ear, nose, and throat, eye, dental, orthopedic, gynecologic, urologic, communicable disease, and psychiatric. Sometimes these various services are not segregated, but segregation usually promotes efficiency of personnel and economy of time and materials. Communicable disease control is aided by segregation of the service. A service might also be designated by the place where service is given, such as the operating room, outpatient department, emergency room, diet kitchen, x-ray laboratory, clinical laboratory, central supply services, and a variety of other departments.

Even though the overall administrative

responsibility for the hospital rests with the administrator, it is impossible for one person to carry the total load of work involved in hospital administration. In the majority of situations he delegates appropriate responsibilities to department heads, who are specialists in their fields.

Nursing department

The nursing department is the organizational structure through which nurses in a hospital or health agency provide nursing care for patients under the jurisdiction of the institution. The primary purpose of the department is to provide comprehensive, safe, effective, and well-organized nursing care through the personnel of the department. The personnel typically consists of the director and assistant director of nursing service, supervisors, head nurses, and staff nurses. All of these are registered nurses who are responsible for the various elements of the process used in planning and directing patient care, in controlling the setting, and in facilitating accomplishment of the total nursing care of the patient.

Other personnel who function in the nursing department may include licensed practical or vocational nurses, nursing assistants who give direct patient care under supervision, and ward secretaries who manage much of the desk routine.

Other hospital departments

Typically, a number of the following service departments are necessary for effective functioning of the hospital.

Admitting department. The purpose of the admitting department is to receive and identify the patient. Pertinent information relative to medical care is obtained, and the choice of the type of room is decided. Often a registered nurse is in charge of this department because she is usually sensitive to the needs of the entering patient.

Cashier and crediting department. Near the admitting department are located the cashier and crediting department, where the patient or relative may make the necessary financial arrangements or pay his final bill on discharge.

Pharmacy. Most hospitals operate a pharmacy. The department head is always a registered pharmacist. In the pharmacy prescribed medications for the patients are obtained and the necessary drugs for hospital use are prepared.

Laboratories. The laboratories are directed by a pathologist, who is a physician specially trained in the methods of detecting changes that take place in the tissues and fluids of the body during disease. Functions of the laboratories consist of the performance of tests and procedures necessary for diagnosis and treatment. The laboratories are considered to be a part of the medical department.

Radiology department. A radiologist, who interprets and reports results of the x-ray films taken and developed by the radiologic technologists, is a medical doctor who heads the department. Other diagnostic measures and radiation therapy procedures are administered under his direction.

Dietary department. One of the departments with which the nurse is closely associated is the dietary department. Its function is to plan, prepare, and serve meals for patients and sometimes for other hospital personnel and visitors. A dietitian is at the head of the department. She may have one or more assistants who have charge of divisions with the department, such as the therapeutic dietitian or the teaching dietitian. A lay person, known as a food manager, may be in charge of the cafeteria for hospital personnel. Other personnel in the dietary department include a chef, a baker, kitchen maids, and dishwashers.

Social service. The social service department assists in obtaining aid for patients and their families. This department serves also as a liaison between the patient and community agencies. Some of its activities might include helping to secure a new type of occupation for a father who has lost a limb, transferring a patient to another institution, directing a mother toward an agency for her retarded child, referring a patient with cancer to an agency or organization that will supply dressings, or helping to place an aged patient in a nursing home.

Physical therapy department. The purpose of the physical therapy department is to treat patients by means of such physical agents as heat, water, light, and exercise. The department head is a physical therapist. Other members of the department who actually work with the patients may be physical therapists or specially trained technicians.

Occupational therapy department. In the occupational therapy department treatment consists of having the patients engaged in some type of occupation or craft. Like physical therapy, its chief objective is to help in the rehabilitation of the patient. It is also used as a form of diversion for a chronically ill person and as therapy for a mentally ill patient.

Chaplain. An important member of the hospital personnel is the chaplain. The nurse may be of assistance to the chaplain in meeting the spiritual needs of the patient. Very often hospitals provide chapels for the use of patients, visitors, and hospital personnel.

Outpatient department. The outpatient department is a connecting link between the hospital and the community through its provision of care to patients who usually are not hospitalized. A great deal of preventive work is accomplished by the clinics as well as by the outpatient department. Examples of clinics connected with outpatient departments are well-baby clinics or ear, nose, and throat clinics.

Medical records. The medical record librarian is responsible for the administration of the medical records department.

The medical records of patients are filed and stored for use in a variety of purposes, including future service to the patient, research, and use as legal documents.

Housekeeping and maintenance departments. Very essential areas in a hospital are the housekeeping and maintenance departments. The chief housekeeper is usually the person who supervises the work of maids and janitors in keeping the hospital clean and in preparing units for patients. The functions of the maintenance department are to repair the building and appliances and to supply such services as heat, power, and electricity. In the maintenance department will be found engineers, carpenters, and electricians.

Purchasing department. The purchasing department is almost always a division of the business or administrative department and is headed by a person known as the purchasing agent, who does the buying for the entire hospital. The products are delivered to a storeroom and then dispensed to the different areas. In some instances, drugs may be purchased directly by the pharmacist, and some special brands of food may be purchased by the dietitian.

Central supply department. The purpose of the central supply department is to prepare and furnish other departments with equipment and supplies needed in patient care, such a sterile dressings, sterile hypodermic syringes and needles, treatment trays, and special mechanical devices. It usually is under the supervision of the nursing department.

Interrelationships of departments

Probably no other enterprise encompasses as many diversified professional services and separate activities as a hospital. The function of patient care and service reaches through all levels of hospital social structure, affecting even those who do not have direct contact with patients. These persons have a feeling of satisfaction that their work contributes to the care of pa-tients. Service to patients provides a unify-ing force at all levels of hospital organiza-tion.

The functions of the hospital are achieved when all departments and all in-dividuals in the hospital organization are able to communicate effectively with other departments and individuals. Effective in-teraction results in increased understand-ing of others and is essential to productive, harmonious functioning. The cohesiveness of the personnel is based on mutual respect of others and of their contributions, on self-respect, on satisfaction with one's own performance, and on the common goal of service.

SUMMARY

This chapter has attempted to give a panoramic view of the complex field of contemporary health care and has sug-gested reasons for the student to develop awareness of the role of nursing in today's total pattern of health care.

Knowledge regarding the control of dis-ease was greatly expanded in the late nineteenth and early twentieth centuries through scientific discoveries in the physi-cal, biologic, social, and medical sciences. Although striking results in disease control were achieved through application of the new scientific knowledge, industrialization and rapid urban growth were accompanied by a host of social ills affecting health and well-being. This was a motivating factor in the beginning of organized efforts by the local, state, and federal governments to promote the public health.

The goal in preventive health care is to maintain equilibrium between health and illness, with the balance in favor of maxi-mum wellness for the individual. Man is viewed as a biopsychosocial being with coping mechanisms for adapting to life situations that are biologic, psychologic, and social in origin. The sum of the mech-anisms that maintain relative constancy of the body's internal environment consti-tutes homeostasis.

Stress, which is thought of in terms of a multiplicity of changes that take place in the body as a result of a stress agent, is always a threat to homeostasis. Selye is credited with developing the stress syn-drome theory through which he identified the three stages of physiological changes in response to stress that he termed the "general adaptation syndrome." In this concept adaptation is used to describe work expended by the body in attempting to maintain homeostasis and to ward off the effect of the stressor. Through the adaptive mechanisms stress is counteracted. When the body is unable to adapt, maladaptation diseases may follow from faulty adaptation to stress.

Understanding of adaptation is signifi-cant in the nursing process. The nurse is concerned about man as a total being, at whatever point he may be along the health-illness continuum. Through assess-ing the patient's responses to stimuli in his position on the continuum, the nurse can more realistically develop intervention that promotes the patient's efforts toward ad-aptation, thus helping to make his adaptive energy more available for the healing process.

Health is described as a positive, dy-namic state leading to physical and mental efficiency and is related to the concept of homeostasis. Disease and trauma are pre-sented as causing disequilibrium that may be too great for the coping mechanisms of the individual unless therapeutic interven-tion is instituted. The ability to maintain personal health is mandatory if the nurse practitioner is to assist others within the community to achieve their full potential.

Basic ideology underlying the role of government in provision of health care is that health promotion and maintenance encompass activities beyond the scope of individual control, that every individual has the right to health and to medical service

31

regardless of ability to pay for service, and that the scientific and technologic resources of the United States and of all other nations are required for the conservation of life and health.

Knowledge of current trends in federal legislation and health care and their implications for nursing are pertinent concerns of today's health team members. The hospital may be described as a complex community health agency organized to facilitate functioning of the health team in meeting the needs of sick and injured persons.

SUGGESTED READINGS

Aradine, Carolyn, and Hansen, Marc: Nursing in a primary health care setting, Nursing Outlook **18**:45, April, 1970.

Duncan, Mary Loue: The hospital as a primitive society, American Journal of Nursing **70**:106, January, 1970.

Eyres, Patricia J.: The role of the nurse in family-centered nursing care, Nursing Clinics of North America **6**:27, March, 1972.

Fischer, G. Valentina, and Connolly, Arlene F.: Promotion of physical comfort and safety, Dubuque, Iowa, 1970, William C. Brown Co., Publishers, pp. 8-86.

Ornstein, Sheldon: Objective—a national policy on aging, American Journal of Nursing **71**:960, May, 1971.

Stokes, Gertrude A.: Extending the role of the psychiatric-mental health nurse in community mental health, Nursing Clinics of North America **5**:635, December, 1970.

Storz, Rita R.: The role of a professional nurse in a health maintenance program, Nursing Clinics of North America **7**:207, June, 1972.

Walker, A. Elizabeth: Primex—the family nurse practitioner program, Nursing Outlook **20**:28, January, 1972.

Wilner, Daniel M., and others: Introduction to public health, New York, 1973, The Macmillan Co.

3 Scientific principles and the nursing process

USING SCIENTIFIC PRINCIPLES IN NURSING

The essence of the nursing process lies in the synthesis of self-sharing with the patient and knowledgeable service to the patient. Experiencing an effective sharing encounter with the patient is the surest way for a nurse to appreciate its significance (or even its existence when it is achieved), yet using scientific knowledge is also essential to provide the intellectual foundation necessary for nursing care. Nursing would be reduced to a mechanical routine devoid of all human qualities if it were a purely scientific procedure without inclusion of regard for the patient's being. Scientific aspects of nursing are inherent in the total nursing process, but it is the person-to-person contact that more often provides the catalyst to strengthen the patient's potential for maximum functioning. Commitment to the use of scientific principles, then, does not preclude the use of one's "self" by becoming involved in close human relationships with patients.

SCIENTIFIC PRINCIPLES DEFINED

Every nurse practitioner is confronted with an increasing flow of data requiring decision making to meet patients' nursing needs. Because these needs are constantly changing, the nurse must vary decisions to adjust to these changes as new information is received for processing. To use this information and arrive at valid decisions, the nurse must formulate or comprehend general scientific principles that govern nursing care, reason from such laws and principles, and direct nursing action in accordance with them.

Scientific principles, which are drawn from all fields of learning, may be defined as *comprehensive and fundamental laws, doctrines, truths, or sets of facts that form the basis for established rules of action.* An example of a scientific principle derived from the social sciences is that all *behavior has a purpose.* The nurse makes continuous use of this principle in planning nursing action to meet the objectives of patient care, and this task is clarified if the nurse realizes that a patient's constant complaining might be an unconscious protest against being physically dependent on others for his care or that similar complaining by another patient might stem from a different source, such as conscious or unconscious fear of impending surgery.

33

Governing the nurse's action in planning nursing care with each patient would be the understanding of the scientific principle that *all behavior is purposeful.* The recognition that similar behavior patterns may be evidence of many dissimilar purposes leads the nurse to adjust nursing action to meet each individual patient's needs. One patient may need reassurance, whereas another might need to provide as much self-care as he is capable of providing.

The physical sciences as well as the social sciences offer many principles useful to the nurse. One principle used in the management of wounds is that *absorption capabilities and wicking action of cotton materials vary with the structure of the material.* In planning care for a patient with a heavily draining wound, a nurse would select a dressing with maxiumum absorption quality and wicking action combined.

As important as knowing what a principle is is knowing what it is not. Many times an isolated rule, such as "No smoking while oxygen is in use," might be mistaken for a principle. Such a rule does *not* include the reason for the action taken and therefore does not constitute a principle. If nursing students relied upon the principle, then, that *oxygen supports combustion* to guide nursing care, they would realize the significance of the "no smoking" rule. Thus they would be provided with a safe guide for action in any situation involving oxygen and patient care and know why the action was indicated. A principle, then, is a fact or basic assumption that is believed and becomes a settled rule of action that gives a reason for the method employed and that provides a safe guide for action.

SCIENTIFIC PRINCIPLES AND PROBLEM SOLVING

The process that the nurse uses in making application of fundamental ideas or scientific methods in the concrete world of nursing requires an approach that is commonly called problem solving. The term "problem" should not suggest a negative or undesirable situation to the student but rather a question to be answered or an issue to be resolved.

Inductive and deductive problem solving

Problem solving is a positive process of step-by-step scientific reasoning that may be inductive or deductive in form. *Inductive* reasoning implies the development of knowledge and the formulation of generalizations or principles. The *deductive* process requires drawing inferences from general principles or applying knowledge already possessed. To arrive at a generally acceptable principle through every inductive reasoning process or research design using the inductive scientific method is not realistic or feasible. Nor is it essential to search for a principle to attach to every nursing action. Scientific knowledge is incomplete in many areas and certain practices are continued on purely empirical grounds because they are known to "work."

However, by proving or disproving the soundness of a given practice through future research or by deducting knowledge from principles known to be applicable to nursing at the present time, the nurse can be guided toward the best possible care for every patient when systematically using scientific problem solving as one component of the nursing process.

The problem-solving process

The terms *scientific* and *systematic* are of key importance in differentiating between effective problem solving and haphazard trial-and-error attempts to meet the patient's nursing needs. Whereas some problems are solved with ease—almost automatically—others require much time and effort. The process, whether it is inductive or deductive, typically involves four major phases:

1. Recognizing and defining the problem
2. Collecting data from observation and experiment
3. Formulating and implementing a solution
4. Evaluating the solution

Often a number of problems occur at the same time, one phase of problem solving occurs simultaneously with another phase, or one step may take longer than another. Nonetheless, in carrying out nursing responsibilities within the health team, the nurse directs each of these steps toward achieving the patient's fullest potential for functioning independently.

STEPS IN PROBLEM SOLVING
Recognizing and defining a problem

Interference with the optimal adjustment of an individual in maintaining homeostasis may often result in the develop-

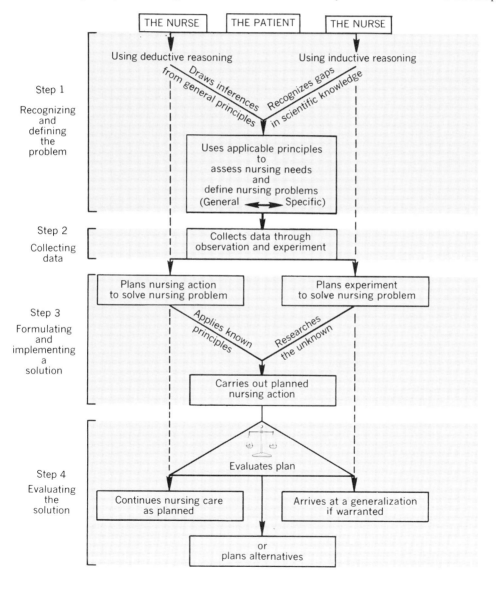

Fig. 3-1. Scientific principles and problem solving in nursing.

ment of actual or potential health needs for that individual. Recognizing these needs and focusing on the related nursing problems is the first phase of the problem-solving process (Fig. 3-1).

A problem may be stated in a general or specific manner. General nursing problems useful as guides in identifying patients' specific problems have been classified by various nursing authorities. For instance, *supplying oxygen to all body cells* is a general problem common to many patients. A variety of more specific problems may be related to this general one. A patient with abnormally high blood pressure from atherosclerosis (a "specific" problem) and a patient with abnormally low blood pressure from internal hemorrhage (also a "specific" problem) will both need active measures to supply oxygen to the tissues (a "general" problem common to both patients).

Whether general or specific, the existence of a problem is closely related to concomitant principles. *Facilitation of the maintenance of oxygen supply to body cells,* for example, becomes a problem only when there is potential or actual interference with the principle that *cells of the body require an adequate supply of oxygen to maintain homeostasis.*

Awareness of these relationships between general and specific nursing problems and related principles will enable the nurse to transfer, adapt, and use what he or she has learned when faced with nursing situations where they are applicable. It will also alert the nurse to the need for research where there are gaps in knowledge and where practices are being carried out on the basis of faulty or ill-defined principles.

Reasoned understanding of observations can then be achieved in the next phases of problem solving, which will be discussed with examples of both inductive and deductive processes. The inductive nature of the development of knowledge will be exemplified by describing how each phase of problem solving might be carried out in a typical research design for testing medication to lower blood pressure, thus facilitating the supply of oxygen to the tissues. The deductive process of using knowledge already possessed will also be followed through each problem-solving step. Scientific principles will be cited to show how the nurse would rely on such principles in alleviating a patient's lack of oxygen from hemorrhage when planning and carrying out nursing measures within the patient's overall medical plan.

Collecting data from observation and experiment

Data or information may be collected through observation and experiment. Observations in turn may be "natural" or "contrived." A contrived situation involves controlled experimentation followed by observation. The problem of maintaining adequate oxygen supply to the body cells in patients with elevated blood pressure might be investigated by testing of an experimental medication given to lower blood pressure. In a typical research design using the inductive approach, three "matched" groups of patients' reactions to the medication would be compared. One group would receive the drug, another would receive an inert substance that appeared to be the prescribed drug, and the third group would receive no medication. Observations would be carefully recorded for analysis leading to warranted conclusions and generalizations. As a member of the research team, the nurse would participate in making observations in contacts with the patients involved.

Natural or nonexperimental observations are more frequently made by the nurse. Observations of the patient's total nursing needs are an essential component of nursing care. As the second step in deductive problem solving, the nurse makes systematic observations of the patient's needs relevant to that problem. Following the patient who lacks oxygen as a result of internal hemorrhage as an example, the nurse would draw inferences from a number of principles in order to distinguish between relevant and nonrelevant data. In assessing the degree of intensity of the problem, the nurse would, for example, make regular observations of the patient's pulse rate and blood pressure. The nurse would know that *the pulse rate varies inversely with the blood pressure* and that *the lower the amount of circulating blood volume, the lower the arterial pressure.* In working within the physician's medical plan, cognizance of these principles and their significance to the patient's condition would lead the nurse to use the data collected through observations in formulating and implementing a tentative solution to the problem as part of the patient's nursing care plan.

Formulating and implementing solutions

The third major step in the problem-solving sequence is to plan and to try a tentative solution to the problem. In analyzing observations from experimental data, such as comparison of the effectiveness of medication to reduce elevated blood pressure, the experimenter induces logical conclusions. These conclusions are made on the basis of whether his hypothesis regarding medication would (or would not) be supported. If his analysis is of a statistical type, the conclusions would lead to a probability statement expressing the degree of confidence the experimenter could place in his acceptance or rejection of the hypothesis. The hypothesis might be stated in terms of how well the medications would (or would not) lower blood pressure or why the medication would be (or would not be) effective. Implementing the solution would depend on the outcome of these factors.

In analyzing collected data about the patient with oxygen lack from internal bleeding, the nurse formulates tentative solutions for solving the problem or preventing the problem from increasing in intensity if possible. The principles noted earlier and related to observations of the patient's blood pressure and pulse rate would be among those the nurse would continue to use in making a judgment upon which to act within the specific area of responsibility. As a member of the health team, the nurse knows how and when to initiate a specified nursing action and knows how and when to seek additional intervention by the physician. Thus using such knowledge constitutes the third step in the problem-solving sequence —that of formulating and implementing a tentative solution to the patient's particular nursing problem within the total nursing care plan.

The solution of any nursing problem is, of course, designed and carried out to alleviate or reduce the patient's need for nursing and medical assistance if this is possible. Although the roles assumed by the nurse and by the doctor are different, no attempt to differentiate sharply between a "nursing" problem and a "medical" problem need be made. The nurse and physician are working together in focusing on the patient's total health needs. As in other steps in the problem-solving process, the nurse is working with other members of the health team in evaluating the solution to the patient's problem.

Evaluating the solution

Whatever the tentative solution or nursing care plan, the problem-solving process is not complete without arriving at some sort of judgment as to whether the problem has been resolved, unresolved, or created new problems. In judgment of the experiment to compare results of the medication to lower blood pressure, for example, many methods of evaluating the solution or validating the conclusions might be useful. Further investigation might be indicated to find out whether the medication would be useful for large numbers of patients over long periods of time without causing unwanted side effects. The probability statement predicting the effectiveness of the medication or how the effectiveness was or was not achieved could be weighed from a broader base of evidence. From such experimental data it is often possible to induce a warranted generalization and thus provide the basis for arriving at a scientific principle applicable in other patient care situations.

Using the *deductive* approach in the case of the patient with internal hemorrhage, the prescribed solution to the problem might be to replace blood loss by means of a transfusion. The nurse would be responsible for pooling the observations of all members of the health team in making an evaluation of the process of supplying adequate oxygen to the patient by means of a blood transfusion.

Among the principles that would guide the nurse in evaluating the administration of the transfusion would be the knowledge that the *fluids flow from an area of higher pressure to one of lower pressure* and that *the pressure gradient is directly related to the rate of flow.* The nurse would be expected to maintain the flow of solution slowly and continuously without raising the intravascular pressure to the point that would cause increased bleeding. Whenever indicated at any point, the nurse would communicate personal evaluations to the physician and other health team members responsible for the medical management of the patient.

Evaluation of the solution to the problem as part of the total nursing care plan is as important as planning the solution to the problem. With careful evaluation the success or failure of the trial solution can be judged. It should be understood, however, that evaluation, as well as other steps in the problem-solving sequence, does not necessarily occur as an isolated activity of that sequence. Rather, it is

usually continuous and may be both formal and informal; nevertheless, evaluation is always essential in measuring the consequences of planned nursing intervention (Fig. 3-1).

SUMMARY

Becoming a nurse who shares close personal communication—or fundamental encounters—with patients is a major component of the nursing process. Using scientific principles and problem solving complements this aspect of the nursing process and helps to ensure that those in nursing today will be prepared to make thoughtful and intelligent decisions affecting the lives and deaths of patients in the unknown world of tomorrow.

The problem-solving process of arriving at generalizations or principles through research-oriented inductive reasoning has been described step by step in this chapter. Experimental testing of a medication to help supply oxygen to the tissues by lowering the blood pressure index was used as an example of how a nurse might be working with the health team in conducting such research.

Deductive reasoning by the nurse through consideration of existing principles in problem solving has also been followed by describing an example of a patient with oxygen lack resulting from internal hemorrhage. Nursing problems common to many patients are related to a variety of more specific problems. The existence of such problems is in turn related to scientific principles, some of which remain to be identified through future research. Each step of systematic problem solving requires decision making. The nurse equipped to deal with nursing problems in a wise and resourceful manner must be able to use knowledge of general laws and reason from them or to formulate new laws through the problem-solving process.

The union of commitment to nursing in

both a personal and a scientific sense may go slowly at first, because the nursing process is not just the lending of oneself, the memorization of facts, or a listing of vaguely understood principles. It is rather a change in the character of the student that results in giving one's self, thinking in a scientific manner, and habitually relating general principles to immediate perceptions as a basis for rational decision making.

QUESTIONS FOR DISCUSSION

1 Define a scientific principle in your own words.
2 What is the difference between a rule and a principle? A procedure and a principle?
3 How is inductive reasoning different from deductive?
4 What is your definition of the scientific method?
5 Trace the stages in problem solving in your own words.
6 How are scientific principles derived?
7 Give an example of how one scientific principle might be applied to several different patient situations.

SUGGESTED READINGS

Abdellah, Faye G., Beland, Irene L., Martin, Almeda, and Matheney, Ruth V.: Patient-centered approaches to nursing, New York, 1970, The Macmillan Co.

Berggren, Helen, and Zagornik, A. Dawn: Teaching nursing process to beginning students, Nursing Outlook 16:32, July, 1968.

Carlson, Carolyn: Behavioral concepts and nursing intervention, Philadelphia, 1970, J. B. Lippincott Co.

Carlson, Sylvia: A practical approach to the nursing process, American Journal of Nursing 72:1589, September, 1972.

Carrieri, Virginia K., and Sitzman, Judith: Components of the nursing process, Nursing Clinics of North America 6:115, March, 1971.

Collins, Rosella D.: Problem solving—a tool for patients, too, American Journal of Nursing 68:1483, July, 1968.

Garant, Carol: A basis for care, American Journal of Nursing 72:699, April, 1972.

Griffith, Elizabeth W.: Nursing process; a patient with respiratory dysfunction, Nursing Clinics of North America 6:145, March, 1971.

Hanebuth, Lorna: The use and abuse of principles, Nursing Forum 7:308, November 3, 1968.

Kraegel, Janet M., Schmidt, Virginia, Shukla, Ramesh K., and Goldsmith, Charles: A system of patient care based on patient needs, Nursing Outlook 20:257, April, 1972.

Zimmerman, Donna S., and Ghorke, Carol: The goal-directed nursing approach: it does work, American Journal of Nursing 70:306, February, 1970.

4 Principles and problem solving applied to body mechanics

RELEVANCY OF SCIENTIFIC PRINCIPLES AND PROBLEM SOLVING

The statement was made in the preceding chapter that the process that the nurse uses in making application of fundamental ideas and scientific methods in the concrete world of nursing requires the problem-solving approach. Awareness of the relationship between general and specific nursing problems and related principles will enable the nurse to transfer, adapt, and use the accumulated knowledge and experience when faced with nursing situations where principles are applicable. Thus organizing ideas and facts into principles enables the nurse to have a clear, organized fund of knowledge ready for use in nursing situations. Principles have relevance only as they are applied to identified nursing problems and used as guides for developing realistic alternatives of action.

UTILIZING PRINCIPLES IN SOLVING NURSING PROBLEMS

The use of principles is a process that facilitates each of the problem-solving steps. It seems incredible that nurses would undertake the complex responsibility of planning individualized patient care, engaging in the assessment and decision-making process that require a systematic and comprehensive approach in meeting the total health needs of the individual, without first identifying and defining the problems. Yet this can happen, with resulting failure to satisfy the needs of the patient without the nurse understanding the cause of failure or, even worse, failing to recognize that there are unsatisfied needs. What are the chances that the patient's problems will be solved unless their presence is first recognized and then clearly identified and defined?

Recognizing and defining the problem. A problem in patient care is generally de-

40

fined as an interruption in the individual's ability to meet a need within the context of health and in which the nurse can be of assistance. The existence of a problem is closely related to concomitant principles. The example given in Chapter 2 can be carried a step further to illustrate the point. Cells of the body require an adequate supply of oxygen to maintain homeostasis. Knowledge of this basic principle leads the nurse to the recognition of problem factors that create interference with the maintenance of oxygen supply to body cells.

For instance, with understanding of the principle regarding cellular need for oxygen, the nurse would immediately recognize the significance of faulty positioning of the patient and prolonged inactivity in relation to the oxygen supply of body cells. Violations of principles of body mechanics in positioning the patient such that there is interference with expansion and effective ventilation of the lungs or prolonged pressure on the skin and underlying tissues will be quickly identified as problems and defined clearly and concisely by the nurse who has developed the habit of using principles in carrying out the mechanics of problem solving. Identified problems are best stated in behavioral terms when possible. For instance, using descriptive terms depicting the observations in the preceding example, the problems may be stated as: "difficulty in breathing when lying in supine position" and "large reddened, abraded area on coccyx." Thus the task of problem identification is facilitated by knowledge of principles drawn from the biologic, physical, and behavioral sciences.

Collecting data from observation and research. Information may be collected through systematic observations of the patient's needs relevant to the problem or problems. Following the example of the patient who lacks oxygen as a result of incorrect positioning and prolonged in activ-

ity, the nurse would draw inferences from a number of principles in order to distinguish between relevant and nonrelevant data. In this instance useful concepts and related principles might include:

1. The functional ability of the body and its various systems is based on activity.
2. Normal cellular activity requires:
   a. A consistent supply of oxygen, nutrients, and other chemicals
   b. Circulating blood as a means of transportation of oxygen, nutrients for cellular utilization, and elimination of metabolic by-products
3. A decrease in the volume and pressure of the circulating blood in a tissue causes a decreased functioning of the tissue.
4. Movement of voluntary muscles assists venous return of blood to the heart by exerting pressure on the veins of the body.
5. Under normal conditions, contraction of skeletal muscles during exercise causes an increase in the blood supply to the muscles involved.
6. The relative concentration of oxygen and carbon dioxide in the body fluids is the principal chemical regulator of the respiratory rate.

These and other related principles coupled with the concepts that efficient body mechanics is the correct poise and control of the body with normal functioning of every part in maintenance of proper alignment and that an etiologic factor involved in deficient respiration is poor posture are helpful in assessing the degree of intensity of the problems. (See further discussion in Chapter 19.)

Cognizance of these principles and their significance to the patient's condition would lead the nurse to use the data collected through observations in formulating and implementing a tentative solution to the problem as a part of the patient's nursing care plan. Such a plan would be congruent with the physician's medical goals.

Formulating and implementing solutions. The third step in the problem-solving sequence is to plan and to try a tentative solution to the problems. In analyzing data about the patient with oxygen deficit associated with incorrect positioning and prolonged inactivity, the nurse formulates tentative solutions for solving the problems or for preventing them from increasing in intensity if possible. The physiologic principles noted earlier are a few examples of those that the nurse could continue to use to make a judgment upon which to act within her area of responsibility.

This step becomes clearer by looking at how the nurse might use these principles in formulating a tentative solution to the patient's particular problems as *a part* of the total nursing plan of patient care. Referring to the first and second stated principles—the functional ability of the body and its various systems is based on activity, and normal cellular activity requires a consistent supply of oxygen, nutrients, and other chemicals—knowledge of these facts would probably lead the nurse to plan at least these measures:

1. Positioning the patient with the various parts of the body in basic physiologic alignment, as nearly as these anatomic relationships can be achieved and maintained (Fig. 4-1)
2. Regular and frequent changes of the patient's position
3. Daily exercise, including full range of motion of the joints unless medically contraindicated
4. Maintaining the joints in a functional position, preventing prolonged hyperextension or contraction of opposing muscle groups

As seen in this illustration, the physiologic principles often suggest the tentative solution to the nursing problems. As in other steps of the problem-solving process, the nurse works with other members of the health team in evaluating the solution to the patient's problems.

Evaluating the solutions. The problem-solving process is not complete until some sort of judgment is made as to whether the problem has been resolved, is unresolved, or has created new problems. Using the *deductive* approach, the nurse would evaluate the success or failure of the measures, the tentative problem solutions, based on the selected principles related to activity. In assessing success or failure the

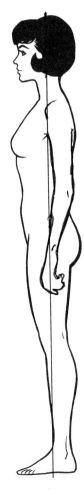

Fig. 4-1. Standing position.

nurse would observe the patient in this example for signs of increasing oxygenation, muscle tone, and range of motion and for the absence of contractures, decubiti, and insufficient respiratory excursion.

The nurse would communicate these evaluative observations to the physician and other health team members responsible for the medical management of the patient. Both the medical plan of treatment and the nurse's plan for patient care would be adjusted according to the evaluation of the tentative solution to the patient's problems. The evaluative process, as well as the other steps in the problem-solving sequence, does not usually occur as an isolated activity in the sequence. Rather it is more often a continuing and on-going activity through which the nurse is aware of the patient's adaptive response at any point and is quickly alerted to the need for adjusting the nursing intervention as the original problem resolves, or is still unresolved, or is made aware of the occurrence of new problems. The usefulness of principles and the scientific method is more precisely outlined in Chapter 6 in relation to assessment of the patient's adaptation level.

Mere memorization of vaguely understood principles is not a sound basis for the utilization of the problem-solving process in a scientific manner. Skill in utilizing the process is fostered by habitually identifying true principles drawn from the biologic, physical, and behavioral sciences and relating them to immediate perceptions as a basis for rational decision making.

PRINCIPLES OF BODY MECHANICS IN NURSING
Selected biologic principles

Some principles selected from anatomy and physiology have been stated earlier in this chapter and have been related to the nursing process. Further application of these same principles is relevant to specific procedures, for example, such as to the preparation of the bed for occupancy by the patient.

The parts of the body with which the nurse is mostly concerned in bedmaking are the vulnerable areas of tissue resting against the mattress. The contact points having very little soft tissue padding over bony structures include the spine, ribs, shoulder blades, hip bones, coccyx, elbows, ankles, and heels. Large areas of soft tissue resting on the bed are the buttocks, thighs, and arms. The body in these various areas exerts uneven points of pressure against the mattress, and the greatest pressure is made at points of prominence or of greater weight. The physical principle regarding gravitation, or weight, stated in the following section on physical principles, accounts for the pressure of the body parts against the bed.

The pressure of body parts against the mattress, especially when the body parts are not in correct alignment, may be so great or continued over so long a period of time that the blood supply becomes depleted, with failure in transportation of oxygen and nutrients needed for cellular utilization and elimination of metabolic by-products. If allowed to continue, this will result in tissue damage and ultimate formation of decubitus ulcers. Application of the foundation bedding so that it is tight and wrinkle free will afford some lessening of discomfrot and pressure on vulnerable tissues. The pressure of tight upper bedding holding the feet in an incorrect position of body alignment will contribute to the development of contractures and decubiti.

These illustrations emphasize the point that the nurse needs to be well informed regarding the principles of activity and of body mechanics that provide reliable guidelines in performing safe and effective manipulative skills in the conduct of patient care.

Posture and body mechanics

Each body system has its own particular function. The musculoskeletal system must provide balance, motion, and stability. The skeletal structure acts as a firm support for the soft body tissues and their movements and also protects certain internal organs by forming a bony cage around them. Movement between the bones is possible to varying degrees because the skeleton is jointed and the bones are held together by specialized connective tissue fibers, the tendons and the ligaments. Ligaments are strong flexible bands that help to hold the bones together at the joints. Tendons are the cords, or bands, that attach the muscles to the bones. Muscles are attached to the jointed skeleton in such a manner that the bones are moved as though they were a series of levers. The type of lever and the efficiency of movement depends on the angle and site of attachment of the muscle to the bone and on muscle tone (Figs. 4-2 and 4-3).

Although each of these elements of body position, or posture, plays its own role in the ability or inability of the person to function, their interrelatedenss must be recognized in maintaining the internal and external equilibrium of the individual and his environment. Because they act together, any factor that interrupts the function of one element affects the others. The

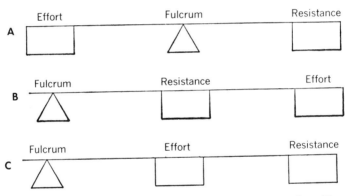

Fig. 4-2. Types of levers. **A,** Class I. **B,** Class II. **C,** Class III.

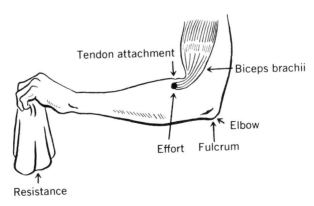

Fig. 4-3. Lever action of the arm.

relationship of internal equilibium and body position, muscle tone, and movement ought not to be overlooked. The importance of this relationship is discussed in Chapter 19.

Body posture, or alignment, is generally defined as the position in which the various parts of the body are held while sitting, standing, walking, and lying. Good posture is then inferred to be efficient posture, which will vary with the individual and the activity. Good body mechanics, by implication, is the correct poise and control of the body with normal functioning of every part in maintenance of proper alignment. Recognition of what constitutes proper body posture in each activity, or inactivity, is important for the nurse and all others who work with patients in the prevention and corrections of deviations.

Proper body alignment

The criteria for proper alignment are usually described with the body in standing position and in relation to physiologic functioning. The standards of proper body alignment may then be applied to the other postures of standing, sitting, or lying.

Since the body is an arrangement of jointed segments, it is in proper alignment in the standing position when these segments are centered over each other in such a way that the center of gravity of each is centered over the body's base of support (Fig. 4-4). This is efficient body posture because in it the body is able to maintain stability and balance with the least effort. When these criteria for efficient posture are not preserved, the relationship between muscles and bones making up the various segments becomes inefficient because these structures are then in positions of functional disadvantage. The malalignment usually causes the center of gravity to shift forward, producing strain upon the involved muscles and bones in

their efforts to maintain stability and support of the body.

Selected physical principles

Background for application of the principles of physics to body mechanics is an understanding of basic anatomic and physiologic concepts of body posture and movement related to the skeletal, muscular, and nervous systems that explain the relationship and functioning of these systems in maintaining posture and producing motion. The reader is urged to review relevant anatomy and physiology content, identifying pertinent concepts while continuing with this chapter. Basic concepts of gravity and force, or energy, should also be reviewed because most body movements involve pulling against the force of gravity in some degree.

Principles derived from physics underlying body posture and movement are

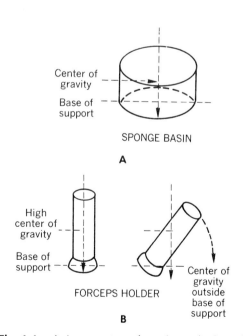

Fig. 4-4. A, Low center of gravity and a broad base of support increase stability. **B,** Stability is lessened when the center of gravity is raised and the base of support is narrowed.

equally applicable for both patient and nurse. Selected principles pertinent to the subject of bedmaking are presented, with emphasis on the point of view that their application is essential for efficient use and positioning of the nurse's body to avoid strain on its various parts during this activity. Physical principles underlying body posture and movement that can serve as guides to the nurse in (1) development of personal habit patterns of efficient body posture and movements and in (2) arrangement of position for the patient that will promote his comfort and well-being include the following statements:

1. All matter has inertia; therefore, a body at rest tends to remain at rest, and a body in motion tends to continue to move in a straight line unless another force of different direction is applied.

2. Force, such as a push or a pull, exerted against the mass of a moving body will produce a change in its velocity. (Force is the effort, or power; mass is the resistance; velocity is speed going in a certain direction.)

3. Gravitation or weight is the force of attraction, or pull, between the earth and an object on or near it. (Gravitational pull accounts for the fact that more force is usually required to lift a heavy body than to push or pull it along a smooth surface.)

4. Torque is the effectiveness of a force producing a rotating motion of a body around a fixed point; as torque increases with the distance of the force from the fulcrum, equilibrium of the body in motion decreases.

5. The center of gravity of a body is considered to be the point at which the mass or weight of the body is concentrated. (The center of gravity can be located by drawing diagonals and finding their midpoint. See Fig. 4-4, A.) The closer the object being moved is held to the center of gravity, the better the control over the object.

6. A body is in equilibrium when a line drawn perpendicularly from its center of gravity passes through its base, so that (a) as long as the center of gravity falls within the base of support, the body is stable; (b) if the center of gravity falls outside the base of support, the body is unstable and will topple over (Fig. 4-4, B); and (c) a low center of gravity and wide base of support increases the stability of a body (Fig. 4-4, A).

7. A lever is a rigid bar, either straight or curved, one part of which (the fulcrum, or axis) is fixed, while the other is freely movable. In a lever the force times the distance from the effort to the fulcrum equals the resistance times the distance from the resistance to the fulcrum.

8. Where there is motion between two contacting surfaces, frictional forces oppose the motion; friction is the resistance caused by the presence of irregularities that tend to interlock when surfaces slide on each other.

Application of physical principles to bedmaking activity. Movements of the body take place by means of the muscles and bones functioning on the principles of mechanical leverage and gravitational pull. The bones and cartilages act as the lever, the muscles supply the force or power that produces movements, and the joints are the fulcrums.

Levers are divided into three classes, class I, class II, and class III, depending on the relative positions of effort, fulcrum, and resistance (Fig. 4-2).

In a lever of class I, the fulcrum lies between the effort and the resistance. The class I lever is rare in the body. The best example is the forward and downward movement of the head in nodding.

In a lever of class II, the fulcrum is at one end and the resistance lies between it and the effort. The outstanding example of this type of lever in action in the body is that of standing on the toes.

The lever of class III is the commonest type found in the body. In a class III lever the effort is applied at a point lying between the resistance and the fulcrum. A typical example of a lever of class III is observed in bending the elbow to lift a weight with the hand (Fig. 4-3). In this type of lever the effort must always be greater than the resistance. Maximum speed is obtained by shortening the effort arm. Practically all levers in the body are arranged so that the distance between the fulcrum and the point of application of effort is short, thus giving maximum speed and control.

Since force must be exerted to change velocity, more effort, or energy, is needed to make many little arm movements than to make one continuous motion; hence, smooth continuous movements are produced with the least amount of effort. The act of raising the arms requires muscle contraction, which eventually produces fatigue. Therefore, when opening or folding linen during bedmaking, articles of linen should be placed on the edge of the bed rather than being held above shoulder level or with arms outstretched, since the latter positions require greater energy output. Changing the position frequently brings different muscle groups into action, thus tending to lessen fatigue while performing a task.

The flexor muscles of the arm (biceps) make third-class levers of the bones to which they are attached. The biceps muscle contracts and draws the hand upward. In a third-class lever the fulcrum is at the end. The fulcrum is the elbow, the effort is exerted by the muscle, and the resistance is the weight being lifted (Fig. 4-3). Obviously then, by sliding a body or object on a smooth surface rather than lifting it up to move it, the nurse is utilizing the pull of gravity rather than working against it. The effect of moving rather than lifting is to reduce the amount of energy required to accomplish the task. An example might be that less effort is required to move a patient up toward the head of the bed by assisting him to slide on the smooth surface of the bed rather than by lifting him to move him upward.

In the type of muscular activity just described, the nurse increases the force applied to the movement by using body weight to assist in accomplishing the sliding movement of the patient. This is done by separating the feet, with the forward foot pointing in the direction of desired movement, and then rocking backward and forward to overcome the initial inertia and to gain velocity in accomplishing the sliding movement of the patient's body. In this way the nurse uses the strength of all of the large leg and thigh muscles in performing the motion, thus avoiding strain on arm, shoulder, and back muscles. The work is further shifted to the long, strong muscles of the thighs by flexing at the knees and hips while keeping the back in straight alignment. The direction of moving the weight is usually straight ahead.

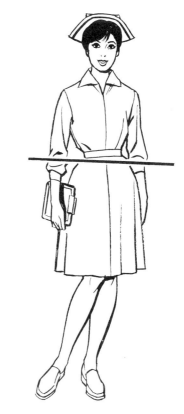

Fig. 4-5. The center of gravity is about at the second sacral vertebra.

If the body is twisted in performance of activities, unnecessary strain is placed on the structures of the back.

In man the center of gravity is located approximately at the level of the second sacral vertebra (Fig. 4-5). Since stability of the body is maintained by keeping the center of gravity over its base, the feet, which form the supporting area of the body, should be separated when it is desirable to provide a wider area of support. In any activity, such as bedmaking, the nurse can apply this principle for main-taining stability of working position by assuming a broad stance and by bending at the knees and hips but keeping the back straight. In doing so the center of gravity can be kept within the base of support. The nurse in Fig. 4-6 is demonstrating this principle as well as the concept that the nearer to the center of gravity a weight is held, the greater the possibility that strain will be reduced. In Fig. 4-7 these concepts of correct body mechanics are illustrated during the motions of tucking the sheets under the mattress.

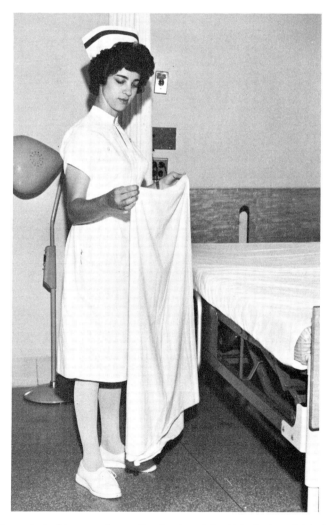

Fig. 4-6. Linen is held away from the body while it is being folded. The feet are separated for greater stability.

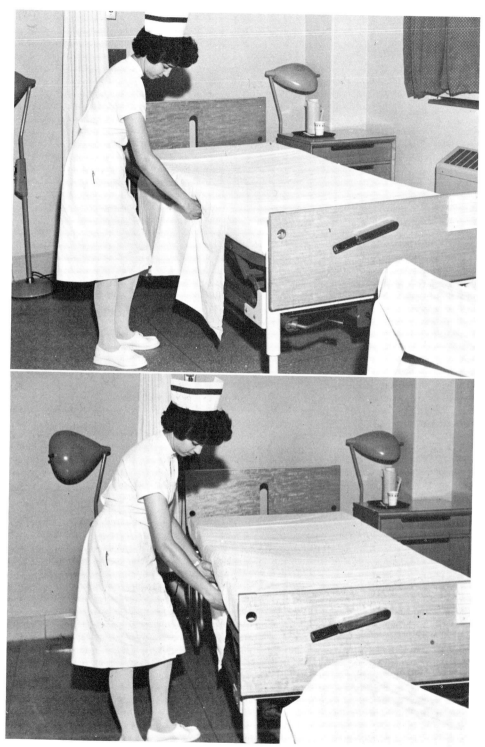

Fig. 4-7. Good body mechanics reduces fatigue and increases efficiency.

INTRODUCTION

Correct body posture keeps the center of gravity as nearly as possible in the same vertical line. When the body is held erect with all parts in proper alignment while standing, walking, or sitting, less muscular force is required to maintain balance (Fig. 4-1). However, such posture faults as protruding abdomen and stooping shoulders will cause the center of gravity to shift forward. The comparatively frail muscles of the back must then exert more force in order to keep the center of gravity in the normal position for maintaining balance.

Movements of specific parts of the body are as follows (Fig. 4-8):

1. Head—flexion, forward, backward, right, and left; extension; rotation to the right or left; circumduction to the right or left
2. Vertebral column—flexion and extension
3. Fingers—flexion and extension; abduction and adduction
4. Thumb—opposition with all fingers
5. Wrist—flexion and extension
6. Elbow—flexion and extension; pronation and supination

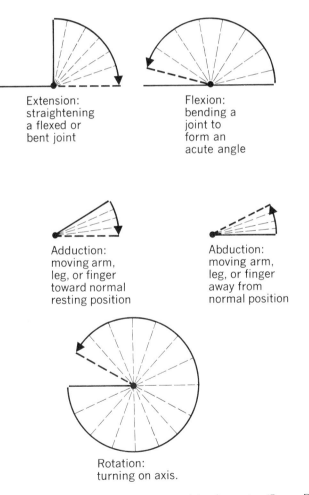

Extension:
straightening
a flexed or
bent joint

Flexion:
bending a
joint to
form an
acute angle

Adduction:
moving arm,
leg, or finger
toward normal
resting position

Abduction:
moving arm,
leg, or finger
away from
normal position

Rotation:
turning on axis.

Fig. 4-8. Descriptive terms used for movements of body parts. (From Drury, John H., Jr.: Handbook of range-of-motion exercises, Jenkintown, Pa., Intermed Communications, Inc.)

50

7. Shoulder—flexion and extension; abduction and adduction; rotation, inward and outward; circumduction
8. Toes—flexion and extension; abduction and adduction
9. Ankle—flexion, dorsal and plantar; extension
10. Knee—flexion and extension
11. Hip—flexion and extension; adduction; rotation, inward and outward; circumduction

The standing position may be thought of as the basic position from which constant changes are being made. Following are characteristics of the normal standing position (Fig. 4-1):

1. Head extended (erect)
2. Normal curves of back reduced to minimum
3. Chin in and back
4. Chest most forward part
5. Shoulders slightly abducted
6. Elbows slightly flexed
7. Wrists extended
8. Fingers flexed
9. Abdomen flat and relaxed
10. Buttocks contracted
11. Thighs extended and slightly abducted
12. Knees slightly flexed
13. Feet pointing straight ahead, parallel, about 3 inches apart, and at right angles to legs

There should be a feeling of tallness, with the top of the head pulling away from the soles of the feet. The standing position varies constantly for comfort and for many purposeful movements. Front and back stability is increased by advancing one foot in front of the other. Lateral stability is increased by separating the feet sideways.

In the basic sitting position, the weight of the trunk rests on the tuberosities of the ischia of the pelvic bones, on the buttocks, and on the thighs. Following are characteristics of the normal sitting position:

1. Head erect
2. Chin in and back
3. Curves of back normal
4. Chest most forward part
5. Shoulders abducted and possibly flexed forward
6. Elbows flexed and supported
7. Wrists extended
8. Fingers flexed
9. Abdomen flat and relaxed
10. Thighs flexed at right angles to trunk
11. Knees flexed at right angles to thighs
12. Feet flexed at right angles to legs and supported on floor or by some other means

These characteristics should be applied to the patient who may sit up in bed with the knees extended, or he may sit on the edge of the bed with the knees flexed and the feet over the edge of the bed, or he may sit out of bed in a straight or comfortable chair or in a wheelchair.

In walking, the center of gravity produces a torque (tendency to twist) as the feet are alternately lifted and placed forward. Reducing the twisting motion to a minimum lessens the energy output in walking.

In the movements already discussed the presence of friction hinders motion by increasing the amount of work required in overcoming the resistance offered, as, for instance, in sliding the weight of the patient along the mattress toward the head of the bed. However, friction is an advantage in other movements. For example, friction is needed between the sole of the shoes and the floor to prevent slipping when walking or in moving heavy objects. When a decrease in friction is necessary, it may be lessened (1) by smoothing the surface, such as in tightening the bottom sheet and draw sheet, (2) by applying a film of lubricant between the two sliding surfaces to act as a cushion between the irregularities of the sliding surfaces, as in the Gatch cranks on the bed, or (3) by rolling a heavy object instead of sliding it. The last point explains why the patient's bed is on wheels.

Many other practical applications of basic physics principles to nursing procedures involving physical activity for the nurse are described in readily available current nursing literature. The reader is encouraged to consider carefully the application of these principles of correct body posture and body mechanics for both nurse and patient as each new procedure is studied and to put them immediately into practice from day to day. In this way correct habit patterns will be established from the beginning, which will result in efficient and esthetic body posture and movements for the nurse.

The nurse will probably be able to internalize pertinent principles more readily if the problem-solving techniques outlined earlier in this chapter are applied to the study of correct body mechanics. For this purpose specific procedures are indicated that can be utilized as situations in which problem-solving techniques may be employed to further the establishment of desired habit patterns. In each situation the following should be identified: (1) movements to be accomplished; (2) principle, or principles, that are applicable; (3) body posture or postures to be assumed in carrying out the movements, using stick figures to illustrate center of gravity and posture; (4) direction of movement; (5) muscles that can be used with greatest efficiency to accomplish the movements; (6) use of devices for assisting in lifting and moving, such as a draw sheet; and (7) muscles or other body structures that are most apt to suffer strain through failure to use effective body mechanics in performing the necessary movements.

Many other procedures and situations could be added to the following suggested examples:

1. Correct body posture while standing and while sitting

2. Working at a lower level, such as bathing a patient in a bathtub, or operating the Gatch cranks on a bed

3. Carrying a heavy object such as a basin of bath water or a stack of clean bed linen

4. Lifting a heavy device, such as a sandbag, from a lower level up to the surface of the bed

5. Repositioning the mattress for the bed patient by moving it toward the head of the bed

6. Assisting the helpless patient to move to the side of the bed

7. Assisting the helpless patient to move up in bed

8. Raising the shoulders of a helpless patient

9. Assisting the helpless patient to turn on his side

10. Placing the helpless patient on the bedpan

11. Assisting the patient to a sitting position on the side of the bed

12. Assisting the patient out of bed to a standing position

13. Assisting the patient from bed into a chair

14. Moving a helpless patient from bed to a stretcher

15. Placing and adjusting pillows under the head of a helpless patient

Positioning in illness

When one is making the occupied bed, the most opportune time to position the patient may be when the foundation of the bed has been completed and before the top covers are placed over the patient. Often the patient is active and able to assume a position for himself that is comfortable and needs little assistance from the nurse in this regard. However, there are many patients who need varying degrees of assistance with positioning, either for comfort or for a variety of therapeutic reasons, such as preventing contracture and decubitus ulcers or for facilitating breathing and promoting drainage and other examples that have already been presented. When a therapeutic position is included in the physician's orders for the patient, the nurse assists the patient with the prescribed positioning to obtain maximum therapeutic benefit from the treatment. When positioning is not a specific order by the physician, it is a nursing responsibility to position the patient according to his priority of needs. The nurse bases judgments on the intelligent assessment of the patient's needs and knowledge of appropriate principles. Techniques for making nursing judgments and decisions have been presented in other chapters.

From the principles already presented, the nurse can appropriately make the following assumptions that will give guidance in carrying out responsibilities for positioning the patient:

1. The various parts of the patient's body should be kept in basic physiologic alignment as nearly as possible. (See Fig. 4-1 and also the description of these anatomic relationships.)

2. Joints should usually be maintained in a functional position, preventing prolonged hyperextension or contraction of opposing muscle groups.

3. Regular and frequent changes of position should be made to prevent excessive pressure on vulnerable tissues, stimulate circulation, and facilitate breathing and for a variety of other reasons that may apply to specific patients. A time schedule for turning, suitable for most patients, is at least every 2 hours.

4. Most patients need some daily exercise, including full range of motion of the joints, unless medically contraindicated.

The fundamentals of positioning the patient as presented here should be viewed as a foundation from which application and modification can be made in any clinical situation, depending on the varying conditions of individual patients.

There are many positions that can be assumed by the patient in meeting his anatomic and physiologic needs when confined to bed. Three lying positions in bed may be assumed: back-lying (dorsal), side-lying (lateral), and face-lying (prone). Correct alignment of the body in any lying position is the same as in the standing position. The difference is that the body is in a horizontal plane instead of in a vertical one. The lying position should be one of ease and comfort, permitting complete relaxation. A firm mattress is essential for correct lying posture. Most patients can maintain themselves in good posture and are able to change position from time to time. Others are not able to maintain proper posture and need to be supported.

Correct back-lying (dorsal) position. The back-lying position is maintained by supporting the *head and cervical curve* of the back with a small pillow. The head should be straight with the vertebral column. If more than one pillow is used, three will be needed for proper support under the head and back (Fig. 4-9).

The *lumbar curve* should be supported with a small pad or pillow. If three pillows are used, one pillow supports the lower back.

The *chest* is the most forward part.

The *arms* should be in slight abduction on pillows.

The *thighs* are extended. Supports such as sandbags or trochanter rolls may be used on either side (Fig. 4-10, *A*).

The *knees* are slightly flexed by a small pad or pillow under them or by raising the knee rest 4 or 5 inches.

The *feet* should be apart about 3 inches and at right angles to the legs by means of a foot support, which may be a box or a footstool turned on its side. The foot support should be 4 or 5 inches above the toes.

The foot support should be placed firmly against the foot of the bed to keep it in place. A bed cradle may be used to keep the covers off the toes.

Correct side-lying (lateral) position.

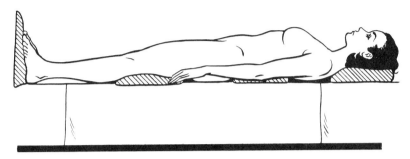

Fig. 4-9. Diagram showing back-lying position.

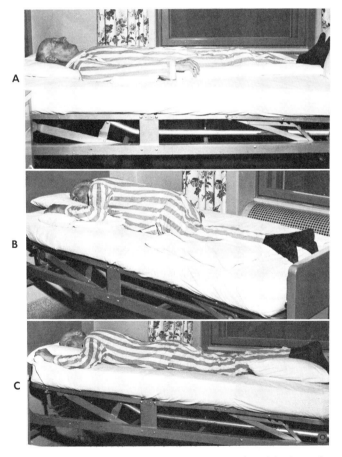

Fig. 4-10. **A,** A comfortable dorsal position. **B,** A comfortable lateral position. **C,** A comfortable prone position.

The side-lying position is maintained in the following manner:

1. By supporting *head* on pillow and aligning it with vertebral column
2. By supporting *curves of back* with stiff pillow
3. By supporting *lower side* with small pad from ribs to ilium
4. By supporting *abdomen* with pillow in front
5. By having *upper arm* in abduction on top of front pillow
6. By having *thighs* in extended position or flexed
7. By having *knees* slightly flexed and abducted by means of pillow placed between legs from above knee to ankles (Fig. 4-10, *B*).

Correct face-lying (prone) position. The face-lying position is maintained in the following manner:

1. By keeping *head* on line with vertebral column but turned to one side
2. By supporting *shoulders* in abduction with small pads or pillows under them
3. By supporting *abdomen,* if necessary, with pillow extending from lowest rib to ilia

4. By having *thighs* extended
5. By supporting *feet* at right angle and toes off bed by pillow under legs or by extending toes and feet over end of mattress
6. By having *knees* flexed by placing pillow under legs (Fig. 4-10, *C*).

A test for good posture in any static position is to compare it to the basic standing position. In all positions the head is on a straight line with the vertebral column, the curves of the back are not exaggerated, the chest is the most forward part of the body, the feet are at right angles to the legs, and the knees and elbows are flexed, more or less. The mattress of the later models of the hospital bed can easily be adjusted (by means of cranks or electric pushbuttons) to the normal body curves.

The patient may rest in a static posture, but frequent moving and turning are necessary for good circulation and respiration. If the patient cannot change his position, the nurse must change it for him. No position will remain comfortable and safe indefinitely.

Correct sitting posture in bed with the knees extended is maintained by supporting the curves of the spine in their normal

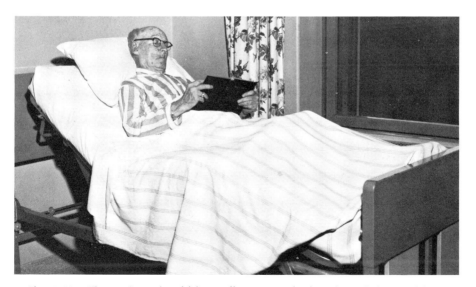

Fig. 4-11. The patient should be well supported when in a sitting position.

position with pillows, by supporting the arms, by slightly raising the knees, or by providing devices to hold the feet at right angles to the legs (Fig. 4-11).

The volume of blood from the heart is less when sitting than when recumbent. Therefore, patients with heart conditions are more comfortable when they are sitting up.

A patient may sit on the side of the bed with the feet unsupported in order to equalize circulation in the legs. This is termed *dangling*. Pressure of the mattress edge against popliteal blood vessels is to be avoided. If support of the trunk is needed, the nurse may stand beside the patient to hold him. Support for the feet may be provided by placing a chair under the feet. Some patients eat their meals in this position (Fig. 4-12).

Wheelchairs are adjustable for comfort and safety of the patient. Correct alignment of the body is provided by pillows at the back. The buttocks are placed well back in the chair. If the knees are flexed, the leg rest is adjusted for comfort. The footrest is placed at right angles to the chair.

PSYCHOSOCIAL ASPECTS

The time spent in bedmaking can often be utilized by the nurse in accomplishing more than just the mere mechanics of bedmaking and positioning of the patient. For the bed patient it can be a time in which an effective nurse-patient relationship is intentionally fostered by the nurse. While supplying environmental and physical comfort, the nurse may be able to interact with the patient in such a way as to help meet these psychologic needs. Some psychologic factors that might be

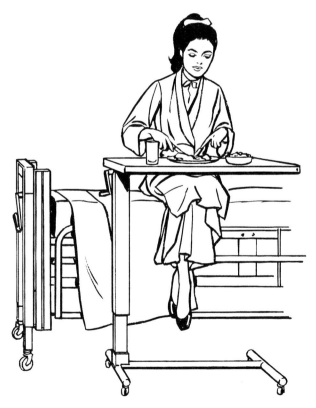

Fig. 4-12. Patient sitting on the side of the bed in good posture.

considered while making an occupied bed might include (1) adopting an appropriate manner of greeting the individual patient, (2) interacting in a meaningful way that leads to establishing rapport with the patient, (3) relieving the patient's uncertainty by explaining the procedure to him and what it entails, (4) providing privacy by screening and draping, and (5) controlling the amount of physical exertion that the procedure will cause for the patient.

The patient is more apt to experience the generally relaxing effect of clean, smooth, linen if the nurse works efficiently and rapidly in handling the bedding, is gentle in lifting and turning him, avoids jarring the bed, lifts the mattress minimally to tuck in the foundation linens, and arranges the articles in his unit for his convenience and preference.

LEARNING SITUATIONS FOR THE PATIENT

While making the occupied bed, the nurse may have an opportunity to explain the importance of correct body posture for the patient and may suggest ways of achieving and maintaining it. While lifting and moving the patient, the nurse should instruct him in how he can cooperate in making the activities safe and efficient. He may also learn a great deal just by watching the skillful nurse carrying out the various procedures.

If the patient needs bed care after dismissal, members of the family may need instruction in the prevention of contractual deformities and decubiti and in how to move, turn, and position him, as well as in how to make the occupied bed at home. Suggestions for improvising materials at home may be given. Information regarding comfort devices that can be purchased or rented for home use may be supplied. It may also be appropriate to encourage the patient and his family to anticipate the services of the visiting nurse or liaison nurse after dismissal from the hospital.

SUGGESTIONS FOR TECHNIQUE IN BEDMAKING

The following may be helpful for both the nurse and the patient in the bedmaking process:

1. Begin work in a systematic order. A little planning will save time and effort.
2. Have all equipment on hand in order of use.
3. Arrange environment for convenience. A chair at the foot of the bed saves many steps. Clean linen may be placed on the seat of the chair, and linen being removed from the bed to be used again may be folded and hung over the back of the chair. It will thus be convenient. Soiled linen should be placed directly into a laundry bag or hamper.
4. Save steps by accomplishing a task with each movement. For example, when placing the bottom sheet on the bed, begin at the foot and smooth to the head of the bed, tuck under the top of the mattress, miter the corner, and tuck under the side as you return to the foot of the bed. You are now near the chair with the linen and are ready to proceed with another piece.
5. It is advisable that the foundation part of the bed be completed before the top bedding is placed. When one is making an occupied bed, the bottom plastic draw sheet, if used, should be well covered by the cotton draw sheet to avoid contact with the patient's skin.
6. Variations may be made with the top bedding, such as the addition of bed cradles, canopies, and other mechanical devices. The upper bedding needs to be well secured across the foot of the bed but loose enough to

provide sufficient space for toe comfort. This looseness may be provided by merely raising the top covers over the toes a few inches and letting them fall again, by a toe pleat, by a cradle, or by bedboards upright against the footboard of the bed. Sometimes the top covers are secured around the footboard by pinning, or they may simply hang loose over the footboard.

SUMMARY

Selected principles of body mechanics have been used as an illustration of the relevancy of principles and problem solving to the planning of patient care that is individualized and directed toward maintaining homeostatic equilibrium between the person and his environment.

The chapter has explored at a basic level the process that the nurse uses in making application of principles in the problem-solving approach to the identification of the patient's needs and to guiding the nurse in decision making when planning and implementing patient care. Positioning in illness and bedmaking are specific activities to which the selected principles of body mechanics are applied.

QUESTIONS FOR DISCUSSION

1 Explain in your own words how use of related scientific principles facilitates identifying and defining the patient's problems.
2 In your next clinical experience observe an example of a nurse using (or could have been using) a physiologic principle in making a judgment upon which to base individualized care in solving a patient's problem.
3 Using the deductive approach, evaluate the success or failure of the tentative solution to the patient's problem observed in the preceding question.
4 What are the criteria for proper body alignment?
5 State in your own words the physical principles that explain each of the following:
   a Why less energy is required to maintain correct body posture than faulty posture.
   b Why friction hinders motion.
   c Why friction is desirable on the sole of the nurse's shoes.
   d How the nurse uses her own body to facilitate moving the patient toward the head of the bed.
   e Why more energy is required to make many little arm movements than to make one continuous smooth motion.
6 Which joints are capable of both adduction and abduction?

SUGGESTED READINGS

Barber, Janet M., Stokes, Lillian G., and Billings, Diane M.: Adult and child care—a client approach to nursing, St. Louis, 1973, The C. V. Mosby Co., pp. 183-188.

Bruner, Lillian S., and others: Textbook of medical-surgical nursing, Philadelphia, 1973, J. B. Lippincott Co., pp. 158-176.

Drury, John H., Jr.: Handbook of range-of-motion exercises, Nursing '72 **72**:19, April, 1972.

Foss, Georgia: The "how to's" of bed positioning, Nursing '72 **72**:14, August, 1972.

Foss, Georgia: Use your head and save your back . . . body mechanics, Nursing '73 **73**:25, May, 1973.

Millen, Helen M.: Physically fit for nursing, American Journal of Nursing **70**:520, March, 1970.

Moidel, Harriet C., and others: Nursing care of the patient with medical-surgical disorders, New York, 1971, McGraw-Hill Book Company, pp. 529-579.

Straud, Fleur L.: Modern physiology, the chemical and structural basis of function, New York, 1965, The Macmillan Co., pp. 555-575.

Stryker, Ruth P.: Rehabilitative aspects of acute and chronic nursing care, Philadelphia, 1972, W. B. Saunders Co., pp. 111-179.

5 Principles of communication and patient teaching

COMMUNICATION
Definition

Communication, in this context, may be defined as a sending-receiving process for channeling messages between individuals in person-to-person relationships. One individual is the transmitter and the other is the receiver of the message. In this exchange of messages, or ideas, the roles of sender and receiver are constantly reversed as a response to the message occurs. Generally, the response is accompanied by a change in the recipient, such as a difference in the way he thinks, feels, or acts. The change in the recipient may or may not be perceived by the transmitter of the message.

The need to communicate is universal. Whenever two or more people are to-

gether, some kind of communication is bound to occur, because individuals depend upon each other for satisfaction of physical, environmental, and psychologic needs. No one of us in today's technologic society and crowded cities could possibly grow all of his own food, build his own house, make cloth and sew his own clothes, provide fuel for cooking and for warmth, or develop a sense of security and of belonging all by himself. Obviously, the satisfaction of many of our human needs comes through interacting with other people, and our success in interacting is dependent upon the ability to communicate.

Through the use of language in the communication process, man expresses himself in order to satisfy his needs and desires, and he is enabled to live and work with other people in a social order.

Forms of communication

Although the spoken word is probably the most frequent mode for transmitting messages between persons, there is a nonverbal language of conveyance through which the message may be perceived. Regardless of its form, communication is satisfying to the individual when he feels that he has really transmitted to others what he wanted to convey. Effective communication promotes productive relationships between individuals.

Verbal communication. The spoken (and/or written) word is a most frequent mode for conveying information and one's ideas, thoughts, and feelings to others. Verbal communication implies the use of words to convey ideas of the sender. The receiver translates the words into ideas again. If the transmission process has been accurate, the ideas of the sender and receiver are the same. When they are different we say that there is a "break in communication."

For example, Mr. M., a possible diabetic patient, is to have a glucose tolerance test. While instructing him about this test, the nurse says, "You should not eat breakfast." On succeeding mornings after the test Mr. M. refuses to eat breakfast. When questioned as to the reason for this refusal, if he states, "Miss Jones told me not to eat breakfast," this could very possibly represent a considerable gap between the message the nurse intended to convey and the idea as perceived by Mr. M., resulting in failure of communication between the nurse and the patient.

The success of verbal communication is affected by a number of variables. The very word symbols used to express an idea may in themselves be a source of misinterpretation. The words represent an idea, or an object, to the sender, but they may have quite a different connotation in the mind of the receiver. When people do not agree as to the exact meaning of a word or words, this constitutes a problem in semantics. An example of this type of communication breakdown might be a situation in which the patient, Mr. B., requests the nurse to get his tablet for him. The nurse, to whom "tablet" means the patient's p.r.n. medication because he has been complaining of pain, responds, "It is not time for it yet, Mr. B." However, Mr. B. is really asking for the writing pad that is just out of his reach. This confusion would be a matter of difference in connotative meaning.

In the preceding illustration, the confusion is easily detected and communication quickly restored. In other situations the break in communication may not be recognized or the problem understood, resulting in misinterpretation not so quickly and easily corrected. One cardiac patient was told that he was to be "taken for an EKG." Thinking that this meant some kind of surgery, he became extremely apprehensive and fought valiantly with the orderly who came to transport him because he did not want to go to the operating room for surgery that he considered to be a terrible mistake. This strong emotional experience originating in a communication failure might well be accompanied by undesirable physical effects.

Other variables that can influence the receiver's perception and interpretation of the sender's verbal message include such things as tone and pitch of voice or word inflection that can evoke emotional responses. Psychologic and physical states as well as cultural factors and past experiences can affect perception and interpretation of the spoken words.

Basically, the aim of communication is to promote productive relationships between individuals or groups of people. This is a person-centered (patient-centered) view of the communication process in which failure in communication becomes a problem in interpersonal relationships.

Nonverbal communication. Seldom is communication entirely verbal, for the attitudes, feelings, and thoughts from which the communication arises may also be conveyed, either intentionally or unintentionally, through such nonverbal media as gestures, facial expression, body posture, and body movements. These forms of communication transmit ideas, modifying the perception and interpretation of both sender and receiver as their roles are constantly reversed in response to the changes resulting from the messages received.

The involved individuals may be largely unaware of the nonverbal process and its effect on the interaction. This does not, however, lessen the effect of these media, which usually evoke degrees of emotion that may not be conveyed by the audible words alone. For example; the patient who blandly says, "I am fine," may reveal other strong indications of distress through such nonverbal communication as facial expression, restless movements, sighing respiration, or poor appetite. The feeling tone that we communicate to others on a nonverbal level is an extension of our attitudes and tends to produce sustained response in others. A patient may react more strongly to the nonverbal cues he senses than to the words actually spoken to him.

Both verbal and nonverbal aspects of communication are significant in maintaining effective interaction with others.

The communication process

The transmitting and receiving of messages is pointless unless *meaning* is present for the individuals involved in the communication process. In literature on the subject, communication has been variously described as a triangle illustrating the three elements of the process. One point of the triangle (A, the sender) represents the *meaning,* or message, that the sender transmits. The second point (B, the symbols used to transmit the message) represents the verbal and/or nonverbal symbols used in transmitting the message. The third point (C, the receiver of the message) represents the one who perceives and interprets the symbols, transposing them back into meaning.

In the communication triangle the line from C back to A represents the *feedback* from the receiver to the transmitter. Kron in *Communication in Nursing* refers to this as the "perpetual triangle of communication." In this view of the communicative process, the relaying of interpretation from the receiver back to the sender is necessary for the sharing of ideas. It is through feedback that the original sender knows whether or not his ideas are accurately perceived and interpreted, and opportunity for clarification of misunderstandings when they occur is provided. For example, you, as team leader, instruct a new aide to make the empty bed on the east side of the four-bed unit. The aide hesitates, looking puzzled. You do not understand the reason for her apparent lack of understanding until feedback from her lets you know that her sense of direction is confused in this new situation. Therefore, she is not sure which direction is east. Because of the feedback to you from her you are able to clarify your original instruction to her.

The ability of the receiver to transpose the message of the communication accurately will be greatly affected by his cultural background, knowledge, attitudes, physical and emotional condition, skill in interpreting the nonverbal cues as well as the verbal symbols, and the context of the situation.

Communication arises out of thought processes. The message of a communication is valueless without the thought processes of the transmitter and receiver functioning to bring ideas and

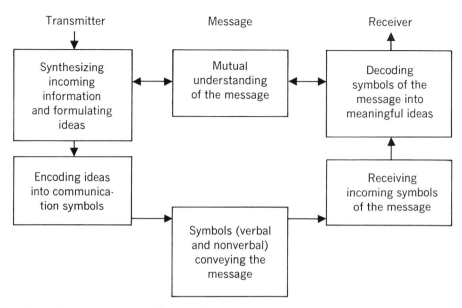

Fig. 5-1. Mutual understanding of the message conveyed in the communication arises out of the thought processes of both the transmitter and the receiver.

words into meaningful relationship between the individuals (Fig. 5-1).

Avoiding communication failures through application of principles

The communication process falls short of its goal unless the decoded message has the same meaning for the receiver as did the original message for the sender. What will help us to be understood by others, and to understand other people?

Through conscious effort, application of the following guiding principles, which are offered as suggestions, may lead to the development of more effective habits in the communication process.

1. Identify clearly what is to be communicated. It is worth taking the time to establish a goal or goals, to think what it is one wants to say, and to formulate the message carefully.

2. Seek to set the climate according to the goals for the intended interaction. Climate includes the factors and influences—physical, emotional, and environmental—in the situation that surrounds

the interacting persons. Recognizing factors within the situation that adversely affect the communication is the basis for action by the nurse. For example, the bedside light glaring in the patient's eyes will certainly detract from the communication process unless the nurse adjusts the light for the patient's comfort. Or the patient may have behaviors that the nurse finds offensive, such that the communication of the nurse with the patient is affected. The nurse would need to first examine her own feeling and objectivity in planning a conversation with this patient. The climate should be perceived as favorable by both the patient and the nurse.

3. Choose words calculated to convey the message accurately. Avoid technical or abstract words, clichés, or words with more than one meaning that are apt to be misinterpreted. Choose familiar words and use them correctly.

4. Consider the other individual and how he may react to the words chosen for the message. Are his cultural background, life style, attitudes and needs such that he

is apt to perceive the message as it is intended to be understood?

5. Be aware of the nonverbal communication being transmitted. The meaning of the message may be altered by tone of voice and inflection, by facial expression, and by gestures and other body movements.

6. Time the message to coincide with the point of most likely receptivity on the part of the other individual.

7. Wait for feedback from the other individual. This will aid in determining whether or not the message has been correctly understood. The response, verbal and/or nonverbal, will give clues regarding the accuracy of transmission and interpretation of the message.

8. Listen and observe, giving full attention to receiving and correctly interpreting the other individual's response without interrupting him.

9. Look for implied meanings of the other individual while trying to understand his point of view.

10. Evaluate the effectiveness of the communication process in achieving the intended goals. This gives the nurse an opportunity to look at the process in retrospect, determine the effectiveness of the verbal and nonverbal exchanges, and identify those responses that helped to clarify the patient's thoughts and feelings and that either furthered the goals or blocked communication. Evaluation leads to the revision of goals and communication approaches.

COMMUNICATION BETWEEN NURSE AND PATIENT
Communication in the nurse-patient relationship

There are numerous channels of communication that must be kept open in health care situations because communication enters into all on-going activities and personal relationships. It is the tool through which cooperative relations within the organization are maintained that are essential in providing effective care of patients—making assignments, planning and giving patient care, teaching, and evaluating. The more complex and specialized nursing becomes, the more necessary are well-developed communication skills and techniques for transmitting ideas.

Important as communication throughout the hospital is in providing the cooperation and understanding among personel so essential for total patient care, the focus here is on the communication process in the nurse-patient relationship.

Greater opportunities are now being recognized by nurses to relate therapeutically with the patient through communication skills utilized throughout the various steps of the nursing process, whenever the nurse is in contact with the patient (Fig. 5-2). Purposeful, goal-directed communication can be in progress with the patient during most nursing activities, for example, while admitting the patient, measuring vital signs, administering prescribed treatments, and teaching the patient. Administering hygienic care measures, particularly bathing the patient, affords the nurse an opportunity to encourage the patient to communicate his ideas and feelings, to assist him in discovering healthy ways of dealing with his emotional needs, and to gather data regarding physical signs and symptoms that are significant in developing the nursing care plan.

As the nurse seeks to increase the effectiveness of the time spent with the individual patient it is usually possible to discover ways of creating a warm, accepting climate to which the patient will respond.

Interviewing in nursing activities

Increasingly, the interviewing process is being used by nurses. The interview is a purposeful, goal-directed conversation be-

63

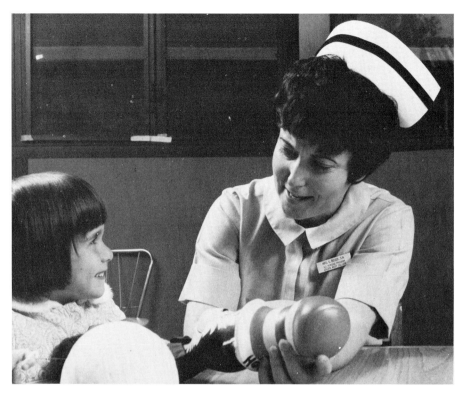

Fig. 5-2. Communication in the nurse-patient relationship is important at all ages.

tween the nurse and patient, his family, or other members of the health team. It is directed toward the maintenance or restoration of health and may be practically indistinguishable from therapeutic communication. It is not limited to a formal counseling situation but may occur wherever the nurse is with the patient. On the part of the nurse it involves the use of "self" in performing "caring" responsibilities. The therapeutic use of the "self" in caring for the patient means first to "care about him" as an individual. This attitude on the part of the nurse creates a warm, accepting climate that makes it possible for directed and progressive changes to occur in the patient. The nurse interacts with the patient to promote and facilitate these changes, which are directed toward improving, promoting, and maintaining health.

Through application of communication principles, the nurse can deepen personal understanding of the interviewing process and can develop skills and techniques that are effective in assisting the patient to change his behavior.

Communication techniques

Emphasis upon developing and refining communication techniques early in one's nursing experience is an advantage not only in administering care concerned with the sick person and his family but also with the promotion and maintenance of health. It is important for the nurse to be comfortable in one-to-one relationships with patients in order to deal with the needs of the whole person.

In face-to-face communication with the patient, everything the nurse says may be considered as either promoting the therapeutic effect or as being therapeutically ineffective in the communication process.

Therapeutically effective communication techniques

Examples of commonly recommended techniques include the following:

Silence. This is an interlude without verbal exchange, although much nonverbal communication may take place. It is the expectant kind of silence that encourages the patient to verbalize. Even though silent, the nurse conveys interest and expectation that the patient will take the initiative and talk about whatever is a pressing problem to him. Silence gives the patient an opportunity to organize his thoughts and to consider his feelings.

Restating the patient's main idea. The patient says, "I didn't eat breakfast. I can't eat." The nurse restates, "You can't eat." The nurse may repeat the patient's comment or question for several reasons, including: (1) to let the patient know his communication has or has not been understood, (2) to encourage the patient to restate and clarify his communication, and (3) to encourage him to continue talking. The patient infers the meaning intended by the nurse through the tone of voice, inflection, facial expression, and other nonverbal communication.

Reflecting his apparent ideas or feelings. Echoing his feelings back to the patient encourages him to examine what he has expressed and to either accept or reject the accuracy of the nurse's reflective echo. This is a suitable approach when the nurse observes that the patient's behavior seems to imply meaning other than the actual words spoken. It offers a way for the nurse to explore perception of the patient's behavior in an effort to determine the correctness of an observation or to gain more information when unsure of the patient's need. For example, the nurse notes Mr. J.'s anxious expression as he says, "I am supposed to have my opera-tion in the morning, but my head aches, and I don't think I can sleep tonight." The nurse responds reflectively, "You are concerned about your operation."

Using an open-ended question or statement. This kind of an offering tends to encourage the patient to continue speaking since it implies that the nurse has been listening and is interested in what follows. The nurse might use such open-ended leads as: "And then . . .", "And after that you will . . .", "Tell me about it."

Accepting. Responses such as merely nodding or saying, "Uh hmm" or "I follow you . . . ," signify to the patient that he is communicating with the nurse. Facial expression, posture, and tone and voice inflection must also convey acceptance if the responses are to be meaningful to the patient as intended by the nurse.

Clarifying. When the meaning is uncertain, the nurse can appropriately seek to discover what the patient is trying to say since he usually senses when he is not being understood. The nurse may ask, "Are you saying that . . .?" or state, "I'm not sure that I follow."

Listening. This means to give full attention to what the patient is saying, with the purpose of grasping the message that the patient is conveying, verbally or nonverbally. The patient may be encouraged to continue by the accepting responses of the nurse.

Ineffective communication

Some common approaches cited here have been selected as examples of techniques that tend to interfere with further effective nurse-patient interaction.

Advising. Telling the patient what to do is usually unwise because the patient may interpret it to mean that the nurse considers him incapable of self-direction. Advising tends to keep the patient from thinking through his problems for himself and arriving at his own solution. It should not, however, be confused with supplying the patient with data that he may need in formulating his own course of action.

Reassurance. Reassuring the patient is to imply he doesn't really have any reason to be anxious. Consequently, it denies the validity of the patient's own feelings and leads him to view the nurse as not understanding. This blocks the patient from exploring his feelings and anxieties with the nurse. Attempts to reassure the patient include such meaningless responses as: "Don't worry. It'll be O.K." "You're doing fine." "There's nothing to worry about." "Just leave it to the doctors." "I wouldn't worry."

Such vague responses are very apt to call forth negative feelings in the patient who will not then discuss his problems and anxieties with the nurse because he doesn't feel he can risk further lack of understanding, which he may feel is actually ridicule. To say glibly, "Keep your chin up," is to exude false cheerfulness that conveys to the patient that the nurse doesn't *really* care about his feelings.

Disagreement and disapproval. Disagreeing and/or disapproving are conveyed by using responses such as "That's not good" or "Don't do that." These are *disapproving* responses that imply a punitive attitude on the part of the nurse. Rather than to say "Don't do that" if the behavior is disturbing another patient, the nurse might say, "I will have to close your door, Mr. J., because you are keeping Mr. L. awake," thus directing attention to the effect of Mr. J.'s behavior on Mr. L. rather than on rebuke for his behavior as judged by the nurse. To respond "I disagree . . ." or "You're wrong . . ." or "I can't believe that . . ." is to imply a judgmental attitude. *Disagreeing* causes the patient to feel that he must somehow defend himself against the nurse.

Probing. Probing may consist of asking too many questions or asking questions that may seem inappropriate to the patient or as though he is being asked for more information than he is willing to give. The patient may respond with silence, evasion, or hostility.

Rejection. Failure to interact with the patient regarding his ideas, or not respecting his ideas, is rejecting him. For example, Mrs. J. says, "I am so worried because my husband hasn't come to see me today. If he really loved me he would come every day." If the nurse were to respond, "You are being very unreasonable to expect your husband to come every day," this would probably close off the subject, leaving the patient feeling rebuffed. Another response apt to produce a similar patient reaction is, "Let's discuss something more pleasant," which again is failure to let the patient reveal his problems.

TEACHING PATIENTS
Learning needs

Teaching has become an increasingly important part of the nurse-patient relationship. It is not uncommon to hear statements implying that teaching is inherent in nursing, or that all nurses function as teachers, or that the nurse is a "role model" of healthful living for the patient. This increasing emphasis on the teaching function of the nurse may be partly explained by the shift toward chronic and long-term illness, creating a need for the patient and his family to learn how to work with their problem and how to live a satisfying life within the restrictions imposed upon them by the health limitations of the problem.

The patient and his family need to be taught how they can cope with the specific problems and the modifications necessary for their particular situation. Provision for this kind of teaching has become a significant component in the planning of patient care, both in the setting of an acute episode of illness in the hospital or in other types of settings in which nurses are involved in patient care in community health agencies or in the patient's home. Teaching activities in this context are concerned with encouraging behavior beneficial to the health of the individual and his family.

The teaching-learning situation

For a teaching-learning situation to exist, there must first be an existing need or problem that motivates the individual to learn and for which information is available and useful to the individual in making appropriate decisions about his behavior. For continued success of the teaching-learning process, support and direction to assist the individual in altering his behavior and in carrying out decisions are often necessary. Reinforcement of learning is helpful in stabilizing the desired behavior change.

The quality of the patient teaching-learning process is directly dependent upon the effectiveness of the nurse's communication skills. Teaching and learning is more than a process of information giving, for the patient (learner) usually needs help in translating the information into behavior. Use of therapeutically effective communication techniques will help to ensure his maximum accuracy in receiving the information and translating it from idea into behavior.

Principles and methodology

While it is true that some teaching is done by the example of the nurse, much more can be accomplished through application of the principles and methodology of the teaching-learning process. The teacher in any situation is often compared to a catalyst because he brings the learner and the information together and stimulates a reaction. The teacher's activities either facilitate or hinder the learner's reaction.

Assessment of the present status of the patient and of the factors that will influence his learning is usually the first step in establishing the existence of need for learning, which then leads to determining the teaching content and methods and to establishing the desired goals or behavior changes. Teaching is facilitating achievement of the desired goals. Evaluation, which is an ongoing part of the teaching-learning process, is assessing whether or not the desired changes have occurred.

Only very fundamental and commonly recommended principles of learning are offered here as a beginning, generalized approach to teaching-learning situations, either in meeting patient needs for instruction or in developing staff members to their fullest potential. Other helpful principles can be readily identified that will be useful in specific situations. Through attention to the application of basic principles of learning, the nurse-teacher can stimulate the occurrence and continued progress of learning and strengthen personal skills in the teaching role.

1. *The learner's personal characteristics, knowledge, and prior experiences influence learning potential and give direction to planning content.* This implies that before developing a teaching plan it is essential to discover as much as possible about the learner from all available sources, but learning directly from him how much he already knows, his understanding of what more he needs to know, and his perception of the urgency for him to learn at this time are essential.

To illustrate the usefulness of this principle, consider the needs of Mrs. Garcia, a 35-year-old Mexican-American who had recently entered the United States and who speaks very little English. She had been admitted to the hospital with a diagnosis of pneumonia, but it was soon discovered that she was also a new diabetic. With treatment her condition began to improve, and the physician suggested that instructions should be given as soon as possible in long-term self-care in all aspects of diabetes. Miss Jones prepared a very complete set of plans for instructing Mrs. Garcia in all aspects of self-care. Knowing that Mrs. Garcia's English usage was limited, Miss Jones arranged for a Spanish-speaking nurse, Mrs. Gonzales, to interpret as necessary. She also had assembled a variety of teaching aids with which to instruct Mrs. Garcia in the basic understanding of diabetes necessary for self-care.

Mrs. Garcia, however, soon became restless and appeared irritated and disinterested. Mrs. Gonzales, observing the patient's reaction, discussed the situation with her and soon discovered that Mrs. Garcia already possessed a working knowledge of diabetes, insulin administration, diet, and skin care because her daughter had been a diabetic since early childhood and had been under her care and supervision.

Prior assessments by Miss Jones before developing her teaching plans for Mrs. Garcia would have helped her to establish a better climate for communication and learning, gain respect for the degree of knowledge and skills already possessed by the patient, develop more realistic teaching content to ensure Mrs. Garcia's understanding of her own specific insulin dosage and dietary needs, and spend her own time more wisely.

2. *The learner's felt need and readiness influence content and rate of learning.* This principle also is illustrated by Miss Jones' experience with Mrs. Garcia.

3. *Learning activities are more meaningful when the learner participates in setting the learning goals.* Goals, or objectives, define what the learner wishes to accomplish and tell the teacher what is to be taught. The objectives help the nurse-teacher to determine what content is realistic and relevant to attainment of the established goals. This is seen in the following example.

Miss Jones, team leader, noted that the nurse aide on her team had recorded a temperature of 39.4° C. (103° F.) for Mr. Smith. Her own observation of the patient led her to question the accuracy of the temperature reading, which upon checking proved to be only 37° C.

In discussing this incident with the aide, Miss Jones learned that Mr. Smith had just finished drinking a cup of hot tea when the aide had come to place the thermometer in his mouth. The aide expressed dismay at her own lack of knowledge not only about this procedure of temperature measurement but also about many other activities to which she had been assigned as a team member. The aide indicated desire to learn about "all these things." Through further discussion Miss Jones and the aide established as a beginning goal *the ability to measure body temperature accurately in any situation.* This situation also illustrates the second principle regarding the influence of the learner's felt need on learning.

4. *Active involvement of the learner is essential if learning is to occur.* Handing the patient a set of instructions for following a diabetic diet upon discharge from the hospital probably will not result in the diet being followed at home. Instruction must begin sufficiently in advance of discharge to allow time not only for active discussion with the patient but for practice in problem-solving situations in planning and preparing his own meals. Real learning will take place when the patient is actively involved in performing the procedures with the guidance of the nurse-teacher, rather than the nurse merely demonstrating the procedure for the patient to observe passively (Fig. 5-3).

5. *Retention of learning is increased by putting it to immediate use.* Referring to the illustration of Miss Jones and the aide, if the aide's assignment include temperature measurement over a period of time and with a variety of patient situations,

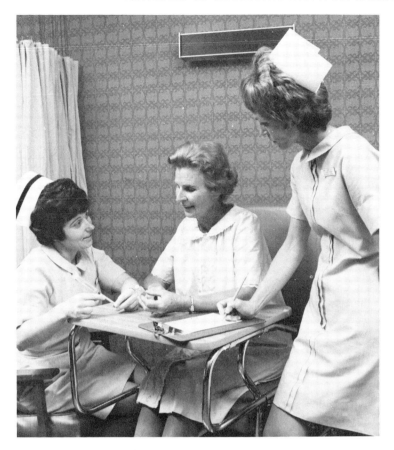

Fig. 5-3. Active involvement of the patient is essential if learning is to occur in patient teaching.

her learning is apt to be retained longer than if several weeks elapse before Miss Jones again assigns this responsibility to her.

6. *Learning is facilitated by relating material to be learned with what the learner already knows.* Looking again at Miss Jones' experience with Mrs. Garcia, the teaching plan should obviously be built upon what Mrs. Garcia had already learned through taking care of her diabetic child.

In general, people today receive a great deal more information about health matters through television and other means than before. The factor of previous knowledge and relating current teaching needs to such prior medical information must always be considered by the nurse in planning patient teaching. However, it is wise to first assess through conversation the accuracy of the patient's understanding of these matters.

7. *Learning is facilitated when the patient is allowed to learn at his own rate with objectives that are adjusted so that he can achieve success, which in turn tends to motivate him to further accomplishment.* Success is in itself a strong motivating factor in undertaking the next task, particularly when it occurs fairly early in the learning process.

8. *Reinforcement of learning rate, amount of retention, and degree of behavior change are facilitated by rewards of recog-*

69

nition, praise, and peer status. There are many ways of reinforcing learning, depending upon the learner's value system. Behavioral objectives enable the learner to quickly identify his own successful behaviors. Commendations may serve as reinforcement for employees. Reward is usually more useful than punishment in reinforcing motivation.

Selection of teaching method

Appropriate methods selected for the chosen content will facilitate the learning process. Learning tasks may be categorized as: (1) acquisition of information, (2) application of acquired knowledge, and (3) acquisition of skills.

In most learning situations some *information serves as a foundation for understanding* of new skills. Teaching techniques suitable for giving information include short talks combined with discussion and questions and programmed materials and other audiovisual teaching aids through which self-pacing may be used. Whatever method is selected, either for individual or for group instruction, it is well to remember that illness tends to shorten the individual's attention span.

Application of the acquired information involves integration of the knowledge into the learner's goal-directed activities. The problem-solving method may be suitable for some patients in applying the knowledge learned. The problem-solving steps outlined in Chapter 3 are useful for this purpose.

In using this method the nurse assumes a supportive role, helping the patient with each step of the problem-solving process as may be necessary in a particular situation. Referring once again to the learning needs of Mrs. Garcia, Miss Jones might prepare a problem-solving situation with the diabetic diet or insulin administration that would stimulate Mrs. Garcia's interest and further motivation.

The acquisition of new skills is a frequent learning need of patients, for example, changing his own colostomy dressing or testing urine for sugar and acetone. The nurse-teacher might appropriately include the demonstration method with skill practice as part of her teaching plan (Fig. 5-4). Sufficient practice should be planned to assure the patient's competency and self-confidence.

Selection of teaching time and place

It is extremely important to time the teaching with readiness on the part of the patient, physically as well as psychologically. The plan of care should definitely include a sufficient amount of time so that the patient and nurse can proceed at a pace suitable for the patient without interruption by other activities. It is well to plan relatively brief teaching periods to avoid tiring the patient.

The choice of place may be varied, but usually the patient's unit is a suitable location, at least in the early instruction periods. In some hospitals conference rooms or classrooms are conveniently located. Such locations would be suitable for group teaching of patients or staff.

An important factor in the effectiveness of teaching is continuity, which is usually best provided by planning for one nurse to accomplish the entire teaching needs of an individual patient.

Evaluation of learning

Evaluation in health teaching should help the learner to ascertain his achievement in terms of the predetermined goals. It helps the nurse-teacher and the learner to determine whether or not the desired behavior has been learned and also how effectively it has been learned. The behavioral objectives are useful in the teaching-learning process when they describe the precise activities necessary to demonstrate that the desired learnings have occurred.

An example of behavioral objective used as a means for measuring achievement can be seen in the situation of Mrs. Cooper, who was being taught to change the

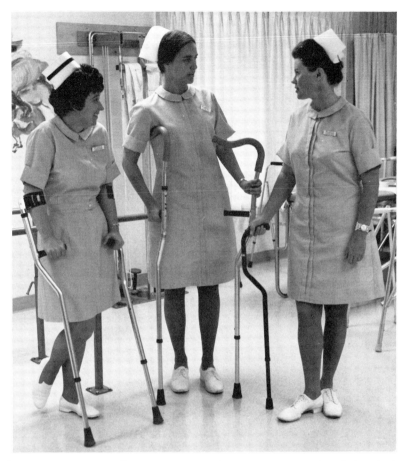

Fig. 5-4. Nursing students prepare to demonstrate use of assistive devices.

dressings on a draining wound for her husband after his discharge from the hospital. Among the objectives might be these: (1) is able to open packages of sterile dressings without contaminating them and (2) always washes hands before and following the dressing change. These are two objectives that tell Mrs. Cooper and the nurse-teacher exactly what behaviors are to be achieved by Mrs. Cooper.

Evaluation carried out in this manner is meaningful and specific in terms of the activity for both the learner and the teacher.

SUMMARY

Communicating with patients through purposeful conversation is an esssential part of total patient care. The purpose of

communication with the patient is to identify and meet his health needs, a process upon which the nurse who is faced with the necessity of developing the plan of patient care must rely.

Communication is defined as a sending-receiving process for channeling messages between individuals in a person-to-person relationship. Both verbal and nonverbal forms are useful to the nurse. Meaning must be present for the individuals involved in the communication process, otherwise communication has not occurred. Through feedback the sender ascertains whether or not his message has been accurately perceived and interpreted by the receiver.

Communication failures may be avoided

71

through application of guiding principles that lead to the development of more effective habits in the communication process.

The central focus is on the communication process in the nurse-patient relationship. Purposeful, goal-directed communication can be in progress with the patient during most nursing activities. The interviewing skills of the nurse may be directed toward the maintenance or restoration of health. Therapeutically effective communication techniques that need to be developed early in one's nursing experience are in sharp contrast to ineffective communication interactions with the patient.

The learning needs of patients are an increasingly important part of the nurse-patient relationship, and their satisfaction may be furthered by application of communication techniques in the teaching-learning process. Through attention to the basic principles of learning, the nurse-teacher can stimulate the occurrence and continued progress of learning and can strengthen her own skills in the teaching role. Selection of suitable teaching methods and the time and place of teaching are important factors in influencing the effectiveness of learning.

In health teaching, evaluation of learning in terms of achieving performance of the activities specified in predetermined goals will serve as a measurement of the competency of the learner in performing the desired behaviors.

QUESTIONS FOR DISCUSSION

1 How does a person's cultural background affect his communication?
2 Listen to nurses talking and list words used that may be misunderstood by patients and visitors unfamiliar with hospital language.
3 Observe your own experiences with communication in the hospital. Identify any breakdowns in communication. Why did they occur? How could they have been prevented?

4 How many of the patient's complaints on your unit may have been caused either directly or indirectly by communication failures?
5 Give examples of nonverbal communication that you have observed.
6 Describe the communication process, identifying the various elements of the process.
7 Why is "feedback" important in the communication process?
8 What is meant by "climate" in the communication process? Why is it important?
9 Can you identify additional principles in communication beyond those given in the chapter?
10 Discuss common blocks to effective communication.
11 Discuss the components of an effective teaching-learning process.
12 Relate the principles of learning to specific patient-teaching situations.

SUGGESTED READINGS

Aiken, Linda H.: Patient's problems are problems in learning, American Journal of Nursing 70:1916, September, 1970.

Amacher, Nancy J.: Touch is a way of caring—and a way of communicating with an aphasic patient, American Journal of Nursing 73:852, May, 1973.

Aradine, Carolyn R., and Hansen, Marc F.: Interdisciplinary teamwork in family health care, Nursing Clinics of North America 5:211, June, 1970.

Drummond, Eleanor E.: Communication and comfort for the dying patient, Nursing Clinics of North America 5:55, March, 1970.

Field, William E., Jr.: Watch your message, American Journal of Nursing 72:1278, July 6, 1972.

Heller, Vera: Handicapped patients talk together, American Journal of Nursing 70:332, February, 1970.

Hershey, Nathan: When is a communication privileged? American Journal of Nursing 70:112, January, 1970.

Kron, Thora: Communication in nursing, Philadelphia, 1972, W. B. Saunders Co.

Muecke, Marjorie A.: Overcoming the language barrier, Nursing Outlook 18:53, April, 1970.

Redman, Barbara K.: The process of patient teaching in nursing, St. Louis, 1972, The C. V. Mosby Co.

Schmidt, Joan: Availability: a concept of nursing practice, American Journal of Nursing 72:1086, June, 1972.

Veninga, Robert: Communications: a patient's eye view, American Journal of Nursing 73:320, February, 1973.

6 Biopsychosocial aspects of patient care

ADAPTATION AS A BASIS FOR PATIENT CARE
Concept of man's integrated wholeness

With the growing emphasis on high-level wellness and the preventive aspects of health care, a holistic approach is needed that will assist the nurse to develop understanding of the behavioral aspects of professional care. A framework for understanding the sources of stress and the psychologic and social influences experienced by the patient becomes increasingly important.

There appears to be general acceptance of the idea that the condition of high-level wellness implies integration of the whole being of the person—his body, mind, and spirit—in the functioning process as an organized whole. The "integrated wholeness" is generally understood to include the biologic, psychologic, and spiritual dimensions of man as viewed against the background of his interaction with a changing environment. These elements are so interrelated that they cannot be separated meaningfully. For example, it is impossible to examine the brain alone and understand its functioning apart from the whole body. One must consider the entire physical organism as a whole in order to gain understanding of the role of the brain in integrated functioning of the body.

Likewise, it is impossible to meaningfully separate the physical aspects of man from the whole being, for the idea of wholeness expresses man's interrelated functioning as a physical, social, psychologic, and spiritual being. Accordingly, man is viewed as a composite of interrelated systems and, in his wholeness, expresses the organization and interrelatedness of these component systems, which have no fine lines of demarcation.

This holistic concept of the person mandates that nursing include concern not only for the physical needs of the individual but that attention be focused on the relevant psychosocial aspects of the pa-

75

tient and his family. The systems are in constant state of interaction with each other in such a way that a change in one system affects the others. Therefore, an approach is needed that will assist the nurse to consider the various possible facets of the *individual* who is ill or who needs assistance with some aspect of health, with the physical needs being considered within the framework of the individual's total integrated being. This approach will influence the entire nursing process, bringing into focus the assessment and intervention for all systems in the provision of more effective patient care. This approach encourages one to recognize that the overt behavior of the individual is influenced by forces included in the theories of all of the merging fields of biologic, psychologic, and social studies and to recognize that no one of these systems controls behavior exclusively.

The term "adaptation" in current usage includes the multiplicity of genetic, physiologic, psychic, and social phenomena through which adjustment (homeostatic balance) is achieved in response to changes within the environment. More specifically, in the context of nursing, adaptation may be understood to include the responses of the body through which it attempts to cope with the elements of the total environment, both internal and external, in order to retain its unity and integrity.

According to this view of adaptation, it is generally understood that *the processes of living are the processes of adaptation.* One might conclude by saying that man's health is judged by his ability to adapt physically, psychologically, and socially to changes in his environment.

Summary of the adaptation level theory

In Chapter 2, health and illness were presented as being the ends of a continuum along which the person can be located at any given time. At whatever point on the continuum man is located, he is in constant interaction with a changing environment. A variety of stimuli (stress agents, referred to as stressors) will impinge on him, and he must respond to these. For instance, the person who is moving toward the illness side of the continuum may encounter strange new stressors such as symptoms, perhaps hospitalization, diagnostic procedures, and the like with which he will need to cope. The coping mechanisms man uses for adapting to these stressors in his changing life situations are biologic, psychologic, and social in origin. An example of a biologic coping mechanism through which the relative constancy of the body's internal environment is maintained is homeostasis. A specific illustration of homeostatic effect is maintenance of body temperature at a relatively constant level because of the balance that exists between heat production and heat loss in response to changes in the environment.

The stress agent is always a threat to the person's homeostatic equilibrium, physical, psychologic, and social. Adaptation is a term used to describe the work expended by the body in warding off the effect of the stressor in its effort to maintain homeostasis. Through the dynamic adaptive mechanisms the effects of the stressors are mitigated and at times are counteracted. A positive response to changing stressors is an outcome of adaptation.

The level of adaptation, and thus the ability to respond to change, fluctuates according to differences in perception, judgment, sensitivity, and performance in an individual at any one time. According to Helsen's concept of adaptation, constant and varied stimuli impinge on each individual at all times.* In every situation con-

*Helsen, Harry: Adaptation-level theory, New York, 1964, Harper and Row, Publishers.

fronting a person there is in existence an adaptation level to impinging stimuli. This level is the mean of the pooled effect from three kinds of stimuli. These are:

1. *Focal stimuli.* These provoking stimuli command the attention of the person. Stimuli become focal because of size, intensity, position, novelty, quality, movement, and internal predisposing factors, such as set and attitude.

2. *Contextual stimuli.* This category includes those stimuli that surround the focal stimulus. They are all other environmental stimuli present— physical surroundings, other people present, and so on.

3. *Residual stimuli.* These are recalled remnants of past experiences that influence the meanings attached to other stimuli. Included are attitudes, values, beliefs, and other factors that influence an individual's behavior in a given situation.

Each kind of stimulus may exert more or less influence upon the pooled effect and subsequent behavioral response.

In determining the pooled effect of focal, contextual, and residual stimuli, it is necessary to weigh the more recent stimuli, with the last stimulus carrying the heaviest weight of all. An adaptive state is the point at which no stimulus is recognized as causing an imbalance between the person and his environment. The further impinging stimuli are from the prevailing adaptation level, the more distinctive they are and the greater the effect they will have on behavior. The less stimuli differ from the adaptation level, the more neutral they are perceived to be. Change in any condition of stimulation results in some change in adaptation level. Every stimulus that impinges on the person pulls his adaptation level more or less in its own direction. Stimuli are modified by other stimuli, and their effectiveness depends upon many innate and acquired biopsychosocial factors affecting the individual.

In this concept of adaptation any inclination to respond arises from the difference between the stimulation and the adaptation level. The *greater the difference, the stronger the response will be.* A simple illustration will help to make the point clear. The fresh scent of baking bread will bring the hungry person quickly to the source of the fragrance. If, however, there is only day-old bread being offered, the magnitude of response will certainly be less. The concept contains the idea that the strength of the response depends also on the *adaptation level.* By longer exposure to the scent of baking bread, the sensation of smell very soon diminishes because the end organs of the sensory cells quickly become adapted to the odoriferous stimulus, which can then be expected to produce a weaker response than it did originally.

The basic premise of the adaptation level theory is that an individual's attitudes, values, ways of structuring his experiences, judgments of physical, esthetic, and symbolic objects, intellectual and emotional behavior, learning, and interpersonal relations all represent modes of adaptation to environmental and organismic forces. All behavior is meaningful, in that all behavior represents man's attempt to adapt to his changing environment.

At whatever point the person is along the health-illness continuum, he must adapt to the variety of stimuli assailing him. A positive response to such stimuli or environmental changes requires adaptation. The behavioral indication of a positive response is a decrease in reaction to the predominant stimulus. Such adaptation frees the person to respond to other complementary stimuli present; for example, relief from pain allows the patient to respond to stimuli indicating need for eating, sleeping, and other activities.

Referring again to Chapter 2, the three stages of response to stresses, the *general adaptation syndrome,* are outlined together with the essential elements in the body's defense against stress. The Roy adaptation model, one of many ways of viewing man's adapting, refers to these defenses as *coping mechanisms.** According to this model the *regulator mechanism* works mainly through the autonomic nervous system, which provides the initial alarm reaction readying the individual for the "fight or flight" response to the focal stimuli. The *cognator mechanism* identifies, stores, and relates stimuli so that symbolic responses can be made. It is described as acting consciously by means of thought and decision and unconsciously through the defense mechanisms.

Assumptions regarding the effectiveness of the coping mechanisms are used to discern when the patient is unable to adapt to a presenting problem. For example, adaptation failure may be recognized through marked autonomic activity (increased heart rate, blood pressure, tension, excitement, and so on) coupled with cognator ineffectiveness (inability to identify the problem, inability to identify a goal for action, and inability to decide upon means for reaching a goal) (Fig. 6-1).

Man's modes of adaptation

In the Roy adaptation theory man is conceptualized as having four modes of adaptation. These four modes appear in the following outline, together with examples of characteristic problems associated with each need.

Basic physiologic needs and problems.† As man responds to environmental changes, he will need to keep in balance the following needs (numbered heads) and problems (subheads):

1. Exercise and rest
   a. Immobility
   b. Hyperactivity
   c. Fatigue and insomnia
2. Nutrition
   a. Malnutrition
   b. Nausea and vomiting
3. Elimination
   a. Retention and hyperexcretion
   b. Constipation and diarrhea
   c. Incontinence
4. Fluid and electrolytes
   a. Dehydration
   b. Edema
   c. Electrolyte imbalance
5. Oxygen
   a. Oxygen deficit
   b. Oxygen excess
6. Circulation
   a. Shock
   b. Overload
7. Regulation
   a. Temperature
      (1) Fever
      (2) Hypothermia
   b. Senses
      (1) Sensory deprivation
      (2) Sensory overload (pain)
   c. Endocrine system
      (1) Endocrine imbalance

Self-concept. The "self" of a person responds to changes in the environment. Self-concept includes all the ideas, feelings, beliefs, and attitudes that a person has about himself and his possessions. To maintain psychologic adaptation, defense mechanisms may be used to protect the ego when the self-concept is threatened. Values that may be threatened during illness include:

1. Physical self: loss—depression following mastectomy
2. Personal self
   a. Moral-ethical-guilt—child with rheumatic fever blames illness on disobeying his mother
   b. Self-consistency–anxiety–patient

---

*Roy, Sister Callista: Adaptation: a conceptual framework for nursing, Nursing Outlook **18**:44, March, 1970.

†Roy, Sister Callista: Adaptation: implications for curriculum change, Nursing Outlook **21**:163, March, 1973.

pacing the floor the night before surgery

c. Self-ideal and expectancy-powerlessness—teen-ager in traction unable to try out for varsity

3. Interpersonal self
   a. Social disengagement—elderly woman refuses to communicate with staff
   b. Aggression—cardiac patient yells at nurse

Role mastery. In this mode of adaptation man is viewed as regulating his performance of duties according to his vary-

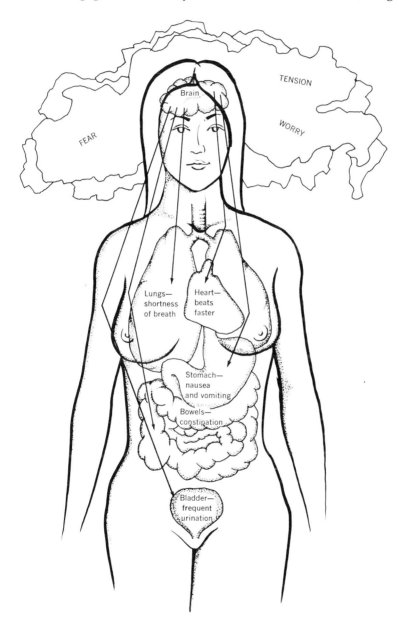

Fig. 6-1. Adaptation failure in stress may be recognized through increased autonomic activity. Sometimes associated are changes in vision, sweaty palms, chilly sensations, and diarrhea or constipation.

ing positions in society. Role change is threatening, and adaptation to the new role is required:

1. Role failure: perceived inability to perform behaviors related to role—amputee, former truck driver, concerned about supporting family
2. Role conflict: perceived expectations of others regarding role behavior differs from own expectations—wife with active pulmonary tuberculosis whose children expect her to take care of them as their mother

Interdependence. Environmental changes may threaten conflict in a person's interactions) with other persons with whom one is interdependent:

1. Dysfunctional independence: insistence on autonomous behavior to detriment of well-being—hospitalized toddler refuses food from nurses
2. Dysfunctional dependence: failure to initiate autonomous behavior when it is feasible for well-being—postoperative patient refuses to participate in self-care

Supportive role of the nurse

The nurse is actively involved in the patient's environment, seeking to support his adaptive mechanisms as he struggles with the forces in the situation. In the conceptual framework of adaptation, *nursing intervention* becomes the means through which the nurse's knowledge and skill are interposed in supporting and promoting the patient's adaptive potential to the highest level of effectiveness. As such, it must be based on understanding and application of relevant scientific knowledge basic to the nurse's recognition of the individual's organismic responses that reveal the nature of the patient's adaptation in progress. *Nursing assessment* is the process through which the nurse perceives how the patient is adapting to maintain or regain a favorable balance on the health-illness continuum. It is the application of

knowledge and understanding in perceiving and evaluating the forces in the situation that are acting on the individual and the effectiveness of his coping mechanisms. The *substance of nursing* lies in perceiving when the individual's (and/or family's) coping mechanisms are no longer effective and using this information as a rational basis for judicious decision making in nursing intervention designed to foster the patient's adaptation, whenever this is possible. The unique role of nursing is conceived of as a therapeutic function through assessment and intervention.

ADAPTATION CONCEPT IN NURSING
The nursing process

As the adaptation concept in nursing is further developed, it becomes apparent that the nurse focuses on the patient as responding to stimuli present because of his position on the health-illness continuum, the goal being to bring about an adapted state in the patient that frees him to respond to other stimuli. To accomplish this goal, the nurse uses the processes of nursing assessment and nursing intervention, through which it is presumed that the patient's conserved energy will be available for the healing responses, thus contributing to the overall goal of the health team.

Assessment and intervention

In the Roy* adaptation model, the nurse making an assessment *first* recognizes the patient's position on the health-illness continuum and then observes the patient's behavior in each of the *four adaptive modes,* identifying and listing the *positive* and *negative behaviors.* As indicated on pp. 77-78, positive and negative behaviors are recognized by answering the

*Roy, Sister Callista: Adaptation: a basis for nursing practice, Nursing Outlook **19**:255, April, 1971.

question: Is the patient free to respond to a variety of factors in the situation, or does his behavior reveal that his bodily reactions and thought processes are concentrated primarily on coping with the predominant stimulus? The nurse evaluates the forces acting on the patient and the effectiveness of his coping mechanisms in dealing with the predominant stressor stimuli and explores the questions: How well is the patient adapting in this situation? Are there negative behaviors?

This type of exploratory questioning of the patient's behavior leads to the *second level of assessment,* in which the nurse seeks to outline the factors influencing the negative behavior. The patient may be included in this process, with the nurse enlisting his verification of the stimuli that are experienced by him as most focal, that is, the stimuli that are predominant to the patient. Focal, contextual, and residual factors influencing the patient's behavior are assessed. Through this phase of the assessment process the interrelatedness of the adaptive modes in the patient's situation may be more clearly identified.

With the needed information available to begin developing the nursing plan for patient care, the nurse moves to the second step of the nursing process, which is *intervention.* With the intent of promoting patient adaptation, the nurse seeks to plan care that will change the patient's response potential. This goal is attained by lowering the intensity of the focal stimulus, if possible, to bring it closer to the level of the patient's coping ability within the context of the situation. This may involve manipulating the focal stimuli, the contextual stimuli, and/or the residual stimuli. The nursing action is based upon the patient's apparent level of adaptation within each of the four adaptive modes.

The problem-solving approach as described in Chapters 3 and 4 is in harmony with most theoretical frameworks and is a useful tool in the Roy adaptation model

for nursing as outlined in this chapter.

As the plan of care is implemented, the nurse continues the assessment process and evaluates the outcomes to determine whether or not the patient's behavior has changed in the direction of the desired goal. Adjustments in the plan of care are based on selection of approaches that appear to have the highest probability of success in promoting patient adaptation. The nursing plan of care as developed in this model is consistent with Chapter 13, and they may be used as complementary approaches.

The following example is an illustration of the nurse focusing on one aspect of the patient's response to a focal stimulus and nursing action taken to promote an adaptive response.

Forty-eight hours after major abdominal surgery, Mrs. K. is still nauseated and vomiting, unable to retain anything by mouth, and is receiving intravenous fluids. The nurse notes that meperidine is still being administered for control of pain and that there is a p.r.n. order for an antiemetic medication. In this *first level of assessment* the nurse observes the patient in the adaptive modes, listing the *positive and negative behaviors* (Table 6-1). The nurse then utilizes the *second level of assessment:* (1) outlining the factors influencing the negative behavior, nausea and vomiting, (2) hypothesizing that meperidine is causing the nausea and is the stimulus that Mrs. K. finds most difficult to cope with, (3) verifying with Mrs. K. that nausea is the most disturbing factor in the immediate situation, although she has not associated the medication with it as actually being the *focal stimulus,* and (4) continuing the assessment process by looking for other relevant *contextual* and *residual stimuli* that may be influencing factors. Together, the nurse and patient identify such *contextual* factors as discomfort from the long-continued intravenous fluids, postoperative pain (described by Mrs. K.

Table 6-1 First level of assessment

	Behavior	
Assessment factors	**Positive**	**Negative**
1. Basic physiologic needs: Nutrition		Inability to retain food or fluids

Table 6-2 Second level of assessment

	Stimuli		
Behavior	**Focal**	**Contextual**	**Residual**
Vomiting Inability to retain fluids or food	Meperidine (most likely cause of the behavior)	Restricted to intravenous fluids Unpleasant odors increase nausea (for example, smoking)	Former experience with postoperative vomiting

as mild), the unpleasant smell of cigarette smoke coming from the other patients in adjoining units, and the contributing *residual* factor of two former experiences that Mrs. K. has had with persistent postoperative vomiting (Table 6-2).

At this point, with the needed information identified, the nurse establishes for Mrs. K.'s *plan of care,* the *goal* of eliminating nausea and vomiting, and unsuccessful efforts to retain oral fluids and food, after having asked the question: Can the focal stimulus be changed to bring it closer to the level that Mrs. K. can handle? The nurse may decide to verify the possibility of a relationship between meperidine and persistence of the nausea and vomiting by observation of the time relationship of giving the drug and the incidence of nausea. The nurse can then consult with the physician to determine whether or not another pain medication could be better tolerated by Mrs. K., if it is needed for further control of pain, together with maxi-

mum use of the prescribed antiemetic medication. It may be also that the nurse will decide to counsel with the patient, exploring the residual influence of Mrs. K.'s former experiences with postoperative nausea and vomiting and the possibility of anticipatory effect in the present situation. And the nurse will make every effort to control unpleasant odors in the environment (Table 6-3 and Fig. 6-2). Using this portion of the total plan of care for Mrs. K., the nurse will *evaluate* its effectiveness in terms of the patient's altered behavior in achieving the goal. The following day, nursing assessment and evaluation reveal that Mrs. K.'s nausea and vomiting have mostly subsided, that intravenous fluid therapy is discontinued, and that oral liquids are being retained. Mrs. K.'s comment to the nurse is that she thinks the "pain medicine" (meperidine) caused her nausea and vomiting.

In this simple illustration one can trace the process employed by the nurse: (1) to

Table 6-3 Plan for patient care

Nursing care plan

Goal	Approach
To eliminate nausea and vomiting and promote ability to retain food	1. Assess possible relationship between nausea and prescribed medications
To prevent dehydration from nausea and vomiting	2. Administer p.r.n. antiemetic medication
	3. Control unpleasant odor of cigarette smoking
	4. Provide fluids when tolerated
	5. Counsel patient regarding psychologic influence of former experiences with postoperative nausea and vomiting

assess the behavior of Mrs. K. in the adaptive mode of the basic physiologic needs (in this example limited to the appetitive system) and the factors influencing the negative behavior of vomiting, (2) to intervene to change the negative behavior by altering the focal, contextual, and residual factors influencing the behavior, and (3) to evaluate as to whether or not the approach has changed the negative behavior of Mrs. K. and promoted her adaptation.

It should not be inferred from this uncomplicated illustration, however, that an identified need always requires a given nursing approach. Rather, this model encourages the nurse to view the need in its total setting, or the complex of stimuli influencing the patient and his ability to cope with the need, and to systematically use all of the data in developing the plan for patient care.

The adaptation model—a stable frame of reference

Many nursing programs are attempting to or have integrated the curriculum, and all are confronted with differing concepts of the career ladder, changing practices,

new roles, and various other kinds of innovations. In these times of rapid change, a stabilizing frame of reference is needed to serve as a guide in developing innovations while promoting a rational system of articulation and progression within the "career ladder" and to delineate the unique function of nursing in relation to other health workers. For example, the physician focuses primarily on the stimuli affecting the patient's position on the health-illness continuum; his focus is on the patient's disease, its diagnosis, and treatment in achieving his goal of moving the patient along the continuum from illness to health. The social worker is concerned primarily with the patient, the family, and social forces affecting them, focusing on the goal of social productivity more than on patient adaptation. Nursing, on the other hand, focuses on the patient as a person responding to the stimuli bombarding him by reason of his position on the continuum. The nursing goal is to promote an adaptive state in the individual that releases him to respond to other stimuli, conserving his energy for the healing process, thus contributing to the overall goal of the total health team. Although

PATIENT CARE ASSIGNMENT

Student:		Date:	
Patient:		Age:	Room:
Diagnosis:			
Diet:	I&O:	Additional information:	
TPR:	B/P:		
Bath:			
Activity:			

Student's self-evaluation (of care given):

Student's self-evaluation (of care given):

ASSESSMENT AREAS	POSITIVE BEHAVIOR (describe)	NEGATIVE BEHAVIOR (describe)
Ventilation		
Circulation		
Fluid and electrolyte		
Regulation		
Exercise and rest		
Nutrition		
Elimination		
Self-concept		
Role mastery		
Interdependence		

Fig. 6-2. Patient care assignment worksheet, suggested for use in developing the patient plan of care. NOTE: These two sample pages may be printed on both sides of one sheet of paper. (Courtesy Nursing Faculty, Golden West College, Huntington Beach, Calif.)

STIMULI

Negative behavior Describe pt's behavior	Focal Cause of behavior	Contextual Environment	Residual Beliefs-attitudes

NEGATIVE BEHAVIOR	NURSING INTERVENTION

Instructor's notes:

Fig. 6-2, cont'd.   For legend see opposite page.

there is some overlapping with other health disciplines, the adaptation model helps the nurse to focus on her specific functions among the other related health care systems.

The question might very well be posed: What is basic nursing and what constitutes preparation for it? The proponents of the adaptation concept of nursing would respond that this theoretical model is based on the philosophic belief that the focal point of nursing is man and his interaction with a changing environment, that it is established upon the thesis that man requires assistance in coping with his changing environment at whatever point on the continuum he finds himself, and, therefore, that the basic level nurse should be prepared to promote man's physiologic and psychosocial adaptation in both health and illness. From this point of view, nursing is a social necessity in that it functions to promote man's adaptation.

Among the advantages of the adaptation concept in the preparation of the nurse are the following outstanding features. It provides for basic adaptation problems through which the nursing process becomes largely a problem-solving experience requiring much depth and breadth of vision on the part of the nurse, rather than emphasizing only the accumulation of knowledge. However, according to the Roy model, assessment and intervention in simple, known adaptation problems could begin at the nursing aide level, the student with potential moving on to other types of programs and progressing to the level at which problem solving in the unknown begins. At the more advanced levels nurses learn to see themselves as change agents in dealing with the patient and families, both in the hospital and in the community. Health teaching and leadership roles are strands of knowledge and practice that continue throughout the appropriate levels of

the curriculum based on the Roy model.*

Since the adaptation concept encourages nursing to look at the assessment and intervention regarding adaptation problems, the nurse practitioner might specialize in a given problem area or in adaptation problems in a specific patient situation. These possibilities seem to be consistent with the presentation of nursing and the total health services concept presented in Chapter 1. The apparent trend is toward independent and/or expanded practitioner roles in nursing, and the adaptation model would provide an appropriate framework for the professional preparation of nurse practitioners functioning in these roles.

SUMMARY

The adaptation model provides a conceptual framework for nursing that helps the nurse to recognize the patient's position on the health-illness continuum, to observe significant behaviors in each of the adaptive modes, and to determine what behaviors require nursing intervention and the factors relevant to resolving the problem, that is, to provide the data for establishing goals and for selecting nursing approaches for achieving the goals of supporting and promoting patient adaptation.

The adaptation concept of nursing can provide for integration of the basic curriculum while providing stability in curriculum change necessary to distinguish levels and roles in nursing that will meet the changing health service needs of our society.

QUESTIONS FOR DISCUSSION

1 What is the meaning of the "holistic" concept of man?
2 In the context of nursing, what is included in the term "adaptation"?
3 What is meant by the statement:"The pro-

*Roy, Sister Callista: Adaptation: a basis for nursing practice, Nursing Outlook 19:165, April, 1971.

cesses of living are the processes of adaptation"?

4 Give an example of a biologic coping mechanism through which relative constancy of the body's internal mechanism is maintained.

5 In Helsen's adaptation level theory, what three kinds of stimuli have a pooled effect and influence behavioral response?

6 What is the behavioral indication of a positive response?

7 What is meant by the expression "general adaptation syndrome"?

8 What is meant by the term "stressor"?

9 In context with the adaptation model, what are the "coping mechanisms"?

10 According to the adaptation model, how does the "regulator mechanism" function?

11 How may adaptive failure be recognized?

12 In the adaptation concept of nursing, what are the processes through which the nurse functions? Describe each process.

13 When and how does the nurse make use of the four adaptive modes?

14 How could the adaptation model serve as a stabilizing influence in nursing education and nursing practice?

SUGGESTED READINGS

Fisher, Valentina G., and Connolly, Arlene F.: Promotion of physical comfort and safety (Foundations of Nursing Series), ed. 1, Dubuque, Iowa, 1970, William C. Brown Company, Publishers, chaps. 2 to 4.

Helsen, Harry: Adaptation-level theory, New York, 1964, Harper and Row, Publishers.

Roy, Sister Callista: Adaptation: a conceptual framework for nursing, Nursing Outlook 18:42, March, 1970.

Roy, Sister Callista: Adaptation: a basis for nursing practice, Nursing Outlook 19:254, April, 1971.

Roy, Sister Callista: Adaptation: implications for curriculum change, Nursing Outlook 21:163, March, 1973.

7 Cultural aspects of patient care

CULTURAL INFLUENCES
Cultural background

Social, cultural, and psychologic factors interact dynamically. Culture may be thought of as the total way of life of a people, the social legacy the individual acquires from his group. Ethnic and social backgrounds influence the way patients see and react to the hospital. The fact that cultural differences exist should be accepted, and the nurse should make an attempt to learn about and view sympathetically the beliefs and customs of all groups.

The culture concept is cardinal to an understanding of ourselves and our world. Every patient belongs to one or more subcultures, depending on his occupation, his income, and his antecedents. Common backgrounds in language, customs, beliefs, habits, diets, and traditions often characterize people in ethnic groups that react in predictable ways.

Variables useful in identifying social classes are education, occupation, income, prestige, interaction, and place of residence.

Custom and group habits are referred to as folkways and mores. Folkways are the accustomed and time-honored ways of doing things, the social habits that become routine and that are often performed without thinking. Mores are customs that are regarded as particularly sacred and necessary to social welfare. These folkways and mores play an important part in the routine of daily living. They carry an emotional impact that makes them resistant to change.

The patient brings with him something from his cultural background that determines the way he perceives his relationship with the physician or nurse and that facilitates or impedes interaction or communication. Knowing about the patient's cultural background enables the physician, nurse, medical social worker, or other health specialist to deal with the patient more realistically and to be more flexible in treatment plans.

The hospital

The hospital also has its social characteristics that tend to stimulate a considerable amount of dread and apprehension on the part of the patient. It represents a way of life that has its own customs, language, and values. It is a unique world in terms of sights, sounds, and smells that are not comparable to everyday experiences outside and to which the patient must make some adjustments.

Categories of troubles that patients bring to the hospital with them include worries about what is happening at home and in the community from which they have been separated, worries about children, husbands, and wives, worries about jobs, and worries about finances. Thus the basic problem faced by the patient in the hospital is anxiety.

Much of the anxiety connected with being ill results from the unknown, and not knowing what to expect builds up anxiety. The patient's fear of the unknown is caused by lack of knowledge of his illness and its complications, by very little knowledge of treatments, by being in a strange place, by being alone and away from his family, by being housed with strangers and cared for by strangers, by lack of achievement, and by having nothing to do or being left to pass the time in whatever way he can with minimum activity, which may mean a kind of tense boredom. It is natural to be afraid of what is strange or unusual, but knowledge sometimes dispels fear. However, the patient may be afraid to ask questions because everyone seems so busy. Or perhaps the patient is afraid to know the answer. Many patients who do not know the nature of hospital procedures are afraid to ask the results. Perhaps the greatest fear of all is the patient's dread of how he will be received as a person. Sharing his feelings with nurses and with other patients may well be a therapeutic process in itself.

A new patient coming into any hospital is unwittingly behaving or misbehaving along culturally determined patterns. This, along with learning the rules of the new small culture into which he is enter-ing, produces stress. Unvarying routine may constitute quite a variation from the patient's accustomed way of living. He is expected to be dependent upon the nurse and to surrender a great deal of his personal freedom. He gives up some of his outside connections within the hospital system.

The patient is likely to have difficulty in adjusting to the average general hospital, where he may well consider himself unnecessarily robbed of independence and the opportunity to make his own decisions.

The patient and his family too are unduly sensitive to experiences of all kinds that occur in a hospital. Their adjustment may range in its effect from matters of the immediate moment that have direct bearing on life and death to future situations that deal with public and community relations.

The patient is an individual member of a family unit of society. The family, the home, and normal community activities seem to furnish a frame of reference against which he measures or seeks to interpret many aspects of his hospital experience. The illness of any member of a family will indirectly affect other members of the family. The patient, in his sickness, has two rights: to be exempt from his normal social role responsibilities and to be cared for since he cannot get well by an act of decision or will. The primary obligation of caring for the sick person falls on members of his family. The patient may or may not accept his sick role, and his family may or may not accept it. Nonacceptance builds up anxiety.

How the patient reacts to his illness may be conditioned by the feelings of members of his family who may be under emotional tension or economic stress that consciously or unconsciously is transmitted to him. Sickness is a time when the family is expected to rally to the patient's side. Sickness frequently disrupts family role relationships, necessitating a shift in responsibility that a family member may not be able to make, or the shift may have consequences that are threatening to the patient.

Satisfying nurse-patient relationships must include the patient's family and be fostered in an atmosphere of mutual confidence, understanding, and trust. Members of the family need to feel accepted and should be given the opportunity to do things for the patient, and they should be given an explanation concerning his care. The families of pediatric, psychiatric, and surgical patients need to be skillfully oriented to the patient's experience and their communication with him. Acute illness, critical debility, and major physical handicaps create problems in communication that the nurse must interpret for the family and friends who visit the patient. The adjustment of the patient and his family to the hospital may affect his willingness to accept the treatment offered him or to stay until it is complete.

Most patients come to the hospital with a positive attitude, a factor that can be utilized by hospital personnel in medical care. Positive attitudes toward hospitals can give psychologic support to both patients and members of the staff. The patient places himself in the hands of hospital personnel hoping that he will receive adequate care, and he thus submits to necessary dependence for recovery from illness. Such willingness is a deterrent to anxiety. The hospital, being committed to good patient care, provides the patient protection against outside tensions and interferences.

The recovery of the patient from his illness is influenced by his relations not only to hospital personnel but also to his family and other nonhospital groups whose contact is usually restricted in terms of number of visitors and hours of visiting.

Except for patients with extensive hospital experience, anxiety may be produced by strange uniforms, equipment, and language. The hospital and its equipment in themselves induce anxiety in many persons, particularly those with limited education and life experience. Good equipment and technical knowledge on the part of the worker are important deterrents to anxiety.

Among the features of the hospital subculture that a patient notices very quickly is a lack of privacy. Illness places a patient in a relatively intimate association with other patients and hospital personnel whom he considers strangers. He is literally forced into regressive relationships he might otherwise never choose.

Adjustment to the hospital is made easier for the patient if the nurse helps him meet his psychologic needs. Needs create tensions, and tensions give rise to anxiety that may hamper recovery.

Every patient has needs that must be satisfied, but he is not always able to identify them, knowing only that he feels the tension they generate. Most actions involve a fusion of several needs. Needs come and go and sometimes conflict with each other. Needs are classified in different ways. However, the great majority of lists of basic psychologic needs include (1) the need for recognition, (2) the need to belong, (3) the need for understanding, (4) the need for stimulation and personal growth, and (5) the need for security.

Everyone wants to be recognized as an individual and to feel that he is important to someone else. The need for attention increases in response to illness. One objective in nursing is to preserve the dignity of the patient. The nurse respects and accepts the patient as a person, addressing the patient by his correct name and title. Respect for the patient includes the right for the patient to have his own feelings and to express them to those who may understand them. Each patient is a particular person with different behavior patterns and will react to his illness differently from anyone else.

The patient has a need to belong. He belongs to his family and briefly to the hospital milieu. He wishes to be accepted in the hospital as well as at home. There is no set rule for making a patient feel at home in a hospital. The nurse gives warmth and sympathy to help him feel more comfortable in a strange place and explains routines and treatments.

The patient has a need for understanding his own illness and problems. He wants to know what the hospital expects of him, what his responsibilities are, and how well he can meet these responsibilities. The nurse should let him know what he is to do and how the hospital is attempting to meet his expectations. Discovery of patients' expectations requires much careful listening and judicious questioning. When patients feel understood, they will have a feeling of trust and confidence. The nurse must take an interest in each patient as an individual in order to understand him and learn the meaning of what he says and does. During the performance of a lengthy procedure, the nurse interacts with the patient during a period long enough to gain some understanding of him.

The patient has a need for stimulation and personal growth. A new experience furnishes stimultion and is important for the patient who finds sameness in the day-after-day activities. New experiences for the patient may take the form of treatments, persons in the environment, and even meal trays. A treatment that a patient is learning to perform on himself can provide much stimulation. Change, such as being moved to a different area, provides new knowledge and understanding and gives the patient something different about which to think and talk.

Security is the greatest need of the patient. The feeling of security is the result of having the needs for recognition, belonging, understanding, and new experiences met. A patient feels secure when he is made to feel welcome and is cared for by a warm, understanding nurse. Patients depend on nurses for what will happen to them, for giving them a comfortable feeling of being in good hands, and for knowing that both the nurses and physicians are concerned with their best interests. The patient may feel insecure because he has no control over what is happening to him and he is surrounded by strangers.

When a patient's needs are satisfied, he has a feeling of comfort and happiness. In satisfying his needs, the nurse inspires a peace of mind that allows the patient to be at rest both mentally and physically and creates through skillful communication an atmosphere acceptable to the patient.

Religious aspects

The patient's attitude toward his illness and his problem of adaptation to the hospital can be facilitated or hampered by his and his family's religious beliefs.

Religion traditionally has focused upon a God beyond the individual and has concerned itself with relating the individual to that God. In times of crisis, such as illness and death, man typically turns to God. In illness people who have not thought of religion for years ask, "Why has this happened to me?" "What is the meaning of this?" Sometimes patients cling to the hand of the nurse and beg, "Pray for me." The resources of religion can be brought to help the patient meet the facts of the situation.

Religious beliefs are seldom held to oneself but are part of group processes, so that there is immediate family support for the patient. There is little doubt about the symbolic indication of group support that prayer presents. It helps the patient's own attitude or belief that he will recover, that there are forces available to facilitate the healing process. Here, religion is not seen as a healing process apart from science but as a cooperating agent. It is important for the nurse to be of help, to understand not only the spiritual needs of the patient but also the means and methods that organized religion has for meeting those needs.

Catholicism. Generally, Catholic patients will desire to see a priest and to receive the sacraments while hospitalized, particularly if the hospitalization is of a serious nature or of long duration. Also, many Catholics desire to see a priest prior to surgery. The nurse should be astute to any expression of spiritual needs or tactfully ask the patient whether he has any desire to have the priest call on him. Of course, his wishes are respected. If the patient is hospitalized where a Catholic chaplain is not in residence or where family members cannot notify a priest, the nurse assumes this responsibility.

Some patients may prefer to visit with their own parish priest, and the nurse helps with these arrangements if necessary. The patient may request the reception of Penance (Confession) and/or Holy Eucharist (Communion). If the patient is to receive the sacrament of Penance, he should be afforded privacy at this time. If he is in a ward, his bed should be screened.

To prepare for Communion, Catholics usually fast from food and liquids (other than water) for 1 hour before the reception of this sacrament. However, this may not be possible for the hospitalized person, who may receive Communion regardless of his fasting status. The Catholic patient will desire to be alone prior to the reception of Communion, during which time he is making his spiritual preparation. No special arrangements are necessary in the patients room, though he may prefer to have the head of the bed elevated. Following the reception of this sacrament, he will again desire a period of privacy.

The sacrament of the Last Anointing may be administered to Catholics who are considered to be seriously ill, who are seriously injured, or who are aged. One should not assume that death is imminent if this sacrament is administered, since the reception of Last Anointing offers special prayers for the recipient as well as the anointing of the senses with holy oil. A Catholic patient may request that he receive this sacrament, and a priest should be notified. No special room preparation is necessary since the priest will bring his own materials for this sacrament. He may anoint the patient's feet (this is optional), and so the bed covers should be loosened at the foot of the bed, and the hands should be on top of the covers.

If death is impending for a Catholic patient, a priest should be notified. Catholics desire that a priest be with them when death is near and that he administer the sacrament of the Last Anointing. This sacrament can also be administered when the patient is unconscious and even up to 2 hours after being pronounced dead by a physician, since the moment of death is uncertain. Because this sacrament offers strength in preparing for death to the Catholic patient and spiritual consolation to his family, it need not be regarded as a frightening experience but rather a strengthening and comforting one.

Protestantism. Protestantism is not one religion or church. Rather it is composed of various faiths or denominations that differ widely in their beliefs or practice. However, there are certain characteristics that they have in common: Christ is the head, the Bible is their guide, and salvation is by faith. Most Protestants practice some form of baptism. However, many reject infant baptism and baptize only adult candidates.

Many Protestant churches sponsor hospitals, and these hospitals usually employ a full-time chaplain who ministers not only to members of his own faith but to anyone who needs help.

Some Protestants have prayer books and may bring them to the hospital. The Gideon Society has graciously supplied most hospitals with translations of the King James version of both Old and New Testaments.

No set rules can be applied to the practice of Protestant ministers in the hospital. For some denominations the sacraments of Communion and Baptism may be administered in a manner quite similar to that of Roman Catholic priests. It should be mentioned here that Protestants usually partake of the wine as well as the bread during Communion. Some Protestants observe Lent by participation in special services. However, they may or may not observe fast days.

The Anglo-Catholic clergyman speaks of himself as "priest" and is addressed as "Father" by his parishioners. His method of administering to the sick is similar to that of the Roman Catholic priest, and he will need the same materials for administering the sacraments as the Roman Catholic priest. Other Protestant ministers may be addressed as Chaplain, Reverend, Brother, Elder, or Pastor. The practice of a pastor in the sickroom may vary from just a casual visit to prayer, reading of the Scriptures, hearing of confessions, and Baptism.

Judaism. It is quite difficult to define Judaism. The religious definition of a Jew is "one who accepts the faith of Judaism." Judaism is also "a civilization" or way of life because Jews share a common history, common prayer, a vast literature, and a common moral and spiritual purpose.

Judaism holds that man can best worship God by imitating those qualities that are godly: (1) as God is merciful, so man must be compassionate; (2) as God is just, so must man deal justly with his neighbor; and (3) as God is slow to anger, so man must be tolerant.

Jews and Christians share many things in common, the most important ones being probably the truths of the Old Testament and the Ten Commandments.

There are three branches of Judaism: Orthodox, Conservative, and Reformed. The Orthodox Jew stems from a faith that has been unaltered for more than 3,000 years. He accepts the Bible as the revealed word of God. He observes the Sabbath (late Friday evening to Saturday evening) strictly, performing no work, conducting no business, and carrying no money. He adheres to every detail of the dietary laws. Conservative and Reformed Jews, as the names imply, are somewhat relaxed in the keeping of some of the traditions and adhere more to the customs of the modern Protestant.

Jews more or less observe "kosher" or dietary laws, which may be found in the Old Testament (Leviticus, Chapter 11): (1) they do not eat the meat of certain animals, such as the pig, horse, and hare; (2) they do not eat any seafoods that do not have fins and scales, hence, no shrimp, lobster, crab, or oysters; (3) meats must be slaughtered by the quickest method possible with the least amount of pain to the animal, and the people who perform the act should be God-fearing men (Jewish men do not indulge in the sport of hunting game); (4) meat, fowl, and dairy products are never eaten together, and cooking vessels must be kept scrupulously clean.

It is almost impossible to provide a complete kosher diet in a non-Jewish hospital. However, the nurse can do much to help the patient make the proper adjustment by giving suggestions to the diet kitchen and making substitutions when possible.

The most important holiday for the Jewish patient is Yom Kippur. It is marked by 24 hours of prayer and fasting and is known as the Day of Atonement. Rosh Hashanah is the Jewish New Year, and the Rosh Hashanah of 1974 is the year

5736 on the Jewish calendar. Jewish religious books are the Talmud and the Torah, which contain codes of ethics, history, and the Mosaic Law.

The center of the Jewish religion is in the home, and some member of the family will usually contact a rabbi for the patient. However, the nurse may do so if requested or if the patient is without family or friends. The religious practices of the rabbi in the hospital are somewhat similar to those of the Protestant minister. The Orthodox Jew should never be left alone when in a dying condition.

Other religions. The Seventh-Day Adventists also keep dietary and health laws similar to those observed by Jews and observe Saturday as their Sabbath.

Other common faiths are Jehovah's Witnesses, Mormons, and Christian Scientists. Since it is impossible to include the practice of every religion, the nurse should be acquainted with unfamiliar faiths.* Resource material is available in all libraries, and all hospital chaplains know how to secure help for members of all religious faiths.

Since only a certain percentage of the population belongs to a church, the nurse will meet patients who have no active church affiliation. Methods of meeting their spiritual needs are found by physician, by nurse, and by social workers. As the nurse observes spiritual needs, he may do one of two things and sometimes both: (1) introduce a clergyman into the situation or (2) attempt to minister to the need. It is important for the nurse to discover from the patient's record whether he has any active church affiliation. For persons who are Ancient and Accepted Freemasons, any member of the order will come to the aid of a brother, and the organization will also conduct a funeral or burial service that is appropriate for anyone who has faith in a Supreme Being.

*For quick reference, consult Routh, E. C.: Who are they? Shawnee, Okla., 1952, The Bison Press.

SUMMARY

Factors to be considered in the adjustment of a patient to the hospital environment include his cultural background, his physical condition, his socioeconomic status, and his methods of communication.

Consideration for the patient's cultural background can often help to make his adjustment therapeutic and to prevent regression. He makes his needs known by communication, and the understanding nurse aids by listening attentively. Most of the time, stress will cause the patient to want to talk even when he would not do so otherwise. In illness, the patient faces many conditions about which he can do nothing but talk. Talking is his way of doing something about the problems. Talking to a clergyman may bring comfort to a patient in distress. Sometimes talking relieves his anxiety about the hospital or about his home conditions. Since the religious faith of the person plays such an important role in his recovery or acceptance of a chronic disease, it is the duty of the nurse to learn about various religious faiths to be able to understand the patient's behavior and to give assistance when necessary. The hospital chaplain has become an important member of the health team and is a source of comfort to the patient.

QUESTIONS FOR DISCUSSION

1 Define "culture," "ethnic," "psychosocial," and "socioeconomic."
2 Consider a person of a particular culture. How do his customs differ from yours?
3 Why does a patient regress in illness? Name three aspects of his adjustment to illness that show regression.
4 Much of a patient's anxiety is caused by fear of the unknown. Name five facts you may give a patient to prevent this fear.
5 Name as many ways as you can in which a person is different from every other person.
6 How would you attempt to meet a patient's

spiritual needs if no clergyman were available?

7 List some denominations that do not practice infant baptism.

SUGGESTED READINGS

Allport, Gordon W.: The individual and his religion, New York, 1961, The Macmillan Company.

Daoust, J. M.: Spiritual care of the sick, L'Hôpital d'Aujourd'hui **16**(7):20, July, 1970.

McKnight, Earle T.: A chaplain interprets his work, Canadian Nurse **57**:1139, December, 1961.

Naiman, H. L.: Nursing in Jewish law, American Journal of Nursing **70**(10):2378, November, 1970.

Pederson, W. Dennis: The broadening role of the hospital chaplain, Hospitals **42**(9):58, May 1, 1968.

Reinhardt, Adina M., and Quinn, Mildred D.: Family-centered community nursing: a sociocultural framework, St. Louis, 1973, The C. V. Mosby Co.

8 Developing a safe and therapeutic environment

THE THERAPEUTIC ENVIRONMENT

Meaning. Environment in this context may be defined as the total of all the external conditions and influences affecting an individual in the illness situation. These "conditions and influences" include the tangible physical factors in the situation, such as the architectural features, furnishings, decor, lighting, ventilation, and the like, and the psychosocial forces exerted upon the patient. The latter include less tangible "feeling tones" created by the customs, routines, cultural values, interpersonal relationships, and prevailing concepts of the appropriate roles and behaviors of the patient and the nurse. These psychosocial factors were introduced in Chapter 6. In other chapters the concept of adaptation and the balance of the internal environment through homeostatic mechanisms has been presented. Here, the focus is on the possibility of modifying the external environment to meet the needs of the patient.

Goal. Clearly, the goal in dealing with external environmental factors is the development and maintenance of a situation that will be favorable for the patient, favorable for both his physical and psychologic well-being. Such a situation is generally referred to as a therapeutic environment. In this concept of the external environment the emphasis is on patient-centered care and on the activities that are geared at one and the same time to promoting (1) his physical welfare and (2) purposeful interaction between the patient and the staff that will foster emotional balance, growth, and recovery of health, within the potential of the individual patient.

CHARACTERISTICS OF A THERAPEUTIC ENVIRONMENT

A therapeutic environment is one that contributes to the well-being of the patient

96

and does not retard his recovery; in other words, it is a health-promoting environment.

Basic characteristics

The distinguishing elements of such an environment include at least the following characteristics:

1. Adequate comfort, food, cleanliness
2. Freedom from injury—mechanical, thermal, chemical, electric, radiational, bacteriologic, allergic, or psychologic
3. Individualization of patient care with the opportunity for the patient to participate in his own plan of care within the limits of his capacity and readiness
4. Friendly, courteous, accepting atmosphere throughout the unit that encourages meaningful cummunication between patient and nurse
5. A feeling of security and self-worth on the part of the nursing personnel
6. Absence of unresolved conflict among personnel
7. Diversional activities available for the patient

Modifying the environment

In recent years knowledge of the impact of the social environment upon human behavior has been applied to understanding the influence of environment upon the patient's behavior and his progress toward recovery. Since the character of the patient's hospital experience is so greatly affected by the personnel and their interrelations with him, the nurse has an essential role in creating and maintaining an environment that will be helpful to the patient.

Attention can be focused on the patient's needs through exploration of such questions as: How does the patient's home environment differ from the hospital environment? How does the patient feel about his illness? How does he feel about hospitalization? How does the patient and his family feel about the nurse and other personnel? How has the hospital environment affected the patient? How has it contributed to his recovery? What unfavorable experiences have occurred? What actions have the nurse and other staff members taken to tailor the patient's environment according to his particular needs? Such questions can serve as a positive force in modifying the various physical and psychologic environmental factors for the patient's benefit.

Through listening to the patient and encouraging him to express his feelings, the nurse can gain knowledge of him that is of assistance in encouraging him toward involvement in planning his own care and in assuming responsibility, within his limitations, for decisions that must be made. Positive adaptation on the part of the patient can thus be encouraged, and he may regain patterns of response that help him handle stress in a manner that is compatible with physical and psychologic balance. In the event of permanent or long-term disability, the patient can also be assisted to accept his limitation and to plan realistically for his future. This process is facilitated by treating the patient as a responsible person who can be informed and consulted about his own therapy and who is allowed to react honestly to the situation and to what is being done for him.

In many situations patients may appropriately be encouraged to assist each other. For instance, a patient who has been experiencing difficulty accepting a colostomy may be greatly helped by another patient who has already adjusted to this limitation. The alert nurse can find many ways of promoting significant patient interaction that may stimulate interest and serve as a form of social therapy where indicated.

Nurses may also add to the therapeutic environment through their approach to the patient's family members and other visitors, who are often emotionally involved in the patient's situation and who therefore sometimes react with anxiety, but who may be able to provide useful information about the patient that may affect his plan of care.

A very important area of nursing influence in developing a therapeutic environment is coordinating with other professionals or groups involved in patient therapy—the physician, dietitian, physical therapist, social worker, for example—so that treatment schedules and routines will be planned for the benefit of the patient. The nurse may also use her knowledge of interpersonal relationships in communicating with aides and orderlies to increase their understanding and ability to assist in meeting the patient's physical and psychologic needs.

Other ways in which nurses can exert leadership in adapting routines and in modifying the value system for the patient's welfare are suggested in Chapters 6 and 7, which discusses the cultural aspects of patient care, and in Chapter 13, in which the focus is on planning nursing care.

SCIENTIFIC PRINCIPLES AND THE PATIENT'S UNIT
Principles selected from microbiology

The following principles that are applicable to the care of the patient's unit have been selected from microbiology:

1. Pathogenic microorganisms may be transferred from the source to a new host (a) *directly* by contaminated objects, called *fomites,* and by insects, called *vectors,* and (b) *indirectly* by *airborne* particles of dust and droplets of moisture.

2. Pathogenic microorganisms require organic food (organic substances such as body discharges and food particles).

3. Growth and reproduction of microorganisms may be prevented by chemicals or heat, which interfere with their life processes. This inhibiting process is called *bacteriostasis.* (In contrast, *sterilization* is

the process of destroying all microorganisms, whereas *disinfection* destroys most nonsporeforming pathogens.) The effectiveness of bacteriostasis by chemicals depends on (a) the type and number of organisms present, (b) the concentration of the chemical solution used in the process, (c) the time allowed for chemical action, and (d) the nature of the material subjected to the chemical action.

Application of principles

These bacteriologic principles should be applied to the cleaning of the unit and equipment between their use by patients. Based on these principles, the following cleaning procedures that are safe and effective in protecting the patient and hospital personnel from infection can be developed for housekeeping.

1. Methods of sweeping and dusting, and other general cleaning, should inhibit airborne transfer of microorganisms.

2. Insects should be eliminated.

3. All organic material should be removed from equipment or surfaces before the disinfection process. Rinsing with cold water first will aid in removing organic materials without coagulating them on the surfaces, thus interfering with their removal.

4. Cleaning and disinfecting chemicals that will not harm surfaces or materials to be treated can be selected.

5. Cleaning and disinfecting solutions should be used in the required concentrations and for the specified length of application, according to the directions, to ensure effectiveness.

6. Use of disposable equipment as much as possible lessens danger of transferring microorganisms. Nondisposable articles used by a patient, such as bedpan, basins, and the like, should be thoroughly cleaned and disinfected after use and before being issued to another patient.

Although much of the cleaning process is actually performed by other personnel, the nurse should be aware of the underlying principles and be able to apply them when necessary or to recognize practices that are unsafe or ineffective in preventing the spread of pathogenic microorganisms. It is the nurse who observes and regulates the patient's physical environment.

With proper application of these principles, the newly admitted patient can be escorted into a clean unit.

The typical patient unit

In the immediate environment of the patient are the things he uses. His unit may consist of an elaborately furnished private room, a section of a semiprivate room, or a ward, in which the minimum equipment is a bed, a bedside stand, and a chair. Many units contain an overbed table. Bedside stand equipment may consist of a basin, soap dish, mouthwash cup, curved basin, bedpan, and urinal if needed. Individual disposable equipment saves labor of cleaning and assures clean utensils for the new patient. Whatever is for the patient's use should be clean, in good working condition, and as attractively arranged as possible. However, the patient's wishes should be respected as much as possible, with belongings easily accessible. The unit should be easy to keep clean and the equipment easy to sterilize after each patient's use. Manufacturers are providing furniture with more color and of different materials to make pleasant and cheerful surroundings for the patient (Fig. 8-1). There is a great deal that can be done through color, decoration, and arrangement of furniture and facilities to reduce the impression of an institution and

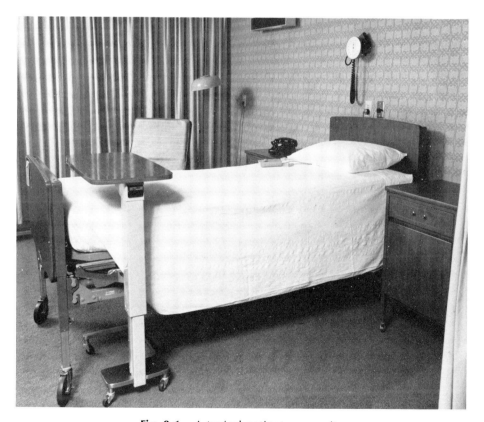

Fig. 8-1. A typical patient care unit.

to heighten the feeling of home. The housekeeping department is responsible for supervising the care given to the patient's unit.

Usually the patient tends to develop possessive feelings regarding his unit and all that it contains. He may even come to regard the unit as his "castle" and resent intrusion or the appropriation of its contents by others, including the nurses. The thoughtful nurse is guided accordingly and, when entering the patient's unit, speaks to him immediately, thus recognizing his presence and his right of possession and privacy in the unit. Explaining to the patient why one is removing an article of equipment from his unit is a matter of common courtesy.

Such environmental factors as noise, odors, safety hazards, cleanliness, and similar things can usually be controlled by the nurse. Adjusting the bed, bedside table, other furnishings, and the patient's possessions in his unit for his comfort and according to his needs can make the surroundings more conducive to rest, comfort, and relaxation.

SAFETY FACTORS IN THE ENVIRONMENT

A safe and comfortable environment is one that contributes to the well-being of the patient and does not retard his recovery. It implies freedom from injury—mechanical, thermal, chemical, electric, radiational, bacteriologic, allergic, or psychologic. It is concerned with quiet, provision of pleasant surroundings, elimination of unpleasant sensations of touch and smell, atmospheric conditions (temperature, humidity, and ventilation), and lighting. The same factor that makes the environment safe may add to the comfort of the patient. Knowledge and judgment must be exerted in order to prevent accidents and to develop an awareness of physiologic reactions and psychologic disturbances that may predispose the patient

to physical trauma. The creating of an immediate environment that is conducive to safety of the patient is a nursing responsibility.

Mechanical injury may be caused by machines as well as by falls and blows. A patient may be injured by a fall from a bed or a window, by a fall while standing or walking, by cords or tubing tangled about him or about equipment, by the movement of a wheelchair or stretcher, or by inadequate protection while being lifted or moved.

Mechanical injury may be prevented by using rails or guards on windows and beds, by having floors dry and floor coverings fixed firmly, by holding stretchers and wheelchairs securely while assisting patients, by having equipment firmly and safely attached in place, by movers of patients lifting together and giving directional signals.

A periodic check of equipment assures that it will be safe and ready for use. Precautions are taken to prevent breakage of glassware and breakage and blunting of needles.

Thermal injury is caused by fires or other sources of heat. The triple hazards of fire are burns, trauma, and asphyxiation. Exclusive of fires, burns may occur from the application of heat, such as a hot-water bottle, electric heating pad or other electric devices, or a steam inhaler. When applied, these devices must be watched carefully. Hot solutions used in treatments should not exceed the degree of heat prescribed for the procedure.

Some possible causes of fires in a hospital are smoking in bed, defective wiring, spontaneous ignition of tincture of benzoin fumes in a steam tent, explosion of gases and x-ray films, and the use of electric hot plates about the bed.

Fires are prevented by good housekeeping, good maintenance, and good discipline. Good housekeeping means avoiding rubbish accumulation, keeping oily rags in metal containers, and closing fire doors and doors of clothes chutes and dumb-waiters. Good maintenance means reporting frayed electric cords and defective electrical equipment, not overloading circuits, preventing escape of flammable liquids or gases, wiping up greases, and having fire extinguishers recharged from time to time. Good discipline means having a practical plan for use in case of fire, having fire drills from time to time, assigning each one a task to perform in the event of fire, obeying signs relating to prevention of fire, such as NO SMOKING, and knowing how to call the fire department. The small number of disastrous hospital fires speaks well for the constant vigilance of nurses and other personnel.

Chemical injury involves the use of too strong chemicals on the skin or taken internally or an overdose of a prescribed drug. Poisonous chemicals should not be left within reach of the patient and should be guarded carefully if used at the bedside. Such chemicals may be those used for disinfection or for treating wounds. They should also be separated in the medicine cabinet from drugs to be given to patients. Many commonly used drugs have toxic effects if given in large doses or concentrations or given at too frequent intervals, hence the need for accurate measurement of drugs and for giving medicines at the stated intervals. The smaller the dose of a drug, the more potent the drug is and the more reason the nurse has for precaution in the calculation of its dose. Drugs are stored in places suitable to preserve their chemical character. They should be discarded upon deterioration, and they should be labeled clearly and accurately.

Electrical injury results in burns from an electric current. Burns may be caused by defective wiring or defective equipment. Sometimes the degree of heat may be increased beyond the point of safety in an electric heating device. Since water is a conductor of electricity, touching an electric connection with wet hands may produce a burn. Static electricity from friction of bedding is seldom harmful, but very often it produces an unpleasant sensation.

Prevention of electrical injury consists of not overloading circuits and of reporting defective wiring or appliances.

Radiation injury occurs from overexposure to x-rays or radium. These injuries are prevented by having trained operators in charge of the machines and devices used for administering these rays. The nurse may prevent further injury by reporting changes in the skin or other tissues under treatment.

Bacteriologic injury is caused by disease-producing microorganisms. Microorganisms cause diseases that can be spread from person to person and also infections. The so-called hospital infection is caused by the *Staphylococcus,* which is normally found on the skin and mucous membranes. It may be transferred by body contact or by discharges.

Bacteriologic safety has to do with elimination of disease-bearing organisms and dirt that harbors them in such a way as not to harm the patient or to cause a cross-infection or a reinfection. A cross-infection means that a patient becomes infected in the hospital with a disease other than that for which he was admitted.

Since harmful microorganisms are spread more by the hands than by any other method, it becomes necessary for physicians, nurses, and other workers to wash their hands frequently and thoroughly before and after the care of each patient and many times while performing different treatments on the same patient. Handwashing removes microorganisms and is best accomplished by using running water, soap, and friction twice, rinsing twice, and drying thoroughly (Fig. 8-2). Handwashing is more effective in removing microorganisms if each soaping is accompanied by friction on all parts of the hands and wrists, including the sur-

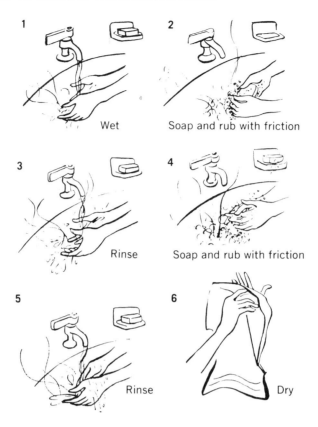

1. Wet
2. Soap and rub with friction
3. Rinse
4. Soap and rub with friction
5. Rinse
6. Dry

Fig. 8-2. An efficient method of handwashing.

faces between the fingers. Soaps recommended for handwashing contain a variety of antibacterial agents. These soaps tend to have a lasting bacteriostatic effect and are not irritating to the skin. They reduce the time of handwashing to about half that required when other soaps are used.

A patient with a communicable disease is separated from other patients not having that disease. During his care, the nurse wears a gown and observes rigid precautions to prevent the transfer of disease organisms. Methods used in caring for a patient with a communicable disease are termed *medical asepsis.* An attempt is made to prevent the organisms from contaminating clean areas. Further discussion of communicable disease technique is given in Chapter 32.

Effective techniques for disinfection and sterilization should be employed. Sterilization is a process whereby all microorganisms are destroyed. Disinfection is a process whereby most pathogenic nonsporeforming forms of microorganisms are destroyed. Bacteriostasis is a process whereby the growth and reproduction of microorganisms are prevented.

Many materials are sterilized or disinfected before being used in treatments. Sterilization and disinfection are accomplished chiefly by means of heat, chemicals, and, in recent years, ultraviolet light. Direct ultraviolet rays will kill many types of pathogenic microorganisms if there is ample exposure. Other methods of destroying bacteria that exist but that are applied in special cases or are rather unreliable are freezing, drying, x-rays, ultrasonic waves, and surface-tension depression. When the normal tension of water of 73 dynes is decreased to 40 or below by the addition of chemicals, such as the quaternary ammonium salts (Zephiran Chloride), certain bacteria are inhibited or destroyed.

Heat is the safest and the usual agent for sterilizing in hospitals. Methods of applying heat for sterilization are exposure to steam under pressure (autoclave), dry heat, boiling, and occasionally flaming. In using heat, consideration is given to the nature of the materials to be sterilized, to the time of exposure to the heat, and, with the autoclave, to pressure. Most pathogenic microorganisms can be killed by a temperature above 140° F. (60° C.), but mature spores may survive many hours of boiling temperature. All living organisms can be killed by exposure to moist heat at a temperature of 250° F. (121° C.) for 15 minutes. Disinfection with heat at home may be accomplished by using the oven, by boiling, by using a pressure cooker, and, for small materials, by ironing with a hot iron or flaming with a match.

The extreme heat necessary for killing bacteria is destructive to some materials, however. It softens rubber, chips enamelware, and dulls sharp instruments. Some equipment, such as thermometers, cannot be exposed to heat. Therefore, chemicals are used for disinfecting such instruments. In using chemicals, consideration is given to the material to be disinfected, the strength of the chemical, and the time of exposure. Chemicals used for disinfection are alcohol, preparations of phenol, and quaternary ammonium salts such as Zephiran Chloride.

The method employed when using sterile equipment and maintaining sterility throughout the treatment is termed *surgical asepsis.* Surgical asepsis is employed in treatments of wounds.

Methods have been devised to make food and water safe to be consumed. Between the inspector and the consumer, food must be handled and stored in a way to prevent contamination. All food, water, milk, and ice should be kept clean. Milk should be kept properly refrigerated at all times. Microorganisms are not readily killed by low temperatures, but their active growth may be prevented. Personnel handling food should always wash their hands before preparing or handling the food. Persons who are known carriers of disease should not be employed in food-handling positions.

Sewage treatment plants have helped to eliminate many diseases. More or less virulent organisms are always present in human excretions, so that care must be used in handling these and disposing of them or of dressings that contain them. If waste material must be disinfected before being emptied into the hospital plumbing, chloride of lime in a 1% solution is an effective disinfectant.

Insects also carry microorganisms. Winged insects are kept out by screening, and other insects are best eliminated by cleanliness and constant alertness. Institutions have contracts with exterminators who make regular inspections and who use their own methods employing chemicals to kill vermin.

Cleanliness is of the utmost importance from the standpoint of preventing and controlling the spread of pathogenic microorganisms. The immediate environment should be free from dust, dirt, and organic material such as food and body discharges. Cleaning is accomplished usually by the use of water, soap, and friction; air; and sunshine. Air aids in drying and carries away odors. Sunshine has disinfecting properties. Water is the universal solvent. Cold water dissolves albumin, which is found in organic material. Soap reduces the surface tension of water, and a reduced surface tension increases the wetting power of the water and causes the water to go into crevices and to slip between particles of dirt and fabric, thus

103

loosening debris. The froth helps to carry off the dislodged dirt. Soap also forms a colloidal suspension with grease and thus aids in its removal. The mechanical action of rubbing aids in removing organisms from surfaces.

The method of cleaning should be adapted to the materials to be cleaned. Methods should be safe, silent, unobtrusive, economical, and odorless. The selection of cleaning materials and equipment should be based on their known efficiency as physical and chemical agents for the removal of dirt and destruction of microorganisms.

Injury from allergens may result from insect bites or from materials in the environment, such as feathers, mattress, food, cosmetics, lotion, powder, or soap. Allergic injury is manifested by skin reactions including a rash, irritation of mucous membranes such as sneezing, coughing, watery eyes, or difficult breathing. Prevention of this type of injury may be accomplished by having plastic covers on pillows and mattresses, by using dustless methods of cleaning, by engaging the services of an exterminator, by using substances that do not cause allergic reactions on the skin, and by screening against insects.

Psychologic safety has to do with preventing emotional upsets when possible. It is known that psychologic disturbances are definite factors in accidents. The patient who is fearful, anxious, angry, or depressed may have impaired judgment and therefore needs particular protection from physical harm. The calm, confident attitude of the nurse, provision of privacy, explanation of procedures to be performed, and encouragement of the patient in the sometimes seemingly slow process of recovery can do much to prevent trauma. The psychologic well-being of the patient is enhanced by providing pleasant environmental factors or at least keeping unpleasant ones at a minimum. A person's senses may be more acute when he is ill.

Sensations that would scarcely be noted when a person is well become of major importance when he is ill.

Unpleasant sights are disturbing. Equipment used for treatments should be removed as soon as possible, and soiled dressings should be disposed of quickly. The appearance of order and harmony in the surroundings gives a cheerful outlook that is an asset to recovery. A room that is free from dust and dirt, has balance, color, and harmony, and at the same time has some things in it from home such as a picture or a clock may be more acceptable to the patient.

Color affects the patient's feelings. Pastel and other light shades break the monotony of the environment. They may appear in the walls, in the furniture, in the bed covering, and in the draperies. Color may also be provided by flowers and other decorations.

Loud or unpleasant sounds may be disturbing; however, few patients desire absolute elimination of all sounds. Sensitivity to noise varies with each individual from day to day, depending on his health, fatigue, and mental attitude. A person who is sick or tired is very sensitive to noise. Noise produces irritability and restlessness in those slightly indisposed and fatigue and exhaustion in acutely ill patients. Sudden, loud, or meaningless sounds are generally disagreeable, even to those in good health. Noise interferes seriously with sleep. Not all noise can be reduced by sound conditioners and soundproof materials. Noise caused by friction may be reduced by lubrication. Metal carriers may be made more soundproof by rubber wheels and bumpers. A conscious effort must be made by workers within a hospital to maintain as quiet an environment as possible in order to conserve the strength of the patient and to promote the efficiency of the personnel.

Unpleasant sensations of touch may come from the roughness of the blanket fibers, from the weight of the bedclothes, or from wrinkles in the bedding. Tactile irritation may come from hardness of the bedpan or other equipment or from the sharpness of the nurse's fingernails. These disagreeable sensations should be reduced as far as possible.

Disagreeable odors inhibit gastric reflexes and sometimes produce nausea. Disagreeable odors may come from soiled dressings, the bedpan, drainage from the patient's body, or any other part of the environment. Odors are best reduced by removing the source of the odor and by proper ventilation. Sometimes fragrant or nonfragrant deodorants are used.

Atmospheric conditions include attention to room temperature, humidity, and ventilation.

Ventilation means movement in the air. Adequate ventilation should be provided according to the individual patient's needs and wishes. Patients vary in their preferences regarding the amount of room ventilation, and these preferences should be respected when feasible. In the modern hospital, air-conditioning usually provides adequate control of atmospheric conditions.

Lighting in the patient's environment is a factor that makes for safety and comfort, and it is provided by natural or artificial light. Sunlight is warming and cheerful and may improve both mental and physical well-being. The eyes, however, should be protected from the direct rays of the sun. Artificial light should be strong enough to prevent eyestrain and diffused enough to prevent glare, which may injure the eyes. The amount of light needed depends on the use of the light and the kind of work being done. The rational bed patient should have within his reach a light that he can control.

INFECTION CONTROL IN THE HOSPITAL

Reference was made in the preceding sections to the problem of bacteriologic safety, methods of handwashing, sterilization, and cleanliness, and selected bacteriologic principles were applied to the care of the patient's immediate environment. The purpose of this section is to consider briefly the seriousness of the problem of hospital-acquired infection in relation to safety of the patient.

Since the advent of antibiotics and chemotherapeutic agents, observance of precise medical and surgical aseptic techniques has become very lax in many hospitals. The general trend during the last 30 years has been to rely increasingly upon the effectiveness of these types of medications to prevent the occurrence of infection, or if an infection did occur to treat it with a variety of these agents. Some of the bacteriostatic agents are more or less specific for infections caused by particular organisms and therefore became widely used for prophylaxis. Sometimes this was without real justification, since the point is supported by literature that in many instances the presence of the organism alone is not sufficient to cause infection unless the resistance of the host is lowered, as it often is in the hospital patient.

The repeated warnings that with indiscriminate use of these agents the adaptive response of microorganisms would result in the development of antibiotic-resistant strains of certain pathogens has come to pass. This is true, for example, of *Staphylococcus,* which is frequently a causative organism in hospital-acquired infections.

The development of antibiotic-resistant strains of pathogens is only one significant aspect of the now worldwide problem of infection control. Currently, solid waste disposal in hospitals is a complex and enormous problem that has become a public health hazard as well as an issue in individual patient care and in providing safety in the patient's immediate environment.

How can a hospital safely rid itself of vast quantities and varieties of contaminated waste materials, including the huge amounts of paper and plastic disposables used throughout the hospital? Some important aspects of this complex environmental quality control problem include:

Increasing use of "disposable" products in the hospital. This accounts for most of the sharp rise in weight and volume of hospital wastes, currently estimated at approximately 34 pounds per day for each patient. The volume of per patient waste will continue to increase if institutions continue the trend toward less of the reusables and more of the disposables. A significant related problem is that an effective disposal method for one kind of material may not be an effective or safe method of disposal for another type of waste.

In-hospital transportation of contaminated waste. The quantity of contaminated objects to be disposed of, and therefore transported through the hospital, has increased in proportion to the total volume of disposables. The transporting of contaminated wastes in the hospital is hazardous, for regardless of the method used there is always danger of spreading infection, either by direct contact of personnel or by airborne contaminants. After waste has been transported to a central facility, the problems of volume, diversity of material, and its infectious property make disposal of these wastes extremely costly and technically very difficult.

Technical problems of disposal. The careless disposal of potentially contaminated (infectious) waste products placed in the hospital waste-disposal system and/or the community disposal system without having been first treated by some method of sterilization increases the danger of cross-infection. Such waste may consist of used surgical dressings, human tissues from the operating room and the pathology laboratory, in fact, everything that has come in contact with the patient is potentially contaminated and becomes a hazard when added to the disposal system. Methods of disposal currently used include incineration, grinding, which reduces waste

for final disposal through the sewage system, and compaction for burial in a landfill. The difficulty with any method is that it may fail to either properly reduce plastics or it fails to render the waste material noninfectious or nontoxic.

Sterilization of wastes. Studies of these problems seem to agree that all waste materials that leave the hospital should be free from infectious agents, although no practical method has yet been found to separate the contaminated from the uncontaminated waste for special treatment. When untreated waste material with disease-spreading potential is collected and transported from the hospital to a landfill, handlers may be exposed to infection and pathogens may survive and be leached back into water supply systems. This is also an undesirable method of disposal for untreated wastes because plastics are not biodegradable. The most generally approved in-hospital method for handling bacteriologically hazardous waste appears to be sterilization by autoclave. Then the treated waste could be ground, incinerated, or compacted and/or placed in plastic bags for final disposal with relative safety. The danger to the patient and staff of cross-infection within the hospital would be greatly reduced.

A summary of generally recommended measures for infection control in the hospital includes:

1. Support of the efforts of the hospital infection control committee to investigate and keep records of all instances of infection and give leadership in developing and implementing infection control measures

2. Informing of all hospital personnel so that each individual understands the pollution problem and the principles involved and can participate effectively in the control measures

3. Application of existing technology to provide for the safe and efficient collection, handling, and disposal of all contaminated material

4. Selective use of disposables

5. Specific measures to reduce or eliminate the sources of infection and to break the contact between the source and the individual host, including:

a. Thorough handwashing technique by all personnel (The role of contaminated hands in spreading infection has been well established.)

b. Strict practice of medical aseptic technique by all personnel

c. Strict practice of surgical aseptic technique by all involved personnel

d. Exclusion of personnel with active staphylococcal lesions or other infections from work in the hospital

e. Thorough concurrent and terminal disinfection for all known or suspected cases of infectious nature

f. Adherence to bacteriologic principles in all housekeeping and maintenance practices

g. Effective pest control

h. Sanitary food service

i. Scrupulous cleanliness throughout the hospital

Because of having acquired in-depth understanding of the basic principles underlying infection control, the nurse may perform a significant role in coordination of the efforts of all personnel in the problem of infection control. For this reason the nurse is often an active participant in the work of the hospital's infection control committee.

Principles of surgical aseptic technique are presented in Chapters 30 and 31 and principles of medical aseptic technique in Chapter 32.

SUMMARY

A therapeutic milieu is described as a dynamic, flexible living environment that is concerned with the specific needs of an individual patient and/or a group of patients to promote positive living experiences and positive health changes. Regardless of environmental influences, the patient is the focus of concern as the personnel seek to maintain a therapeutic environment that will help the patient in his progress toward recovery.

Selected principles from microbiology are applied to the care of the patient's unit. The environment of the patient should be safe and comfortable in order to promote his early recovery. Both safety and comfort may be obtained through some of the same factors used for proper atmospheric conditions, cleanliness, effective techniques for prevention of disease, and control of the psychologic aspects of the environment. Disinfection by the use of chemicals cannot compensate for want of cleanliness or ventilation. Routine housekeeping does not come under the duties of the nurse, but in an emergency anything pertaining to the comfort and well-being of the patient becomes the responsibility of the nurse. The provision of a proper physical environment, one that is clean, comfortable, and pleasant, is an essential aspect of care because of the interrelationship between the physical constitution and mental states.

The seriousness of hospital-acquired infection is presented in relation to the safety of the patient. The problems of transporting, collecting, and disposing of vast quantities of contaminated hospital waste are discussed. A summary outline of generally recommended measures for infection control in the hospital is included, with emphasis on restraining sources of infection if the patient is to be protected from cross-infection. The success of infection control depends in a great measure upon the degree of effectiveness with which patients, nurses, physicians, and ancillary personnel maintain the basic principles of medical and surgical aseptic technique.

QUESTIONS FOR DISCUSSION

1 Identify at least three of the related scientific principles that are basic to the statement: "Cleanliness is of the utmost importance from the standpoint of preventing and con-

trolling the spread of pathogenic microorganisms."

2 What is the meaning of therapeutic milieu in a general hospital?

3 What ways can you suggest to modify hospital routines that would improve the patient's feeling of acceptance?

4 Discuss the psychologic effects various colors may have on the patient.

5 If a fire broke out in your ward of four patients, what would be the appropriate action to take?

6 What criteria would you suggest for the "selective use" of disposables in the hospital?

SUGGESTED READINGS

Conti, Mary L.: The loneliness of old age, Nursing Outlook **18**:28, August, 1970.

Donn, Richard: Responsibility for sterility isn't disposable, Hospitals **46**:123, March 16, 1972.

Duncan, Mary Lou: The hospital as a primitive society, American Journal of Nursing **70**:106, January, 1970.

Frenay, Sister Agnes C., and Pierce, Gloria L.: The climate of care for a geriatric patient, American Journal of Nursing **71**:1747, September, 1971.

Haslam, Pamela: Caring for the total patient-noise in hospitals: its effect on the patient, Nursing Clinics of North America **5**:715, December, 1970.

Litsky, Bertha Yanis: Germs make trouble when nurses make beds, Modern Hospital **116**:61, May, 1971.

Litsky, Bertha Yanis: Scientific housekeeping and the professional nurse, Nursing Clinics of North America **5**:99, March, 1970.

Litsky, Warren, and others: Solid waste: a hospital dilemma, American Journal of Nursing **72**:1841, October, 1972.

Sovie, Margaret D., and Fruehan, Thomas: Protecting the patient from electrical hazards, Nursing Clinics of North America **7**:469, September, 1972.

Waste disposal creating a problem for hospitals, New York Times, October 25, 1971, p. 65.

Wenzel, Kathryn: The role of the infection control nurse, Nursing Clinics of North America **5**:99, March, 1970.

Wilkinson, Laura: Praise as a therapeutic tool, RN **34**:58, June, 1971.

9 The patient's admission

PROCESS OF ADMISSION

In Chapter 2 the hospital was presented as a community health agency, an institution with a function of service. The patient usually enters a hospital of his own free will following the advice of his physician or may, when suffering from a mental illness, be committed through a legal process.

The usual procedure for admission to a general hospital is for the physician to advise the patient of his need for hospitalization and then to call the hospital for a reservation. This advice may be given in the patient's home, in the physician's office, in a clinic, or in the emergency room. The news that hospitalization is necessary is usually disconcerting since it means an interruption in the patient's life routine. In some instances the patient must go to the hospital at once. In others he may have a little time to do some thinking and planning about his work, his family, his home, and his finances. Perhaps he will need aid from social agencies. Hospitalization insurance or health and accident insurance carried by at least three fourths of the population helps to lessen the feeling of financial insecurity for the one who possesses it.

Patients may be transported to the hospital by ambulance or by automobile or may even walk. Usually they are accompanied by a relative or a friend. The patient is received at the hospital by an admitting officer who has been expecting him because in most instances the physician called beforehand to arrange the admission. The reception of the patient is now recognized to be of so much importance that hospitals seek to employ admitting personnel who are especially qualified by virtue of their general poise and courteous manner. The admitting officer secures the necessary data, which should be accurate since further records will depend upon the admission record. The name should be spelled correctly, and the age should be accurately recorded. The necessary data obtained from the patient concerns name and address, age, occupation, religion, and hospitalization insurance. Signatures are obtained for the consent of some types of care, and an Addressograph plate usually is made. Blood may be drawn for the routine blood tests, and a chest

109

x-ray film may be taken. An identification bracelet may be put on the patient's wrist. Sometimes when the physician calls for the reservation, the admitting office mails an admission blank to the patient for obtaining initial data. This procedure saves the patient much time in the admitting office.

The admitting record, signed permits, and perhaps also other pages of the chart are taken to the nursing unit with the patient. The admitting clerk, an aide, a volunteer worker, or a nurse accompanies the patient to his unit.

Everyone concerned with a patient's admission—the receptionist in the admitting office, the person who transports him to his room, the head nurse, the bedside nurse assigned to his care, the physician who takes the preliminary medical data—should relate to him in a warm, supportive manner. It is everyone's responsibility to make the adjustment of admission as easy as possible (Fig. 9-1).

NURSING RESPONSIBILITIES

Every hospital has its own specific admission routines and procedures, but there are general factors and nursing responsibilities that are almost always applicable and that should be considered.

The arrival of the patient in his unit automatically starts the machinery of diagnostic and therapeutic measures and nurs-

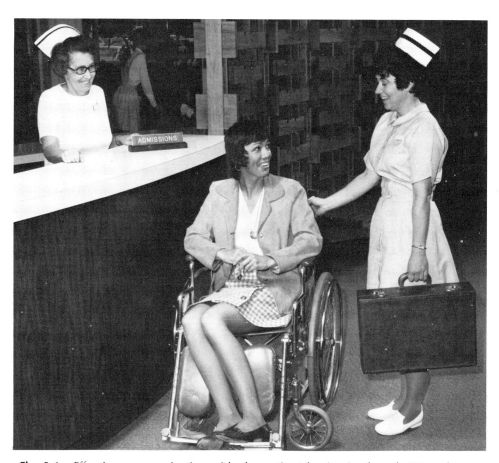

Fig. 9-1. Effective communication with the patient begins in the admitting department. (Hoag Hospital Presbyterian, Newport Beach, Calif.)

ing care. He may be provided with a hospital gown, or he may wear his own sleeping garments. He may or may not be put to bed at once. Temperature, pulse, respiration, and blood pressure are taken. If a urine specimen has not yet been sent to the laboratory, it is obtained at this time. Clothing and valuables are cared for according to hospital policy. Money, except for a small amount, and valuables may be sent home or placed in the hospital safe. Patients who are not seriously ill or who do not require special treatments or nursing care are encouraged to wear their own gowns and pajamas.

The nurse who admits the patient begins his chart. In addition to the admission data, which have already been made out, two other important sheets are the graphic chart and the nurses' record. Temperature, pulse, respiration, and blood pressure are recorded on the graphic chart. On the nurses' record, notations are made of the time and the mode of admission, which may be by walking, wheelchair, or stretcher (gurney). Also recorded are objective and subjective symptoms. Objective symptoms are those that the nurse can see, hear, feel, and smell, whereas subjective symptoms are those that the patient tells about but that may not be detected by the nurse. Notations are also made of any specimens or requests sent to the laboratory, visits of the

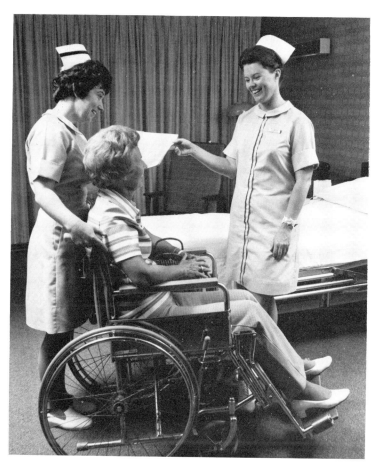

Fig. 9-2. Welcoming a new patient into the unit prepared for her arrival.

intern or attending physician, and any medications or treatments given.

The Kardex is also begun, and nursing care cards are made out so that the care of the patient may be carried along smoothly.

A history is taken and a physical examination made by the attending physician or intern immediately on admission or sometime within the first 24 hours, depending on the condition of the patient. The nurse prepares the patient for the physical examination by explaining its purpose and obtains equipment and otherwise assists as much as is needed.

It is very important that the new patient be greeted by the nurse, who will introduce him to the other patients in the immediate area and to other personnel (Fig. 9-2). This initial courtesy may serve as an opening for the beginning of a useful nurse-patient relationship as well as assist the patient to develop a feeling of belonging. This is also an opportunity for beginning orientation of the patient to his new hospital environment.

The patient's orientation might include explanation of hospital routines for visiting hours, meals, awakening, and retiring; how to use the call signal; location of the bathroom, or how to request the bedpan and/or urinal if restricted to bed rest; and the role of the various personnel who may be expected to visit the patient.

The nurse will also want to spend time in acquainting the patient with what is expected of him and what will probably occur at specific times. It is important that the nurse also try to assist the patient's family members in developing confidence and to feel as comfortable as possible in the situation. The experiences early in the first few hours of hospitalization can have a powerful effect on the patient. They may favorably affect his adaptive adjustment to hospitalization, or, if stressful, they may delay or prevent his successful adjustment in the illness situation. Even though the

diagnosis may not yet be known, there is much that the nurse can do to begin developing a plan of care and to help the patient maintain his individuality and independence from the beginning of his hospitalization.

Examples of relevant principles drawn from the social sciences can be found in other chapters, Chapter 6, for example. It should be noted that many of the basic scientific principles are useful to the nurse in a variety of different contexts and may be applied repeatedly in understanding patient needs and in solving patient care problems. In the following section some applications are made to the nurse's interaction with the in-coming patient.

PSYCHOSOCIAL ASPECTS

Every patient leaves his family, his friends, and his familiar safe habits of life and enters a strange place with strange customs where he does not know anyone, where he may think he will surely suffer, and where he might even die. There are few moves in life that are more ominous than the move from the home to the hospital.

Every patient, just by virtue of being sick, is threatened, insecure, and full of anxiety. The patient fears his present condition, what caused it, what it may become, how long it will last, and sometimes what people will think of him. Very few approach an operation without fear.

At the onset of the illness, the patient will react as he would to any other serious stress situation. Individuals who have had difficulty in adjusting to the usual stresses of life manifest more anxiety during illness than the person who is more flexible to daily changes.

The adjustment of the patient to the hospital may affect his willingness to accept the treatment offered him. One unaccustomed to illness may appear apprehensive of treatment and fearful of complications, and he may make many complaints even though his illness or disability is of a minor nature. In the hospital the patient is one of many, whereas at home he had a definite individual role.

One feature of the hospital that the patient notices very quickly is the lack of privacy. Intimate details of his life are collected and written into his record to be read by people he does not know. If he is in a multiple bed unit and is confined to bed, he is housed with strangers and carries out certain intimate life processes in the presence of these strangers.

The expense of illness is naturally a matter of concern to most people, and when the family at home suffers from loss of income also, the patient becomes more distressed. Interruption of work is a source of constant worry, especially to business and professional people who hold positions of responsibility. Inactivity and dependence upon others for the simplest physical needs are irritating to many patients. Uncertainty exists regarding the seriousness of one's illness or the meaning of various tests and treatments.

Insecurity may develop because of the strangeness of the place and of attending persons. In this new environment the patient meets many new people, and he is expected to relate and communicate with them. As many as twenty or more different persons may enter a patient's room in one day, and each of these has a varying degree of responsibility for and a different role in the patient's care.

In the hospital a patient must not only adjust to a strange bed, to strange food, and to strange sounds, but he must also be ready to cooperate with anyone who enters his room at any unexpected time to give him treatment or medication.

Isolation from one's family and friends sometimes causes more suffering than does the physical malady. The patient is not able to order his social relationships in his own way as he might at home.

Since first impressions are often lasting, special effort should be made to show interest, kindness, and understanding during the first moments of the patient's admission. The support given in the admitting office should be further enhanced by the nurse's interaction with the patient. The initial approach to the patient should be one of friendly helpfulness. The nurse should explain, in terms the patient can understand, the general hospital routine and other information that the patient would appreciate. Assisting the patient to feel at ease and inspiring his confidence in the hospital are part of the admission procedure. A feeling of security may be imparted by the presence of a warm, understanding nurse who has a genuine desire to assist the patient to achieve emotional and physical comfort.

It is important to establish an effective rapport with the patient before beginning his care in order to obtain his cooperation. When a patient is admitted to a ward or to a semiprivate room, courtesy demands that he be introduced to at least those patients who are in nearby beds.

If the patient is isolated, the nurse should explain the purpose of the isolation and provide him with sufficient diversion when he is ready for it.

There is a vast difference in the physical and mental condition of patients entering the hospital, and an individual plan of care needs to be made out for each one. The patient needs to be prepared psychologically for treatments in order to reduce his apprehension. Apprehension and fear are tensing emotions, and in order to derive the most benefit from treatments the patient should be as relaxed as possible. For these reasons the patient is told why his possessions may be taken from him, why a physical examination is done and what it will involve, and why certain diagnostic tests are made and how he can cooperate. During the physical examination he should be protected from embarrassment by draping, screening, and the quiet, matter-of-fact attitude of the physician and the nurse.

Sometimes illness is associated with a

social problem such as poor housing, insufficient clothing, or inadequate food. Sometimes illness brings social problems. A strain is put on the family income and involves such matters as whether the patient is the wage earner, the nature and duration of the illness, and the resources for meeting expenses.

In some instances the patient has been referred to the hospital through a social agency, of which the nurse should have some knowledge. Social problems are also presented by patients who do not speak English, by deaf patients, and by blind patients. Methods of helping these individuals should be sought (Fig. 9-3).

LEARNING SITUATIONS FOR THE PATIENT

The patient can learn much from the nurse through skillfully directed questions and answers. He can acquire appropriate

information about his condition, diagnostic tests, and treatments. Through careful explanation by the nurse he may be prepared to cooperate in the physical examination.

SUMMARY

The patient's adaptation to hospitalization depends upon various factors—his age, sex, cultural background, intellectual capacity, past experiences, and the nature of his health problem. His first contact with the hospital is usually in the admitting department, where lasting impressions may be formed. Because the patient in admission is undoubtedly experiencing feelings of dread and insecurity, the character of his reception by the staff is of the utmost importance.

Some of the nurse's concerns are to help the patient to feel at ease in a new and different environment, through listen-

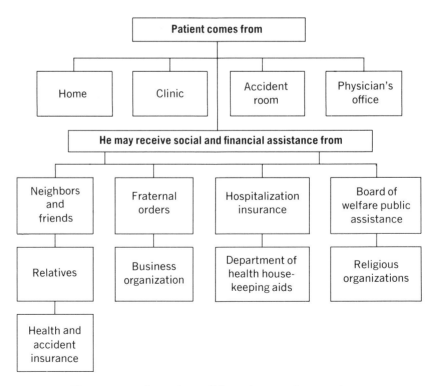

Fig. 9-3. Outline of possible assistance for a patient.

ing and communicating with the patient to help him identify and accept his feelings in regard to his health problem, and to maintain the patient's individuality and independence from the beginning of hospitalization. It is important that thought be given to the orientation of both the patient and his family during the process of admission.

QUESTIONS FOR DISCUSSION

1 Select a particular patient. Find out all you can about his social and family background. What social problems does he present? What type of friends does he have? What about his home? his customs? his speech? his education? his standard of living? What other possible problems could he present? What social agencies are concerned with him? What social agencies could possibly be concerned with him?

2 Does the patient seem nervous? tense? excited? Or is he cheerful and relaxed? Does he seem apathetic and depressed or alert and stable?

3 What methods might a nurse use to secure cooperation from a patient?

4 How does illness affect the behavior of an individual?

5 Why is it very important for the nurse to meet the family of the patient?

6 List the members of the health team (for a particular patient) who might be concerned with this patient's needs, either directly or indirectly.

LIFE SITUATION

Mrs. Osborne, a young mother of three school-aged children, has entered the emergency room of a local hospital. She complains of severe abdominal pain. The physician has diagnosed the condition as acute appendicitis and has ordered her to be admitted. She expresses great concern for the welfare of her children, who soon will be coming home from school. She tells the nurse that since her husband is out of town on a business trip there will be no one at home to care for the children. She refuses admission and says that she must leave immediately and go to her children. How can you, as the nurse, help Mrs. Osborne?

SUGGESTED PERFORMANCE CHECKLIST

Comfort

1 Is the bed opened before the arrival of the patient?
2 Is the nurse competent and courteous?
3 Does the nurse explain the hospital routine?
4 Is needed assistance given in undressing?
5 Is the patient made physically comfortable in regard to light, warmth, back rest, and the like?
6 Is explanation made before procedures?
7 Is physical exposure avoided?
8 Is opportunity provided for voiding before the physical examination?
9 Are the patient's relatives given consideration?

Therapeutic effectiveness

1 Is care adapted to the needs of the patient?
2 Are the necessary laboratory examinations initiated?
3 Are cardinal symptoms checked at once?
4 Is good rapport instituted?
5 Is adequate assistance given the physician?
6 Is a definite plan begun for the patient's care?
7 Does the patient show evidence of a positive adaptation to his new role as a patient?
8 Is charting accurate and pertinent?

Economy

1 Is the unit checked for completeness before the arrival of the patient?
2 Is the energy of the patient conserved?
3 Are all materials to be used in the admission routines at hand?
4 Is the nurse aware of the plan of treatment?
5 Does the nurse save time and effort?

Safety

1 Is the patient properly transported to his room?
2 Is consideration given to the patient's physical and mental condition?
3 Are valuables and other belongings properly cared for?
4 Is proper draping supplied for the physical examination?
5 Is instruction given to the patient in the use of the signal system?

6 Is the signal placed within the patient's reach?

SUGGESTED READINGS

Ammon, Lillian Louise: Surviving enucleation, American Journal of Nursing **72:**1817, October, 1972.

Canaday, Mary E.: SSPE—helping the family cope, American Journal of Nursing **72:**94, January, 1972.

Robinson, Lisa: Psychological aspects of the care of hospitalized patients, Philadelphia, 1968, F. A. Davis Co., pp. 1-9. In the author's own words this section "is written in such a way as to demonstrate the negative aspects of admissions procedures."

10 Assessing health-illness status and needs

SKILLS IN PATIENT ASSESSMENT

The individual patient entering the impersonal, complicated hospital environment brings with him all those characteristics that make him a unique person with his own unique needs. The hospital is a community composed of many unique sick persons. It is charged with the responsibility of providing services and care for the many members of its community in the safest and most economical way.

By its very nature the hospital becomes a complex, impersonal organization with administrative policies and routines in order to accomplish the responsibility with which it is charged. The very framework that provides a well-planned, smoothly functioning institution for the benefit of the patient also provides an environment in which it is highly possible that the patient will be "lost in the shuffle" and thus become depersonalized, unless the nursing staff is able to recognize and face the reality of the uniqueness of each and every patient in the hospital community and provide a patient-centered (that is, individualized) plan for meeting the unique needs of each patient.

Individualized nursing intervention is dependent upon the ability of the nurse to make an accurate observation and assessment of the individual patient's health-illness status and his unique needs and, through consideration of all the relevant factors, to formulate a dynamic, ongoing plan of care that is continuously updated in sensitive response to the inevitable changes. Alterations in the patient's physical and emotional condition and the effects of his interaction with the composite environmental factors impinging on him must be registered and accounted for in the plan of care.

Basic skills available to the nurse in the data gathering and assessment phases of the nursing process include the following.

117

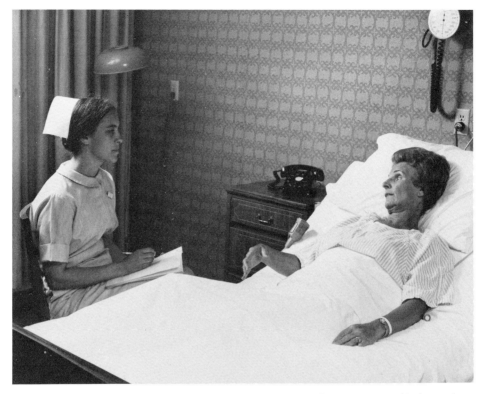

Fig. 10-1. The assessment interview with the patient is a basic source of information.

1. *Communication* skills lead to meaningful nurse-patient interaction, through which relevant and essential information about the patient as an individual, his condition, and his medical problem is gathered directly from the patient. When a trusting relationship is established, the patient is often able to discuss with the nurse the problems he may consider too confidential to share with others. Such interactions may occur coincidentally as the nurse listens to the patient while administering physical nursing care. Structured interviews with the patient may also provide the source of information related to specific needs of the individual patient (Fig. 10-1). Chapter 5 is relevant in this context.

2. *Observation* skills, which are dependent upon developing the acuity of the senses, are essential because it is through sensory impressions that we gain information about the world in which we live and the people with whom we are associated. The nurse must become selective in the observation process, learning what to see, hear, feel, and smell and what is relevant in the patient's interaction with his environment, recognizing that observations are relevant when they fit into a pattern of organized relationships.

3. *Objectivity,* which may be thought of as skillful viewing of data, events, and phenomena in an impersonal, unprejudiced manner, is a characterisitic of professional performance in the use of problem solving in application of the scientific method.

4. *Specific procedures and techniques* are used in observation of the patient, for ex-

ample, measurement of vital signs. The skills in performing such techniques with accuracy must be mastered.

The focus in this chapter is primarily on the skill of observation, which leads the nurse to initiate activity in behalf of the patient.

OBSERVATION—FIRST STEP IN NURSING PROCESS
Definition

Observation is the gathering of data by recognizing and noting facts or occurrences. In this context observation refers to the gathering of information about the patient and his situation. The data thus gathered are needed to develop the plan of care for the patient.

Observation, which is fundamental in scientific work and all intelligent and effective action, is based on knowledge, interest, attention, and the development of skill in this method of gathering information. In observing, the nurse should know what to observe, how to describe and record what has been observed, and how to interpret and draw inferences from the data gathered through observation.

Not only is nursing observation important in the patient's plan of care, but the physician also often utilizes the nurse's observations in arriving at a diagnosis and in prescribing treatment. Data obtained by observation might be the deciding factor between life and death. Observation data are used to regulate the activity of the patient in accord with his strength and to plan nursing care in a way that will produce the maximum benefit and comfort. The quality of the hospital's service may be evaluated through analyzing a variety of carefully recorded observations.

Developing skill in observation

Skill in observation is the result of deliberate concentration on developing the art of seeing perceptively, that is, to see accu-

rately and in detail, to understand the meaning of what is seen, and to use purposefully the data thus gained. It is developed through systematic and regular practice. Essential to developing skill in observation is basic understanding of normal body functioning, of human behavior, and of abnormal changes that may occur. The observer needs to have a fund of accurate knowledge against which to test information that may be obtained through experienced use of the senses—seeing, hearing, touching, and smelling—in assessing health-illness status.

Indications that variations from the normal anatomy and physiology of the human body are present will usually be referred to as signs and symptoms. *Signs* are objective evidences of abnormal changes that may be recognized by the observer apart from the patient's impressions, for example, cyanosis, edema, and mydriasis. *Symptoms* are defined as perceptible changes in the body or in its functioning that indicate an abnormal condition. Signs are sometimes classified as *objective symptoms. Subjective symptoms* are those that are perceptible primarily to the patient, such as pain or mental and emotional reactions. The observer may or may not see indications that subjective symptoms are present. A patient may experience pain without manifesting outward change; conversely, he may grimace and clutch at a body part as though in pain but may not actually be experiencing pain. Temperature, pulse, and respiration are often referred to as *cardinal symptoms* or vital signs, and those affecting the whole body as *general* or *constitutional symptoms. Prodromal symptoms* are those that occur in the initial stages of a disease. A complex of symptoms that make up a characteristic picture of a particular disease is called a *syndrome.*

The nurse develops skill in observing signs and symptoms presented by the patient and in describing and reporting the observations using correct terminology. However, it is well to remember that although it may be inferred that the patient's symptoms indicate urgency of treatment or present a picture of a particular disease entity, the nurse would not make a medical diagnosis but might summon the physician, if necessary.

METHODS OF DIRECT OBSERVATION

Observation by sight. Through sight one observes such physical indications as facial expressions and mannerisms; state of alertness or apathy; color and condition of the skin and mucous membranes; appearance of mouth and teeth; presence of rashes, scars, bruises, wounds, and wound dressings; swollen areas; shape, position, and movement of body parts; shivering; position and activity of the patient; gait and build; drainage and discharges from body cavities and wounds; absence of a body part; prostheses, braces, and supports; color and condition of fingernails and toenails; reading on a thermometer; amount and kind of food presented and eaten; kind of clothing and personal articles that may reveal something about cultural background and occupation. Other examples of visual observation may be cited.

The nurse makes many inspections of the patient in assisting with the physician's examinations. Equipment that may be used by the physician, nurse, or other health workers to observe by sight includes many common items. A flashlight is used to cast more light on a part, but sometimes it is placed behind a part to cast shadows, as in transillumination. A head mirror also reflects light. Other instruments include the following: a tongue blade, a thermometer, manometers for measuring pressures of arterial and venous blood and spinal fluid, a tonometer for measuring pressure in the eyeball, specula of various sizes and shapes to fit

the different orifices of the body (ears, nose, vaginal canal, and rectum), a laryngeal or dental mirror for examining the throat or teeth, a skin pencil for marking the skin, a tape measure or ruler or caliper for measuring parts.

Endoscopes are instruments used in many cases to straighten canals and in all cases to provide a light for looking into body cavities. The otoscope is used for the ear canal; the ophthalmoscope, for the eye; the proctoscope, for the rectum; the gastroscope, for the stomach; the bronchoscope, for the trachea and the bronchial tubes; and the cystoscope, for the bladder. The fluoroscope employs x-rays for making a part visible; the x-ray machine records permanent pictures; the electroencephalograph and the electrocardiograph record tracings useful in diagnosis.

Observation by hearing. The nurse may be able to tell much about the patient's condition through the sense of hearing. The alert nurse will note many sounds that reveal the patient's positive or negative adaptation in the illness situation, for example, changes in sounds of breathing that may indicate interference with a patient's patent airway, restlessness, pain, or any situation requiring intervention. The patient's voice reveals something about his general condition and his emotional status. Observation through the sense of hearing is usually done without the aid of instruments. However, the stethoscope is a useful instrument that conveys sounds produced in the body to the ear of the listener.

Observation through sense of touch. To examine by the sense of touch is to palpate. Through the sense of touch, texture, irregularities, enlargements, movements of the pulse or of the chest wall, or other movements may be detected. Touching the patient may also reveal something about his temperature, turgor of tissues, and strength of grasp. The significant observations of cold, clammy skin or hot, dry skin may be noted. The patient may reveal something about his emotional status when he touches the nurse.

Observation through sense of smell. Although the sense of smell, and also taste, probably have more limited usefulness in observation than the other senses, these may enable the nurse to become aware of certain physical or environmental problems pertaining to the patient. Some medical conditions are accompanied by characteristic odors. For example, the urine of a patient with phenylketonuria is said to be quite distinctive; the breath of the person in diabetic acidosis has a characteristic "fruity" odor resulting from the high acetone level; certain types of discharges may be identified by odor. Unpleasant odors in the environment alert the nurse to the need for appropriate corrective measures and ventilation. By knowing tastes of various foods and drugs, the nurse may be able to judge whether the patient has a normal sense of taste.

PLAN FOR OBSERVATION
Observation checklist

A nurse's plan for observation in assessing the patient's health-illness status and needs for nursing might include the following steps.

1. A general impression of the patient's physical state noting age, body build, obvious symptoms and apparent degree of illness, mental status, and state of consciousness should be acquired. If there is opportunity, information should be gathered through verbal communications with the patient and family members regarding the patient's illness and his habits of personal hygiene, exercise, sleep, eating, elimination, role and place in the family, and family perception of his illness and how he should be treated.

2. The various senses and measuring

devices are used in direct observation, asking oneself such questions as: What significant details can I see? What clues are suggested by the facial expression? body posture or position? What are the cardinal symptoms? What can be learned through the sense of touch? Are there any significant sounds? If there is an odor, what is it? What does it mean? What mannerisms, attitudes, and difficulties in adjustment are discernible? What medications has the patient been taking? Does he have any known allergies? Any other observations indicated for a particular patient may be added to this list.

An example of a very detailed nursing observation checklist appears in Beland's *Clinical Nursing: Pathophysiological and Psychosocial Approaches.** Using this type of outline the nurse can prepare a suitable observation checklist for her use with an individual patient's situation.

Nothing is insignificant in clinical observation. Closer, more frequent observations are needed in the care of a very ill patient, elderly patients, infants and children, and all patients in whom complications are feared. The sicker or the more helpless the patient, the greater is his need for skillful observation by the nurse.

3. From the information thus gathered pertinent observations should be recorded and nursing needs of the patient identified. This is the basis for beginning the development of a nursing care plan.

Recording observations

Observations that are relevant to assessing the patient's symptoms and needs are communicated both verbally and in written form. A concise but complete verbal report is given to the team leader and/or head nurse. The patient's chart contains the forms used for the complete record of

*Beland, Irene L.: Clinical nursing: pathophysiological and psychosocial approaches, New York, 1970, The Macmillan Company, pp. 18-22.

his progress, including those on which the written nursing observations and comments are recorded. Clinical recording should be documentation of adequate nursing care received by the patient.

Symptoms and observations should be recorded in accepted medical terms using correct grammar. All entries on the chart should be significant and dignified and couched in the proper medical terminology. Regardless of whether printing or writing is used in entering nursing notes, legibility is of utmost importance.

Facts are charted in order to keep the physician, nurses, and other workers informed of the reactions and progress of the patient. The chart is used many times in medical research. It may also be used in legal suits.

Aids to the nurse's own observations are the admission record, medical history, laboratory reports, progress notes of the physician, and notes made by other nurses. However, one should be familiar with the entire record and have an understanding of the notes from other clinical departments.

In any circumstance the physician is notified of pertinent changes in the patient's condition, and notes are made on the appropriate chart forms. Each hospital has its own established chart forms and charting procedures that should be followed meticulously.

OBSERVATIONS RELATED TO CHANGES RESULTING FROM ILLNESS

When observing a sick person one looks for changes related to the illness. Observation may be directed toward specific aspects of body structure or functioning that may be altered as a result of the disease process or injury. These changes are referred to as signs and symptoms of either positive or negative adaptation as the body strives to deal with the associated pathophysiology. According to the con-

cept of adaptation, the living organism (person) may respond to the pathophysiology and psychopathology in such a manner that the damage is repaired, although individuals vary in their capacity to adapt.

Nursing observation begins in considerable detail with the admission of the patient, and thereafter it is a process that is continued while other nursing activities are in progress. This gives an opportunity for the plan of care first to be formulated and then to be adjusted with the patient's changing needs.

The nurse bases assessment of the patient's needs on all that has been learned through observation and communication with him and on the information that has been gathered from other available sources. The process of recognizing the patient's needs and identifying the related problems, often called the *nursing diagnosis,* is an important preliminary to developing the plan of nursing care. The process of planning nursing care is the subject of Chapter 13.

SPECIFIC OBSERVATIONS

The nurse's observation and appraisal techniques become increasingly skillful when they are directed toward a purposeful consideration of what is to be perceived about the patient. Using an outline of specific observations to be considered is of assistance in gathering and organizing significant data about the patient.

Observation of the patient as a person

In the illness situation one looks for characteristics that indicate the patient's state of adaptation or maladaptation. The following points are suggested as a guide in observation of the patient in the early interaction while the nurse is seeking to establish rapport.

Body posture, movements, and gait often tell the observer a great deal about how the patient feels, both physically and mentally. Certain body postures are generally considered to portray typical moods; for example, head up, shoulders thrown back, and spritely walk presumably indicate an alert, gay frame of mind, whereas stooped posture with head and shoulders slumped forward, knees bent, and shuffling walk are supposed to depict depression and melancholy. A person in pain usually assumes a position that is most favorable for the affected part. Skeletal defects may sometimes be noted through faulty posture. It is also important to note the body alignment for every patient in order to maintain the principles of body mechanics that facilitate such functions as respiration, circulation, and muscle balance. The nurse should be able to recognize at once when the patient is unable to maintain posture that facilitates body functioning.

Facial expression and demeanor will usually convey some impression of the patient's frame of mind. Is the patient's expression sad, serious, smiling? However, it is well to keep in mind that the effect of illness on the patient's attitude may be difficult to evaluate, partly because in most instances the nurse is unaware of the patient's usual affect and also because people often tend to put on a "front," trying to look and act according to their perception of what they think may be expected of them. A primary objective at this point is to assume the patient's point of view.

Speech may be noted in terms of degree of talkativeness, general tone of voice, clear or slurred speech, language barrier, anxious expressions, hoarseness, or loss of voice. Does the patient speak in a well-controlled and modulated manner?

Eyes generally are an important part of the facial expression. They reflect moods of gaity, anxiety, or apprehension that the nurse can soon learn to recognize with some accuracy.

Skin color and condition are quickly noted, giving additional clues regarding the patient as a person.

Nutritional status in general is relatively evident to the observer just by the appearance of the patient. Problems of obesity and underweight are readily recognized. The nurse may soon develop some skill in appraising nutritional status through color and turgor of the skin and condition of the hair in addition to obviously aberrant body weight. As the nurse interviews the patient, clues can be recognized that give insight regarding the patient's dietary habits, appetite, likes and dislikes, and fluid intake. Artificial dentures or dental problems interfering with the ability to cope with food should be noted.

Elimination patterns can be appraised through inquiry and observation. Provision for supporting the patient's established habits can be incorporated into the plan of care.

Personal hygiene, or lack of it, is usually obvious to the observer but should always be described in acceptable terms. Are there significant odors or halitosis? Are the hair and scalp clean and healthy? Is the hair oily and disheveled? Is there a general appearance of neatness and cleanliness?

Sleep habits may also be assessed through interviewing and observation. It is important that specific information be obtained so that the patient's sleep needs can be recognized and provided for in his plan of care.

Prostheses of any sort should be noted and provision for assisting the patient with necessary care should be included in the plan of care. Not only the presence of the prosthesis should be observed but also its fit. Any problems associated with it should be recorded.

Observation of signs and symptoms

The medical history and physical examination, which together furnish information leading to diagnosis and a program of therapy, are the physician's responsibility. The physical examination is a systematic and exhaustive search for any significant deviation from the normal. While the eliciting of signs and symptoms is an important part of the physical examination, it is not solely the physician's responsibility to recognize the occurrence of variations from the normal. Symptoms may change or entirely new ones may develop during the absence of the physician. Therefore, it is a nursing responsibility to recognize changes in the patient's presenting symptoms that can be noted by the practiced observer, to receive the patient's complaints, to evaluate the significance of the observations and complaints, to record accurately and objectively the characteristics of what has been observed, and to report immediately those significant changes in symptoms, or new symptoms, through proper channels of communication.

In describing, evaluating, and recording signs and symptoms, it is helpful to look for certain characteristics: time of onset, character of onset, constancy, location, intensity, and previous occurrence.

The eliciting and reporting of the following commonly occurring signs and symptoms are within the scope of nursing practice. This listing is not intended to be exhaustive.

Vital signs are among the most frequently requested observations. The significance of findings is discussed in Chapter 11.

Chills usually occur as an adaptive response resulting from stimulation of the hypothalamic heat center by a pyrogen (or other factor such as intracranial pressure), which is analogous to setting the thermostat of an automatic heating system to a higher level. Heat is produced until the set level of temperature is reached. With a sudden stimulation of the center, the patient has a chill, shivers, and feels cold, even though his body temperature may already be above normal. Peripheral vasoconstriction causes the skin to be pale and cold to the touch. The shivering causes increased muscular activity with increased heat production. The chill lasts until the temperature climbs to the level set through stimulation of the hypothalamic heat center by the pyrogen. A balance between heat production and dissipation maintains the temperature at this higher level as long as the pyrogen is effective. As the chill subsides the skin becomes hot and flushed, and the patient complains of feeling hot. When the pyrogenic factor is removed, peripheral vasodilation occurs with diaphoresis and rapid loss of heat by radiation and vaporization, and the body temperature returns to normal.

Bleeding, its source and amount, should always be carefully observed and evaluated. Small amounts of bleeding may or may not be significant, depending on the source and associated symptoms. Excessive bleeding constitutes hemorrhage. External bleeding is easily detected by the observer. Internal bleeding, however, often first recognized by general symptoms and changes in the vital signs, is less easily detected but is usually of serious import.

Drainage and body discharges should always be observed and accurately described. Drainage refers to the material coming from a wound, and the word "discharge" is generally used to indicate abnormal material excreted from a body orifice.

Pain does not produce outwardly recognizable manifestations; therefore, a patient's complaint of the presence of pain should always be respected. Some patients may not mention having pain, but its presence may be inferred through such behaviors as restlessness, position assumed, changes in facial expression, or, in some patients, simply lying quietly but appearing tense. When reporting pain, in addition to the characteristics already suggested, descriptive adjectives may be used, including such terms as dull, throbbing, sharp, aching, cramping, constant, intermittent, localized, generalized, and radiating.

Anorexia, nausea, and vomiting may occur together or separately, and retching may or may not accompany nausea and/or vomiting. Significant observations regarding vomiting include: Is the onset preceded by nausea or is it sudden and without warning? Is it projectile? prolonged? What is the character of the vomitus? mucous? watery? Is it undigested food? Is it like coffee grounds? Is there a fecal odor? Is it bloody? What is the amount? Prolonged vomiting may result in dehydration and electrolyte imbalance. Aspiration is a possibility and should always be considered to be a danger for weak, helpless, or unconscious patients.

Abdominal distension may be the result of a variety of causes, but it is usually associated with accumulated gas or fluid in the intestine, with ascites (accumulated fluid in the peritoneal cavity), or with urinary retention. Distension causes discomfort and, depending on the cause and degree, may be a threat to the patient's well-being. Therefore, it should be recognized and evaluated promptly.

Edema, accumulation of fluid in the tissue spaces, is usually a symptom of some other primary condition. It is easily recognized by increase in size when it involves a visible part of the body. When the imprint of light finger pressure remains in the edematous tissue, it is referred to as pitting edema. Edema occurring within the cranium results in a serious increase in intracranial pressure. When pulmonary edema develops, its presence may be suspected by shortness of breath and cough with frothy, blood-tinged sputum. This is a condition that requires immediate medical treatment.

Cough is a protective reflex essential for life because it keeps the respiratory pas-sages free of foreign particles that would obstruct the airway and predispose to pulmonary infection. Coughing is also the mechanism by which secretions are moved from the air passageways of the respiratory tract. While the cough is essential, persistent coughing may be exhausting to the patient and therefore requires management. Terms used to describe the cough are dry, productive, hacking, harsh, rasping, wheezing, whooping, and paroxysmal. Sputum may be clear, yellow, green, rusty, streaked with blood (hemoptysis), frothy, copious, or offensive in odor.

Pruritus is generalized or localized itching, a common subjective complaint in skin disorders. Frequently, it accompanies rashes and urticaria. These problems should always be reported since it is important that the causative factor be identified and eliminated if possible. In any case, therapy that will bring relief to the patient should be instituted.

Sensory changes may be caused by neurologic abnormalities. These effects may be characterized by a change in the intensity of one or more of the senses. For example, decreased sensations of pain, temperature, and touch may be noted. Impairment of sense of position and movement may be demonstrated by the patient's inability to perceive passive movement of a limb. The implications of sensory loss in relation to nursing needs should be carefully considered for the individual patient. The presence of numbness and tingling might suggest pressure and circulatory interference from a cast, tight bandage, or other appliance or from improper positioning.

Dizziness, a feeling of lightheadedness, may also be a neurologic symptom, or it may be related to circulatory changes, hypotension, emotional hyperventilation, or anoxia of the brain from any cause. It may result in fainting (syncope). Safety of the patient should be one of the first considerations, particularly if he is in an upright position.

NURSING ROLE IN THE PHYSICAL EXAMINATION

Methods used by the physician and sometimes by the nurse in observing the patient include inspection, palpation, percussion, and auscultation. *Inspection* means observing with the eye, and it is associated with light and seeing. It is the method probably of the greatest usefulness. *Mensuration* is really a comparative inspection in that it aims to make comparative measurements of corresponding parts of the body. *Palpation* is the art of feeling with the hand. Some organs are always palpable. Others are palpable only when enlarged or displaced. *Percussion* and *auscultation* are procedures that depend on the production of sound. Percussion is tapping an area to elicit sounds, whereas auscultation is listening to sounds within the body with a stethoscope. Percussion is based on the fact that a hollow organ, such as the lungs when filled with air, will give a characteristic sound when tapped, and if that organ is filled with fluid, a duller sound is produced.

Special techniques have been devised to

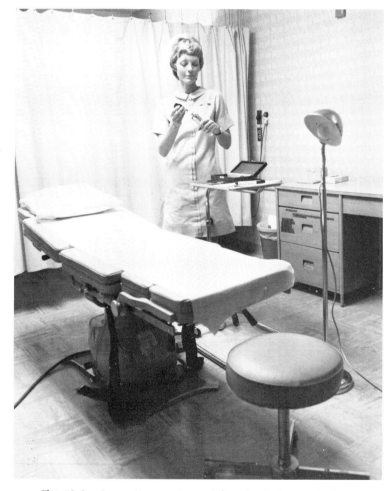

Fig. 10-2. Preparing equipment for physical examination.

note certain signs such as temperature, pulse, respiration, and blood pressure. Laboratory and x-ray facilities are available for observation of body functions, cavities, and excretions. The anatomic changes noted on examination constitute the physical signs of disease.

Some signs of illness can be detected only by scientific apparatus in the hands of a skilled physician or a nurse. Some instruments, such as the stethoscope, the ophthalmoscope, and the speculum, are accessory to the senses, to which they give a farther reach and a finer accuracy.

One of the chief methods of determin-

ing a patient's condition is by means of a physical examination. For this reason, one usually is done within the first 24 hours of a patient's hospitalization. Information gained at this time helps in understanding the patient's complaints and aids in making the final diagnosis.

The chief duties of the nurse in relation to the physical examination are (1) to have the necessary equipment in readiness (Fig. 10-2), (2) to drape and place the patient in the proper positions, and (3) to give moral support to the patient by giving simple explanations and avoiding unnecessary exposure (Fig. 10-3). Undue emo-

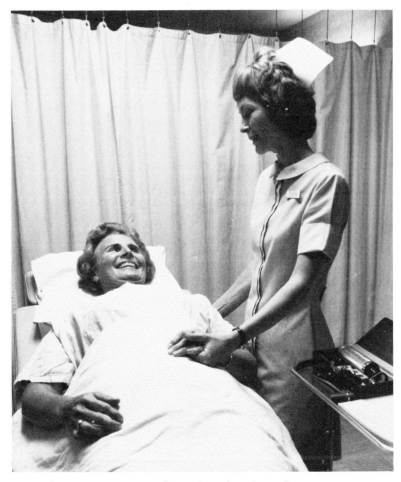

Fig. 10-3. Preparing the patient for physical examination.

tional strain and rigidity of certain muscles may interfere with the examination. Providing opportunity for the patient to void before the examination will aid in relaxing the abdominal muscles. Through the use of nonverbal communication, the patient may be assisted to become calm and relaxed.

Under the most favorable circumstances, a complete physical examination is a lengthy and tiring procedure. The nurse can do much to expedite matters by becoming familiar with routine techniques and the purpose for which they are used. The following routine is typical of the general procedure.

The physician usually begins by taking a history in order to become acquainted with the patient and to help put him at ease.

Clothing should be removed and the patient covered with a sheet or treatment blanket to facilitate exposure of the parts necessary for the examination.

The examination usually is begun with a general observation of the entire body for general build and state of nutrition and then is followed by close-ups for details, beginning at the head and proceeding to the feet. Good light is essential, preferably daylight. Special instruments, such as the otoscope or the ophthalmoscope, are used for examining open cavities.

The anterior and posterior chest walls are examined through use of the stethoscope to detect sounds not audible to the unaided ear. The presence of fluid in the chest may be detected by percussion (tapping).

Palpation is the chief method of examining the internal organs. Size, misplacement, and many other conditions may be determined.

The extremities are observed for deformities, circulatory disturbances, and skin lesions. Reflexes are tested by means of the percussion hammer.

If indicated, the general physical examination is followed by a special examination or a more thorough examination of one specific area, such as eye, ear, pelvic, rectal, or cystoscopic examination.

Laboratory tests and x-ray examinations are often used to confirm physical findings. These are discussed in Chapter 12.

PROBLEM-ORIENTED MEDICAL RECORDS
Basic premise

The problem-oriented medical record is a relatively new system of structuring patient care records. The system was introduced by Dr. Lawrence Weed, based upon the theory that a *core of behavior* should be taught rather than a core of knowledge requiring a memory-dependent system. The sheer volume and variety of medical knowledge make dependence upon the recall of facts increasingly unrealistic for effective functioning of today's health practitioner. POMR (problem-oriented medical records), in contrast, is based on developing the practitioner's capacity to extract data from source material and to analyze the data in a systematic, thorough, analytically sound, and efficient mode, which leads to the development and achievement of specific, attainable goals. Through the management of medical records the performance of those providing patient care is subject to review, which is comparable to the findings of one scientific researcher being open to the scrutiny of other researchers. Critical assessment of records tends to promote professional growth.

This system is envisioned by its proponents as having powerful implications for all health care disciplines, including nursing. For this reason, nursing personnel should have some acquaintance with the concept. The system, as introduced by its originator, is comprehensive, applicable to the hospital setting, or easily adopted in a community health service. However, this model is of interest to nursing because it supports the systematic planning of patient care, which is a nursing responsibility of mounting importance. The focus of this section is on the application of the system to problem-oriented charting, which is a modification of the Weed system.

The four basic elements of POMR, when properly implemented, cause the nurse to focus on the patient rather than on the task. It helps nursing to justify what it does in that the nursing care plan is incorporated into the patient's progress record in conjuction with the physician's therapeutic plan and the plan of other health care personnel concerned with solving the patient's problems.

POMR elements

In Dr. Weed's system there are four main elements: (1) a data base, (2) a problem list, (3) an assessment and plan for each problem, and (4) progress notes and related data.

The *data base* includes the same basic information obtained in the admission workup—initial history, physical examination, and laboratory tests—but the information is standardized. Standardization in this context means that the personnel concerned with the delivery of health care to a given segment of population have defined the data base content that they believe essential to providing efficient, comprehensive health care to the given population. This is a preliminary to implementing the POMR system.

Patient problems are identified from the data base. Each problem is numbered, titled, and listed on a sheet in the front of the patient's chart. It is emphasized that (1) all the patient's known problems are listed, physiologic, psychologic, and social, (2) any member of the patient care team (patient, physician, nurse, dietitian, or other) updates the problem list as additional information is obtained, new problems are iden-

tified, or a problem becomes inactive, and (3) the patient shares in the responsibility of the team for maintaining an accurate, comprehensive problem list.

Assessment and planning for individual problems are developed. Each problem is described and evaluated and an initial plan devised for each problem, which is recorded in the body of the patient's chart under the number and titled problem to which it is related. This includes such things as the orders, plan progress notes, and so forth. A logical format for this process has evolved under the easily remembered initials of *SOAP model*, which includes the following components:

Subjective data: the problem as the patient views it and feels about it

Objective data: physical and laboratory findings and other relevant findings and developments about the problem

Assessment: the continuous, ongoing evaluation of the problem, noting changes as they occur and using established criteria for assessment

Plan: the plans developed for diagnosis, therapy, and patient teaching

The purpose of this system of handling data regarding the patient is to develop records that show whether there was or was not an orderly observation of symptoms, to determine what they mean, and to see what was done about them. In other words, the SOAP model encourages the development and use of sound logic in problem analysis and patient care plan formulation. It also encourages communication among the members of the team.

Progress notes and related data as made by the various members of the health team are recorded together—physician's notes, nurses' notes, physical therapy notes, consultation, or other notes entered in a continuing sequence. When the problems are complex, flow sheets may be used to record specific parameters to ensure proper interpretation and management of the problems, particularly when they are changing rapidly.

Advantages of the POMR system

Those in situations where the POMR system is used generally report the following advantages:

1. It promotes a logical, specific listing of the patient's problems, the current treatment for each, and the plans of the health care team for each.

2. The record produced provides meaningful feedback for evaluating the quality of patient care. The audit of such records is an instrument for quality control of the patient care services and for promoting the educational experience of health care personnel.

3. The system has potential for change and improvement in health care.

Implications for nursing

Using Dr. Weed's theory that a *core of behavior* rather than a core of knowlege should be taught, preparation for nursing could include a core of behavior applicable to a lifetime of health care performance, rather than the learning of a set of facts that are outdated in a few years. This system can serve as a tool for developing that core of behavior that the student would learn from real data in the actual patient care situation. It is applicable not only to basic nursing education but also to continuing education and to the daily intellectual stimulation of nurse practitioners, increasing their ability to explicitly define and assess patient problems, and to the planning, implementation, and evaluation of patient care in close coordination with the total interdisciplinary team. In the process, areas for clinical nursing research would be recognizable.

Referring to the current nursing issues discussed in Chapter 1, it would appear that this system could be of assistance in attacking such problems as accountability in nursing, peer review, and continued competency of the practitioner.

Problem-oriented charting

This system of charting does not differ basically from the charting generally advocated. However, its value is that it does make essential data more obvious to the reader: what has been done for the patient, the *reason* for what has been done, and the outcome of the intervention in terms of patient response. In this context, a problem is defined as anything that interferes with the patient's needs, for example, the need for food or the need for elimination. The associated problems might be nausea, vomiting, constipation, or anuria.

This system of charting is extremely relevant to use of the adaptation model described in Chapter 6, and it is enhanced by use of the problem-solving method and application of scientific principles outlined in Chapters 3 and 4.

The essential steps in problem-oriented charting may be outlined as follows:

1. State in one or two words the problem identified.

2. Indent and underline the problem statement for ease in reading the chart.

3. Write a narrative description for further explanation of the problem as necessary to convey the complete message.

4. Describe the action taken using these questions: Was the problem solved by the action taken? If not, what else is being done?

5. Repeat these steps until the problem is satisfactorily resolved.

Fig. 10-4 is a comparison between traditional chart comments and problem-oriented chart entries.

It should be remembered that problem-oriented charting is *not* intended to replace any of the following: (1) factual charting (for such basic things as bath, side rails, and the like, a checklist may be posted at the foot of the bed), (2) patient care plans, (3) patient interview forms, or (4) informed nursing judgment based on

Traditional comments		Problem-oriented chart entries
C/O being cold	Coldness	*States feels cold. Temp. 98.4°. Blanket placed over patient. States feels more comfortable.*
Ambulated in room	Ambulation	*Ambulation in room with assistance, for second time after surgery. Able to walk full length of room & back to bed. Denies dizziness or excessive pain. States feels some weakness.*
C/O dizziness	Vertigo	*States feels dizzy even though is in bed. V/S 136/72, 82, 14. Medicated for vertigo. Relief obtained in approx. 20 min.*
Itches all over body	Itching	*States itching sensation present over entire skin surface. Is on med. for itching which she feels is not helpful. Dr. X notified. Topical hydrocortisone lotion applied as ordered. States feels much relief from lotion.*
Unable to sleep	Sleep	*States unable to sleep because of pain in abdomen at incision site. Med. for pain by Polly, R.N. Asleep in about 40 min.—slept remainder of night.*
Requested sleeper for insomnia. No further complaints at this time.	Insomnia	*States cannot sleep because of "strange surroundings" of hospital (is first hospitalization). Requested med. for sleep. Slept 6 hours after hypnotic given.*
States mod. amt. formed light brown stool with flatus after suppository	Constipation	*States no BM in 2 days. Glycerine supp. inserted. States had mod. amt. light brown, formed stool with flatus & indicates feels "relieved."*
Medicated for pain in rt. side	Pain	*States has pain in rt. side at area of abrasions & contusions. Indicates pain is of dull, throbbing type & extends from lower ribs to iliac crest. Med. given. Indicated relief obtained in approx. 30 min.*
Became confused. Posey restraint applied. Restless	Confusion and restlessness	*Appears to be confused & restless (e.g. does not know where he is, date, or year; talking about spiders on "wall & ceiling." Electrolytes and other lab data reviewed—normal. No history of drug or chronic alcohol use according to family. Restrained with Posey belt and wrist restraints. Dr. Rigmon notified. Medicated for restlessness per order. Appeared to be resting but awake in about 45 min. Asleep after about 1½ hr.*
Refused supper. Took some nourishment at H.S.	Appetite	*States did not feel hungry at dinner. Denies nausea. Was able to take approx. 6 oz. milk and cup custard at H.S.*
Up & voided in BR	Voiding	*Amb. with assistance to BR. Voided 300 ml. light straw-colored, clear urine. Assisted back to bed & rails up. Tolerated activity without discomfort.*

Continued.

Fig. 10-4. A comparison of the traditional chart comments and problem-oriented chart entries (From unpublished materials; by permission of Jane Ann Caruso, Patricia Dunbar, and Mike Gilliam, Beverly Hospital, Montebello, Calif.)

Traditional comments — cont'd		Problem-oriented chart entries — cont'd
Complains of leg pain — right leg. Medicated for pain	Pain	Indicates has pain in rt. lower posterior leg. States is burning-type pain. Onset about midmorning but not severe until this evening. Slight redness & swelling noted in area. Dr. Zlinka notified. Hot moist compresses & K-pad with temp. set at 98° applied to affected leg. Med. for pain. Heparin 40,000 U. given. Indicated comfort obtained in about 45 min.
Rash noted on body. Dr. Sikey notified. Med. given	Skin rash	Has slightly raised, red rash over trunk, extremities, & face. Onset abrupt following inj. of penicillin. V/S stable @ 120/70, 84, 16. Alert & responsive. Dr. Sikey notified. Benadryl 100 mg. IM given. Appears comfortable. Skin rash less noticeable after about 2 hr.
C/O K-pad being too warm. CSR notified		States K-pad is too warm. Area inspected & appears reddened. CSR notified to check temp. CSR technician here, temp. adjusted. Pt. states comfortable now.

Fig. 10-4, cont'd. For legend see p. 131.

scientific knowledge, which must precede the implementation of nursing action for a given patient problem.

Problem-oriented charting is useful in nursing because it provides a framework for synthesizing data from which to make nursing decisions.

LEARNING SITUATIONS FOR THE PATIENT

The patient and his family should gain accurate and appropriate information and understanding about his condition as a basis for acceptance of needed therapy. He should be encouraged to discuss any worries he may have or anything he views as a problem. Assisting the individual to begin thinking through his problems as groundwork for developing acceptable ways of working with his physical and/or psychologic problems leads to more mature levels of adaptation.

SUMMARY

Observational skills of the nurse are directed toward gathering information about the patient as a person, toward eliciting data intended to assist in developing awareness of the patient as a human being and a member of a family, toward taking a "closeup" picture of the psychosocial features of the patient as well as of his physical state, and toward utilizing the holistic view of man in the provision of nursing care.

The importance of observation as a nursing skill is presented as a means through which the nurse contributes to the care and well-being of her patients. Observation encompasses gathering information about the patient through the unaided senses as well as through the use of special equipment and techniques of examination.

QUESTIONS FOR DISCUSSION

1 Someone has said that nursing is three-fourths observation. Justify this statement.
2 How does a nurse observe?
3 How does a physician observe?
4 Define diagnosis and prognosis.
5 Define subjective symptoms, objective symptoms, and cardinal symptoms.

NURSING PROGRESS NOTES

DATE & TIME		NOTES
10/18 8 A.M.	Pain	Having severe left sided chest pain radiating down left arm. Skin warm and diaphoretic. B.P. 108/62, A.P. 118 R. 24. Very apprehensive. Medicated for pain. Color slightly cyanotic. O₂ started at 6 L/min via cannula.
8:30 A.M.	Change in pattern	Having frequent P.V.C.'s 10-12 min. P.B. of Xylocaine started at 2 mg/min. Doctor notified.
8:45 A.M.	Pain	States pain has eased up. Color improved and he seems much more relaxed. B.P. 118/66 A.P. 90 R. 18. Skin still slightly diaphoretic.
9:30 A.M.	Monitor pattern	Only a rare P.V.C. now. P.B. Xylocaine slowed to 1 mg/min.
10:00 A.M.	Elimination	Urine output low — only 25 cc since 6 a.m. Has pitting edema of both legs and has moist nonproductive cough. Doctor notified and orders received. Lasix given IV. Hourly output started.
11:00 A.M.		Has had 350 cc output following Lasix.
12:00 P.M.	Rest	Asleep. Allowed to rest as much as possible. A. Wright, R.N.
10/24 11:00 A.M.	Activity	Moves from chair to bed slowly. States he is "too weak" to move. Assisted into bed. Instructed to ring call light for assistance before getting out of bed. C. White, R.N.
11:30 A.M.	Coughing	Has a dry hacking non-productive cough. Coughs more when speaking. States he has been taking cough medicine for several days but it's only helpful for a short time. Advised that doctor has ordered a different medication for his cough. B. Jones, LVN
8:00 P.M.	Appetite	Stated did not feel hungry at dinner. Denies nausea. Has able to take approximately 6 oz. milk and a cup of custard at 7:45 p.m. L. Smith, NA
9:00 P.M.	Pain	Indicated pain in right lower posterior leg. States is burning type pain. Onset about mid-morning but not severe until this evening. Slight redness and swelling noted in area. Dr. Jones notified @ 9:05 p.m. Hot moist compresses and K pad with temp set at 98° applied to affected leg at 9:15 p.m. Medicated for pain at 9:10 p.m. Anticoagulant therapy started as ordered.
9:45 P.M.		Indicates comfort obtained; pain in right lower leg has almost gone. S. Camp, R.N.

Fig. 10-5. Example of problem-oriented nursing and dietary progress notes (From unpublished material; by permission of Ruth Magness and Kay Barrera, Beverly Hospital, Montebello, Calif.)

6 List in detail what you would note while you admit a patient.

7 What are the advantages of the problem-oriented medical records system?

8 What social problems of the patient may you observe?

LIFE SITUATION

Mr. Jones, 35 years of age and not acutely ill, is being admitted for an appendectomy. He has never been hospitalized before and assumes a false and unconvincing air of lightheartedness and jokes about his independence. What fears is he attempting to conceal? What will your approach be? How will you record this in your admission notation?

SUGGESTED READINGS

Bloom, Judith T., and others: Problem-oriented charting, American Journal of Nursing 71:2144, November, 1971.

Byers, Virginia: Nursing observation, Dubuque, Iowa, 1968, William C. Brown Co., Publishers.

Fowkes, Virginia, and Hunn, Virginia K.: Clinical assessment for the nurse practitioner, St. Louis, 1973, The C. V. Mosby Co.

Gane, Donna: Sparky: a success story, American Journal of Nursing 73:1176, July, 1973.

Gardner, M. Arlene Martin: Responsiveness as a measure of consciousness, American Journal of Nursing 68:1035, May, 1968.

Kalkman, Marion E.: Recognizing emotional problems, American Journal of Nursing 68:536, March, 1972.

MacBryde, Cyril, and others: Signs and symptoms, Philadelphia, 1970, J. B. Lippincott Co.

Mayeroff, Milton: On caring, ed. 1, New York, 1971, Harper and Row, Publishers.

Moses, Dorothy V.: Assessing behavior in the elderly, Nursing Clinics of North America 7:225, June, 1972.

Robinson, Lisa: The crying patient, Nursing '72 2:16, December, 1972.

Roy, Sister Callista: Adaptation: a basis for nursing practice, Nursing Outlook 19:254, April, 1971.

Schell, Pamela L., and Campbell, Alla T.: POMR—not just another way to chart, Nursing Outlook 72:510, August, 1972.

Weed, Lawrence: Medical record, medical education, and patient care, Chicago, 1970, Year Book Medical Publishers, Inc.

Woody, Mary, and Mallison, Mary: The problem-oriented system for patient-centered care, American Journal of Nursing 73:1168, July, 1973.

11 Vital signs in assessing adaptive response

VITAL SIGNS

One of the most common observations made by the nurse in relation to a patient's condition or progress is that of assessing his temperature, pulse, and respiration. These findings, along with blood pressure readings, are known as the vital signs. Because these findings are governed by the vital organs and often disclose even the slightest deviation from normal body functioning, assessment of the vital signs is the most critical of observations regarding the patient's condition. Significant variation in these findings may indicate problems relating to insufficient consumption or overconsumption of oxygen, blood depletion, electrolyte imbalance, bacterial invasion, or emotional distress.

A patient's vital signs are usually checked immediately upon admission to a hospital or clinic and are usually repeated at regular intervals during any acute stage and probably twice a day during the remainder of his stay in the hospital.

Because of the frequent repetition of taking a patient's temperature, pulse, or respiration, the procedure sometimes tends to become automatic, and unless the mechanisms that control these signs and the need for accuracy are thoroughly understood, observations and charting may have limited usefulness to others who are concerned with the patient. Therefore, understanding of the scientific principles involved as a basis for interpreting the symptoms is very important.

BODY TEMPERATURE

Temperature is a measurement of heat expressed in degrees. Body temperature may be defined as the degree of heat

135

maintained by the body; it is the balance between the heat produced and the heat lost (Fig. 11-1).

The center for heat regulation in the body is in the hypothalamus, a portion of the brain. An intricate adjustment of physiologic reflexes maintains the body temperature at nearly constant level. Because of this factor, man is known as a warm-blooded animal (Fig. 11-2).

The regulation of the body temperature is brought about in two ways: by chemical regulation of production of heat, termed *thermogenesis,* and by the physical regulation of heat loss, termed *thermolysis.*

Principles from biologic and physical sciences

A fairly definite range of body temperature must be maintained for efficient cellular and enzymatic activity.

1. The range in body temperature within which the cells can function efficiently is approximately 34° to 41° C. (94° to approximately 106° F.).

2. Body cells vary in their ability to withstand the extremes of temperature; central nervous system cells usually cannot function efficiently above 41° C.

3. There is a normal variation in temperature between morning and evening hours. The minimum temperature occurs in the early morning hours. The maximum temperature is reached in the late afternoon or early evening. A slight rise in temperature from the time of ovulation until menstruation is normal in the female.

4. Body temperature is controlled by regulation of the rate at which the tissues produce heat and the rate at which heat is lost from the body.

5. The amount of heat produced by the body can be *decreased* to prevent overheating by:

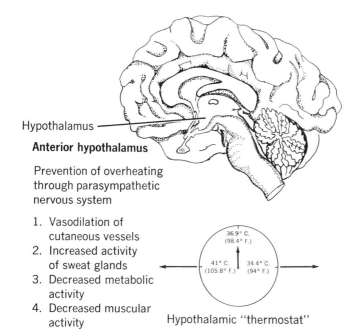

Hypothalamus

Anterior hypothalamus

Prevention of overheating through parasympathetic nervous system

1. Vasodilation of cutaneous vessels
2. Increased activity of sweat glands
3. Decreased metabolic activity
4. Decreased muscular activity

36.9° C. (98.4° F.)

41° C. (105.8° F.) ← → 34.4° C. (94° F.)

Hypothalamic "thermostat"

Posterior hypothalamus

Conservation of body heat through sympathetic nervous system

1. Vasoconstriction of cutaneous vessels
2. Decreased activity of sweat glands
3. Increased metabolic activity
4. Increased muscular activity (shivering—through stimulation of the reticular system)

Fig. 11-1. Hypothalamic mechanism for control of body temperature.

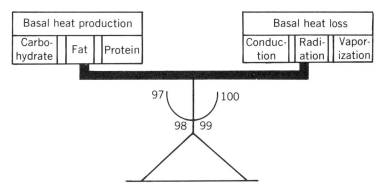

Fig. 11-2. Body temperature is the balance between heat production and heat loss.

a. Decreasing the cellular metabolic activity. Heat is a part of the energy produced when the tissues oxidize carbohydrates, fats, and proteins. When the nutrients oxidized are decreased, the heat output is also decreased. This decreased metabolic rate means decreased work output. The decrease is effected through the thyroid gland and the medulla of the adrenal gland.

b. Decreasing muscle activity. Maintenance of muscle tonus involves production of heat. Tonus is decreased by heat. Muscles in a warm environment tend to be relaxed, so a feeling of lethargy is experienced.

c. Increasing circulatory activity in the skin. Heat is lost to the environment through radiation from the skin surface. As a result of vasodilation of the capillaries in the skin bringing increased blood to the surface, more heat will be lost to the atomsphere by radiation. The external environmental temperature must be lower than that of the body in order for radiation of heat from the body to occur.

d. Increasing perspiration and respiration. Body heat is decreased through water molecules constantly diffusing through the skin and through the alveoli of the lungs to form water vapor.

6. The amount of heat produced by the body can be *increased* by:

a. Increasing cellular metabolic activity. The heat liberated is increased as the amount of nutrient oxidized by the tissues is increased. Thyroxin also increases tissue oxidation.

b. Increasing muscle activity. Heat liberated by maintenance of muscle tonus can be increased by involuntary tensing of the muscles, as in shivering, and also by voluntary exercise.

c. Decreasing circulatory activity in the skin. By peripheral vasoconstriction, the amount of blood circulating to the surface of the body is decreased, resulting in less heat lost by radiation.

7. The hypothalamus is a coordinating center for the autonomic nervous system. Therefore, it influences such involuntary actions as changes in arterial pressure, vasoconstriction and vasodilation, and sweating, which are important in preventing external temperatures from affecting the temperature of the tissues and fluids of the body. The function of physiologic regulation of body temperature is located in the specialized receptor center of the hypothalamus. (See Fig. 11-1.)

8. Mechanisms for hypothalamic control of body temperature in prevention of overheating (anterior part of hypothalamus) include:

a. Stimulation of the thermostatic mechanism by slight changes in temperature of the circulating blood. A change of 0.01° C. will result in an adaptive response.

b. Stimulation of the parasympathetic nerves through the axons of the specialized receptor cells that ultimately synapse on the cell bodies of the parasympathetic nerves. Stimulation results in: (1) vasodilation of peripheral blood vessels, which causes more heat to be lost by radiation, and (2) increased activity of the sweat glands.

9. Mechanisms for hypothalamic control of body temperature for conservation of body heat through the sympathetic nervous system (posterior part of hypothalamus) include:

a. Vasoconstriction of peripheral blood vessels, decreasing heat lost by evaporation.

b. Decreasing activity of the sweat glands by direct inhibition through the sympathetic nerves.

c. Increased metabolic rate of the tissues. The sympathetic nervous system stimulates the adrenal medulla, causing it to secrete more epinephrine into the circulation, which in turn increases the rate of tissue oxidation.

d. Shivering. Through stimulation originating in the hypothalamus, rhythmic contraction of the muscles occurs, increasing the heat liberated.

10. Circulatory changes and loss of subcutaneous tissue occurring in old age may influence the effectiveness of the mechanisms for temperature control.

11. Pyrogens act (directly or indirectly) by "resetting" the hypothalamic temperature regulating centers so that temperature regulation is at a higher level for mechanisms operating to increase heat loss.

a. Peripheral vasoconstriction and a sensation of chilling occur with loss of body heat.

b. As heat production is then increased, it is accompanied by vasodilation, flushing, and uncomfortable sensation of warmth, until the body fluids and tissues reach the elevated temperature of the hypothalamic "thermostat."

Principles from behavioral sciences

An individual is more likely to experience satisfaction in relationships with nursing personnel when he has been prepared for specific situations before they occur.

1. Some knowledge of the facts about the situation has been supplied to him.

2. Some instructions about his goals and behavior in the situation have been given.

Additional pertinent statements may be selected from related chapters that can be applied in this context.

Homeostasis

Heat is produced in the body by the oxidation of food. Because the muscles and glands are the most active tissues, more oxidation takes place in them than in any other tissues.

Activities concerned with the production and loss of heat include vasoconstriction, vasodilation, sweating, shivering, and panting. Anything that interferes with normal heat balance interferes with the functions of the whole body. Receptors for the sensations of heat and cold are of different structure and of slightly different distribution. They are placed about 0.1 to 0.3 mm. below the surface of the skin. There is a narrow zone of environmental air between 82.4° and 86° F. (28° and 30° C.), in which the heat production and heat loss are practically identical. Above 86° F. (30° C.) the skin vessels dilate, and there is a slight secretion of sweat. Below 82.4° F. (28° C.) the vessels constrict, thus preventing heat loss.

Vasoconstriction and dilation affect

chiefly the loss of heat by radiation, but both also influence moistness of the skin as well as losses by convection. Unless heat elimination keeps pace with heat production, the average body temperature must rise. Heat is lost from the skin by radiation, vaporization, convection, and conduction. The proportion of heat lost in these different ways varies with the condition of the body and with the temperature and humidity of the environment.

Radiation means the transfer of heat from the surface of one object to that of another that is not in contact by way of electromagnetic waves. These waves travel through space without causing any appreciable change in the temperature of the air. Radiative heat interchange is dependent on four factors: the radiative characteristics of the body itself, the radiation area, the surface temperature, and the mean temperature of surrounding objects. The human body, as a result of heat produced by metabolism, radiates energy through the air to other objects.

Loss of heat by radiation constitutes 60% to 65% of the total loss of heat. At low environmental temperatures radiation is the main method of heat loss. At temperatures of 93° to 95° F. (33.8° to 35° C.), evaporation is the main factor.

If the body is immersed in water that has a temperature higher than that of the body, the body temperature tends to become equal to that of the water because radiation cannot take place. This rise may occur in a hot tub bath.

The amount of radiation from the body is in proportion to the radiating surface area, which amounts to about 85%. There is no effective radiation between the opposing aspects of the legs or between the arms and the body. Nonconducting clothes reduce radiation.

Evaporation is the process whereby a substance in liquid state is changed to a vapor state; such a process requires heat. As moisture on the skin evaporates, the body is cooled. Evaporation

accounts for 20% to 30% of heat loss. Vaporization of water removes heat from the surface of the skin and respiratory tract because with the human body each gram of water takes up 580 calories from its surroundings when it passes from a liquid to a vapor state. Insensible perspiration (sweat before it becomes visible) accounts for a constant proportion of heat loss. Approximately 300 ml. of water are vaporized from the skin daily, and about 500 ml. of water are vaporized from the lungs daily.

The amount of vaporization depends on several variables: the surface area, the amount of sweat produced, the temperature of the skin and corresponding vapor pressure of sweat, the vapor pressure of the air, and the velocity of air movement.

Convection is the method of transferring heat by circulating air or liquid, and it depends on the temperature of the atmosphere. The most important factor influencing heat loss by convection is air movement. A breeze or a wind increases loss of heat by convection. Convection is dependent on the relative densities of air or fluid at different temperatures, the warmer and lighter air or fluid rising and the cooler air or fluid falling.

Conduction is the transfer of heat directly through a substance from the hot part to the cold part, from one molecule to another in gases, liquids, and solids, by direct contact. It is the least important means of heat loss from the body. Heat is transferred by conduction from the body to any substance in contact with the body—tidal air, clothing, foodstuffs, and water. Man seldom loses much heat by conduction.

A body temperature usually above 99° F. (37.2° C.) is spoken of as an elevation of temperature, or fever. In fever, heat production is increased out of porportion to heat elimination. It is caused by a disturbance of the thermoregulating center in the hypothalamus, which is set at a higher level; therefore, the level of body temperature rises uniformly. Dehydration may also cause fever.

Normally heat is produced in the body by the slow combustion of food in the presence of oxygen. The heat thus produced in the muscles and glands is distributed to all parts of the body. Vital processes of the body depend on the maintenance of a certain degree of heat, which varies in different areas of the body. Fever is usually caused by abnormal proteins released into the body fluids during disease processes. These proteins have a direct effect on the hypothalamic thermostat to reset its normal operating range at the higher temperature level. The condition is referred to as *pyrexia. Hyperpyrexia* and *hyperthermia* usually refer to high temperature, 105° F. (40.5° C.) or more. Temperatures below the normal range are spoken of as subnormal temperatures.

In fever the skin is pale because of constriction of the peripheral blood vessels. After the fever temperature is established, heat loss keeps pace with heat production more by vasodiliation than by stimulation of sweat. Prolonged periods of fever are always significant. However, fever may be beneficial in some infections because of its destructive effect on the causative organism.

The beginning of fever is termed *onset,* and may be sudden or gradual. The decline of fever, which may be sudden or gradual, is called the *defervescence.* Sudden decline of fever is termed *crisis.* Gradual decline is called *lysis.* The course of fever is referred to as *fastigium* or *stadium.*

Types of fever are constant, intermittent, and remittent (Fig. 11-3). A *constant* fever is one that does not vary more than 2° C., and the temperature does not come down to normal during the day. An *intermittent* fever shows large variations on a graphic sheet far above and below normal during the same day. A *remittent* fever is one in which the changes may be wider than 2° C., but the temperature does not come to normal. A *hectic* fever is an intermittent fever in which the daily changes are very wide. It is often associated with chills and sweating. A *relapsing* fever is one in which short febrile periods are interspersed by periods of 1 or more days of normal temperature.

Some symptoms of fever are flushed face, hot and dry skin, thirst, rapid pulse, headache, nausea, vomiting, constipation or diarrhea, and general aching over the entire body. Sometimes when a temperature of 105° F. (40.5° C.) occurs, delirium exists and convulsions may follow, after

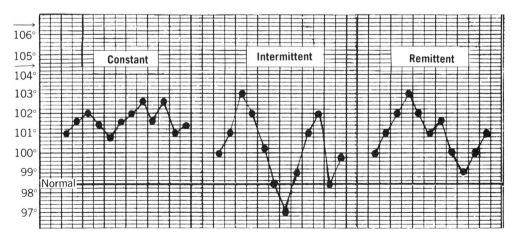

Fig. 11-3. Temperature graphs showing different types of fever.

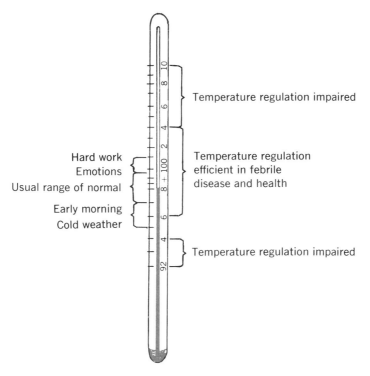

Temperature regulation impaired

Temperature regulation
efficient in febrile
disease and health

Hard work
Emotions
Usual range of normal

Early morning
Cold weather

Temperature regulation impaired

Fig. 11-4. Significance of ranges of temperatures.

which the patient goes into a coma and soon dies.

The temperature curve used to be an aid in diagnosing certain diseases that were accompanied by a rise in temperature (Fig. 11-3). However, with modern methods of diagnosis, early treatment many times prevents the characteristic rise in temperature.

A temperature below 97° F. (36.1° C.) is called a *subnormal* temperature. An extremely low temperature is one of the greatest depressants to vital functions. Subnormal temperatures may be caused by excessive heat elimination, lessened heat production, and depression of the nervous system, such as in shock. A warm environment, rest, and warm drinks usually will raise a subnormal temperature to normal.

A person's temperature is not the same all the time, and the normal temperature of two persons may not be the same. Body temperature varies with the time of the day, the time of the month (for females), and the age of the person. It is lowest in the early morning when activity is low, and highest in the afternoon when activity is increased. The reverse is often true of night workers. A daily variation of 1° or 2° often is found in a single individual. The temperature is not the same in various parts of the body. Under the tongue, the temperature may be 98° F. (36.6° C.), while blood temperature may be 100° F. (37.7° C.) and the liver (the highest in the body) may be 102° F. (38.8° C.). Menstruation produces a sudden fall in temperature, which slowly rises again after ovulation to a maximum just before the next menstrual period.

Human life may exist within a temperature range of 77° to 113° F. (25° to 45° C.), but extreme temperatures within this range are serious (Fig. 11-4). There is no one normal temperature, but instead a

141

fairly wide zone from 97° to 100° F. (36.1° to 37.7° C.). (See also Fig. 11-1.)

Within certain limits heat production can be controlled in several ways: by eating more protein food, by stimulation of the adrenal glands, by cold, or by involuntary activity.

With heavy clothing and cold air, water vaporized from the skin condenses in the clothing, giving back some of the heat of condensation to the body but losing most to the outside air.

Severe exercise causes a rise in temperature because heat is produced faster than it is eliminated. Unconscious tensing of muscles, such as in shivering and cold, increases heat. During fever, more blood is sent to the skin, thus helping the body to reduce its temperature.

The skin acts as an enormous dam with many sluiceways placed across the stream of internal heat that can be opened or closed as occasion demands. Heat is lost from the body by three channels: skin, lungs, and excretions. The most important is the skin, through which about 85% of heat is lost.

The human skin is well adapted to eliminating heat by three mechanisms: (1) an extremely delicate apparatus for detecting temperature changes, (2) an efficient vasomotor control of its blood supply, and (3) its sweat glands.

In cold weather the cutaneous blood vessels constrict and redistribute the blood so that a greater portion of heat is found in the internal organs, and heat loss from the skin is minimized. In a warm environment the cutaneous blood vessels dilate, thus bringing more blood to the surface, which increases radiation and evaporation of heat. The sweat glands keep the skin moist so that cooling results from evaporation. When heat production is excessive or when the atmospheric surroundings are too warm, evaporation speeds up.

When the body temperature is abnormally high, a cold bath or a cold environment may produce comfort, but after about an hour constriction from cold changes to vasodilation and the skin becomes warm again. Exercise should be limited, and the diet should contain much liquid. When the fever declines, heat loss exceeds heat production.

To lower body temperature, cool-water sponges may be used. They remove heat by vaporization of moisture from the skin.

To raise body temperature, blankets are applied. Blankets, being full of air spaces, serve as insulation and keep the body heat from escaping. A hot-water bottle conducts heat to the body. Hot drinks increase body temperature by conduction. Rubbing the body surface increases heat in the skin by friction, which changes mechanical energy to thermal energy.

Drugs used to produce fever are called pyretics. Stimulants produce more body heat by increasing metabolism. The sweat glands can be stimulated directly by pilocarpine, acetylcholine, and adrenalin. Atropine produces fever by blocking the cholinergic fibers to the sweat glands.

Drugs that decrease temperature are called antipyretics. Among these are the coal-tar analgesics and quinine. They increase heat elimination by the skin by depressing the brain and heat-regulating center. Depressants such as morphine and alcohol lessen the activity of the nervous system and lower the temperature of the body.

The antibiotics, such as penicillin and streptomycin, lower temperature by preventing bacterial action.

Measurement

The clinical thermometer is used in measuring body temperature and is available in both Fahrenheit and centigrade scales (Fig. 11-5).

The principle on which the thermometer is constructed is the expansion of mercury when subjected to heat. The thermometer is made of glass and consists of

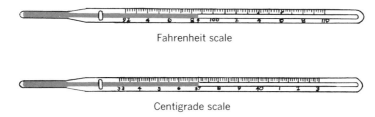

Fahrenheit scale

Centigrade scale

Fig. 11-5. Comparison of Fahrenheit and centigrade scales.

an end bulb containing mercury and a stem in which the mercury rises. This column of mercury remains at the height to which it rises and must be shaken down. A constriction near the bulb prevents the mercury from receding and thus provides a more accurate reading.

Bulbs vary in size and shape to fit the different orifices. Colored bulbs are available to designate rectal or isolated thermometers. The mouth, rectum, and axilla areas are used chiefly because they simulate the inside of the body.

A good blood supply under the tongue and the fact that the thermometer can be held in place by the tongue while the mouth is closed makes the mouth a convenient place for taking temperature. Also containing a plentiful blood supply is the rectum, which is not influenced by external air temperature. Rectal temperature is nearer the temperature of the inside of the body than is mouth temperature. The axilla usually is moist from perspiration, and even if it is dried, enough moisture and air may be present to prevent an accurate body temperature reading.

The range of scale on a clinical thermometer may be either from 90° to 110° F. divided into 0.2° intervals or from 34° to 43° C. divided into 0.1° intervals.

Readings are usually taken at the nearest tenth. Temperature readings are usually graphed and may be recorded in the bedside notes and on other special sheets when indicated.

Sometimes it becomes necessary for the nurse to convert a temperature reading from one scale to another. This can be done by following a very simple formula:

	C.	F.	
Boiling point—	-100°	212°-	—Boiling point
Freezing point—	-0°	32°-	—Freezing point

From these facts it can be seen that water boils at 212° and freezes at 32° on the Fahrenheit scale, whereas it boils at 100° and freezes at 0° on the centigrade scale. Between the boiling points and freezing points there are 180 and 100 degrees, respectively. To have both scales start at 0, it will be necessary to subtract 32 degrees from the Fahrenheit scale, which gives the following relationship:

$$C : (F - 32) :: 100 : 180$$

This equation reduces to:

$$C : (F - 32) :: 5 : 9$$

If one desires to find the centigrade equivalent when given the Fahrenheit reading, it can be done easily by solving for C. and vice versa by solving for F. when given centigrade.

EXAMPLE: Find C. when the Fahrenheit reading is 98.6°.

Substituting:

$$C : (F - 32) :: 5 : 9$$
$$C : (98.6 - 32) :: 5 : 9$$
$$C : 66.6 :: 5 : 9$$

Multiply the extremes together and multiply the means together:

$$9 C = 333.0$$
$$C = 37°$$

143

EXAMPLE: Find F. when the centigrade reading is 40°.

Substituting:

$$C : (F - 32) :: 5 : 9$$
$$40 : (F - 32) :: 5 : 9$$

Multiply the extremes together and multiply the means together:

$$5 (F - 32) = 9 \times 40$$
$$5 F - 160 = 360$$
$$5 F = 360 + 160$$
$$5 F = 520$$
$$F = 104°$$

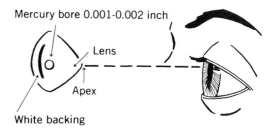

Fig. 11-6. Cross section of a thermometer showing how to read a thermometer by looking through the apex.

Clinical thermometers are easily broken and should be handled with care. They should be held by the upper stem and shaken down by a quick turn of the wrist. Mechanical devices that can shake down a dozen or more at one time are available. This is a time-saving process and also prevents breakage.

A clinical thermometer should neither be subjected to high temperature nor rinsed in warm water. Mechanical cleansing and chemicals are used for sterilization.

To read a thermometer, one should hold it at the upper end of the stem with one hand. Standing with the back to the light, slightly rotate thermometer back and forth until the markings on the graduated scale can be seen. The reading is taken at the point on the scale where the column of mercury ends. The fine bore is difficult to see, and magnification is provided in front by the shape of the thermometer, which acts as a lens (Fig. 11-6).

When the thermometer is removed from the mouth, it is wiped toward the tip to avoid contaminating the fingers of the worker. During the drying process, it is wiped from the tip to avoid contaminating the cleaned area.

Rectal thermometers are lubricated to reduce friction between the thermometer and the mucous membrane of the anal canal.

In taking oral temperature, the nurse places a watch within range of vision in order to assume an erect position. In taking rectal temperature, the patient should be near the edge of the bed to prevent reaching and stretching on the part of the nurse. After the thermometer is inserted into the anal canal, the nurse may assume an upright position while holding the thermometer.

In taking temperatures, individual thermometers may be kept at the bedside, or a tray containing several thermometers may be carried from patient to patient. The cleaning and shaking down of thermometers is usually done in the central supply room.

There are now available electrical thermometers that have proved to be more sensitive and more accurate than the standard glass thermometer, and they are also economical since there is little breakage. However, the public has been slow in accepting them.

The patient should understand what is being done for him in order to give his cooperation. He needs to understand that the mouth should be kept closed while an oral thermometer is in place. The nurse should not leave the thermometer in the mouth any longer than necessary because the patient may become uncomfortable. It is best not to leave the room while a patient's temperature is being taken. A few patients fake their temperature if they have a chance. Some may read the thermometer if they are left alone and may become unduly alarmed. If the nurse remains near and removes the thermometer as soon as it has registered, the patient will be comfortable and more willing to cooperate.

Since exposure of the anal region is not pleasant, the patient is screened and kept covered by the top bedding as well as possible while the nurse holds the thermometer in place.

Since exciting emotions may cause the temperature to rise, the environment is kept quiet and psychologic upsets are prevented.

In some situations the patient may not be informed of his temperature reading, so that he will not become unduly alarmed. Sometimes a patient thinks something is wrong if his temperature varies as much as 0.2° from 98.6° F. (37.0° C.). If it is high, he may feel prostrate and sense the fact that the temperature is not normal. Sometimes insufficient knowledge produces more harm in a patient than if he knew the true facts concerning his condition. However, the physician's wishes should be considered and also the patient's level of awareness. It is usually possible to find answers to a patient's questions concerning his temperature that will be honest, reasonable, and nonalarming. One should never "talk down to" the patient nor should the nurse use jokes or other trite conversation about a patient's temperature.

Taking a temperature involves cooperation between the patient and the nurse. The task is sometimes delegated to a practical nurse or aide. Cooperation is necessary also between the nurse and the central supply room in order to have the trays ready for use at stated intervals. The team leader or head nurse is informed at once of patients whose temperatures are above 100° F., or 38° C. Patients with elevated temperatures usually require more planned nursing care. The physician

depends on accurate temperature taking and recording in diagnosis and treatment of the patient.

Public health nurses carry a rectal and an oral thermometer in their bags and usually take the temperature of patients they visit.

Suggested points

1. Body temperature should be evaluated in relation to the patient's usual temperature, emotional state, time of day, activity, and method used.

2. Elderly persons react sluggishly, so that a small rise in their temperature may be of much more significance than a higher temperature in an infant. Infants have poor temperature control and, hence, irregular temperatures and exaggerated responses.

3. Almost everyone thinks in terms of the oral temperature. It may be affected by hot and cold drinks, mouth breathing, and other factors, and is used mostly for convenience. The rectal method is preferred for a more accurate reading and should be used for children and unconscious and irresponsible patients.

4. Oral temperatures should not be taken within 30 minutes following the intake of hot or cold food or fluids. Smoking and gum chewing may also affect temperature readings.

5. Rectal temperatures are contraindicated in rectal or perineal surgery, diarrhea, and other diseases of the rectum.

6. A high humid environmental temperature may produce a fever because heat cannot be eliminated by either radiation or evaporation.

7. When a thermometer is removed from the patient, it is wiped toward the tip to avoid contaminating the fingers of the worker.

8. Friction is necessary to ensure cleanliness of a thermometer.

9. Body temperature may be lowered by removing the patient's clothing and plac-

ing him in a cool environment, by the application of alcohol or a tepid sponge, or by the use of antipyretic drugs.

10. Typical temperature curves that were formerly diagnostic are less frequently seen because of the effective use of antibiotics and chemotherapeutic drugs.

11. A subnormal temperature may be just as significant as a high one, as it may indicate shock, hemorrhage, or decreased body functioning.

12. The rectal temperature is considered to be the most accurate because the rectum most nearly simulates the inside of the body.

13. Most conscious patients usually are aware of the fact that their temperatures are elevated. The cooperation of the patient is necessary for obtaining accurate readings, and therefore thermometers should not be left in place for longer periods of time than is necessary.

14. The delegation of taking the patient's temperature to a nonprofessional worker does not relieve the nurse from the responsibility of evaluating and reporting to the proper authority.

Summary

Body temperature is one of the first symptoms reported in illnesses. Temperature of the body depends on the delicate balance between heat production and heat loss, and any interference with either changes the temperature reading. Heat is produced in the body by oxidation of food. It is lost chiefly by radiation and vaporization from the skin. It may be retained in the body by heavy clothing and increased temperature of the environment. It may be more quickly dissipated by light clothing and air in motion.

Temperature is a measurement of heat expressed in degrees. Body temperature means the degree of heat of the body. The normal body temperature is the balance maintained between the heat produced and the heat lost.

The temperature of the body is measured by placing a clinical thermometer in the mouth, the axilla, or the rectum. The rectal temperature is considered to be the most accurate temperature. Temperatures are taken by rectum on babies, children, and irrational patients. Taking temperatures by mouth is the most usual and convenient method. Axillary temperature is the least reliable, although occasionally it is used when mouth and rectal temperatures cannot be taken. Placing the hand on the forehead will reveal whether the skin is warmer than usual.

The temperature of the body is a diagnostic aid. It is so important that, along with the pulse and respiration, it is called a cardinal symptom. Many conditions are characterized by an elevation of body temperature and some by a fall.

Temperature readings are graphed on a special form so that comparison with previous and subsequent ones can be easily seen.

Modern methods of treatment prevent the temperature curve that used to be typical of many diseases.

PULSE AND BLOOD PRESSURE

Pulse and blood pressure are phenomena that concern the circulatory system. *Pulse* may be defined as the alternate expansion (rise) and recoil (fall) of an artery as the wave of blood is forced through it by the contraction of the left ventricle. *Blood pressure* is the pressure the blood exerts against the walls of the vessels in which it is contained. *Systolic pressure* is the greatest pressure that the contraction of the heart causes. *Diastolic pressure* is the lowest pressure that occurs between the contractions of the ventricles. *Pulse pressure* is the difference between the systolic and the diastolic pressures. Pulse is one of the cardinal symptoms. It gives an indication of the manner in which the heart is functioning. Since the pulse is greatly influenced by the blood pressure, they usually are considered together.

Principles from biologic and physical sciences

The circulatory system consists of the heart, arteries, veins, and capillaries and is a closed transportation system. The following principles selected from the biologic and physical sciences are mainly related to variations in pressure in this closed system.

1. The greater the force and volume of the blood propelled into the arteries by ventricular contraction, the greater will be the blood pressure.

2. The amount of peripheral resistance affecting the arterial pressure is dependent on:

   a. The caliber of the blood vessels. The larger the caliber, the lower the pressure in the system.
   b. The elasticity of the blood vessel walls. The more rigid the walls, the greater the pressure in the system.
   c. The viscosity (resistance to flow) of the blood. The greater the viscosity of the blood, the higher the pressure will be in the system.

3. Postural changes affect the arterial blood pressure. The pressure increases immediately when changing from lying to sitting or standing position.

4. Physical activity causes a rise in blood pressure.

5. The emotional state of an individual influences the blood pressure through the relationship of the emotions and the autonomic nervous system.

6. During sleep the blood pressure falls, reaching the lowest point during the early portion of the sleep period and rising slowly until the time of waking.

7. Excess weight raises the blood pressure through the resulting increase in blood capillaries, which in turn places more work on the heart.

8. Chemicals, such as hormones and drugs, that cause vasoconstriction or vasodilation affect the blood pressure.

Physiology of the pulse

The heart muscle is involuntary and is innervated by the autonomic nervous system. The sympathetic nerves accelerate the heartbeat, whereas the parasympathetic nerves, through the vagus, slow the heartbeat. The heart pumps blood in sufficient amount and force to meet the needs of the body and maintain the circulation. The two atria contract at the same time. As they relax, the ventricles contract. As the left ventricle contracts, it forces about 60 ml. of blood into the aorta and on into other arteries. The walls of the arteries, being elastic, expand as an added amount of blood is forced into them. The arteries relax as the wave of blood passes, only to expand again with the next wave of blood. This expansion and recoil of the arteries is the pulse and serves as an indication of the frequency of the heartbeat.

Pulse is present in all arteries but can best be felt in the radial, carotid, facial, temporal, femoral, or dorsalis pedis arteries, which may be pressed against a bone. The most common site for counting the pulse is over the radial artery. The average frequency or rate of the pulse is between 60 and 90 a minute.

As the blood leaves the arteries and enters the capillaries, the pulse wave is lost. Pulse may be found in the large veins as a result of pressure occurring in the heart or large arteries, which is transmitted to the large veins.

Arrhythmia is a technical term that means any variation from normal rhythm. *Tachycardia* means a fast heartbeat. *Bradycardia* means a slow heartbeat. An irregular pulse is one whose rhythm is not the same for succeeding beats or whose pulsations vary in force. An *intermittent* pulse is one in which a beat is dropped occasionally at regular or irregular intervals. It is not always serious, for it may

147

be caused by tension, indigestion, or excessive use of tea or coffee. *Extrasystole* is an extra beat at intervals. It is seldom serious. *Waterhammer* pulse or *Corrigan's* pulse is a very forceful beat, with the artery falling away very quickly. In a *dicrotic* pulse there is one heartbeat for two arterial pulsations, giving the sensation of a double beat.

The pulse gives an indication of the manner in which the heart is functioning. Pulse is felt with two or three fingers placed over a superficial artery that has a bone behind it. The heartbeat or apex beat is counted over the apex of the heart with a stethoscope. *Pulse deficit* is the difference between the heart rate and the pulse rate. Besides the rate of pulse, the volume, rhythm, and tension are also noted. Volume refers to the fullness of the artery and is described as full, weak, or thin. *Rhythm* refers to the regularity of the beats. A pulse may be termed regular or irregular. *Tension* refers to the force against the arterial walls and is described as high or low.

Factors that increase the pulse rate include exercise, posture, eating, stimulants, exciting emotions, extremes of heat and cold, sights, odors, and sometimes even thoughts. Factors that decrease the pulse rate include rest, fasting, depressants, quieting emotions, and moderate temperatures.

The pulse should be evaluated in relation to the patient's temperature, since the pulse rate must increase in fever to compensate for the greater need for oxygen— usually about ten beats per Fahrenheit degree.

In observing a patient's pulse, one should note the quality and volume as well as the rate, since the rate usually increases to compensate for blood loss, oxygen needs, and the like.

A decreased cardiac output results in a decrease in pulse volume.

The pulse rate usually decreases in the presence of intracranial pressure as a compensation for increased blood pressure.

Drugs such as digitalis are often given to strengthen the heart muscle, thereby increasing the cardiac output, which results in a slower and more normal pulse rate. Heart stimulants and vasoconstrictors increase blood pressure while heart depressants and vasodilators decrease blood pressure. Vasoconstrictors may slow the pulse rate by increasing the force of the heartbeat; likewise, vasodilators increase the pulse rate by releasing the force of pressure against the walls of the arteries.

Physiology of blood pressure

The pressure of blood is dependent on the force of contraction of the ventricles, cardiac output, and resistance to its flow through the vessels. The heart under resting conditions pumps a little over 4 liters of blood a minute. This amount may be increased during strenuous exercise to 30 or 40 liters a minute. The greater the force of the heartbeat and the faster the rate, the higher the arterial pressure will be. If the volume of blood is increased, as with transfusions, the blood pressure is increased. If the volume of blood is decreased, as in hemorrhage, the blood pressure is decreased. When the arteries become less elastic, as in arteriosclerosis, more resistance is offered to the blood flow, and the blood pressure becomes higher. If the arteries relax more than usual, as in shock, the blood pressure falls. *Hypertension* means abnormally high blood pressure. *Hypotension* refers to abnormally low blood pressure. A sudden drop in blood pressure is usually a grave sign, since it may be indicative of hemorrhage or shock.

Normally blood pressure may be affected by the same factors that affect the pulse rate: posture, exercise, eating, emotions, rest, temperature of the environment, and weight. Gravity affects arterial pressure. When a person is standing, pressure in the femoral artery, or any artery below the heart, is greater than in the brachial artery.

Also affecting blood pressure are a noisy environment and the presence of others in the room. For an accurate blood pressure reading, the patient should be mentally and physically relaxed and the muscles in the arm should be relaxed. Generally the blood pressure is recorded in the arm, with the patient in the sitting or recumbent position. The vessel over which blood pressure is recorded should be at the level of the heart.

The term "blood pressure" usually refers to arterial pressure. However, there is a low pressure in the capillaries and a still lower one in the veins. Important factors that influence venous pressure are posture, muscular activity, and respiratory activity.

Arterial blood pressure is measured with a sphygmomanometer (*sphygmos,* pulse) that operates by means of a mercury manometer or a spring. The mercury manometer consists of a glass tube continuous with a reservoir containing mercury. The aneroid (spring) manometer consists of a bellows, the inside of which is connected to the compression cuff. Variations in pressure within the system cause the bellows to expand and collapse, moving a needle across a calibrated dial. The aneroid manometer is standardized against a mercury manometer. The compression bladder is enclosed in a cloth cuff. One type of cuff wraps around the arm, another has metal hooks, and the most recent has overlapping interlocking surfaces. A stethoscope is also needed.

Blood pressure usually is taken over the brachial artery. Nurses take arterial pressure often. The systolic pressure may be obtained without the stethoscope by palpating the radial artery while the cuff of the sphygmomanometer is applied to the arm. However, a stethoscope will be needed for finding the diastolic pressure.

The average arterial pressure of an adult in the sitting or recumbent position mea-

Table 11-1 Variations in blood pressure

	Systolic	Diastolic
Subnormal	Below 90	Below 50
Normal	90-140	50-100
Slight hyper- tension	150	110
Moderate hy- pertension	180-190	115-120
High	200-250	130-160

sured by the sphygmomanometer cuff over the brachial artery in millimeters of mercury (mm. Hg) is 90 to 140 systolic and 50 to 100 diastolic. A systolic pressure below 90 or above 150 may be regarded as abnormal. A diastolic pressure of 110 or over is almost always pathologic (Table 11-1). Systolic pressure is that point at which the blood in the brachial artery is first able to force its way through against the pressure exerted on the vessel by the cuff of the manometer. As pressure in the compression cuff drops, a regular distinct repeating thud is heard with the stethoscope for each beat of the heart, soft at first and increasing in intensity, and rather suddenly it either stops or changes quickly to a soft dull thud. This point is the diastolic pressure. As the cuff is further deflated, the murmur disappears completely, because after the pressure is below the diastolic and blood flows throughout the cardiac cycle, there is no turbulence and hence no sound. *Systolic pressure* corresponds to the highest pressure on the sphygmomanometer that will allow the pulse to be noted during the systolic peak. *Diastolic pressure* corresponds to the lowest pressure on the sphygmomanometer that will allow the pulse to be noted during the cardiac cycle (Fig. 11-7).

Pulse pressure, the difference between the systolic and diastolic pressures, represents the volume output of the left ventricle. Two factors affecting the pulse pressure are the cardiac stroke volume output and the distensibility of the arterial system.

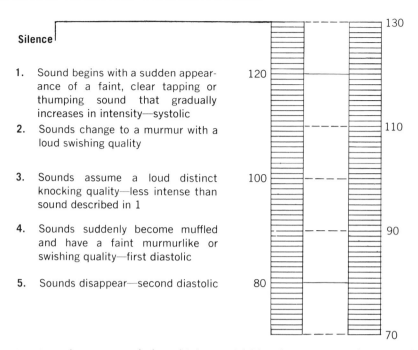

Silence

1. Sound begins with a sudden appearance of a faint, clear tapping or thumping sound that gradually increases in intensity—systolic
2. Sounds change to a murmur with a loud swishing quality
3. Sounds assume a loud distinct knocking quality—less intense than sound described in 1
4. Sounds suddenly become muffled and have a faint murmurlike or swishing quality—first diastolic
5. Sounds disappear—second diastolic

Fig. 11-7. Auscultatory sounds by which arterial blood pressure is determined, assuming that the normal pressure is 120/80.

In man the pulse pressure averages about 40 mm. Hg. The farther the number is from 40, either below or above, the greater significance is attached to the pulse pressure. Pulse pressure varies under certain conditions in which the ability of the heart to act as a pump is impaired.

Pressure in the venous system is determined mainly by the pressure in the right atrium, where the pressure normally is approximately zero. The right atrial pressure tells how well the heart is pumping. Since blood flows toward the heart, the pressure in any peripheral vein of a person in the lying position must be as great or greater than the pressure in the right atrium. For measuring peripheral venous pressure, a catheter or needle can be inserted directly into a peripheral vein and connected to a water manometer. Blood flows into the manometer, and the point at which it stops is taken as the measure. The vein chosen is usually the median basilic. The physician carries out the procedure for venous pressure, with the nurse preparing the equipment and assisting. Venous pressure in an arm or leg of a person lying down is approximately 6 to 8 mm. Hg (91 to 108 mm. or 9.1 to 10.8 cm. water). Normally, venous pressure does not exceed 10 mm. Hg. An estimate of peripheral venous pressure can be obtained from the recumbent patient who lowers and raises the arm below and above the level of the heart. Below the heart the veins are full of blood. As the arm is raised, the veins collapse at a level about 9 cm. above the level of the heart because of the hydrostatic pressure difference between the two levels. This means the pressure in the arm veins is about 9 cm. water. The value of venous pressure may change in cases of cardiac abnormalities.

Physical principles relating to blood pressure

The ventricles of the heart act like pumps. They keep the blood flowing continuously in one direction. Blood flows in the blood vessels because of differences in pressure, called pressure gradient, in them. Fluids flow from a region of high pressure to one of low pressure. The highest pressure occurs upon the contraction of the left ventricle. As the wave of blood passes through the aorta into the smaller arteries, its force is gradually lost because of resistance of the walls of the smaller blood vessels. When the blood reaches the capillaries, the surface is increased greatly and friction is increased (Fig. 11-8). The result is a decided drop in pressure. Blood is drawn into the atria because the pressure in them, as they relax, is less than the pressure in the veins. When blood flows out of the blood vessels, a drop in pressure occurs. A sudden drop in pressure may be indicative of internal hemorrhage. Bodily movements produce pressure on the soft veins and so force the blood onward in the direction of the heart. In breathing, the pressure in the thoracic cavity is changing constantly. A decrease in pressure allows blood to flow from the smaller veins into the larger veins of the trunk.

Gravity affects arterial blood pressure. When a person is standing, pressure in the femoral artery, or in any artery below the heart, is greater than that in the brachial artery. Gravity also affects venous pressure. Therefore, an average reading of venous pressure is taken with the subject lying down.

The principle upon which the sphygmomanometer operates is to balance the pressure in the artery with an externally applied air pressure. The pressure confined in the cuff is transmitted undiminished in all directions. The same pressure that is acting in the artery is acting on the dial spring or on the mercury column to cause it to oscillate. The cuff should be applied snugly and smoothly but not too tightly. If applied improperly, it may cut off the blood supply to the hand, thus causing discomfort to the patient.

The principle underlying liquid manometers used for venous pressure is that the pressure beneath the free surface of a liquid is equal to the vertical height of the liquid times its density. Blood rises in the glass tube until the air pressure downward is equalized by the pressure of the blood upward.

Transmission of sounds through a stethoscope is possible because sound waves pass through glass, liquids, and solids. The sound of the heart passes through the tissues to the diaphragm of the stethoscope, to the column of air in the rubber tubing, and to the tympanic membrane of the ear.

The environment should be quiet when a stethoscope is being used since extraneous sounds interfere with listening to the soft sounds of the heart. Garments also rustle. Therefore, the stethoscope is put directly on the skin.

Psychosocial aspects

The patient should be comfortable and calm before the pulse is taken. Few physiologic phenomena are as profoundly influenced by psychologic factors as is the arterial blood pressure. The recording of

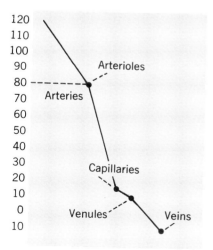

Fig. 11-8. The force of blood is lost as it passes from the arteries.

blood pressure involves physical contact between nurse and patient, which may arouse apprehension, fear, and anxiety in many patients. Much of the anxiety can be reduced or eliminated by the skillful and thoughtful nurse who records the blood pressure smoothly, deliberately, and without ceremony.

Hypertension has been so widely publicized in the news media that it is natural for patients to be concerned about their blood pressure level. The nurse should avoid facial gestures or utterances that the patient might interpret as an indication that his blood pressure is abnormal.

The pulse rate and the blood pressure reading may or may not be given to the patient. If the blood pressure is high, the patient may feel tense and not normal. A patient with high blood pressure may be highly excitable, and his disposition is part of his condition and must be treated as such.

As a rule, the apex beat is taken only on the order of a physician or when the pulse cannot be perceived or in severe irregularities, because of the effect it may have upon the patient. To avoid exciting the patient, special care should be taken in explaining the procedure.

Although the physician may take the pulse rate and blood pressure reading, he very often depends on the nurse's record in determining the direction of diagnosis or treatment.

The patient may have a blood pressure reading made at home, in the clinic, in the physician's office, or in the hospital. A public health nurse may take the reading in a home.

Summary

The pulse and blood pressure are valuable and readily accessible indicators of the state of vital function because they measure physiologic activity and pathophysiologic change. Selected principles from the biologic and physical sciences have been included that are useful in explaining some of the variations in pulse and blood pressure.

Accuracy in measurement of vital signs is essential because the information obtained is indicative of patient progress and is utilized in planning nursing intervention and in evaluating response to therapy. Attention to safety and comfort of the patient during measurement of vital signs is a factor in obtaining accurate observations of the individual patient.

Appropriate reporting and recording makes available the essential information concerning the patient's progress. Experience in evaluating the individual patient's measurements is important in developing the ability to recognize changes in the vital signs that indicate need for urgent medical and nursing intervention.

RESPIRATION

The respiratory system is one of the most vital systems of the body. It is the avenue for the entrance of oxygen and the expulsion of carbon dioxide.

Man can live only a few minutes without oxygen. A deficiency of oxygen in the blood may result from interference with the normal rate of circulation or interference with the normal exchange of carbon dioxide and oxygen, or it may be caused by the condition of the blood itself. The rate and type of respirations are important diagnostic observations. It is possible to increase or decrease the rate within certain limits. Factors that normally increase the respiratory rate include exercise, eating, posture, and extremes of body temperature or environmental temperature. Sensory impulses from all parts of the body can affect respiration. Entering a cold shower causes an intense gasp followed by a period of prolonged inspiration and then by rapid forceful breathing. Elation, anger, and fear increase the respiratory rate. Speech centers of the brain control respiration at times. Opposite factors decrease the rate.

The respiratory tract is also a means of administering medications for both their local and general effects. Oxygen is replaced by this route and many anesthetics are also given by inhalation. By the accidental intake of carbon monoxide and other poisonous gases, toxic effects may be produced.

Principles from biologic sciences

Oxygen in adequate amounts is an element essential to maintaining the oxidative reactions involved in the anabolic processes of the body. The respiratory system provides for the exchange of oxygen and carbon dioxide between the atmosphere and the circulating blood. Since the tissue requirements for oxygen vary, homeostatic mechanisms bring about adjustments, thereby maintaining the exchange of oxygen and carbon dioxide between the external atmosphere and the tissues under normal circumstances. Principles that are helpful in understanding the neural and chemical control of the rate and depth of respiration include:

1. The centers for basic regulation of rhythmic respiration are located in the hindbrain.

    a. The inspiratory center for nervous control of depth and frequency of respiration (amount of air moved through the lungs) is located in the medulla oblongata. These cells stimulate the respiratory muscles.

    b. The expiratory center is also located in the medulla. Expiratory neurons inhibit the inspiratory neurons and produce contraction of muscles of expiration, the result being rhythmic inspiration and expiration.

    c. The pneumotaxic center in the pons is thought to regulate the alternate stimulation of inspiratory and expiratory centers, which further results in rhythmic breathing.

    d. Incoming nerve impulses from the cerebral cortex, the periphery, and the vasomotor and cardiac centers are received by the respiratory center and affect the rhythmicity of respiration. For example, the Hering-Breuer reflex, the stimulus elicited by the pressure of the inflated alveoli sending impulses inhibiting the inspiratory center, prevent overinflation of the lungs and permit the inspiration-expiration cycle to continue in rhythm.

2. The chief chemical regulator of ventilatory rate is the carbon dioxide level (acidity) in the body fluids.

    a. Increasing the concentration of carbon dioxide stimulates the cells of the respiratory centers, mainly the inspiratory center, thus increasing the ventilatory rate, with more rapid passage of carbon dioxide from the lungs. This in turn lowers the carbon dioxide concentration of the blood and diminishes the respiratory activity.

    b. Chemoreceptors in the walls of the aortic arch and the carotid artery respond to hypoxia, low pH, and high carbon dioxide level by reflexly stimulating the respiratory centers.

Voluntary control of respiration is possible for only a short time because the resulting chemical changes in the blood stimulate the respiratory centers, which are more powerful in controlling breathing than are the higher centers. The breath may be held until the accumulated carbon dioxide reaches a level at which the stimulation of the inspiratory center is so powerful that the higher centers can no longer inhibit it. Hyperventilation is also automatically terminated when carbon dioxide is reduced to the level of producing unconsciousness, at which point inactivation of both the higher centers and the respiratory centers causes apnea. Since the carbon dioxide level is again restored during apnea, stimulation of the inspiratory center causes respiration to be resumed.

The respiratory tract is lined with ciliated mucous membrane. The cilia maintain a constant flow of fluid from the sinuses into the nose and down the pharynx. Vaporization of moisture from the mucous membrane helps to eliminate some of the body heat.

In the thin-walled permeable alveoli, the interchange of carbon dioxide and oxygen takes place. The average diameter of an air sac is 0.2 mm., with a volume of 0.004 cu. mm. Behind the surface epithelium lie capillaries of such small bore that the red blood corpuscles are distorted in their passage through them. The area of the enormous number of air sacs is over fifty times the surface area of the body. The red blood corpuscles carry oxygen from the alveoli to the tissues of the body (Fig. 11-9).

The lungs serve also to remove some volatile substances such as alcohol, acetone, and gases that are absorbed into the blood from the intestine.

Respiration is a physical and chemical process, and breathing is the physical and mechanical part of respiration. Breathing goes on in a normal person without his being conscious of it. The factors that regulate and maintain rhythmic respiration are the respiratory center in the medulla, nerve fibers of the autonomic nervous system, and the chemical composition of the blood, all of which respond to the needs of cells in relation to oxygen requirements and elimination of carbon dioxide.

The work of inhaling and exhaling is done by the action of the diaphragm and the ribs. Besides the diaphragm, muscles that are concerned with breathing include the quadratus lumborum, the deep costal muscles, and the muscles of the abdominal wall.

Microbiology

The respiratory tract has many protective mechanisms. The nasal passages constitute the first line of defense against the entrance of harmful substances into the lungs. The cilia of the mucosa entrap bacteria and dust, surround them with fluid, and impel them upward or down the pharynx. Sneezing and coughing are reflexes that protect the nose and throat from irritants. Passage of solids or liquids or irritant gases down the pulmonary tract is blocked by a spasm of the glottis. Toxins from disease-producing organisms may cause an increase in respirations.

Chemistry

Oxygen is a colorless, odorless, tasteless gas that is slightly heavier than air. On this last characteristic of oxygen depends the operation of the open-top tent. Oxygen is

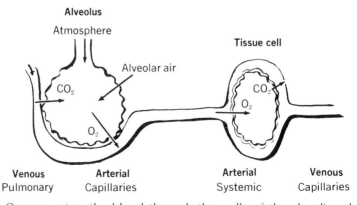

Fig. 11-9. Oxygen enters the blood through the walls of the alveoli and is carried to the tissue cells.

slightly soluble. It comprises 20% of the air and is essential to all animal life. Even when the body is perfectly quiet and there is no food to be oxidized, the average person requires some 15 to 18 ml. of oxygen in each inspiration. Since oxygen cannot be stored in the body, there must be a continuous supply of it. Oxygen is diffused into the blood by means of the respiratory system. Oxygen from the air combines with the hemoglobin in the red blood corpuscles, although a small portion is held in solution in the plasma. At 38° C. and at atmospheric pressure, 1 liter of blood contains 200 ml. of oxygen carried in hemoglobin and only 3 ml. in the plasma. The oxygen is carried throughout the tissues where it oxidizes the foodstuffs that have been absorbed during digestion. The important product of oxidation is heat, which keeps the body warm.

On leaving the pulmonary capillaries, the arterial blood carries from 94% to 96% oxygen. About half of the oxyhemoglobin is reduced, giving its oxygen to tissue cells while the blood is in the tissue capillaries. The blood does not give up all of its oxygen to the tissues nor all of its carbon dioxide to the lungs.

For a normal man the oxygen consumption varies from about 250 ml. per minute at rest to 4,000 ml. or more per minute with extreme physical exertion.

Carbon dioxide is a colorless, odorless, almost tasteless gas, one half heavier than air. The inspired air contains about 0.04% carbon dioxide. The exhaled air contains about 4.5%. Carbon dioxide is produced in the body during the oxidation of food and then carried back to the lungs by the blood.

Carbon dioxide stimulates the respiratory center by increasing the hydrogen-ion concentration of the cells in that center. Chemically the pH of the blood expresses the balance of the acids and bases of the body, which balance is one of the most exactly controlled equilibria in the body. The chief acid and chief alkali in the blood are carbonic acid (H_2CO_3) and sodium bicarbonate ($NaHCO_3$), respectively, so balanced that the ratio $H_2CO_3:NaHCO_3$ equals a constant or nearly so. A comparatively small deviation of the blood to the acid side or to the alkali side may soon result in death.

Carbonic anhydrase, an enzyme present in red blood cells, converts cellular carbon dioxide to carbonic acid at tissue level and carbonic acid to carbon dioxide at the pulmonary capillary level.

The lungs are the chief channel of elimination of volatile acids, the most important of which is carbonic acid.

Physics

The diffusion of oxygen through the alveolar wall into the bloodstream and the diffusion of carbon dioxide from the bloodstream into the alveoli depend on a difference in pressure of these gases. As oxygen goes from the inspired air to the alveoli to the arterial blood and into the venous blood, the pressure decreases. As carbon dioxide passes from the venous blood to the arterial blood to the alveoli to the expired air, its pressure increases (Table 11-2).

Oxygen passes from the air to the tissues. Carbon dioxide passes from the tissues to the air.

Although normal breathing depends chiefly on the partial pressure of gases,

Table 11-2 Gas pressures in millimeters of mercury

	Oxygen pressure	Carbon dioxide pressure
Inspired air	159	0.2
Alveoli	106	40.0
Arterial blood	100	40.0
Venous blood	40	46.0

lung inflation is also a result of a difference of pressure in the atmosphere and in the lungs (intrapulmonic pressure). During inspiration the diaphragm lowers and the chest wall expands, thus reducing the intrapulmonic pressure about 2 or 3 mm. Hg. Air rushes into the lungs. Intrapleural pressure in the adult is 4 or 5 mm. Hg below the atmosphere. It may result from the fact that the thorax increases in size more rapidly than the lungs. The intrapleural pressure is a measure of the elastic force of the lungs. It prevents collapse of the lungs. Upon inspiration the intrapleural pressure increases, and when air is expelled from the lungs the intrapleural pressure decreases.

The ribs are a series of bent levers (Fig. 11-10). The fulcrums are the joints between the ribs and the spine. The effort applied differs according to whether inspiration or expiration is being performed. The resistance is different in inspiration and in expiration.

A very moderate compression of the chest moves at least 500 cc. of air with each breath. This amount of air can easily be supplied by the mouth-to-mouth method of artificial respiration (Fig. 11-11), which is carried out by breathing directly into the patient's mouth, repeating the cycles rhythmically about twelve times a minute. The force of the breathed-in air causes the chest to expand. When the force is released, air goes out of the lungs and the chest goes down. When artificial respiration is used, external cardiac compression is recommended at the same time. Pressure on the sternum pushes the blood out of the heart, and as pressure is released, blood again fills the heart. This cycle is repeated once a second for an adult.

When respirators are used, the air pressure in the chamber is reduced, and the chest wall expands so that air is drawn into the lungs. When normal air pressure is restored in the respirator, the air in the

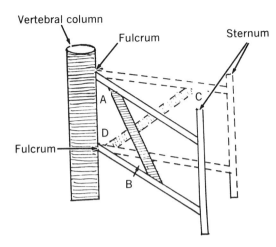

Fig. 11-10. The ribs are bent levers.

lungs is forced out by the natural elasticity of the chest walls.

Observation and recording

True respiration cannot be observed. What one sees is movement of the chest or diaphragm, which is termed *breathing.* By observing these movements and other physical signs, many factors concerning the condition of the patient's oxygen supply can be deduced.

The normal adult breathes about fourteen to eighteen times per minute. A cycle consists of one inspiration and one expiration. Either the inspirations or the expirations may be counted. Breathing may be so quiet that one can scarcely detect chest movements and sometimes so noisy that the respiration can be heard several feet away from the patient. The character of respiration is influenced by pain and other emotions. When a patient's respiration is very shallow, it may be counted by placing the hand across the chest. Since respiration can be affected by voluntary control, it should be counted, if possible, without awareness on the part of the patient. In evaluating respiration, one should consider rate, rhythm, depth, position, and color of the patient. The ratio of respiration to

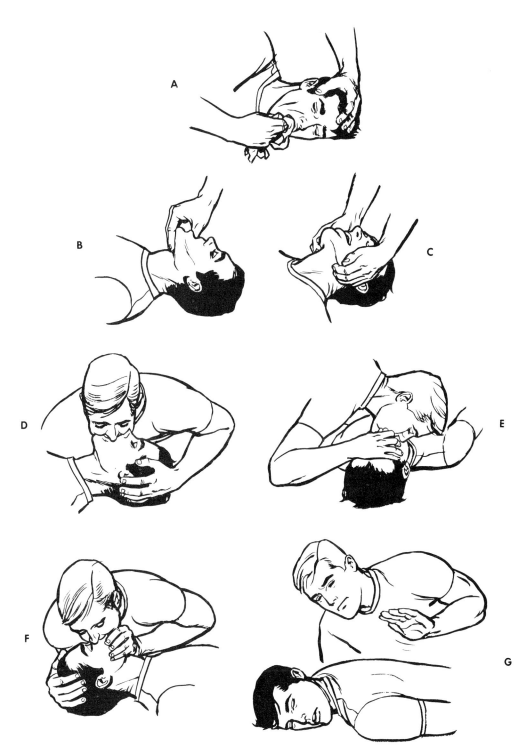

Fig. 11-11. Mouth-to-mouth (or mouth-to-nose) resuscitation by the following steps (repeat cycle twelve times per minute). **A,** Clear passageway by wiping out any foreign material. **B** and **C,** Tilt head and push or pull jaw into jutting-out position. **D** and **E,** Breathe into mouth (closing nose with cheek or fingers). Or, **F,** close mouth and breathe into nose. **G,** If no air exchange, slap on back several times to dislodge any possible foreign material.

157

pulse is 1:4 or 1:5. In illness this ratio may not be maintained. Pallor and cyanosis indicate insufficient oxygenation, regardless of the rate and depth of breathing; a patient receiving oxygen may have a pink skin and yet appear to be having labored respirations.

In order not to excite the patient, respirations are counted while the fingers are on the wrist (Fig. 11-12), after or before the pulse rate is observed. The nurse may feel the rise and fall of the chest wall with the hand and so will not need to watch the movements so intently. In this way she can avoid making the patient feel uncomfortable by very close observation. Sudden or abnormal changes should be reported at once.

Several terms have been used to de-scribe respiration. *Dyspnea* (*dys-,* painful or labored; *-pnea,* breathing) means difficult respirations. *Eupnea* means normal respirations. *Apnea* (*a-,* absence or lack of) means a lack of breathing. It is a term used to indicate the pauses between the cycles of Cheyne-Stokes respirations, which is a series of respirations that gradually become deeper and noisier until a climax is reached when a pause occurs and then the series is repeated. *Stertorous breathing* is noisy breathing. *Orthopnea* is a condition in which the patient breathes easier in a sitting position because the vital capacity is greater in the sitting position than in the recumbent position. *Hyperpnea* (*hyper-,* above) and *polypnea* (*poly-,* many) are terms that refer to fast breathing. *Anoxia* is a term that means

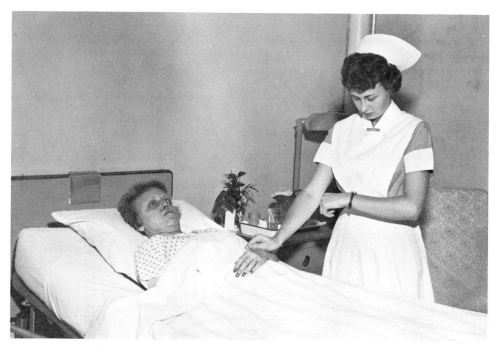

Fig. 11-12. Following the taking of the pulse rate, the nurse continues to hold the wrist until respiration is counted. Respiration may be felt by the rise and fall of the chest as well as by observing chest movements.

lack of oxygen in the tissues. *Anoxemia* is a term that means lack of oxygen in the bloodstream. *Acapnia* means a deficiency of carbon dioxide from want of oxygen. *Hypercapnia* means excess of carbon dioxide in the blood. *Asphyxia* is a condition produced by prolonged interference with a sufficient supply of oxygen. *Cyanosis* is a slate blue color of the skin and mucosa, especially of the lips, cheeks, ears, and extremities, caused by circulation of an unduly large amount of reduced hemoglobin.

Summary

Respiration is a vital function, primarily involuntary, that is subject to neural and chemical regulatory mechanisms. Breathing is the mechanical side of respiration and depends on pressures of the atmosphere, of the alveolar air, and in the intrapleural space. Observation of the respirations provides a measure of how well the respiratory system is functioning.

LEARNING SITUATIONS FOR THE PATIENT

It may be necessary to teach the patient or a family member how to measure and record the vital signs at home. Such instruction should include not only the mechanics of these procedures but also some interpretation of the purpose of the measurements for this particular patient, as well as the general significance of variations. For example, a mother may be taught how to take the pulse of her children and that the normal varies with the age and activity of the child. A patient may be told that one blood pressure reading may not have any significance but that a series of readings may indicate a trend toward high or low blood pressure. Too, the blood pressure is to be considered with other symptoms. It may be explained that blood pressure readings have more significance in some conditions than in others. The patient may learn that chronic high

blood pressure may be controlled, in a measure, by regulating one's life. Abstinence from worry and business cares, moderation in eating, drinking, and smoking, and avoidance of all but the milder forms of exercise may be important practices for a person with high blood pressure.

QUESTIONS FOR DISCUSSION

1 The next time your patient has abnormal vital signs, what further observations will you want to make?
2 What precautions will you need to observe in handling and using clinical thermometers?
3 Explain how you would interpret the sounds you hear in measuring blood pressure.
4 What factors may affect the patient's blood pressure during the process of measuring it?
5 What observations are made while feeling the patient's pulse? While counting respiration?
6 Distinguish between breathing and respiration.
7 What nursing measures will probably be indicated for the patient having a chill?
8 What nursing measures will probably be indicated for the patient with fever? What are his fluid and food needs? What is the condition of his mouth?

LIFE SITUATIONS

1. It is the policy of your health agency to use centigrade thermometers. Upon admission, a patient tells you that her temperature on her "home thermometer" was 102°. How would you interpret this in centigrade readings?

2. Jane Roda, a patient 17 years of age, admitted for observation, was assigned to you this morning for the first time. You learned from her chart that during the past 3 days she occasionally had an elevated temperature and that she had an order for a heating pad if she needed it for back pain. As you approached to take her temperature, she did not seem acutely ill but gave the impression of wanting a great deal of attention. Having put the thermometer in her mouth, you went to the window to raise

159

the shade. As you did so, you caught a glimpse of Jane removing the thermometer and after about 2 seconds returning it to her mouth. When you finally removed the thermometer, the reading was 104° F. How would you proceed?

SUGGESTED PERFORMANCE CHECKLIST
Temperature, pulse, and respirations
Comfort

1 Is the patient in a comfortable position?
2 Are the nurse's hands warm?
3 Is secure hold taken of the wrist?
4 Is the patient screened for rectal temperature?
5 Is the patient's condition considered?
6 Are respirations counted by feeling rather than by watching?
7 Are emotional upsets avoided?

Therapeutic effectiveness

1 Is the thermometer left in place long enough for accurate recording?
2 If abnormal, are the pulse and respirations counted for 1 minute?
3 Are temperature, pulse, and respirations rechecked if uncertain?
4 Is the mouth closed over the thermometer?
5 Are abnormalities reported at once?

Economy

1 Is exposure to high temperature avoided for thermometers?
2 Is the length of time of taking temperature, pulse, and respiration minimum for the method used?
3 Is breakage of thermometer prevented in preparation for use or aftercare?
4 Are temperature, pulse, and respiration taken at appropriate times?

Safety

1 Are the nurse's hands clean?
2 Is the thermometer adequately disinfected?
3 Does the nurse remain with the patient during the recording?
4 Is the rectal thermometer held in place?
5 When removed from the mouth, is the thermometer wiped from the stem toward the bulb?
6 Is the rectal thermometer lubricated?

Blood pressure
Comfort

1 Is an explanation given to the patient?
2 Is the arm relaxed and resting on something?
3 Is the patient in a comfortable position?
4 Are the nurse's hands warm?
5 Is air released from the cuff before rechecking the pressure?
6 Is the reading taken as quickly as possible?

Therapeutic effectiveness

1 Are two readings taken that check to within 5 mm. of each other?
2 Is the cuff applied to the bare arm?
3 Is the brachial artery located before inflating the cuff?
4 If a mercury manometer is used, is it placed on a flat surface?
5 Is the spring or mercury column kept out of the patient's view?
6 Is the pressure reported at once if there is a wide variation from the last reading?
7 Is the charting correct?

Economy

1 Is noise in the surroundings reduced to a minimum?
2 Is the cuff applied high enough to allow placement of the stethoscope?
3 Is air expelled from the cuff before placing it on the arm?
4 Is air in the cuff released slowly?
5 Is equipment returned in order to its proper place?

Safety

1 Is the cuff applied snugly and smoothly?
2 Are the nurse's hands clean?
3 Is the cloth part of the cuff removed and washed?
4 Is the stethoscope adequately cleaned?

SUGGESTED READINGS

Betson, Carol, and Ude, Linda: Central venous pressure, American Journal of Nursing **69**:1466, July, 1969.

Bucholz, Patricia, and Gilbert, Gloria: Understanding the ECG, RN **35**:38, February, 1972.

Butler, Herbert H.: How to read an ECG, RN **36**:35, January, 1973.

Lee, Richard V., and Atkins, Elisha: Spurious fever, American Journal of Nursing **72**:1094, June, 1972.

Littman, David: Stethoscopes and auscultation, American Journal of Nursing **72**:1238, July, 1972.

McInnes, Elizabeth: The vital signs—a programmed presentation including material on the apical beat, St. Louis, 1970, The C. V. Mosby Co.

Nichols, Glennadee A., and Kucha, Deloros H.: Oral measurement, American Journal of Nursing **72**:1091, June, 1972.

Parsons, L. Claire: Respiratory changes in head injury, American Journal of Nursing **71**:2186, November, 1971.

Tate, G. V., Gohrke, C., and Mansfield, L. W.: Correct use of electric thermometers, American Journal of Nursing **70**:1898, September, 1970.

12 Diagnostic tests and measures

CURRENT STATUS

The number of diagnostic tests in current usage is now reaching nearly astronomical proportions. In most hospitals, "blood work" is as much a part of the morning routine as is the giving of medications, bathing, or bedmaking. Because of this continued increase, some authorities feel that physicians are depending too heavily on laboratory tests to diagnose instead of using their eyes, ears, hands, and common sense judgment.

However, because of past valuable experience, diagnostic tests will always hold an important place in the diagnosis and guidance of therapy for the patient. For this reason it becomes necessary for the nurse practitioner to be aware of the common tests ordered and to understand the various roles played in preparing and caring for the patient, assisting the physician, and carrying out agency and laboratory policies.

UNDERSTANDING OF DIAGNOSTIC MEASURES

Diagnostic tests include scientific examinations made in the clinical laboratory, in the x-ray laboratory, and in other special departments. The results help the physician to make a diagnosis and to prescribe the appropriate treatment. Satisfactory results depend on cooperation among the physician, the patient, the nurse, the medical technologist, and the x-ray technologist.

Laboratory examinations include tests made on samples or specimens of body fluids, blood, and excretions, metabolic tests, tests of electrical impulses (electrocardiogram and encephalogram), x-ray examinations, tests on the reproductive tract, and tests using radioactive drugs. Common tests done are routine admission tests, biochemical blood tests, and tests for kidney, liver, and metabolic functions. Along with these also often are ordered

162

x-ray examinations that parallel the corresponding anatomic organ.

As more and more laboratory tests and procedures are developed to pinpoint diagnosis and refine therapy, it is quite possible that within a few short years, ways will be found to diagnose accurately such puzzling diseases as cancer, muscular dystrophy, or emotional disorders. As researchers develop more aids for evaluating patient responses to drugs and therapy, it is hoped that the treatments for these diseases will also become possible.

SCIENTIFIC RATIONALE FOR DIAGNOSTIC TESTS

The rationale for the effective use of diagnostic tests is based on the principle of the human body's adaptive response to maintain or restore homeostasis. The principle of homeostasis is one of the most fundamental of all the physiologic principles. It affirms that the body must maintain a relative constancy of its internal environment in order to survive. Homeostasis is a condition that changes but yet stays about the same—a condition that stays within the same narrow range. Health and survival virtually depend upon the body's mechanism to maintain or restore homeostasis.

Practically all body structures play some role in the various states of the body. It is a job for all the organs; however, the ones most commonly dealt with in diagnostic tests are the liver, lungs, and kidneys.

All body functions in reality are cell functions. Cellular environment is not synonymous with body environment. The body is surrounded by the gaseous atmosphere of the external world. Body cells are surrounded by a liquid atmosphere of an internal world. This liquid environment around the cells is called extracellular fluid since it lies exterior to cells and occupies two main locations—the microscopic spaces between cells, called *intercellular*

or *interstitial* fluids, and the fluid that flows through blood vessels, *blood plasma.*

When body cells become diseased or injured, they are unable to perform their normal functions of maintaining a homeostatic environment. A common example of this is the kidney, whose function is to eliminate the substance urea from the body. In kidney disease or damage, the functions cannot be properly performed, therefore the percentage of urea in the blood will gradually rise. For this reason blood chemistry examinations are often ordered for patients who have circulatory or kidney malfunctions.

One must also remember that body composition and functions change gradually over the years. Blood constituents for a child vary greatly from that of the adult, and those of elderly persons vary greatly from the average adult. Thus gradual changes often result from the process of aging, and they are very significant in determining normal values in diagnostic results.

NURSING IMPLICATIONS

Diagnostic tests are usually performed in the laboratory by a specially trained technician. However, it is often a nurse who must assume the responsibility of seeing that the specimens are collected under controlled conditions and that they are properly handled. The nurse also assumes equal responsibility in seeing that the patient fully understands why the test is being done, the procedure to be followed, and how he is to cooperate.

Probably one of the greatest responsibilities is that of reassuring and supporting the patient, who may be made quite uncomfortable by a test. By the use of simple measures, the nurse may turn an ordeal into a simple procedure, such as when the nurse remembers to place the patient in high Fowler's position to facilitate passage of a Levin tube or to encourage the patient to drink sufficient fluids prior to the collection of urine specimens.

Since the efficiency of a diagnostic test depends upon the condition of the patient and the manner of collecting the specimen, the nurse also becomes responsible for observing and reporting the patient's emotional state and other adaptive responses as in the care of a basal metabolism test (BMR), which would be influenced by both excitement and a rise in body temperature.

The duties and responsibilities of the nurse vary with the different diagnostic tests but usually include those discussed in the following paragraphs.

The nurse prepares the patient mentally by explaining the procedure to be done, why it may be necessary for food or fluid to be withheld, and how he can help in the test. The nurse notifies the laboratory of the physician's orders and is careful that names are spelled correctly. The nurse also cooperates with the technician in carrying out the procedure and obtains the proper type of container and other equipment necessary. The container should be intact and clean, sometimes sterile. Sometimes the nurse needs to prepare a drug or a solution to be used in the test, which may require careful reading and calculating.

The nurse may collect the specimen of urine, stool, or sputum or may assign the collecting of these specimens to a practical nurse or aide. The nurse may assist the physician in placing the patient in position for collecting the specimen or may help to hold him in position during the collection of the specimen. If assisting a physician, the nurse arranges the equipment for the convenience of the physician, perhaps cleanses the skin and drapes the area, observes the reaction of the patient during the procedure, and assists with equipment and materials as needed (Figs. 12-4 to 12-6). After the procedure the nurse helps the patient assume a more comfortable posi-

tion and, if the bedding has been disarranged during the procedure, straightens it and removes equipment.

The nurse labels the specimen according to hospital regulations and fills in the correct form, identifying the patient, the specimen, and the type of test to be performed. Again, it is very important that the patient's name and the name of the test be spelled correctly. The specimen is sent to the proper laboratory. The nurse may care for equipment after use or may direct an aide in its care. The equipment should be cleaned as soon as possible to prevent coagulation of blood or other secretions, and caution should be exercised in the handling of sharp instruments.

The recording on the chart includes the time, the type of test, the solution or drug used, the nature and amount of material withdrawn, the name of the physician who withdrew the fluid, and the reaction of the patient. If a specimen was obtained, this, along with the name of the laboratory to which it was sent, is also recorded. Afterward, the nurse observes the patient for symptoms indicating any untoward effects of the procedure, which may not appear for 24 to 48 hours. The report should be placed on the chart where the physician can see it. In many institutions the responsibility of reporting special tests and recording them on the chart is delegated to the ward secretary or laboratory personnel involved. However, this does not relieve the nurse of the responsibilities of seeing that this service is performed. The physician interprets the findings of the various tests and fits them into his total study in making a diagnosis.

Since breakfast is omitted or delayed before some tests, the patient should be told why, and, in case of delay, it should be served as promptly as possible.

Secretions and excretions, except for wound discharges, come from the mucous and serous membranes. Mucous and serous membranes are lined with epithelium and endothelium, which are formed of simple squamous epithelial tissue or of one layer of thin, flat cells. These cells are constantly being shed from the surface, and they appear in the fluids that bathe the cavities. The normal amounts of serous fluids depend on the size of the cavity.

The nurse should know how to interpret all laboratory reports in terms of normal and abnormal so that more intelligent nursing care can be given (Table 12-2).

SCIENTIFIC PRINCIPLES
Secretions and excretions
Urine

Anatomy and physiology. Urine is formed from the noncolloidal constituents (water, salts, and so on) of blood plasma that filter out from the glomerular capillaries into the renal capsules and are concentrated into urine in other parts of the renal tubules. Elimination of urine plays a large part in maintaining uniform concentration of the normal constituents of the blood. The function of the kidneys is to keep the body fluids at their normal constancy in composition and volume. The kidneys extract almost all the protein waste, the greater part of the salts not needed, and about one half of the excess water.

The rate of secretion of urine is influenced by three factors: (1) the supply of water in the body, (2) the volume or pressure of the blood passing through the kidney, and (3) the activity of the secretory and absorptive processes in the kidneys.

The volume of urine is low in warm weather because of increased perspiration. The amount of urine excreted by a normal adult in 24 hours varies from 1,000 to 1,800 ml. A marked decrease in the normal amount voided may be caused by a small fluid intake, by the loss of body fluids through other avenues, by free perspiration, and by retention.

Microbiology. Equipment for the collection of urine is either clean or sterile. For the usual examination of a voided specimen, the bedpan and the specimen bottle are clean. Sterile containers are used when the urine is obtained by catheter. The catheter also is sterile, and the area around and over the meatus is cleansed with either soap and water or an antiseptic solution. Urine is obtained by catheter to eliminate contamination by vaginal discharges or by organisms on the skin. The specimen should be labeled "Catheterized."

The nurse's hands and the outside of the specimen bottle, which someone else may handle, should not be contaminated by urine.

Disease organisms are often identified in urine. Those commonly looked for include organisms that cause infections in the kidneys or bladder.

Since cold inhibits the growth and action of bacteria, specimens of urine not to be examined at once are put in the refrigerator.

Chemistry. Urine is a complex watery solution of organic and inorganic substances. It normally contains creatine, creatinine, and urea. Urea is the principal waste product of metabolism and constitutes about one half of all solids excreted. Sugar is not normally present in the urine. The level at which sugar spills into the urine is spoken of as the renal threshold, which is about 140 to 180 mg. of sugar in 100 ml. of whole blood. The chemical action of copper sulfate with urine determines the presence of glucose. Many other tests on urine depend on chemical reaction of reagents with the urine.

Sometimes blood cannot be seen unless a chemical that reacts with the blood and proves its presence is added. Such blood is called occult.

Pharmacology. Many drugs are used in laboratory examinations of urine. Some are given to the patient to be excreted, whereas others are used for their reaction with urine. Water is a diuretic, although it is not considered to be a drug. In some instances it is forced in order to obtain an adequate amount of or to dilute urine, and in other instances it may be withheld when the physician wishes to obtain a concentrated urine specimen.

Sodium benzoate, usually administered intravenously in a dose of 1.77 Gm., is used to test liver function. The liver synthesizes benzoic acid and glycine (aminoacetic acid), and the resulting hippuric acid is excreted in the urine. The amount present in the urine gives an indication of how well the liver is functioning.

Glucose for glucose tolerance tests comes in powder form to be mixed with water or in liquid form ready for use.*

Physics. Specific gravity of urine is the ratio it bears to the weight of water. It is measured by an apparatus called a urinometer.

To separate the solids from the liquid portion, urine is placed in a centrifuge that operates on the principle that the solid particles are thrown to the outside (Fig. 12-1).

Psychology. All procedures and tests

*Glucola, a carbonated drink that tastes like cola.

should be fully explained to the patient with a word of assurance and encouragement. The physician may explain the meaning of the test in order to secure the patient's cooperation. During the procedure, diverting conversation can be used to overcome anxiety, which may produce a trace of sugar in the urine.

If a drug is necessary for the test to be made, the patient should be told about its effect. In the case of phenolsulfonphthalein, the patient should be warned about the appearance of the urine.

Blood

Definitions. Red blood cells are called erythrocytes (*erythro-*, red; *-cyte,* cell) and white blood cells are called leukocytes (*leuko-,* white). An increase in red cells is called erythrocytosis or polycythemia (*poly-*, many; *cyt-,* cell; *hem-,* blood; + *-ia,* condition). An increase in white cells, a symptom of many conditions, is called leukocytosis. A marked increase in white cells constituting a disease is leukemia. A decrease in red cells or a decrease in hemoglobin is called anemia (*an-,* lack of). A decrease in white cells is called leukopenia (Gr. *penia,* poverty). Hemoglobin, a protein compound found in the

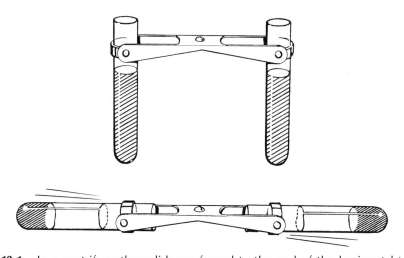

Fig. 12-1. In a centrifuge the solids are forced to the end of the horizontal tubes.

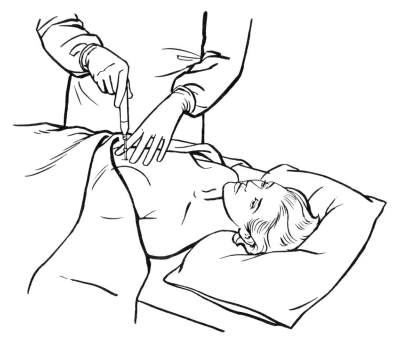

Fig. 12-2. Sternal puncture. A vacuum is created in the syringe by which the soft bone marrow is pulled out.

red cell, has great affinity for oxygen.

Anatomy and physiology. Blood is composed of formed elements, red and white cells and platelets, and the plasma, which is a nutritive, balanced physiologic saline solution in which the plasma proteins are dissolved.

Blood is formed in the bone marrow and spleen, and the bloodstream transports nourishment, gases, hormones, and enzymes to the places they are needed. An examination of the red bone marrow (usually taken from the sternum) will reveal the amount of normal and abnormal constituents. Normally, blood varies slightly, but in certain diseases significant changes are produced.

A complete blood count is a written picture of red cells, white cells, and hemoglobin.

If a small amount of blood is needed, the skin is pierced because the blood is very close to the skin. If a large amount is needed, it is removed from a vein,

usually the median vein because it is most accessible.

For a red or white cell count, blood is diluted and placed in a counting chamber under a microscope. Since it is diluted and only a small amount is examined, an estimation is made of the number of cells in 1 cu. mm.

Sternal puncture is used almost always for diagnostic purposes in blood dyscrasias. Specimens of the cellular elements of the bone marrow may easily be secured by the introduction of a needle into the sternum (Fig. 12-2). The cells present in order of importance are red blood cells, neutrophil band forms, neutrophil segmented forms, and normoblasts. The number of these will vary in the different blood conditions.

Microbiology. The pipettes and the counting chamber for blood counts are clean. If blood is obtained for chemical or bacteriologic tests, sterile disposable syringes and test tubes are used.

Many bacteria are found on the skin. Therefore, before a needle or other instrument is introduced through the skin to obtain a specimen of blood, the skin is wiped with an antiseptic, usually alcohol. Blood for cultures is taken by venipuncture under careful aseptic conditions. The outside of the container should not be contaminated with the blood in order not to expose any person who handles the container to possible infection.

Organisms commonly looked for in blood are those that cause pneumonia, typhoid, and malaria.

Blood withdrawn for serology or for chemical analysis and not examined at once is put in a refrigerator. Blood for cultures should be placed in an incubator. Blood for other tests may be left at room temperature.

An examination of the blood may reveal hemorrhage, inflammation, or a disease process present in the body or may indicate the direction of treatment.

Chemistry. Examinations of the blood may be morphologic, chemical, physical, bacteriologic, and serologic. Chemical tests made on blood are listed in Table 12-1.

For chemical tests, blood is collected before breakfast, since the blood is then most chemically uniform. Absorption of food may alter many of the blood constituents. If fats are absorbed, their presence in the blood (lipemia) may interfere with some of the tests.

The hydrogen ion concentration of the blood remains close to pH 7.4.

For the development of the red blood cells there are chemical substances of known composition (vitamins, iron, copper, thyroxin) and some substances of unknown composition. Among the products of wornout red blood cells are the hemoglobin derivatives—the iron-containing hemosiderin and the iron-free bilirubin. These products are carried to the liver, the former to be returned to the bone marrow and the latter excreted in the bile.

Table 12-1 Chemical tests made on blood

Test	Normal amounts, in milligrams in 100 ml. of blood
Nonprotein nitrogen	25-40
Uric acid	2-4
Creatinine	1-2
Urea nitrogen	15-20
Blood sugar	80-120
Cholesterol	160-200
Chlorides	450-500
Carbon dioxide–combining power	50-70
Calcium	9-11
Phosphorus	2-5
Total base	360
Sodium in serum	310-340
Potassium in red blood cells	420
Potassium in serum	16-22
Van den Bergh test	0.25-1.5
Total plasma proteins	6.5-7.5
Albumin	3.5-5.0
Globulin	2.0-3.0
Fibrinogen	0.2-0.3

The hemoglobin-oxyhemoglobin mechanism is important in the regulation of the reaction of the blood and in the transport of carbon dioxide and oxygen.

The proteins of plasma include, in ascending order of molecular weight, the albumins, the globulins, and fibrinogen. The ratio of the albumin to globulin is spoken of as the A-G ratio and averages 1.75:1. Variations in the ratio are caused mostly by albumins. Colloid osmotic pressure depends principally on the albumin content of the plasma. The average normal colloid osmotic pressure of 37 cm. of water may drop to 20 cm. if albumin concentration falls to 2 Gm. per 100 ml. of plasma.

Pharmacology. Many reagents are used in the laboratory in making examinations on blood. Acetic acid is used to dissolve red blood cells when a white cell count is made. Gower's solution (a solution of glacial acetic acid and sodium sulfate) is used to dilute blood when a red count is made. Bromsulphalein is a dye taken out of the blood by the liver. It is given as a test of liver function and is administered in a dose of 2 to 5 mg. per kilogram of body weight.

Physics. Withdrawal of blood by venipuncture depends on differences of pressure. Blood in a vein is put under greater than normal pressure by the damming action of the tourniquet. Also, the negative pressure in the syringe pulls the blood out of the vein.

Friction removes dirt containing microorganisms from the skin.

Coagulation time may be measured by a tube of fine bore, called a capillary tube, in which the blood rises because it is adhesive to the glass (Fig. 12-3). This phenomenon is called capillary attraction.

Psychology. The nurse should make a careful explanation to the patient when a blood test has been ordered, including what the test is and something of its value. Any misconceived ideas the patient may have about the test should be clarified. A patient may feel more comfortable, both mentally and physically, if he sits or lies down while the blood is being withdrawn.

Gastrointestinal excretions

Anatomy and physiology. During the digestive process, digestive juices flow from the glands that secrete them into the digestive tract. Gastric juice comes from the gastric glands in a daily amount of 1,200 to 1,500 ml. About 1,000 ml. of bile is formed in the liver each day and is concentrated to 100 ml. by the gallbladder. The bile then empties into the duodenum. About 500 to 800 ml. a day of pancreatic juice is also excreted into the duodenum. Besides these fluids, there are some formed in the walls of the small intestines. An examination of the gastrointestinal fluids or of stool will reveal amounts and proper functioning of digestive juices.

Microbiology. The stomach normally

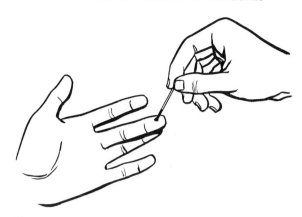

Fig. 12-3. Blood is adhesive to the glass of a capillary tube.

contains very few live bacteria because of the disinfecting action of the gastric juice. However, gastric contents may show tubercle bacilli when repeated sputum examinations have proved negative. The gastric juice is sometimes examined for the Boas-Oppler bacillus, which may appear in patients with gastric cancer.

Microorganisms looked for in epecimens of stool include chiefly those causing typhoid and dysentery. Stool may also be examined in diagnosing undulant fever, food poisoning, and bubonic plague.

Examinations to discover parasitic organisms or their ova are ordered sometimes. Parasites that infect the intestinal tract include the pinworm, roundworm, tapeworm, and hookworm.

No disinfectant should be mixed with a stool specimen.

If a specimen of gastric contents cannot be examined at once, it should be placed in the refrigerator to prevent chemical changes. A sample of bile or of stool may remain at room temperature, with the exception of a stool to be examined for amebas, in which case it is maintained at body temperature until it is examined.

Chemistry. The contents of the gastrointestinal tract may be examined chemically to discover occult blood or to test the degree of acidity or alkalinity. The reaction of the gastric contents is normally acid. The pH of freshly secreted gastric juice is about 1. Gastric juice cannot perform its function if the pH is too high. Chemical tests are performed on gastric juice to determine free hydrochloric acid, blood, rennin, pepsin, and bile.

A tubeless method of determining whether free hydrochloric acid is present in the stomach is in use. It is based on the fact that free hydrochloric acid will displace certain materials from combination with other substances. A compound of azure A dye with an Amberlite cation-exchange resin in the form of granules has been prepared. This is ingested by the patient following gastric stimulation with caffeine given in tablet form. When the gastric contents have a pH of 3 or less, the dye is released from the resin complex and is promptly absorbed and excreted into the urine, imparting a blue or green color to the urine. If the color of the test sample is darker than that of 0.6 mg. standard, it may be concluded that the patient secretes free hydrochloric acid.

The reaction of bile from the gallbladder is slightly acid and that from the liver is alkaline. Pancreatic juice is alkaline because of the presence of sodium bicarbonate.

The chloride content of the gastric juice is about 40% greater than that of blood plasma, while that of intestinal secretion is about 7% greater than that of blood plasma.

Pharmacology. Sometimes a mild laxative is ordered so that a specimen of stool may be obtained quickly.

To stimulate the flow of gastric juice so that a sufficient specimen may be obtained, 50 ml. of alcohol, 7%, may be given through the tube, or histamine phosphate in a dose of 0.85 mg. in a 1:1,000 solution may be given intravenously. The best-known chemical stimulant is histamine, which elicits from the parietal cells a large amount of hydrochloric acid and relatively small amounts of pepsin and mucus. However, since histamine may produce allergic reactions (flushing, headache, drop in blood pressure) in some patients, a skin test is done. If there is no reaction on the skin, the usual dose is given. Histamine also causes hypersecretion of saliva, so wipes or a basin is needed. Reaction to the drug comes on quickly. Adrenalin and a syringe should be on hand in case of reaction to histamine.

Magnesium sulfate, 25%, is used in a dose of 50 ml. in gallbladder drainage to relax the sphincters of the bile ducts and to allow the bile to flow more freely into the duodenum, from which it can be aspirated. Sometimes atropine sulfate is ordered to relax the pyloric sphincter to aid in the passage of the tube. Atropine checks saliva and intestinal secretions but not the gastric secretions.

In the aspiration of pancreatic fluid, secretin is injected intravenously in a dose of 0.75 mg. per kilogram of body weight. It stimulates the flow of pancreatic juice and bile, but the bile is not increased until 3 or 4 hours after the injection of the secretin.

Physics. The stomach tube is used for aspirating stomach or duodenal contents. A smooth, slippery surface is produced on the tube before introducing it very far. Oil, water, or mucus in the passage may serve as the lubricant. Since cold hardens rubber, the tube is placed on ice or in the refrigerator before it is introduced.

Suction is applied with a syringe to the end of the Levin tube, thus reducing air pressure and causing the fluid to flow out of the stomach.

Psychology. If a stool is to be examined, the patient's cooperation is needed. When a tube is being passed into the stomach, the patient needs to be reassured and encouraged (Fig. 12-4). There should be no hurry. The patient should be allowed to express his feelings. He may feel angry while the tube is being passed because it

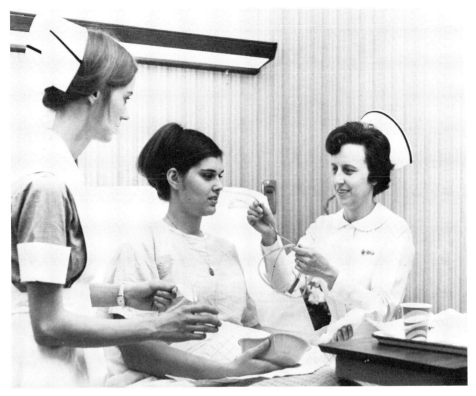

Fig. 12-4. Reassuring the patient prior to intubation.

is most uncomfortable. During the ordeal, privacy should be provided. The patient should be told that histamine may cause flushing and a warm feeling. He may be embarrassed with drooling saliva. During the duodenal drainage procedure, the patient should have nursing support and he should understand the importance of maintaining the various positions that aid in the passage of the tube. If breakfast is to be delayed, the patient should be given an explanation the evening before the test.

Sputum

Anatomy and physiology. Sputum is material from the mucous lining of the bronchial tubes and trachea. Its consistency varies from a thin, watery fluid to thick, purulent material, and it has a pH of 6.6 to 7.1.

Microbiology. An examination of sputum is made chiefly to reveal the presence of bacteria. Bacteria commonly looked for in sputum include those that cause tuberculosis or pneumonia.

If not examined at once, sputum is kept at room temperature until it is examined.

The most favorable time to collect a sputum specimen is early in the morning to avoid having food particles mixed with it. Also, there is more sputum in the morning, because it has not been coughed up during the night. The mouth may be rinsed out before the sputum is coughed up, but strong antiseptics should not be used.

The container most commonly used for the collection is a waxed paper cup. If a sterile specimen is needed, a wide-mouthed glass jar may be used, and care should be taken to prevent contamination of the outside of it to prevent infection from spreading.

Psychology. A patient who expectorates frequently may feel that he is offensive to others and thay they avoid him in order not to catch anything from him. So he may feel rejected.

He may fear too that examination of his sputum may reveal that he has tuberculosis or cancer. The nurse will appreciate his fears and treat him understandingly.

Discharges from wounds or body cavities

Anatomy and physiology. A wound is a break in the skin or mucous membrane. Sometimes healing is delayed because of infection. A report from a smear or culture directs proper treatment.

Microbiology. Smears and cultures are made from excretions of wounds or from any normal fluid anywhere in the body. A smear is a sample of material on a glass slide that is examined under the microscope. A culture is a sample of material planted on culture media, incubated, and microscopically examined.

Smears and cultures are made chiefly from discharges from the nose, throat, eye, vagina, urethra, and wounds. Organisms looked for are those responsible for infections in these various areas. Often, a smear is made to look for cancer cells. Exfoliative cytology is a study of surface cells from an area. The most common example of this kind of smear is the Pap smear (named for Dr. George N. Papanicolaou), in which material is obtained from the vaginal or cervical canal. Care must be taken in handling slides and culture tubes in order not to contaminate the hands.

If slides with smears cannot be examined at once, they are kept at room temperature. Culture tubes are put into the bacteriologic incubator.

Psychology. A smear or culture is made in order to discover the cause of the patient's condition so that treatment can be more effective. The patient may be anxious until the report is available.

Serous fluids

Definitions. Paracentesis or aspiration is the withdrawal of fluid from a cavity to relieve pressure, to treat the cavity, or to obtain information for diagnostic purposes. Fluids found in serous cavities are exudates or transudates. An exudate is a fluid found in inflammations on a surface. An exudate has a specific gravity above 1.018 and serum protein over 4% . A transudate has less than 3% of protein and a specific gravity less than 1.012.

Pneumothorax means air in the pleural sac. The term "open pneumothorax" is used when there is a wound to the outside, whereas the term "closed pneumothorax" is used when there is no wound. Hydrothorax means excess fluid in the pleural sac; hemothorax, blood in the pleural sac; and pyothorax, pus in the pleural sac. Chylothorax means that milky chyle from the thoracic duct has entered the pleural sac.

Edema is any condition in which the water in the intercellular spaces sufficiently exceeds the normal 15% so as to be clinically detectable. The opposite of edema is dehydration. Ascites or hydroperitoneum means excess fluid in the peritoneal cavity. Anasarca refers to general edema of the skin and subcutaneous tissues, the parts becoming swollen and puffy and piting on pressure.

Hydropericardium means excess fluid in the pericardial sac.

Anatomy and physiology. The cerebrospinal fluid is formed in the cells of the choroid plexus, which is a network of capillaries in the ventricles. The fluid is watery, clear, and colorless, the amount varying from 80 to 100 ml. About half of it is around the brain and about half in the spinal canal. It is being constantly formed and drained off. The average specific gravity is 1.006. Traces of protein and a few white blood cells are present. The composition varies with disease, so that an analysis of the fluid is essential in disease of the central nervous system.

A spinal puncture is usually made at the junction of the third and fourth lumbar vertebrae in order to prevent injury to the spinal cord (Fig. 12-5). Headache may follow spinal puncture because of a reduction in spinal fluid. The brain, deprived of a portion of its supporting cushion, settles to the base of the skull when the erect position is assumed, and pain results from pressure on the nerves.

The thorax is lined by a membrane called the pleura, which secretes a small amount of fluid to act as a lubricant between its visceral and parietal layers. An examination of the pleural fluid may be of diagnostic significance (Fig. 12-6).

The peritoneal lining of the abdominal cavity secretes a fluid that accumulates in excess when irritation or obstruction is present (Fig. 12-7).

The pericardium and synovial sacs secrete small quantities of fluid that prevents friction. Pressure of increased fluid in the serous cavities may cause pain by pressure on the nerve endings.

Microbiology. The presence or absence of bacteria or antibodies formed in specific diseases may be shown by tests on body fluids. Organisms commonly looked for in cerebrospinal fluid are those causing meningitis and tuberculosis. The organism commonly looked for in pleural and peritoneal fluid is chiefly that of tuberculosis.

Serous membranes are highly susceptible to bacterial invasions. Techniques designed to remove serous fluids (pleural,

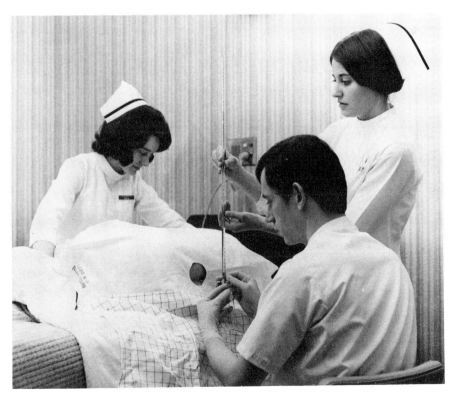

Fig. 12-5. Lumbar puncture. During a spinal tap the nurse keeps the patient in the proper position and measures the pressure.

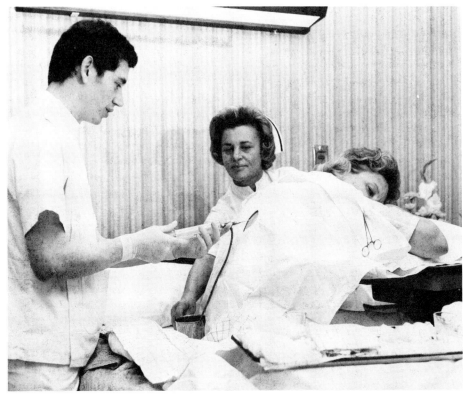

Fig. 12-6. Thoracocentesis. A vacuum is created in the syringe, which exerts a pull on the fluid in the pleural cavity.

spinal, pericardial, peritoneal, or synovial) are sterile techniques. Sterile gloves are worn, sterile drapes are used, the skin is prepared with an antiseptic, and the instruments are sterile.

Chemistry. Fluids of the serous cavities, with the exception of cerebrospinal fluid, contain sugar in the form of glucose in practically the same concentration as that of the blood. The cerebrospinal fluid contains roughly one half as much glucose as is present in the blood.

Pharmacology. In aspiration of serous fluids the site of puncture is prepared with an antiseptic, such as alcohol, thimerosal (Merthiolate), or benzalkonium (Zephiran Chloride), and is anesthetized by a local anesthetic, usually procaine, 0.25% to 0.5%.

Drugs may be injected into the serous cavities for treatment or into the spinal canal to produce general anesthesia.

Physics. Serous and synovial membranes protect against friction of moving parts.

Withdrawal of fluids from the body depends on differences in pressure. All body tissue is constantly exerting a certain pressure that is different for different tissues. All confined body fluids, except pleural fluid, are under pressure greater than atmospheric pressure. When a needle or trocar is introduced into a cavity, the fluid will flow out to an area of less pressure. Since pressure in the pleural space is subatmospheric, a device such as a syringe or suction apparatus or vacuum bottle (for example, a blood donor's bottle) is used to produce less pressure outside in order for the fluid to flow out.

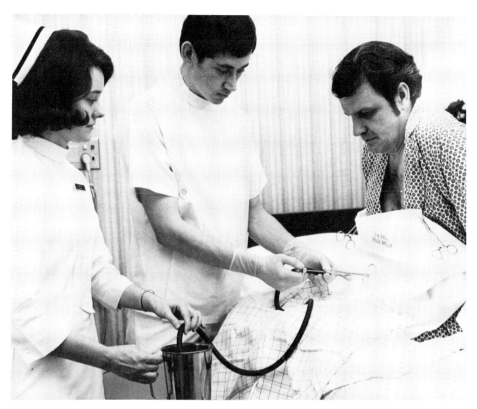

Fig. 12-7. Abdominal paracentesis. Peritoneal fluid flows out since fluid in the peritoneal cavity is under pressure greater than atmospheric pressure.

Pressure within a cavity is measured in millimeters of mercury or in centimeters of water. Since mercury is thirteen times heavier than water, one measurement can be converted easily into the other.

The Queckenstedt test depends on an increased volume in the capillaries of the brain, thus transferring increased pressure to the spinal fluid. Manual force is applied to the jugular veins, and this pressure prevents blood from leaving the brain. However, more blood comes to the brain, and the pressure of the spinal fluid rises. This test is performed with the manometer attached to the spinal needle, and the increased pressure is registered.

The position of the patient profoundly affects the pressure of cerebrospinal fluid. If the pressure of the fluid is 100 to 200 mm. of water in the recumbent position,

it may be 400 to 500 mm. of water in the upright position.

Psychology. Before an aspirating procedure is begun, the nurse should explain to the patient how he may cooperate and why his cooperation is necessary. During the procedure, diverting conversation may be employed. While assisting and speaking with the physician during a procedure, the nurse should be careful of comments and remember that the patient is conscious and very sensitive to conversation. Many patients fear a spinal puncture and need to be reassured.

Basal metabolism test

Anatomy and physiology. Basal metabolism is metabolism of the body at complete rest—comfortable, warm, and relaxed, physically and mentally. Basal me-

175

tabolism may be increased by abnormal occurrences as well as by diseases such as those of thyroid gland. The thyroid gland is a stabilizing influence in the regulation of basal metabolism. Thyroxin in excess of body needs increases the rate of metabolism. The thyroid gland controls in some way the amount of oxygen that an individual uses. The oxygen may be measured by a metabolism tester. The result of the test will aid in making a diagnosis of thyroid conditions.

Psychology. For any test the patient needs to be relaxed and unafraid, but more so for a basal metabolism test. Since the nose is clamped and the mouth is filled with the end of the oxygen tube, the patient fears he will not be able to breathe. The nurse should understand this chief fear and should prepare the patient mentally well in advance of the test by explaining what will be done.

Electrical impulses

Anatomy and physiology. The electrocardiograph makes use of the fact that when a heartbeat wave moves through the heart, it generates a weak but distinct electric current of 1/500 to 1/100 of a volt at the surface of the chest. These changes can be amplified and recorded as an electrocardiogram, from which a cardiologist can tell whether the heart is beating normally. From the report, a diagnosis of heart condition is made.

Minute currents resulting from brain activity are popularly known as brain waves. They can be detected on the scalp and recorded in amplified form as an electroencephalogram. They are valuable clues in detecting damage to the brain and have recently been put to use in learning whether messages intended to instruct deaf children are actually getting into the child's mind and being recognized. A physician interprets the encephalograph.

Psychology. The nurse should explain what is to be done and should tell the patient that there will be no discomfort during the test. Many patients fear these tests because they are associated with electricity.

X-ray examinations

Anatomy and physiology. X-ray examinations are used daily in the practice of medicine and surgery. Hard tissues of the body cast dense shadows on the x-ray plate. In order for soft tissues, such as the intestines, the gallbladder, and the kidney pelvis, to be visualized, a substance opaque to x-rays must be used to fill the organs and to cause them to cast an outline shadow on the film.

Pharmacology. Barium sulfate, a fine, white, odorless, tasteless, bulky powder, insoluble in water and impermeable to the x-ray beam, is used to outline the gastrointestinal tract. It is given by mouth for films of the esophagus, stomach, and small intestines and by rectum for films of the colon. Since it is heavy and insoluble, sometimes a laxative or cleansing enema may be needed to aid in its removal after the examination is completed to prevent constipation or obstruction.

To cause the gallbladder to be seen in an x-ray film, a dye containing iodine (which is opaque to x-rays) is administered either by mouth or intravenously. Several hours (15 to 18) after the dye is given, a film is taken. A normal gallbladder should be well outlined. The usual oral preparations are in white tablet form. The dose is usually calculated according to body weight. The oral dose is 0.5 Gm. and the intravenous dose is 0.3 Gm. for each 10 kg. of body weight. Because iodine is irritating to the gastrointestinal tract, a drug may be ordered to prevent nausea, vomiting, and diarrhea. The concentration of the drug in the gallbladder depends on the rate of absorption, the rate of excretion, and the rate of removal of water by the gallbladder.

The urinary tract may be visualized by the injection of an opaque dye. The dye may be introduced by catheter (called retrograde pyelography) or may be given by vein (called intravenous pyelography). Dyes for pyelograms contain about 50% iodine. The dye, given intravenously, may appear in the urine in 5 minutes.

Physics. X-rays are a form of radiant energy, with a wavelength shorter than that of light. X-rays will penetrate tissue according to the density of the tissue. Calcium in bone offers more resistance to the passage of x-rays than do soft tissues, and bones show well on an x-ray plate.

Psychology. Tests involving apparatus for x-rays and electricity are likely to be feared because of the power of these agents. The nurse needs to be familiar with these devices so as to speak with assurance when telling the patient there is no pain connected with these procedures. Some people fear that radiation will injure them in some way. They need to have their questions answered and to understand that there is no danger, since the amount of radiation used is not sufficient to cause harm.

Tests on reproductive tract

Tests on the female reproductive organs include the introduction of air and iodized oils in order to determine patency of the tubes. The tests are best carried out a few days before the menstrual period.

Microbiology. The skin of the patient is cleaned thoroughly before the instruments are introduced. Sterile sheets are used for draping, and sterile technique is maintained throughout the procedure.

Pharmacology. Carbon dioxide is used in Rubin's test because it is easily eliminated by the body and gives little discomfort to the patient. Iodized oils are used to cast shadows of the genital tract.

Physics. A mercury manometer registers the pressure of gas being introduced. A pressure of 200 ml. is seldom exceeded because of the danger of rupturing the tubes. If the fallopian tubes are occluded,

the pressure will remain high. If the tubes are open, the gas will flow into the abdominal cavity and the pressure will drop.

Psychology. The patient is anxious and hopeful that the cause of sterility can be found and corrected. Sometimes there may be feelings of guilt.

Tests using radioactive drugs

Pharmacology. The radioactive drug most frequently used in diagnostic tests is radioactive iodine ^{131}I. The thyroid gland has an affinity for iodine, and if the iodine is made radioactive, it can be measured with a detector. From the amount of iodine found in the thyroid gland, a diagnosis can be made of the overfunctioning or underfunctioning of the gland.

The tracer dose of radioactive iodine is given as a capsule of 50 μc. After about 2 hours a detector is used.

The method requires the use of relatively expensive apparatus for the measurement of the radioactivity and training in the use of radioactive materials approved by the Atomic Energy Commission.

Psychology. Some people fear any type of radioactivity and need to be told that the small amount of radioactivity in the tracer dose does no harm, since after the test it is rather quickly eliminated from the body, especially in the urine.

PSYCHOSOCIAL ASPECTS

A patient expects the physician to carry out and order whatever test is necessary for his recovery (see Table 12-2). He expects the nurse and the technician to show skill and gentleness in collecting specimens. The nurse must explain to each patient something of the nature of the tests he will undergo, prepare him for them, and call the physician's attention to the reported results.

In diagnostic tests much cooperation is needed. Cooperation is needed between the physician and the nurse, between the nurse and the technician, between the

Text continued on p. 202.

Table 12-2 Diagnostic tests

Name of test	Examination made or purpose	Normal range	Abnormally low value may indicate	Abnormally high value may indicate
I SECRETIONS AND EXCRETIONS				

A. *Urine*
  1. Urinalysis
    (routine single
    specimen)
	Specific gravity	1.006-1.025	Diabetes insipidus;
			overhydration;
			kidney disease
				Dehydration;
				glycosuria

	pH Protein (albumin)	4.5-7.5 None present		Kidney disease; hyper- tension; heart failure; drug posion- ing; toxemia of pregnancy
	Glucose Microscopic Cells	None present		Diabetes mellitus
	Epithelial	None to a few		Kidney and urinary tract disease
	White blood	None to a few		Kidney and urinary tract disease
	Casts	None present		Kidney disease
2. 24-hour specimen	Quantity Specific gravity Sugar, albumin, or bacteria	1,000-1,800 ml. per 24 hours 1.012-1.024 Negative		
3. Acetone	Presence in urine	Negative		Severe disturbance in metabolism

4. Addis
    (addis count)
	Count of red blood
	cells, white blood
	cells, casts,
	epithelial cells
		RBC: 0-450,000
		WBC: 30,000-1,000,000
		Hyaline casts: 0-5,000
		  (in a 24-hour total
		  specimen)		

Preparation of patient and method of procedure	Special equipment	Amount of specimen	Care of specimen	Precautions and comments
See that request slip is completely and correctly prepared. Instruct patient or relative to collect or save first urine voided in the morning; if possible have patient void directly into specimen container. Impress ancillary personnel with importance of proper care of specimen. Send to proper laboratory with request slip as soon as possible. Chart collection of specimen and note that it was sent to laboratory. Receive report and place on chart where can easily be seen by physician.	Litmus Urinometer Acetic acid Copper sulfate Microscope Centrifuge Widemouth specimen bottle	100-200 ml.	Send to laboratory within 2 hours; if specimen cannot be tested within 2 hours, refrigerate.	Normally a voided specimen is satisfactory; in certain conditions—menstruation, for example—catheterization may be necessary to obtain a clean specimen. pH should be measured as soon as possible because urine becomes alkaline on standing.
Instruct patient or relative as to purpose and routine of procedure. Give supportive care as indicated. Have patient void, discard urine, and note time. Save all urine voided in next 24 hours and place in same bottle. Measure all urine and send to laboratory with request. (Have patient empty bladder at end of 24 hours unless a voiding has just preceded this.) Continue as in 1.	Large bottle	Total 24-hour voidings	Add preservative if agency policy. Store in cool place. Send to laboratory on completion of specimen.	
Random specimen Continue as in 1.	Specimen bottle Reacting solution		As in 1 Procedure is usually performed on ward laboratory.	
Explain why and how test is to be done. Give regular diet (except fruit, which may alkalinize urine), but hold all fluid for 24 hours. After 12 hours without fluid, have patient void in clean bedpan. Discard urine. During next 12 hours save all urine voided and place in bottle. Send total urine to laboratory. Continue as in 2.	Large, clean, dry urine specimen bottles Centrifuge Microscope	All urine voided in a 12-hour period	As in 2	This test aids in pinpointing the type of kidney disease present. Cells and casts in urine sediment obtained from a 12-hour total specimen are counted and the amounts of each compared.

Continued.

179

Table 12-2   Diagnostic tests, cont'd

Name of test	Examination made or purpose	Normal range	Abnormally low value may indicate	Abnormally high value may indicate
5. Chlorides, quantitive	To evaluate urinary excretion of chlorides	9 Gm. per liter (depends on intake)		
6. Dilution and concentration test	Measures the capacity of the kidneys to concentrate urine	Concentration: a specific gravity of 1.026 or greater; at least one specimen with a specific gravity of 1.030	Kidney tubule disease	
7. Glucose and blood tolerance or galactose tolerance test	For glucose For galactose	*Oral method:* Blood: peak of not more than 150 mg. per 100 ml. of serum; return to fasting level within 2 hours Urine: Negative *Intravenous method:* Blood: return to fasting level within 1 hour Urine: Negative	Hyperinsulinism; Addison's disease	Diabetes mellitus; liver disease; hyperthyroidism
8. Guaiac test	For blood	Negative		
9. Estrogens	Presence in urine specimen	Male: 4-25 μg. in 24 hours Female: 4-60 μg. in 24 hours Pregnancy: to 45,000 μg. in 24 hours		
10. Friedman's, Aschheim-Zondek, or Hogben test	For pregnancy			
11. Hippuric acid liver function test	For hippuric acid	After 1 hour: 0.7-0.95 Gm. benzoic acid Hippuric acid over 1 Gm.		
12. Ketone bodies	Presence in urine specimen	Negative		

Preparation of patient and method of procedure	Special equipment	Amount of specimen	Care of specimen	Precautions and comments
As in 2	As in 2	As in 2	As in 2	Useful in the management of cardiac patients on low salt diets and in adjusting fluid and ion balance in postoperative cases. A simplified test, using a manufactured table, is now replacing the more complex analytic chemical technique.
Explain why test is being done and the procedure to be followed: 1. Withhold food and all fluid after the evening meal or 12 hours before start of test. 2. Discard urine voided during the evening and night. 3. Collect urine voided 12 hours after fasting begins; collect urine voided 1 and 2 hours later (usually at 7, 8, and 9 A.M.).	Stated amounts of water Clean, dry urine specimen bottles Urinometer Graduate	All urine voided each time specimen is collected	Keep each specimen covered and in a cool place until all are collected. Send to laboratory as soon as test is completed.	Note and record time of each voiding. See that each specimen label includes this information. Impress ancillary personnel with the importance of proper collection, handling, and care of specimens.
Send request to laboratory. Instruct and support patient. Give glucose or galactose as ordered. Collect urine specimens at stated . intervals. Laboratory technician will collect blood specimen. Continue as in 1.	Glucose or galactose (powder or Glucola)	Entire voiding		Helps detect glucose metabolism disorders that are not severe enough to appear in fasting blood glucose levels.
Random specimen	None	100-200 ml.		Catheterize if external bleeding is present.
This is a 24-hour specimen. Proceed as under 2.	As in 2	As in 2	As in 2	
Collect early morning specimen. Continue as in 1.	Rabbit, mouse, or frog Clean specimen bottle	As in 1	As in 1	
Assist with intravenous administration of sodium benzoate. Collect urine 1 hour after injection. Continue as in 1.	Sodium benzoate, 1.77 Gm. given intravenously	Total voiding	As in 1	
Random specimen Continue as in 1.	Clean specimen bottle	As in 1	As in 1	

Continued.

Table 12-2   Diagnostic tests, cont'd

Name of test	Examination made or purpose	Normal range	Abnormally low value may indicate	Abnormally high value may indicate
13. Phenolsulfonphthalein test	Amount of dye excreted	First 15 minutes: 25% or more of injected dye excreted First 30 minutes: 40% of injected dye excreted Within 2 hours: 60%-80% of injected dye excreted	Kidney disease: urinary tract obstruction	
14. Phenylketonuria (PKU)	To diagnose phenylketonuria	Negative		Phenylpyruvic oligophrenia
15. Urine culture	For presence of specific organisms	None		
16. Urea and blood clearance test	For urea	Urea in urine 10% that in blood		

Preparation of patient and method of procedure	Special equipment	Amount of specimen	Care of specimen	Precautions and comments
Explain procedure as necessary. Give water as indicated. Physician or technician will administer dye. Collect specimen as ordered, usually at 15, 30, 60, and 120 minutes after injection of dye.	Clean, dry urine specimen bottles Vial or ampule of dye Sponges Disinfectant Tourniquet Sterile syringe and intravenous needle	All urine voided each time specimen is collected	As in 2	Record time the dye is injected. Be sure patient understands that dye will temporarily affect urine color (pink to red). Record time of each voiding. See that each specimen is numbered in sequence and that each label includes the time.
Explain procedure to mother if indicated. Collect freshly voided specimen according to procedure of hospital's pediatric department, or place absorbent paper in infant's diaper, remove when wet with urine, and allow to dry. For immediate testing: place a drop of ferric chloride solution on wet diaper (or place reagent strip on it); green indicates a positive reaction.	Clean, dry, urine specimen bottle or absorbent paper If test is to be done at once: urine-soaked diaper, 10% ferric chloride solution or special reagent strip	Random voiding	Check to see whether specimen is to be sent to laboratory for testing. If absorbent paper is used to obtain it, place dried paper in an envelope and send to laboratory at once; be sure it is correctly labeled. In many states, the law requires that every infant be tested for phenylketonuria between the fourth and tenth weeks of life. Positive results must be reported to the Board of Health.	Check to see whether infant's mother is to be taught test technique for followup study when the infant is older.
Explain procedure. Catheterize patient. Allow some urine to flow through catheter, then place end of catheter into specimen bottle or sterile basin. Do not contaminate inside of basin or specimen bottle.	Catheterization set Sterile specimen bottle	100-200 ml.	Prevent contamination. Send to laboratory at once.	
Explain procedure and instruct patient. Technician will collect blood specimen or collect urine specimen as ordered. Note and record time of each voiding. See that each specimen of urine and blood is correctly and completely labeled. Continue as in 1.		Urine: all urine voided each time specimen is collected Blood: 5 ml. each time		This test is seldom performed because it has been replaced by more effective tests.

Continued.

183

Table 12-2   Diagnostic tests, cont'd

Name of test	Examination made or purpose	Normal range	Abnormally low value may indicate	Abnormally high value may indicate
B. *Gastrointestinal excretions* 1. Stool: gross microscopic	For parasites For fat, bacteria (especially typhoid bacillus), ova of parasites, amebas For blood	Negative Negative Negative		
2. Gastric fluid (analysis)	Basal acid output (1 hour) Fasting residual volume Maximal histamine stimulation pH	0-6 mEq. per hour Up to 50 ml. Males: 10-40 mEq. per hour Females: 5-30 mEq. per hour Less than 2.0	Pernicious anemia; severe chronic gastritis; gastric carcinoma; pellagra	Peptic ulcer; certain types of gastritis; certain endocrine disorders
3. Diagnex blue (tubeless gastric analysis, Azure A)	For free hydrochloric acid	Positive for free gastric hydrochloric acid of 0.6 mg. or more of the dye is found in urine within 2 hours		
4. Biliary drainage	For volume Color Viscosity Bacteria Cholesterol crystals	Varies Varies from light to dark Varies from thin to thick Negative 20-200 mg. per 100 ml.		
5. Pancreatic drainage	For volume Bicarbonate Amylase Trypsin Lipase	135-250 ml. in 1 hour 90-130 mEq. per liter 300-1,200 units in 1 hour 20-40 units in 1 hour 7,000-14,000 units in 1 hour		

Preparation of patient and method of procedure	Special equipment	Amount of specimen	Care of specimen	Precautions and comments
Gain patient's cooperation by explaining procedure. To prevent contamination of specimen with urine, instruct patient to void first, then to defecate. If enema must be given, explain why and how patient can cooperate. Collect specimen. Send specimen and request to laboratory. Receive report and place on chart where it can easily be seen by physician.	Specimen container with cover Wooden spatula (or tongue blade) Tincture of guaiac	According to agency policy	Transfer stool from bedpan to container. Cover specimen container tightly; send to laboratory at once since feces decompose rapidly. Keep warm for amebas.	When stool is to be collected for such tests as ova and parasites and/or chemical substances, check hospital laboratory's instructions for procedure to be followed.
Delay breakfast. Assemble equipment. Give or assist with test meal. Assist physician in passing tube. Assist or withdraw specimens. Send specimens and request to laboratory. Continue as in 1.	Intubation set Test meal or histamine phosphate, 1:1,000, or 50 ml. alcohol 7%	Entire amount of stomach contents aspirated each time unless otherwise ordered	Label each specimen in proper time sequence; send to laboratory as soon as test is completed.	Intubation is an unpleasant experience. To ease procedure, have patient sit up; encourage him to swallow as tube is advanced to help reduce gagging and nausea. Observe patient closely for untoward reactions to histamine. Emergency drug tray and resuscitation equipment should be available. Patients with a history of allergic conditions such as asthma should not receive histamine. Record time of injection and amount given. Explain to patient that drug may make him feel flushed and warm.
Follow agency policy for giving dye and collecting urine specimen.	Caffeine sodium benzoate for oral use Dye Clean, dry specimen bottles	All urine voided each time specimen is collected		Record time of each voiding, time patient receives caffeine sodium benzoate and dye. Explain that dye will temporarily color urine (green or blue).
As in 2 except tube passed into duodenum Contents withdrawn at certain intervals	Intubation set Magnesium sulfate	As ordered	As in 2	
As in 4	Intubation set Secretin	As ordered	As in 2	

Continued.

Table 12-2 Diagnostic tests, cont'd

Name of test	Examination made or purpose	Normal range	Abnormally low value may indicate	Abnormally high value may indicate
6. Sputum	For bacteria (especially tubercle bacillus and pneumo-cocci) For cancer cells	None		Presence of disease
C. *Discharges from wounds or body cavities*				
1. Smear	For bacteria	Negative		
2. Culture	For bacteria	Negative		
3. Papanicolaou smear	For cancer cells	Negative		
D. *Serous fluids*				
1. Lumbar puncture	For bacteria, especially *Meningococcus Pneumococcus Streptococcus* Tubercle bacillus	Negative		
	Reaction	pH 7.4-7.6		
	Specific gravity	1.001-1.010		
	Cell count	0-10		
	Pressure	100-200 mm. water		
	Glucose	40-70 mg. per 100 ml. spinal fluid		
	Protein	15-45 mg. per 100 ml. spinal fluid		
2. Thoracocentesis	For bacteria (especially tuber-cle bacillus)	Negative		
	Pressure	−4 to −5 cm. of water		
3. Abdominal paracentesis	For bacteria	Negative		
4. Pericardial aspiration	For bacteria	Negative		
E. *Synovial fluid*	Blood-synovial glucose difference	Less than 10 mg. per 100 ml.		
	Differential cell count	Granulocytes less than 25% of nucleated cells		
	Fibrin clot	Absent		
	Mucin clot	Abundant		
	Nucleated cell count	Less than 200 cells per cu. mm.		
	Viscosity	High		
	Volume	Less than 3.5 ml.		

Preparation of patient and method of procedure	Special equipment	Amount of specimen	Care of specimen	Precautions and comments
Instruct patient as to purpose of test and method of collection. Usually in early morning patient coughs and expectorates into container. Sometimes it may be necessary to pass a gastric tube and collect stomach washings as in the case of children or in patients having tuberculosis.	Wide-mouth glass bottle or waxed paper cup with cover	5-30 ml.	Keep covered and send to laboratory as soon as possible.	Make certain patient understands the difference between saliva and real sputum. Instruct patient not to use a mouthwash prior to collection of specimen.
Explain procedure as necessary. Assemble equipment. Drape or position patient if necessary. Assist physician with collection of specimen. Send specimen to laboratory with proper requisition slip. Place report on chart, calling attention to physician if indicated.	Slides Applicators Culture media Alcohol fixing solution for Papanicolaou slide	Dependent upon physician or technician	Maintain sterility. Send to laboratory immediately.	Dispose of applicators and other equipment so as not to infect personnel and other workers.
As in 1 under Discharges from wounds or body cavities. Lumbar puncture is performed by physician.	Sterile lumbar or cisternal puncture set (usually available in a prepackaged unit) Special test tubes Water manometer Skin preparation set Sterile gloves	2-5 ml.	Label specimens in order if more than one. Prevent contamination. Send to laboratory immediately.	This is a surgical procedure. Check hospital policy for permission. Watch patient for untoward reaction. Apply sterile dressing.
As in 1 Thoracocentesis is performed by physician.	Thoracocentesis set	Varies according to physician	As in 1	As in 1
As in 1 Have patient void prior to treatment. Paracentesis is performed by physician.	Paracentesis set Abdominal binder (possibly necessary)	As in 1	As in 1	As in 1
As in 1 Aspiration is performed by physician.	Aspirating set	As in 1	As in 1	As in 1
As in 1	As in 1	As in 1	As in 1	As in 1

Continued.

Table 12-2 Diagnostic tests, cont'd

Name of test	Examination made or purpose	Normal range	Abnormally low value may indicate	Abnormally high value may indicate
II BLOOD				
A. *Hematology*				
1. Hemogram				
a. Red cell count	Red cells counted	4,500,000-5,000,000 per cu. mm. blood	Anemia	Dehydration; polycythemia
b. White cell count	White cells counted	5,000-10,000 per cu. mm. blood		
c. Differential count	Percentage of different kinds of white cells	Neutrophil: 54%-62% of total white cell count		Bacterial infection
		Eosinophil: 0.5%-4% of total white cell count		Parasitic infection; allergic reaction
		Basophil: up to 2% of total white cell count		Certain blood dyscrasias
		Lymphocyte: 25%-35% of total white cell count		Virus infection; leukemia; mononucleosis
		Monocyte: 4%-10% of total white cell count		Hodgkin's disease
d. Hematocrit (HCT)	Comparison of cells to volume of blood	Male: 40-50 vol./100 ml. of blood	Anemia from hemorrhage; defective red cell formation or excessive red cell destruction	Dehydration; polycythemia
		Female: 35-40 vol./100 ml. of blood		
e. Hemoglobin (HB)	Quantity of hemoglobin estimated	12-18 Gm./100 ml. of blood		Same as HCT
		Male: 14.5-16.5 Gm./100 ml. of blood		
		Female: 13.0-15.5 Gm./100 ml. of blood		
f. Platelet	Platelets counted	200,000-500,000 per cu. mm. of blood	Thrombocytopenic purpura; aplastic anemia; Gaucher's disease; septicemia	
g. Reticulocyte	Reticulocytes counted	0.1-1.5 per 100 red blood cells		
2. Coagulation time	Time it takes for blood to clot after removal from a vein	Depends on method used: 9-12 minutes (Lee-White method)		Liver disease; hemophilia; afibrinogenemia
3. Bleeding time	Time for a cut to stop bleeding	2-3 minutes		Thrombocytopenia; allergic purpura; scurvy; uremia

Preparation of patient and method of procedure	Special equipment	Amount of specimen	Care of specimen	Precautions and comments
Send request to laboratory. Assist technician in collection of blood. Explain why tests are being done. Reassure patient that amount of blood to be drawn is not excessive. Have patient sit or lie down. For venipuncture, show patient: 1. How to hold arm 2. After tourniquet is applied, how to open and close fist 3. After blood is drawn, how to apply pressure over puncture site Have patient hold his arm straight up above his head for a time. Chart collection of specimen. Place report on chart where it can easily be seen by physician. Notify physician if necessary.	Clean specimen container (test tube, slides, or pipette, depending on the amount of blood drawn) Sponges Disinfectant For venipuncture: 20-gauge needle; dry, sterile syringe (size depends on the amount of blood to be drawn) Tourniquet or lancet for skin puncture	Sufficient for amount of anti-coagulant used	Usually performed by laboratory technician	Be sure that request slips are completely and correctly made out. Impress ancillary personnel with importance of proper care of specimens.
As in a	As in a	As in a	As in a	As in a
As in a	As in a	As in a	As in a	This test differentiates types of white blood cells; the proportions of specific cells to all white cells have diagnostic signifi-cance.
Venipuncture Continue as in a.	As in a	As in a	As in a	This is the most satisfactory screening test for anemia.
Skin puncture Continue as in a.	As in a	As in a	As in a	Capillary blood is employed. Ear may be punctured instead of finger.
As in d	As in a	As in a	As in a	
Skin puncture	As in a	As in a	As in a	Determines activity of bone marrow.
Depends on test method used Continue as in a.	Venipuncture set Lancet	4 ml.	As in a	Various test methods are used to determine coagulation time; check on method and procedure used by hospital's laboratory.
	Lancet	A few drops	As in a	

Continued.

Table 12-2 Diagnostic tests, cont'd

Name of test	Examination made or purpose	Normal range	Abnormally low value may indicate	Abnormally high value may indicate
4. Sedimentation rate	Time for solid materials in blood to settle	10-13 mm. in 1 hour (Westergren)		
B. *Chemistries* 　1. Acetone 　　a. Qualitative 　　b. Quantitative	Determine presence in body	Negative 0.3-2.0 mg. per 100 ml.		
2. Amino acid nitrogen	As in 1*	4-6 mg. per 100 ml.		
3. Alcohol (ethyl)	As in 1	Negative		
4. Amylase	As in 1	60-150 Somogyi units per 100 ml.		
5. Ascorbic acid (vitamin C)	As in 1	0.7-1.4 mg. per 100 ml. of serum	Vitamin C (ascorbic acid) deficiency	
6. Barbiturates	As in 1	Negative		
7. Base, total	As in 1	145-160 mEq. per liter		
8. Bilirubin 　a. Direct 　b. Indirect 　c. Total	As in 1	Up to 0.4 mg. per 100 ml. 0.4-0.8 mg. per 100 ml. 0.5-1.4 mg. per 100 ml.		
9. Bromsulphalein	To determine amount of dye in bloodstream at end of 45 minutes	Less than 0.4 mg. of Bromsulphalein per 100 ml. of blood	As in 1	
10. Calcium 　a. Total 　b. Ionized	As in 1 As in 1	4.5-5.3 mEq. per liter 9.0-10.6 mg. per 100 ml. Infants: 11-13 mg. per 100 ml. 2.1-2.6 mEq. per liter 4.2-5.2 mg. per 100 ml.	Hypoparathyroidism; acidosis; celiac disease; vitamin D deficiency; kidney disease; osteomalacia; rickets; sprue	Hyperparathyroidism; multiple myeloma; sarcoidosis; vitamin D intoxication
11. Carbon dioxide (CO_2)	As in 1	Adults: 24-30 mM. per liter Infants: 20-28 mM. per liter	Diabetic and other forms of acidosis; kidney dysfunction; severe diarrhea; intestinal-fluid loss; hyperventilation	Alkalosis; excessive intake of sodium bicarbonate; overtreatment with ACTH; present in persistent vomiting or hypoventilation
12. Carbon dioxide pressure	As in 1	35-45 mm. Hg		
13. Cephalin cholesterol flocculation	As in 1	Negative or 1+ after 24 hours 2+ or less after 48 hours		Cirrhosis; hepatitis

*"As in 1" means 1 under *Blood—chemistries.*

190

Preparation of patient and method of procedure	Special equipment	Amount of specimen	Care of specimen	Precautions and comments
As in a	As in a	5 ml.	As in a	
Explain procedure as necessary. Send request slip to proper laboratory. Withhold food or fluid as indicated. Assist technician in collection of specimen. Place report on chart where it can easily be seen by physician. Notify physician if necessary.	Venipuncture set	5 ml.	Performed by laboratory technician	Check agency policy since procedures vary according to locality.
As in 1	As in 1	As in 1	As in 1	
As in 1	As in 1	As in 1	As in 1	
As in 1	As in 1	As in 1	As in 1	
As in 1	As in 1	As in 1	As in 1	
As in 1	As in 1	As in 1	As in 1	
As in 1	As in 1	As in 1	As in 1	
As in 1	As in 1	As in 1	As in 1	
As in 1 and bromsulphalein, 5 mg. per kg. of body weight	As in 1	As in 1	As in 1	Delay breakfast. May give water. Continue as in 1.
As in 1	As in 1	As in 1	As in 1	
As in 1	As in 1	As in 1	As in 1	This a measure of acidity or alkalinity of the blood.
As in 1	As in 1	As in 1	As in 1	
As in 1	As in 1	As in 1	As in a	Some nonhepatic disease as rheumatoid arthritis may produce a plus reaction.

Continued.

Table 12-2 Diagnostic tests, cont'd

Name of test	Examination made or purpose	Normal range	Abnormally low value may indicate	Abnormally high value may indicate
14. Chloride	As in 1	95-103 mEq. per liter	Common in severe vomiting or diarrhea; acidosis; heat exhaustion	Various kidney disorders; Cushing's syndrome; hyperventilation
15. Cholesterol: total esters	As in 1	150-250 mg. per 100 ml. 65%-75% of total		
16. Creatine	As in 1	Males: 0.2-0.6 mg. per 100 ml. Females: 0.6-1.0 mg. per 100 ml.		
17. Creatinine	As in 1	0.5-1.2 mg. per 100 ml.		
18. Fatty acids, total	As in 1	9-15 mM. per liter		
19. Fibrinogen	As in 1	0.2-0.4 Gm. per 100 ml.		
20. Gamma globulin Globulin, total	As in 1	0.5-1.6 Gm. per 100 ml. 2.3-3.5 Gm. per 100 ml.		
21. Glucose tolerance, oral	As in 1	Fasting: 70-110 mg. per 100 ml. 30 minutes: 30-60 mg. above fasting 1 hour: 20-50 mg. above fasting 2 hours: 5-15 mg. above fasting 3 hours: fasting level or below		
22. Glucose	As in 1	80-120 mg. per 100 ml. of serum 70-105 mg. per 100 ml. of whole blood		
23. Insulin tolerance	Differentiation between hypopituitarism and primary hypothyroidism	Fasting: 70-110 mg. per 100 ml. 30 minutes: falls to 50% 90 minutes: fasting level		
24. Iodine, protein bound (PBI)	To determine function of thyroid gland	4.0-8.0 μg. per 100 ml.	Hypothyroidism	Hyperthyroidism
25. Lupus erythematosus (LE prep)	As in 1	Negative		Disseminated lupus erythematosus

Preparation of patient and method of procedure	Special equipment	Amount of specimen	Care of specimen	Precautions and comments
As in 1	As in 1	As in 1	As in 1	Indicates electrolyte balance of the blood. The body tolerates only slight deviation from normal range.
				This is useful in assessing cellular damage in the liver.
As in 1	As in 1	As in 1	As in 1	
As in 1	As in 1	As in 1	As in 1	
As in 1	As in 1	As in 1	As in 1	
As in 1	As in 1	As in 1	As in 1	
As in 1	As in 1	As in 1	As in 1	
Give glucose according to agency policy. Continue as in 1.	As in 1	As in 1	As in 1	
The physician injects 0.1 unit of insulin intravenously. Continue as in 1.	As in 1	As in 1	As in 1	Have on hand a concentrated glucose solution in a sterile syringe in case of reaction. Test is of no value in the diagnosis of hyperinsulinism. This is less sensitive than glucose tolerance.
As in 1	As in 1	8 ml.	As in 1	Patient should not receive iodides for at least 2 weeks prior to test or take iodine-containing contrast-medium substances for x-ray for at least 6 months prior to test.
As in 1	As in 1	As in 1	As in 1	Test is not conclusive, characteristic lupus cells are seen in about 60% of cases. Repeat tests may be necessary.

Continued.

Table 12-2 Diagnostic tests, cont'd

Name of test	Examination made or purpose	Normal range	Abnormally low value may indicate	Abnormally high value may indicate
26. Magnesium	As in 1	1.5-2.5 mEq. per liter		
27. Nonprotein nitrogen (NPN)	As in 1	15-35 mg. per 100 ml.	Severe liver disease	Kidney disease; urinary obstruction; dehydration
28. Osmolity	As in 1	280-290 mOsm. per kg.		
29. Oxygen pressure	As in 1	80-90 mm. Hg		
30. Oxygen saturation	As in 1	96%-97%		
31. pH	As in 1	7.35-7.45	Diabetic acidosis; uremia; lung disorders	
32. Phosphatase, acid	As in 1	0-1.1 Bodansky units 1-4 King-Armstrong units 0.13-0.63 Bessey-Lowry units		Cushing's disease; hyperventilation; excessive sodium bicarbonate intake
33. Phosphatase, alkaline	As in 1	Adults: 1.8-2.6 mEq. per liter 3.0-4.5 mg. per 100 ml. Children: 2.3-4.1 mEq. per liter 4.0-7.0 mg. per 100 ml.		
34. Potassium (K)	As in 1	4.0-5.4 mEq. per liter of serum	Kidney disease; Cushing's disease; prolonged vomiting	Shock; adrenal cortical deficiency, hypoventilation; impaired kidney function
35. Rheumatoid arthritis rapid screening or Latex agglutination test (RA test)	For agglutination			Rheumatoid arthritis
36. Serologic test for syphilis (STS)	To determine presence of antibodies	Negative		
37. Sodium (Na)	As in 1	138-148 mEq. per liter of serum	Kidney disease; diabetic acidosis; excessive hydration; diuretics; Addison's disease	Dehydration; hypothalamic injury; diabetes insipidus

Preparation of patient and method of procedure	Special equipment	Amount of specimen	Care of specimen	Precautions and comments
As in 1	As in 1	As in 1	As in 1	
As in 1	As in 1	As in 1	As in 1	This is a widely used test for renal function. Measures nonprotein substances in serum such as urea, uric acid, creatinine, ammonia, and so on.
As in 1	As in 1	As in 1	As in 1	
As in 1	As in 1	As in 1	As in 1	
As in 1	As in 1	As in 1	As in 1	
As in 1	As in 1	As in 1	As in 1	Indicates hydrogen-ion concentration. The body tolerates only slight deviation from normal range.
As in 1	As in 1	As in 1	As in 1	
As in 1	As in 1	As in 1	As in 1	
As in 1	As in 1	As in 1	As in 1	Indicates electrolyte balance of the blood. Deviation from normal range may produce serious changes in heart rhythm, muscle function. Potassium intoxication may cause death.
As in 1	As in 1	As in 1	As in 1	Test is reasonably specific. An element in the serum of rheumatoid arthritics causes clumping of latex and globulin emulsion.
Use caution about explaining test since some patients become upset if told purpose. Continue as in 1.	As in 1	As in 1	As in 1	A variety of tests, such as Wasserman, Kolmer, Kline, Kohn, and Mazzini, may be used. Since some diseases may cause a false-positive result, these tests are used to confirm diagnosis rather than to establish it.
As in 1	As in 1	As in 1	As in 1	Indicates electrolyte balance of the blood. The body tolerates only slight deviation from normal range.

Continued.

Table 12-2   Diagnostic tests, cont'd

Name of test	Examination made or purpose	Normal range	Abnormally low value may indicate	Abnormally high value may indicate
38. Sulfonamides	As in 1	Negative		
39. Transaminase (SGOT or SGPT)	As in 1	SGOT: 10-40 units SGPT: 5-35 units		For SGOT: myocardial infarction For SGPT: hepatitis; other liver diseases
40. Urea clearance	As in 1	Maximum clearance: 64-99 ml. per minute Standard clearance: 41-65 ml. per minute or more than 75% of normal clearance		
41. Urea nitrogen (BUN)	As in 1	8-20 mg. per 100 ml.	Severe liver disease	Kidney malfunction; urinary obstruction; dehydration
42. Uric acid	As in 1	Male: 2.1-7.8 mg. per 100 ml. Female: 2.0-6.4 mg. per 100 ml.		
C. *Miscellaneous* 1. Blood cultures	To determine presence of specific organisms	None		Specific bacterial organism causing disease
2. Blood grouping (typing)	To determine type of blood	Landsteiner Group distribution in the white population: O, 45%; A, 38%; B, 12%; AB, 5%.		
3. Crossmatching	To determine compatibility of two bloods	Cells agglutinate: AB → A, B → O (diagram) Serum agglutinates: AB ← A, B ← O (diagram)		

196

Preparation of patient and method of procedure	Special equipment	Amount of specimen	Care of specimen	Precautions and comments
As in 1	As in 1	As in 1	As in 1	
As in 1	As in 1	As in 1	As in 1	Transaminases are enzymes that catalyze transfer of amino acids to alpha keto acids. Glutamic oxaloacetic transaminase (SGOT) is released into circulation in abnormal amounts in heart injury. Glutamic pyruvic transaminase (SGPT) is released into circulation in abnormal amounts in liver damage.
As in 1	As in 1	As in 1	As in 1	This test is seldom performed today because it has been replaced by less cumbersome, more useful tests of kidney function.
As in 1	As in 1	As in 1	As in 1	This is considered a more precise test of renal function than NPN.
As in 1	As in 1	As in 1	As in 1	
As in 1	Tourniquet Test tube Culture media Continue as in 1.	As in 1	10 ml.	Culture identifies organism by character of bacterial colony and its reaction to various media.
As in 1	Tourniquet Test tube Continue as in 1.	As in 1	As in 1	Be *certain* specimen is accurately labeled and that requisition slip is correctly made out.
As in 1		As in 1	As in 1	

Continued.

Table 12-2 Diagnostic tests, cont'd

Name of test	Examination made or purpose	Normal range	Abnormally low value may indicate	Abnormally high value may indicate
4. Bone marrow examination	To examine blood cells		Granulocytopenia or increased erythropoiesis from blood loss; polycythemia or macrocytic anemia	Leukocytosis; leukemia; leukemoid reaction
5. Blood smear	To test for malaria and species of causative parasite	Negative		
6. Prothrombin time (PT or Pro time)	To indicate ability of blood to form intravascular clots.	12-15 seconds	Acute thrombo-phlebitis	Liver disease; vita-min K deficiency
7. Rh typing (Rh factor)	As in 2	Rh positive when Rho (D) factor is present; Rh negative when Rho (D) factor is absent		

III BASAL METABOLISM TEST

	Amount of oxygen consumed in given time	−20% to +20%	Hypothyroidism	Hyperthyroidism

IV ELECTRIC IMPULSES

1. Electrocardiogram	Electric impulses of heart contraction	Decided by cardiologist		

Preparation of patient and method of procedure	Special equipment	Amount of specimen	Care of specimen	Precautions and comments
Explain purpose or method of procedure. Reassure patient. Administer sedative, if ordered (usually about ½ hour before). Place patient in bed in supine position, shoulders on a firm pillow and head lower than shoulders. Drape for comfort. (Physician usually proceeds with preparation of puncture site and the administration of a local anesthetic.)	Sterile sternal puncture set (usually available in a pre-packaged unit) Glass slides Cover slips test tubes, plain and heparinized	For smears; 1-2 ml. Additional amounts depending on number of tests to be done	Send to laboratory at once. Apply sterile dressing to site.	This is a minor surgical procedure. Check hospital policy on permission procedure. Offer nursing support throughout. Some pain will be experienced when marrow is aspirated. Valuable in differential diagnosis, especially of blood dyscrasias. Sternum and iliac crest are most readily accessible sites for obtaining bone marrow in which blood cells are formed.
Observe patient carefully for optimum time to collect specimen. Continue as in 1.	Technician usually supplies own equipment.	As in 1	Technician usually assumes responsibility for prompt handling.	Parasites are found in greatest number when specimen is taken at peak of chills or fever.
	As in 1	As in 1	As in 1	Frequent evaluation of prothrombin time is necessary for determining dosage of anticoagulant.
As in 1		As in 1	As in 1	Most important of the twelve Rh phenotypes is the Rho (D) type. Typing is essential for pregnant women and before administering blood.
Send request to laboratory. Explain procedure as necessary. Delay breakfast. May have water ad lib. Give minimum nursing care. Patient is to remain quiet prior to treatment. No smoking or gum chewing is allowed. Provide proper transportation. Receive report and place on chart where it can be seen by physician.	Metabolism tester			Patient lies relaxed and quiet and breathes oxygen. Breathing is recorded on graph.
Send request slip to proper department. Follow agency policy. Explain procedure as necessary. This procedure is usually done at the bedside by a specially trained technician. Give supportive care if indicated since some patients fear electrical equipment. Receive report and place on chart where it can be seen by physician.	Electrocardiograph and jelly			Fasten leads to patient's body. Record impulses on graph.

Continued.

Table 12-2 Diagnostic tests, cont'd

Name of test	Examination made or purpose	Normal range	Abnormally low value may indicate	Abnormally high value may indicate
2. Electroencephalogram	Electric impulses of brain	Decided by neurologist		

V X-RAY EXAMINATIONS

Name of test	Examination made or purpose	Normal range	Abnormally low value may indicate	Abnormally high value may indicate
1. Gastrointestinal series	Motor functions and contour of stomach and intestines	Normal outline of stomach		
2. Gallbladder series	Filling and emptying time of gall-bladder	Gallbladder should be seen in first film and not seen after fatty meal		
3. Chest x-ray film	Clearness of lungs	Clear		
4. X-ray film of urinary tract	Outline of urinary tract	Normal outline		
5. X-ray film of trachea, bronchial tubes, or genital tract	Outline of tracts	Normal outline		
6. X-ray film of bones	Outline of bones	Normal outline		
7. Encephalogram	Outline of ventricles of brain	Normal outline		

VI TESTS ON REPRODUCTIVE TRACT

Name of test	Examination made or purpose	Normal range	Abnormally low value may indicate	Abnormally high value may indicate
1. Rubin's test 2. Iodized oils	Patency of fallopian tubes	Fallopian tubes open and gas allowed to go through		
3. Seminal fluid	Liquefaction Morphology Motility pH Sperm count Volume	Within 20 minutes Greater than 70% normal, mature spermatozoa Greater than 60% Greater than 7.0 (average, 7.7) 60-150 million per 1 ml. 1.5-5.0 ml.		

VII TESTS WITH RADIOACTIVE DRUGS

Name of test	Examination made or purpose	Normal range	Abnormally low value may indicate	Abnormally high value may indicate
1. ^{131}I uptake	Thyroid function	15%-35% of tracer dose in 24 hours		

200

Preparation of patient and method of procedure	Special equipment	Amount of specimen	Care of specimen	Precautions and comments
As in 1 May be necessary to shampoo hair in some instances. Provide proper transportation.	Electroencephalo-graph Bentonite (sulfur) ointment			Fasten electrodes to head. Record impulses on graph.
Send request to x-ray department. Delay breakfast and fluids. Withhold medications. Give supportive care as indicated. Provide proper transportation. Administer barium by mouth or rectum. Make fluoroscopic examination. Take x-ray film. Continue as in IV-1.	X-ray machine Fluoroscope Barium sulfate			
Send request to x-ray department. Assist with administration or give dye. Delay breakfast. Provide proper transportation. Continue as in IV-1.	X-ray machine Gallbladder dye (iodine), 3 Gm. Fatty meal			Give dye several hours before film is to be taken. Take film. After fatty meal take second film.
Send request to x-ray department. Provide proper transportation. Continue as in IV-1.	X-ray machine or fluoroscope			Patient stands against machine and holds breath.
As in 3	X-ray machine Opaque dye (iodine)			Dye given intrave-nously or injected through catheter. Take film.
As in 3	X-ray machine Opaque dye (iodine)			Inject opaque dye into area. Take film.
As in 3	X-ray machine Fluoroscope			Take film.
As in 3	Air X-ray machine			Take film.
As in 3 in X-ray examinations Test is performed by physician.	Air Special apparatus X-ray machine Radiopaque sub-stance (iodine)			
Send request to laboratory. Physician usually instructs patients. Take specimen to laboratory at once. Continue as in 1.	Clean container		Fresh specimen; must remain warm	
Continue as in V-3. This is usually carried out by technician.	Tracer dose of ra-dioactive iodine Scanner			

Continued.

nurse and the patient, and between the nurse and the patient's relatives. The nurse's function to collect a urine, stool, or sputum specimen may be delegated to a practical nurse or an aide. The nurse needs to impress the auxiliary personnel with the importance of prompt collection and proper handling of the specimen.

Relatives or visitors may be of assistance to the nurse in calming a patient while a specimen for laboratory examination is being collected. Sometimes one patient may do much to overcome the fears of another patient.

The nurse needs to be considerate of the patient's stay in the hospital and not prolong it more than necessary because of an oversight of an order for laboratory tests or because of discard of a secretion needed for examination. The request for the examination should be made as soon as the order is left. The laboratory may be reminded if the specimen is not collected or if the report is not received within a reasonable time. The cost of tests may be of consideration to a patient. Laboratory examinations are expensive, and the patient should be warned of the fees before he gets the bill. The physician is notified at once by the laboratory if there is any indication the report shows a great deviation from normal condition.

Diagnostic tests may be carried out in the hospital, in a clinic, in a physician's office, or in a special laboratory. Sometimes the patient takes a specimen to the place of testing. Sometimes the specimen is collected when the patient arrives.

Specimens may be sent through the mails to state or local departments of health. Special regulations govern sending specimens through the mails. There are free clinics for some laboratory tests; the United States Public Health Service maintains some. State and local agencies may operate others. Many boards of health require that food handlers have stool examinations to exclude typhoid carriers from passing on the disease. Many cities and states require Wassermann or Kahn tests before marriage. The nurse should be aware of all facilities for laboratory tests.

LEARNING SITUATIONS FOR THE PATIENT

The test needs to be explained to the patient sufficiently so that he understands why it is important and what he may do to help with it. He may be told how to collect a specimen of urine, sputum, or stool for examination. If the patient must bring urine, sputum, or stool specimen to the laboratory, the nurse will advise him on the kinds of containers to use and caution him that the outside of containers should not be contaminated with the material.

A diabetic patient may need to be shown how to examine the urine for sugar. The nurse will tell him where he may obtain the powders, tablets, or tape for testing urine and will observe the patient as he tests his own urine in the hospital or clinic to be sure he understands how to do it. The visiting nurse may examine a patient's urine in the home.

SUMMARY

Laboratory examinations are indispensable in correct diagnoses. The nurse should understand the methods of collecting specimens and the purposes of the tests so that he may help as much as possible. Types of containers vary with the type of material to be collected. They are either clean or sterile, depending on their use. The nurse needs to explain the tests to the patient so that he will cooperate and will know why his routine varies during the test. Familiarity with laboratory tests will aid the nurse in understanding the patient and his illness and thus will facilitate better nursing care.

QUESTIONS FOR DISCUSSION

1 List the responsibilities of the nurse if the physician's order reads: urinalysis; complete blood count.

2 If a technician collects blood for a blood sugar, what responsibility does the nurse have?

3 How would you prepare a patient for a basal metabolism test?

4 How may nurses and other workers become infected in collecting specimens?

5 Explain the words "occult," "gross," and "urinalysis."

6 In gastric analysis, what is the action of alcohol? histamine phosphate?

7 In biliary drainage, what is the purpose of magnesium sulfate?

8 What drug outlines the gastrointestinal tract for x-ray films?

9 What is the active drug in the dyes used for gallbladder films?

10 In what part is pressure the greatest: spinal canal, pleural cavity, artery, vein? In what part is it the least?

11 Describe what happens in the Queckenstedt test.

12 What is meant by capillary attraction?

13 How is capillary attraction employed in laboratory examinations?

14 Why do patients fear having blood taken for a blood test?

15 What is the chief fear of the patient who is to have a basal metabolism test, and what can you do about it?

16 Why are tests involving x-ray feared by the patient?

17 What persons cooperate in carrying out laboratory examinations?

18 How is a specimen of sputum mailed to a laboratory of a state board of health?

19 Describe a rapid method of testing urine for sugar.

20 When is sterile technique used in collecting specimens?

LIFE SITUATION

Mrs. Austin returned about 11 A.M. from the x-ray department where she had had a gallbladder series. When the nurse came in to check her, Mrs. Austin said, "I wish you would tell me what happened upstairs."

The nurse inquired, "Didn't you have pictures taken of your gallbladder?"

Mrs. Austin said, "I suppose so. That's what they said. I didn't get any breakfast this morning. When I was taken upstairs, they put me on a table and told me to hold my breath and

took a picture. They let me get up and they told me to sit in the dressing room. Someone brought me what they said was an eggnog but it tasted like very thick cream. Then they told me to wait a while longer and they would call me. After about an hour, they took a couple more pictures. I had to hold my breath again. Since I wasn't having pictures taken of my lungs, why did I have to hold my breath so much? There were many patients, and everybody was so busy they didn't have time to explain anything. Now just what did they x-ray —my lungs or my gallbladder?" What explanation would you give Mrs. Austin?

SUGGESTED PERFORMANCE CHECKLIST
Comfort

1 Is privacy provided?

2 Is the procedure explained to the patient?

3 If a meal is delayed, is it served as soon as possible?

4 If instruments are used, are they kept from the patient's view?

Therapeutic effectiveness

1 Is sufficient excretion obtained?

2 Are food and fluid withheld as needed?

3 Is the patient quiet in the morning before a basal metabolism test?

4 Is the patient watched carefully after aspiration?

5 Is the charting pertinent and accurate?

6 Is the patient observed carefully during the collection of the specimen or the examination?

7 Does the nurse show skill?

8 Does the nurse show tact?

Economy

1 Is the specimen labeled properly?

2 Is needed equipment at hand?

3 Is a request sent to the laboratory as soon as possible?

4 Is proper care taken of specimens until examination?

Safety

1 Is the physician's order checked?

2 Is the bedpan clean?

3 Is the specimen sent to the laboratory while fresh?

203

4 Is the container kept clean on the outside?

5 Is proper transportation provided?

6 Is the patient offered the bedpan before aspirations are done?

7 Is the position of the patient secure during aspirations?

8 Is sterile equipment used for specimens taken for bacteriologic study?

SUGGESTED READINGS

Derr, Susan D.: Testing for glycosuria, American Journal of Nursing 70:1513, July, 1970.

Foley, Mary F.: Pulmonary function testing, American Journal of Nursing 71:1134, June, 1971.

Garb, Solomon: Laboratory tests in common use, ed. 5, New York, 1971, Springer Publishing Company, Inc.

Given, Barbara, and Simmons, Sandra: Acute pancreatitis, American Journal of Nursing 71:934, May, 1971.

Harmon, Marna, and Waye, Jerome: Fiber optics: photography in the stomach, RN 34:46, July, 1971.

Lab people tell you what they don't like (and do like) about nurses, RN 35:36, August, 1972.

Laboratory review, Nursing Clinics of North America 5:361, June, 1970.

Nitowsky, Harold M.: Prenatal diagnosis of genetic abnormality, American Journal of Nursing 71:1551, August, 1971.

Shaw, Bernice L.: Emergency care for near-drowning victims, RN 33:49, July, 1970.

Tate, Gayle, Gohrke, Carol, and Mansfield, Louise: Correct use of electric thermometers, American Journal of Nursing 70:1898, September, 1970.

Wallach, Jacques: Interpretation of diagnostic tests, Boston, 1970, Little, Brown and Co.

13 Planning nursing care

THE NURSING CARE PLAN

The position is taken in Chapter 3, *Scientific Principles and the Nursing Process,* that the use of scientific knowledge is essential to provide the intellectual foundation necessary for nursing care. The process that the nurse uses in making application of scientific knowledge and methods in actual planning of patient care is the problem-solving approach. The steps in problem solving are there enumerated and illustrated as a means of arriving at valid nursing decisions. Three excerpts are emphasized here.

1. The nurse equipped to deal with nursing problems in a wise and resourceful manner must be able to use knowledge of general laws and reason from them or formulate new laws through the problem-solving process.

2. The nursing process is not just the memorization of facts or a listing of vaguely understood principles. It is rather a change in the character of the nurse that causes the involved giving of the "self," thinking in a scientific manner, and habitually relating general principles to immediate perceptions as a basis for rational decision making.

3. Nursing would be reduced to a me-

chanical routine devoid of all human qualities if it were a purely scientific procedure without inclusion of regard for the patient's being. Scientific aspects of nursing are inherent in the total nursing process, but it is the person-to-person contact that more often provides the catalyst to strengthen the patient's potential for maximum functioning. Commitment to the use of scientific principles, then, does not preclude the nurse's use of "self" by becoming involved in close human relationships with patients.

The philosophy underlying these statements relating to the planning of nursing care is that there is a dual commitment to nursing. The first is to commit one's "self" to the sharing of close personal communication with the patient as a major portion of the nursing process. The second is commitment to the comprehension and application of general scientific principles that govern nursing care, reason from such laws and principles, and direct nursing action in accordance with them.

It is the melding of these two commitments in nursing that ideally leads to establishing a satisfying nurse-patient relationship in which the "whole person" of

205

the patient is nursed. It leads the nurse to discover the individuality of each patient, to contribute to the alleviaton of his stress, and to enable him to act responsibly in participation with the formulating and achieving of his health goals. In essence, it means *planning with the patient.*

Definition of a nursing care plan. Planning nursing care with the patient, his family, and other members of the health team requires drawing up a written outline to include (1) preventive, diagnostic, or therapeutic activities prescribed by the physician, (2) nursing measures designed to prevent or alleviate related nursing problems, and (3) other special care needed by the individual patient. The plan may be revised as the patient's recognized needs are met or changed or as new needs are identified, but it continues to be the instrument that guides the nurse in taking nursing action.

Purpose of planning care. The purpose of the plan of care is to ensure that the best possible care be made available to the patient and to foresee and help solve future problems relating to his health. Outlining the plan of care in writing assists various workers involved to work cooperatively in providing continuity of care and in being aware of both short-term and long-term goals of that care. For example, the patient's health habits and how they may need modification must be considered, along with the patient's understanding of his condition and the level of self-care that he may achieve.

Personnel planning or providing care. The prescribed activities listed as part of the nursing care plan may be carried out by a team of which the patient is an active member, participating in each step of the process when physically able. Other members of the team may include the physician, nurse, nursing assistant, nutritionist, physical therapist, speech therapist, occupational therapist, medical technologist, psychologist, social worker, or other allied health workers. Activities regarding the patient's hygiene and comfort concern the patient's physical, mental, and spiritual well-being. Such activities include methods by which the environment, both physical and psychologic, is regulated safely and comfortably and methods by which personal care is provided. They involve diet, fluid requirements, personal hygiene, and physical activity. They are dependent on the patient's general condition and may or may not be governed by the physician's orders. Most of these activities are carried out or supervised by the nurse and are usually considered to be a part of general nursing care.

Planning as a phase of problem solving. Planning nursing care is one aspect of the nursing process that is carried out during the third major phase of the problem-solving sequence. As described in Chapter 3, that phase requires the formulation of tentative solutions to given nursing problems after the patient's health needs and related nursing problems have been identified and appropriate data collected (Fig. 13-1). These tentative solutions then become part of the total nursing care plan, which may be implemented, evaluated, and revised as necessary.

Once the patient's needs and related nursing problems have been recognized, the initial step in preparing a nursing care plan is to write down the objectives of the plan of care. These objectives, or goals, express the nature of the patient's health needs and problems in that they indicate *why* nursing action is needed. The nursing action planned indicates in turn *what, how often, when* or *how* the nursing action is to be carried out. Related principles indicate on what bases the nursing action is needed and can be expected to meet the stated objectives. These principles are not usually enumerated as part of the summarized nursing care plan outline. However, the nurse should be able to explain the bases for existing nursing problems and

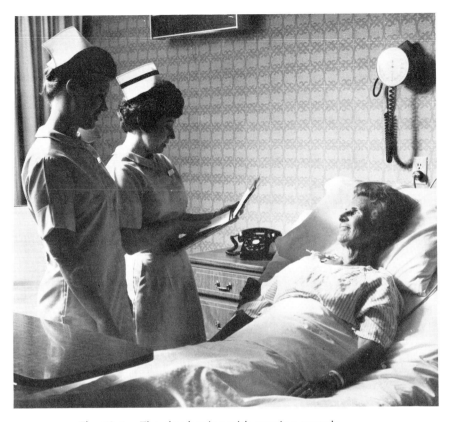

Fig. 13-1. The day begins with nursing rounds.

nursing measures, and the nursing student is usually encouraged to develop the ability to do so by being required to cite identifiable relevant principles when preparing, evaluating, or revising a nursing care plan (Fig. 13-2).

Plan-of-care format and staffing. A nursing care plan may be written in a variety of forms and can be adapted to a variety of situations. Nursing service members usually develop or adopt a nursing care format most suitable to their particular patient needs and agency staffing patterns. One example of a nursing care plan prepared by a nursing student is given in Table 13-1. The nursing staffing patterns commonly found in hospitals may affect the actual implementation of the plan. Three typical methods of assigning patient care responsibilities in nursing are the case method, the functional method, and the team method.

The *case method* means that one nurse performs all nursing services for the patient. The important advantage of this method is that the nurse has close contact with the patient and is able to provide complete nursing care over a longer period of time than with other staffing patterns. The case method gives the nurse a greater opportunity to directly assess patient progress, since the plan of nursing care is compiled and carried it out from day to day by the same person. Often nursing students (as well as "private duty" nurses) assume this type of patient care responsibility. It is usually not administratively or economically feasible, however, for general adoption in most hospital agencies.

The *functional method* of care relieves

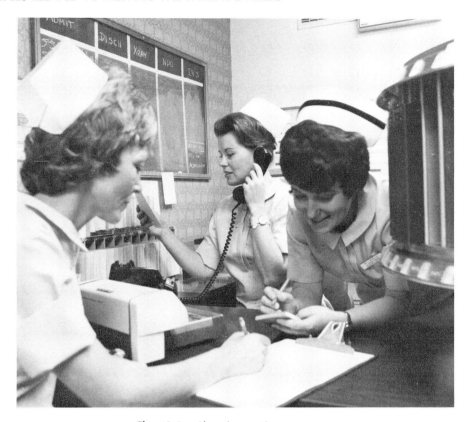

Fig. 13-2. Planning patient care.

the professional nurse of many tasks. The professional nurse may, for instance, give medicines or treatments to several patients but does not give all the nursing care to any one patient. Nursing assistants may carry out measures relating to personal hygiene, observing vital signs, moving patients, and administering treatments.

One advantage of the functional method of dividing the nursing tasks is that a nurse may become expert or very "efficient" in one phase of nursing, such as administration of medications. Such a nurse does not usually have opportunity for more than fleeting contacts with patients, however, and must rely a great deal on others for assessing patient needs and for evaluating the nursing care planned and provided.

The *team method* of care is patient centered even if several persons give the care. The professional nurse directs the care and may give some of it. The direction of care makes the professional nurse the leader of the nursing team. This nurse makes decisions and must be able to understand and communicate with others effectively and be able to help the team work out the organized plan. Other team members may be other professional nurses, nursing assistants, or student nurses. Every team member should have some knowledge of the patient's condition, including his problems and suggested methods of helping him, as well as of his treatment and progress.

A report will give each person this information quickly. Communication with other team members may be by means of complete and concise oral reports, written reports, and charts. The purpose of the report is to impart information about the patient and his problems. The team works together and evaluates the plan in conference at scheduled intervals and as needed. The nursing team leader or supervisor may in turn serve as a member of the health team, as shown in Fig. 13-3.

The student nurse may function in any of these methods, contributing care according to her knowledge and ability. A team relationship implies a desire to cooperate with others in working toward a common goal, the good of the patient, with the team of workers in a closely knit group. The cohesiveness of a team is based on mutual respect and recognition of the contribution of others, self-respect and security in this relationship, satisfaction with one's own needs, and contributions and acceptance of a common goal.

INFORMATION USEFUL
FOR PLANNING NURSING CARE

To plan care effectively, the nurse will need to know much about the patient. The patient is the source of much pertinent information that may or may not be gleaned

from his chart. The admission record reveals the patient's name, address, age, marital status, occupation, nationality, sex, religion, and citizenship. It also contains the employer's name and the name of the person responsible for the patient. The physician's name is included on the admission record. These data provide background material that will help to understand the patient. An example of an admission record is shown in Fig. 13-4.*

Besides the admission record, the nurse should read the patient's history and findings of the physical examination. The information from these records serves to bring into focus the needs of the patient. An example of a patient's history is shown in Fig. 13-5 and that of the findings of the physical examination in Fig. 13-6.

The physician's orders are an essential part of the plan of care and include prescribed diagnostic procedures, treatments, nutrients, medications, and activities. These orders give great leeway to the nurse. The nurse needs to interpret the

*The data included in Figs. 13-4 to 13-7 are based on an actual case, but the names and addresses are fictitious.

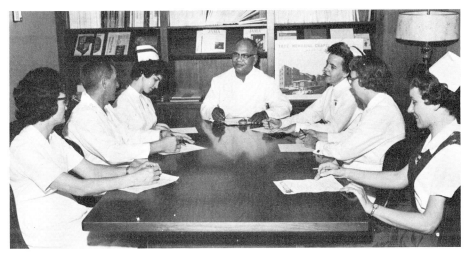

Fig. 13-3. A health team plans and evaluates nursing care.

General Hospital

Name Mrs. L. R.	Date March 5, 1974	Hour 10:30 A.M.	Room 268 B
Street 9673 Frigate St.	City and state Detroit, Mich.	Zipcode 48224	Case No. 2650
Age S (M) W D (W) C 66	Phone 426-5894	Occupation Homemaker	
Religion Catholic		Birthplace Canada	
Diagnosis Diabetes with perineal dermatitis	Previous admission 1971-72	Discharge ☐	Date Hour
Intern Dr. J. Henderson	Service Medical	Died ☐	
Referring doctor Dr. B. Russell	Attending doctor Dr. B. Russell		
Nearest relative Mr. J. R.	Address 9673 Frigate St.		
Responsible party Mr. J. R.	Address 9673 Frigate St.		
Employed by Retired	Address		

Fig. 13-4. Example of a hospital admission record.

orders in relation to the patient's total needs and to plan a program of care to meet these needs. The nurse should be able to read reports from other departments and learn the patient's condition from them. An example of physician's orders is shown in Fig. 13-7, with standard abbreviations indicating many of the details of the necessary medical care.

The plan of care includes a consideration of hygienic activities essential to the patient's recovery or maintenance of health. Aspects of normal health care for which the nurse must provide are (1) cleanliness and care of the skin, (2) sufficient rest and sleep, (3) exercise adapted to the patient's capacity, (4) proper elimi-

nation, (5) proper nutrition, (6) proper posture, (7) suitable diversion, and (8) aid in adjusting to situations. Factors regarding the environment, such as heat, light, and ventilation, must also be considered. Time must be provided for instructing the patient in ways of helping himself, for interpreting the physician's directions, and for checking the patient's performance of procedures that he has learned. The nurse will include in the plan of care time to talk to the relatives and friends of the patient to exchange information about the patient, to discover their attitudes toward the patient, and to help them in adjusting to the patient's condition. It is important to keep in mind, however, that the patient needs to feel that he has control of the situation.

THE NURSING PROCESS

Popular terminology for the various phases of what the nurse does in providing patient care—the *nursing process*—has not been used to this point. For the sake of avoiding confusion, however, common terms as they have been generally used in this connection are here defined.

After data gathering the next step in the nursing process is often called the *assessment phase*. In this phase the nurse relates the information about the patient to scientific knowledge regarding normal functioning and pathophysiology to arrive at a definition of the patient's problem (sometimes called the nursing diagnosis). With the patient's problem identified, the nurse may then move to the final consideration in the assessment phase, which is the statement of objectives to be achieved. This leads to the next phase, called *nurs-*

General Hospital

Surname R		Given names Mrs. L.	(W) C M (F)	Ward 268	Bed No. B	Case No. 2650
Age 66	Nativity Canada	Occupation Homemaker	S (M) W D		Admitted March 5, 1974	
Residence 9673 Frigate St.		Height 5 ft. 6 in.	Weight 159 lb.		Discharged	

Primary diagnosis
Diabetes with perineal dermatitis.

Present complaint
Severe itching in perineal area.

Present illness
Itching began about three weeks ago.

Family history
No tuberculosis.
No family history of diabetes.
Father died of cancer at age of 79.
Mother died of heart disease at age of 80.

Past history
Had one child who was killed at age 3 in an auto accident.
At 26 had uterine fibroids removed.
At 28 had an appendectomy.
At 40 had a tonsillectomy.
At 45 diabetes was discovered. Was treated with insulin and diabetic diet.
At 48 had a bladder suspension.
At 56 had a hemorrhoidectomy performed by an osteopath.
At 64 had cystoscopic and proctoscopic examinations.
At 64 also had digestive troubles.
At 65 was hospitalized for diabetes with vaginitis.
At 65 was hospitalized for diabetes with ureterocele.

Physician or surgeon Dr. B. Russell	Intern Dr. J. Henderson

Fig. 13-5. Example of a patient's history.

211

General Hospital

Surname R		*Given names* Mrs. L.	(W) C. M (F)	*Ward* 268	*Bed No.* B	*Case No.* 2650
Age 66		*Occupation* Homemaker	S (M) W D		*Admitted* March 5, 1974	
Residence 9673 Frigate St.		*Height* 5 ft. 6 in.		*Weight* 159 lb.	*Discharged*	

General condition: Slightly obese woman lying in bed complaining of severe itching in perineum.
Head and neck: Negative.
Eyes: React to light and distance. Glasses.
Mouth: Dentures.
Chest: Lungs clear.
Heart: Pulse 80 strong. Blood pressure 135/82.
Genitourinary: Occasional frequency.
Skin: Negative except in perineal area — covered with numerous condylomas.
Bones and joints: Negative.
Glandular: Negative.
Neuromuscular: Negative.
Impression: Diabetes with perineal dermatitis.

Examined by Henderson

Fig. 13-6. Example of the findings of a physical examination.

General Hospital
Physician's Orders

Date	*Medications and treatments*
March 5, 1974	Benadryl, 50 mg. b.i.d.
	Periactin, 1 tab. (4 mg.) t.i.d.
	Fulvicin, 250 mg. q.i.d.
	Gantricin, 2 tab. (1 Gm.) b.i.d.
	Petroleum jelly to vulva t.i.d.
	Diabetic diet.
	NPH insulin 30 U. o.d.
	Orinase tab., 1(0.5 Gm.) o.d.
	Clinitest and Acetest, q.i.d.
March 6, 1974	Aq. gentian violet 2%. Paint perineum o.d. Potassium permanganate sitz bath for 10 min. o.d.
	Calamine lotion, t.i.d. p.r.n. to perineum.
March 19, 1974	NPH insulin 35 U.
	Dismiss tomorrow.

Fig. 13-7. Example of a physician's orders.

ing intervention. In this phase the nurse implements the stated objective through the plan of care. This is the action phase. The final phase of the nursing process is *evaluation,* in which the nurse seeks to determine the effectiveness of the intervention in achieving the desired goals of nursing care.

SAMPLE PLAN OF NURSING CARE

The following nursing care study is cited as an example of information used by the nurse in preparing and using the nursing care plan.

Nursing care study*

Mrs. L. R. is a delightful 66-year-old woman whose features and actions do not betray her age. She is 5 feet 6 inches tall and weighs 159 pounds. Although she is slightly obese, it becomes her. Her personality could best be summed up in the fact that it just seems she cannot do enough for people. Consideration guides all her actions as she makes an extra effort to do little things for the other patients and the nurses.

This care study is made with following objectives: (1) to better understand Mrs. L. R. and her condition, (2) to view the manifestations of diabetes mellitus in a particular individual and thus have a basis for a better understanding of diabetes and its therapy, (3) to develop an awareness of the complications of diabetes, with their treatment and nursing care, (4) to learn to formulate nursing action according to a particular individual's needs, (5) to develop a knowledge of efficient nursing care for a diabetic patient, and (6) to acquire a better understanding of the reaction and response of an aged patient to diabetes.

Family and culture. Mrs. L. R. was born in Canada on June 17, 1908. She is a Caucasian of the Roman Catholic faith. Through discussion with her, it was

*This nursing care study was compiled by a nursing student.

learned that she came from a medium-sized family and that her education was typical of that received at that time, which means that she did not complete high school and had no special training in a particular field. This has never presented a problem, however, since her husband has always preferred to have her at home. Mrs. R. is presently, and has been since her marriage, a housewife. She had only one child who was killed at an early age in an automobile accident.

The fact that her husband is retired limits their income considerably. He formerly was employed as a bricklayer. After stating that they previously had an average income, she said, "There are only two of us," which probably indicates they manage fairly well. Too, they are insured under a construction worker's organization. The party responsible for her is her husband.

The patient's feeling about hospitalization. Mrs. L. R. was hospitalized for medical treatment of perineal dermatitis. She had been trying to carry out the physician's instructions and treating herself at home for several weeks but with poor results. Being hospitalized caused her to be upset and disturbed at times. She felt that her condition could still be treated just as well at home, where she could be with her husband. Too, her attitude may have been influenced by her previous hospitalizations during which complications developed. Mrs. R's main goal was to have her discomforts relieved with cure of the dermatitis so she could return to her husband, friends, and home environment.

Past history. Mrs. L. R.'s past illnesses are numerous and varied.

1. At the age of 26 she had uterine fibroids that required surgery. This may have been the reason she did not have any more children.

2. At the age of 28 she had appendicitis, necessitating an appendectomy.

213

3. At the age of 40 she had a tonsillectomy.

4. When she was 45, it was discovered that she had diabetes mellitus. There had been no family history of it. She had also had a history of obesity. Obesity is said to be a possible cause of diabetes since it presents an increased demand for insulin, exhausting the cells of the pancreas. Mrs. R. stated that she was treated at that time with regular insulin and a diabetic diet, which she continued for several years.

5. At the age of 48 Mrs. R. needed a bladder suspension. Control of diabetes is often disturbed by the apprehension and trauma associated with conditions such as incontinence, examinations, and surgery. No disturbance was noted in Mrs. R.'s case, however.

6. At the age of 56 Mrs. R. had a hemorrhoidectomy. Rectal incontinence followed the operation for 1 year. It is stated on her chart that the cause of the condition was repaired and cured by surgery in 1965. Nothing indicates that her diabetes was out of control during this treatment.

7. Cystoscopic and proctoscopic examinations were performed at varying intervals, perhaps in the diagnosis and during treatment of the bladder suspension and the hemorrhoidectomy.

8. Mrs. R. had trouble with digestion that was alleviated in 1969. Inadequate digestion hinders normal absorption of food. This could have presented a problem because in order for the regulated diet and insulin administration to control diabetes, the food must be absorbed. If it is not absorbed, an insulin excess will occur, resulting in hypoglycemia or insulin shock. Happily this did not occur with Mrs. R.

9. At the age of 65 Mrs. R. was hospitalized with a diagnosis of diabetes mellitus with marked vaginitis. Since the diabetes was not under control, she entered for better regulation of her diet and insulin. She was placed on a 1,400-calorie diet, and insulin was given according to the Clinitest results. If the Clinitest showed a 4+ or 3+, 15 units of regular insulin were given; if 2+, 10 units; if 1+, 5 units.

Trigonitis and ureterocele were presumed responsible for the lower abdominal discomfort rather than the vaginitis. It was stated on the chart that the vagina showed no evidence of thrush or irritation. Mrs. R's complaint of dysuria and burning on urination for 3 weeks suggested a bladder infection.

An acute infection, probably the flu, was responsible for the diabetes getting out of control. Infection places a great stress on the body, altering carbohydrate metabolism and decreasing appetite, thus changing the insulin requirement. Careful regulation of diet and insulin was necessary for Mrs. R's diabetes to be controlled during this time. It was during this hospitalization that Mrs. R. was instructed about her diabetic condition.

10. During the following year Mrs. R. was admitted again with the diagnosis of ureterocele and diabetes. Her primary complaint was burning on urination. The ureterocele was repaired. The 1,400-calorie diet was stressed again, and she was instructed in the need for maintaining it after she went home. It was stated on the chart that she had been on regular insulin, 20 units three times a day, later on Orinase, 0.5 Gm. once a day, and was now on both. Upon admission she was placed on NPH insulin and regular insulin as well as Orinase. Her blood sugar level dropped, and she was instructed to consult her doctor to regulate the control of the diabetes.

Present admission. Mrs. L. R. was hospitalized again on March 5, 1974, with a diagnosis of diabetes mellitus with perineal dermatitis. Her complaints upon admission were redness, pain, swelling, and itching of the perineum. From her past history and present symptoms, the doctor's impressions were (1) diabetes mellitus and (2) perineal dermatitis probably monilial in origin.

The physical examination showed that

the external genitals and surrounding area were swollen and covered with numerous condylomas (wartlike skin lesions). In Mrs. R.'s case the dermatitis was presumed to be monilial in origin. No tests were performed to prove this fact, but immediate treatment was started.

Pruritus vulvae commonly associated with diabetes occurs without any apparent primary dermatitis. Pruritus, devoid of local pathology at its inception, as the result of scratching, rapidly induces local skin changes, for example, condylomas, which themselves produce itching. The causes are manifold, extending from local irritants to constitutional conditions. With Mrs. R. the possible underlying pathology would be candidiasis (moniliasis) and the constitutional condition the diabetes. It has been proved that the skin of a patient with diabetes is more easily affected by *Candida (Monilia)* than that of a person without diabetes. *Candida (Monilia)* is a genus of fungi.

Often pruritus vulvae in a diabetic patient is considered to be caused by a vitamin deficiency, especially nicotinic acid. Too, in this condition, the vulnerability to any kind of irritation, mechanical, chemical, or microbial, is greatly increased. The increased sugar in the urine serves to irritate further the perineal area, predisposing it to dermatitis.

Treatment. The treatment of Mrs. R.'s perineal dermatitis was directed toward removing the underlying candidiasis (moniliasis) as well as promoting comfort. The therapy was both systemic and local. Several drugs were prescribed for systemic effect.

Benadryl, 50 mg., to be administered once in the morning and once in the evening, is an antihistamine. Antihistamines are useful in treating allergic conditions such as pruritus by preventing the physiologic action of histamine. In full therapeutic doses, if given four times a day, it causes sedation.

Periactin, one tablet (4 mg.), was administered three times a day. Periactin is a potent antagonist of histamine. Periactin is particularly recommended for suppression of pruritus associated with an allergic reaction such as pruritus vulvae.

Fulvicin, 250 mg., was administered orally four times a day. It is an effective antifungal antibiotic for treatment of superficial fungous infections. Decrease of itching and inflammation is generally manifest within a few days.

Gantricin, two tablets (1 Gm.), was administered twice a day. Gantricin is a single, soluble, wide-spectrum sulfonamide particularly useful in systemic and urinary tract infections. Since Mrs. R.'s urinalysis revealed bacterial cells in the urine, Gantricin was indicated.

The topical application of various substances constituted local treatment.

Petroleum jelly was ordered to be applied to the vulva three times a day. It was indicated since the free use of an ointment prevents irritation during micturition. Mrs. R. refused the ointment application, continually stating, "It makes me burn more."

Calamine lotion was applied for complaints of mild discomfort. It contains calamine, zinc oxide, bentonite magma, glycerin, and calcium hydroxide solution, all of which act to produce a soothing effect. It is patted on the involved area with cotton. This lotion provided some relief for Mrs. R., and she requested it about three times a day.

Aqueous gentian violet solution, 2%, was used to paint the perineum once a day. Gentian violet is an antifungal agent especially effective in treating pruritus caused by *Candida (Monilia).* The usual solution is 1% dye in alcohol or water solvent. It stains the clothing. Mrs. R. stated that it seemed to help.

Potassium permanganate solution sitz baths were taken by Mrs. R. for 10 minutes every day at 10 A.M. and 6 P.M. Potassium permanganate is used as an antiseptic since it is a very efficient oxidizing

215

agent. When it comes in contact with the skin, it is reduced to brown manganese dioxide, leaving a brown stain.

Warm water, by dilating blood vessels, increases circulation to the area, bringing white blood cells and other valuable blood constituents to counteract the underlying pathology. Ten minutes is an adequate length of time to obtain the effect of heat. The sitz bath provides for thorough cleansing of the perineum and also the application of the potassium permanganate. Mrs. R. received considerable relief from the baths, her only complaint being about the brown stain that remained on the skin.

Psychologic aspects. Mrs. R.'s emotional reaction to her perineal dermatitis was one of distress and unrest. The perineal discomfort was obviously the most distressing. The itching caused her to scratch the area, resulting in further eruption and pain. The tenderness and swelling of the perineum increased its susceptibility to irritation from urine and from friction of linen. Realizing that she must break the habit of scratching perhaps further placed the discomfort foremost in her mind. The fact of being hospitalized and leaving her husband also upset her. She displayed this by showing signs of depression several times. Otherwise she appeared to be a jolly, considerate elderly woman.

Laboratory diagnosis. The diagnostic studies pertaining to the dermatitis were general. No cultures, smears, or stains were done because of perineal treatment before admission. The admitting urinalysis was normal except for the presence of a few bacterial cells. No albumin or sugar was noted in the urine, although the Clinitest performed four times a day indicated the presence of sugar in ranges of a trace to 4+.

The hematology report indicated the hemoglobin to be 14.1 Gm. per 100 ml. of blood; red blood cells, 4.2 million; hemat-

ocrit, 40%; and white blood cells, 5,100 per cubic millimeter of blood. Generally there is no change in the number of either red or white blood cells in diabetes. The blood sugar level was increased, ranging from 165 to 253 mg. per 100 ml. of blood. Mrs. R.'s temperature remained normal, except for a single recording of 99.6° F. (37.5° C.) on the fifth day after admission. No cause was noted for it.

Result of treatment. During the first 5 days Mrs. R. showed a gradual improvement. The swelling and tenderness decreased. Mrs. R.'s remarks of discomfort and itchiness were lessened. However, considerably more treatment was necessary to clear the condylomas and return the skin to normal. Important, too, were measures to prevent recurrence.

Mrs. R. had been known to have diabetes for approximately 21 years. To understand the relation of diabetes mellitus to Mrs. R. as an individual, it is necessary to have a basic understanding of the disease itself.

DIABETES. Diabetes mellitus is a hereditary disease characterized by an increased amount of glucose in the blood and excretion of this glucose in the urine. It is a chronic metabolic disease involving a disorder of carbohydrate metabolism and subsequent derangement of protein and fat metabolism. Disturbance in the production, action, or metabolic fate of insulin, a hormone secreted by the islands of Langerhans in the pancreas, is the basic defect.

PHYSIOLOGY. Carbohydrate metabolism is defective because the cells are unable to oxidize glucose without insulin. Carbohydrate metabolism does not come to a standstill; it just decreases. Protein metabolism is affected since insulin increases the rate of protein synthesis and alters its ability to be stored. Fat burns in the fire of carbohydrates. Incomplete fat oxidation caused by retardation in metabolism of carbohydrates produces ketone bodies. Excessive ketone bodies are neutralized by blood buffers and are excreted as sodium salts, leading to considerable loss of base in the blood, and consequently acidosis results.

Accordingly, gross changes in body physiology occur. First, the most evident change is hyperglycemia because the glucose remains in the bloodstream unable to be oxidized and converted to the glycogen. Normally after 14 hours of fasting the blood sugar level contains from 80 to 120 mg. of glucose in 100 ml. of blood. The blood sugar level in diabetic patients may range from 120 to 800 mg. of glucose in 100 ml. of blood. The severity of diabetes increases with the amount of glucose.

Second, glycosuria occurs as the blood sugar level rises above the renal threshold of 140 to 180 mg. in 100 ml. blood and the excess overflows into the urine. The renal threshold may be unusually high in some individuals, and the diabetes may be present but not evident from urine findings.

Third, polyuria results because the excretion of glucose carries with it a large amount of water. This results from the osmotic phenomena that water moves from an area of lesser concentration. The urine output may vary from 3 to 10 liters a day.

Typically the three major symptoms are (1) polyuria, (2) polydipsia, resulting from an attempt of the body to restore water loss and prevent dehydration, and (3) polyphagia (excessive eating), resulting from the body's inability to metabolize glucose for energy.

Other symptoms of diabetes are diaphoresis, weakness, fatigue, tremors, weight loss from sugar loss, and trophic changes of the skin.

The principles of management are diet, insulin, and possibly Orinase therapy—all necessitating patient teaching. Severe distrubances in this regime may predispose the patient to insulin shock or diabetic coma.

Diabetic coma is a complication of undiagnosed or neglected diabetes, and it is the result of prolonged and increasing acidosis. The blood sugar level is well above 120. Acidosis is a decrease in the pH of the blood caused by the increased alkali excretion.

The symptoms of acidosis are (1) excretion of large amounts of urine, (2) increased thirst, (3) hyperglycemia, (4) anorexia, (5) nausea and vomiting, (6) vertigo, (7) weakness and drowsiness, (8) ringing in the ears, (9) visual disturbances, and (10) excitement.

Coma is ushered in with (1) Kussmaul's breathing and air hunger, (2) dehydration (dry skin, anuria, soft eyeballs, and elevated temperature), (3) acetone odor on the breath, (4) disorientation, and (5) coma.

A complication of insulin overdosage or too little food is hypoglycemia or alkalosis, in which the blood sugar level is below 40. The alkalosis is a result of the increase in the pH of the blood because carbonic acid is less than normal and the bicarbonates of the blood are increased above normal.

The symptoms of early alkalosis are (1) unusual hunger, (2) nervousness, (3) cold, moist skin with sweating, (4) headache, and (5) faintness. Progressing symptoms are (1) confused slurred speech, (2) numbness of the lips and blueness of the skin resulting from dysfunction of the cranial nerve, and (3) convulsions.

CONTROL. There are two schools of thought on the control of diabetes. One medical group believes that the patient's urine must be kept sugar free and the blood sugar at a normal level. The other believes that the diabetes can be controlled in the presence of an above-normal blood sugar and of sugar in the urine provided enough insulin is taken and enough food is eaten to meet metabolic needs. Apparently Mrs. R. is being controlled from the intermediate standpoint since her blood sugar level previous to admission ranged around 165. The presence of sugar in the urine occurred generally in the early afternoon. Her past charts indicated the same range. Her blood sugar level is being maintained in this range by the NPH insulin 30 units, one Orinase tablet (0.5 Gm.), and diet.

Since Mrs. R.'s blood sugar is still considerably above the normal level, fluctuations would most likely tend toward hyperglycemia, and, if severe, progress to diabetic coma. During this hospitalization, Mrs. R.'s blood sugar rose from 163 to 253, with the 11:30 A.M. Clinitests ranging from a trace to 4+. No characteristic symptoms of a progressing hyperglycemic state were noted. The increase in blood sugar and the glyosuria followed corresponding to the interval decrease of insulin dosage as ordered by the physician, possibly to retest her insulin requirements in diabetic control. On her last day of this hospitalization Mrs. R.'s blood sugar level was 187, so her maintenance dose of NPH was increased 5 units. Her new diabetic control regime consisted of 35 units of NPH insulin in the morning, one Orinase tablet (0.5 Gm.), and a regulated diabetic diet.

NPH insulin is an intermediate-acting insulin preparation. It may be referred to as isophane insulin suspension. The N indicates that it is a neutral solution, the P stands for protamine zinc insulin, and the H means that it originated in Hagedorn's laboratory. Its action places it between globin insulin and protamine zinc insulin. The onset of action is within 1 to 4 hours, and the duration is from 28 to 30 hours.

Orinase is generally used in the treatment of middle-aged or elderly patients with stable uncomplicated diabetes, commonly referred to as mild-adult, maturity-onset diabetes. Orinase lowers the blood sugar level by stimulating beta cells of the pancreas to produce insulin and by decreasing the amount of sugar released from the liver into the bloodstream. It is also helpful in controlling glycosuria, polyuria, and pruritus associated with diabetes. When Mrs. R. received Orinase, its effectiveness indicated some functioning beta cells in the pancreas.

Emotional aspects. Mrs. R.'s emotional reaction to her diabetic condition at present is one of acceptance and understanding. In discussing her diet, she

217

seemed well acquainted with various possible food exchanges and charts. Upon being administered insulin, she stated, "Oh, that is old stuff to me." Proof of her acceptance came when she displayed efficiently the complete technique of taking her own insulin the next day. She was quite familiar with the performance of the Clinitest, although her insulin dosage was not regulated by it.

Diagnostic tests. The diagnosis of diabetes is assumed in patients exhibiting a combination of chronic glycosuria and hyperglycemia. The diagnostic studies performed in relation to Mrs. R.'s diabetic condition were the admitting usinalysis, blood tests, Clinitest, and Acetest. Her urinalysis displayed a reaction of 6.0 and a specific gravity of 1.016, and the sugar and albumin were negative. Highly acid urine with a specific gravity of 1.025 to 1.045 and positive sugar are characteristics of uncontrolled diabetes.

Concerning blood tests, the white blood cells and red blood cells are generally normal in the diabetic patient. Of greater clinical importance is the blood sugar level. A fasting blood sugar was taken every morning to check Mrs. R.'s blood sugar level. It showed her progress and indicated whether adequate coverage was being given by the insulin administered. Her increase in the blood sugar during the decrease in insulin therapy displayed the necessity of more insulin for coverage. Her final maintenance dose was determined.

Urine specimens were required four times a day for the performance of a Clinitest and Acetest. The Clinitest is of clinical importance since it indicates the amount of sugar in the urine. Thus it may be presumed that the NPH insulin received at 8 A.M. taking effect in 1 to 4 hours did not give full breakfast coverage. The Orinase stimulation of insulin was efficient, depending on the presence of functioning beta cells.

The Acetest, in which 1 drop of urine is placed on an acetone tablet, varies in purple shades, depending on the concentration of ketone bodies. The finding is indicative of incomplete fat metabolism. It promptly detects both ketonuria and ketonemia, providing prompt warning of ketosis. Mrs. R.'s Acetests were all negative.

Prognosis. Mrs. R.'s prognosis is good. Although there is no conclusive evidence that diabetes mellitus is ever cured, she may anticipate a normal life expectancy. Although her underlying metabolic disorder may persist, she can compensate for it satisfactorily by means of balancing her activity level, dietary intake, insulin regimen, and Orinase therapy.

Plan of nursing care

Sample format. A plan of care was formulated on the day Mrs. R. was admitted (Table 13-1). It was evaluated, maintained, or modified from day to day to meet her changing needs and responses. The plan focused on the patient's therapeutic, physical, and psychologic needs and related nursing problems, both general and specific. Under therapeutic needs, nursing problems involving control of diabetes mellitus in the presence of infection were identified; under physical needs, relief of discomfort and elimination of infection were stressed; and under psychologic needs, emotional and intellectual processes were considered. Objectives of nursing measures were listed with nursing actions designed to meet these objectives, together with representative principles on which nursing action may be based.

The sample nursing care plan is by no means meant to be an exhaustive one, with all of the patient's nursing needs, problems, measures, and related principles included. Nor is the format meant to suggest any order of priority to be followed by the nursing team in meeting these needs. Rather, it is presented here as a sample or model that incorporates several phases of the problem-solving

Table 13-1 Sample nursing care plan

Identified needs and nursing problems	Objectives of nursing measures	Nursing measures	Applicable principles
THERAPEUTIC NEEDS *General problem* Control of maturity onset diabetes mellitus of 21 years' duration	To establish and maintain better control of Mrs. R.'s diabetes by adhering to prescribed regimen so that 1. Symptoms will be alleviated 2. Further complications will be prevented or delayed 3. Mrs. R. will be able to live within limitations imposed by diabetes after she leaves hospital	Observe patient for signs and symptoms of diabetic acidosis and hyperinsulinism	Insulin must be present for glucose to pass through cell wall to participate in cellular metabolism; hyperinsulinism results in hypoglycemia, hypoinsulinism in hyperglycemia
		Provide diabetic drug therapy, adjusting dosage according to dietary intake, activity, and prescribed control	Balance between dietary intake, activity, and available effective insulin promotes prescribed control of diabetes; infections increase insulin requirements but physical activities reduce it Insulin requirement is directly correlated with total caloric requirement
Specific problem Control of hyperglycemia, glycosuria, and perineal infection of 3 weeks' duration	To assist in control of hyperglycemia and glycosuria within prescribed ranges so that current and future need for diet and insulin can be regulated	Provide prescribed diet; observe and record type and amount of intake	Caloric requirements of the diabetic are same as the nondiabetic of same sex, size, and activity level Carbohydrate intake is matched to type and timing of insulin action to achieve maximum carbohydrate utilization
		Observe daily fasting blood sugar levels	Faulty glucose metabolism results in glucose accumulation in blood
		Administer intermediate-action insulin rotating site of hypodermic injection: NPH insulin 30 or 35 units o.d. as prescribed	Insulin facilitates entry of glucose into body cells; duration of action varies in individuals, depending on rates of absorption and unknown factors

Continued.

219

Table 13-1 Sample nursing care plan, cont'd

Identified needs and nursing problems	Objectives of nursing measures	Nursing measures	Applicable principles
		Administer Orinase orally: one Orinase tablet (0.5 Gm.) o.d.	Orinase lowers blood sugar by stimulating beta cells of pancreas to release insulin or by inhibiting glucose formation from liver glycogen
		Collect voided urine specimen, perform Clinitest and Acetest q.i.d.; observe and record results	Glycosuria, detected by Clinitest, indicates blood sugar level is above renal threshold Ketosis, detected by Acetest, indicates incomplete fat metabolism and impending acidosis and coma
PHYSICAL NEEDS *General problem* Relief of physical discomfort	To promote physical comfort by identifying, reducing, or removing underlying causes of discomfort when possible	Assess or estimate degree of discomfort perceived by patient by listening, observing, and recording changes as they occur	Sensations of physical discomfort indicate trauma or threat of trauma to body Levels of tolerance for pain and discomfort vary among individuals
Specific problem Relief of pain, swelling, itching of perineum caused by monilial perineal dermatitis associated with diabetes mellitus	To prevent further irritation to perineum from friction or micturition by relieving pruritus and eliminating infection present	Discourage scratching by providing diversional activities for Mrs. R.	Vulnerability to mechanical, chemical, or microbial irritation is increased in a diabetic individual
		Avoid unnecessary friction to area while applying medication or bathing	Friction to skin increases irritation Invasion of skin by microorganisms is likely to occur when normal protective mechanisms are broken down
		Apply topical agents to perineal area as prescribed by physician: Petroleum jelly, t.i.d. Calamine lotion, t.i.d. Aqueous gentian violet, 2%, o.d.	Topical agents affect skin locally by providing a protective coating; by acting as emollients and relieving symptoms of itching or burning; and by counteracting infection

		Fulvicin, 250 mg., q.i.d. Benadryl, 50 mg., b.i.d. Periactin, 4 mg., t.i.d.	effects by preventing fungus growth in new skin cells and by preventing physiologic action of antihistamine
		Observe and record effects and side effects of medications	Adjustments in types or amounts of medications may be indicated when desired effects are not achieved or when undesirable side effects occur
		Give potassium permanganate warm sitz bath twice daily, mornings and evenings	Application of heat assists in anti-inflammatory process and relieves discomfort by increasing metabolic rate and relaxing immersed muscles. Raising temperature of a liquid and adding a disinfectant lower surface tension of solution; the lower the surface tension, the better the penetrating power for cleaning
PSYCHOLOGIC NEEDS *General problem* Patient's negative attitude	To establish a therapeutic environment in which Mrs. R. will be able to change her attitude toward a more positive one	Demonstrate an accepting attitude toward expression of negative feelings; avoid direct contradictions of patient's statements	A nonjudgmental climate tends to facilitate communication. Hostile feelings tend to increase or be reinforced if met with further hostility
Specific problem Mrs. R.'s resistance toward being hospitalized for present illness	To identify cause of Mrs. R.'s resistance, if possible, and to identify related learning needs, if present; to help Mrs. R. recognize and accept her hospitalization so that she will be able to gain increased benefit from it and possibly decrease length of her present hospitalization	Listen attentively and attempt to find out how Mrs. R. perceives her situation and what she knows about her diabetic condition	Emotional reactions and organic illnesses interrelated; negative or hostile feelings may interfere with keeping desired control of metabolic process in diabetes
		Make pertinent explanations by building upon Mrs. R.'s present knowledge of her diabetic condition, its relation to her present illness, and her previous experiences with hospitalization	When an individual recognizes the need to learn, in relation to his personal situation and previous knowledge, learning tends to increase. Anticipation that desired effects will result from new behavior motivates desired changes in behavior

Identified needs and nursing problems	Objectives of nursing measures	Nursing measures	Applicable principles	Evaluation

Fig. 13-8. Sample nursing care plan (form).

process using the deductive scientific method. Any number of formats could serve equally well in developing a comprehensive nursing care plan (Fig. 13-8).

Establishing priorities. The nursing student who is learning to develop realistic and useful nursing care plans may often observe a tendency among nursing practitioners to list only the nursing action in a written plan. The unwritten nursing problems, objectives, and principles are presumably understood by the nursing staff, and very often they are not delineated for this or other reasons. The nursing student, on the other hand, is usually encouraged to form the habit of writing comprehensive plans as a student so that she will develop the habit of thinking in terms of comprehensive nursing care as a graduate.

Among other values accrued by the student in formulating nursing care plans is practice in establishing priorities in providing patient care. Many times a day, for one patient or a group of patients, the nurse must decide which aspect of nursing care takes precedence over another—which patient need requires immediate attention and which need can safely wait. Nursing care plans can contribute a great deal toward arriving at these decisions, particularly when they include written objectives and principles as well as nursing tasks. Thus the nursing instructor may frequently use a nursing care plan format designed to serve as a tool in guiding the student to select priorities, or to "put first things first" when providing nursing care.

SUMMARY

A nursing care plan is a detailed program of action, usually written, that is designed to achieve the objectives of care for a given patient. Formulated during the problem-solving process, a nursing care plan is based on recognized nursing needs or problems and related scientific principles. A typical plan, written or unwritten, includes the objectives of patient care and an outline of medical and nursing measures designed to meet these objectives. The plan involves the patient, a variety of health team members, and a variety of forms. It may be adapted to a variety of nursing service situations, and it may have more than one purpose. In addition to giving direction to patient care, a plan may be used to give direction to students' learning needs. A sample nursing care plan incorporating these dual purposes is given in Table 13-1, based on the data collected in the nursing care study of Mrs. R., the patient discussed earlier in this chapter.

QUESTIONS FOR DISCUSSION

1 What is a nursing care plan?
2 What are the purposes of a nursing care plan?
3 Who is involved in preparing and carrying out a nursing care plan?
4 How is a nursing care plan related to the objectives of nursing care? to scientific principles? to the problem-solving process? to establishing priorities of nursing care?
5 What are the sources of information a nurse can rely upon for initial development of a plan of nursing care?
6 How may a nursing care plan be affected by hospital staffing patterns such as team, case, or function? By the evaluation process as it is being carried out?
7 Using the format in Table 13-1, develop a brief written nursing care plan for a patient for whom you will provide care in the near future.

LIFE SITUATION

You are a nursing student who is acting as a member of a nursing team with two nursing assistants, one licensed practical nurse, and one registered nurse who is the team leader. The team members represent varying degrees of ability and levels of responsibility. In planning nursing care during team conferences, what is your attitude toward those having more ability than yourself? those with less? How do various levels of responsibility expected of group members affect your planning? How do you assist the group to establish priorities of nursing care? to evaluate the nursing care plan?

SUGGESTED READINGS

Aiken, Linda H.: Patient problems are problems in learning, American Journal of Nursing 70:1916, September, 1970.

Bower, Fay L.: The process of planning nursing care, St. Louis, 1972, The C. V. Mosby Co.

Cornell, Sudie A., and Brush, Frances: Systems approach to nursing care plans, American Journal of Nursing 71:1376, July, 1971.

Goldsborough, Judith: Involvement, American Journal of Nursing 69:66, January, 1969.

Haferkorn, Virginia: Assessing individual learning needs as a basis for patient teaching, Nursing Clinics of North America 6:199, March, 1971.

Hallburg, Jeanne C.: Teaching patients self-care, Nursing Clinics of North America 5:223, June, 1970.

Harris, Barbara L.: Who needs written care plans anyway? American Journal of Nursing 70:2136, October, 1970.

Mayers, Marlene G.: A systematic approach to the nursing care plan, New York, 1972, Meredith Corporation.

McPhetridge, L. M.: Nursing history: one means to personalize care, American Journal of Nursing 68:62, January, 1968.

Robinson, Lisa: Sick doctors and nurses are sick human beings, American Journal of Nursing 71:1728, September, 1971.

Schmidt, Joan: Availability: a concept of nursing practice, American Journal of Nursing 72:1086, June, 1972.

Sweet, Philothea R., and Stark, Irmagene: The circle nursing care plan, American Journal of Nursing 70:1300, June, 1970.

Vincent, Pauline A.: Do we want patients to conform? Nursing Outlook 18:54, January, 1970.

14 The patient's dismissal

PREPARATION FOR DISMISSAL

Dismissal from the hospital in most cases is initiated through formal permission written by the physician when the patient no longer requires hospital services. In a few instances a patient may wish to leave against the advice of his physician. To do so, he should sign a formal statement releasing the hospital and the physician from the responsibility for any complications that might result from his leaving. A patient may wish to leave in this way when he feels he cannot afford to remain in the hospital because of social or economic conditions or for other reasons.

The aim of hospitalization is to help the patient recover and return to his role as a contributing member of society. Upon departure from the hospital, the patient may have progressed sufficiently so that he may leave ready to resume his usual way of living. Or his condition may be such that he (1) may be transferred to another institution, (2) may need a private nurse at home or the services of a visiting nurse, (3) may depend on his family for nursing care, or (4) may depend on another social or health agency for help.

Very early in the patient's hospitalization, thought should be given as to what will be entailed in his dismissal. Some patients may be faced with a period of convalescence or an extended time of limited activity. Needs pertinent to the individual patient's dismissal should be identified soon enough to assure that a complete plan of care will be ready for his departure. In any case, however, the following appropriate questions are to be investigated:

1. Will he need special equipment or devices such as a brace?

2. If special items are needed, must they be ready by the time of his departure?

3. Will he need such items far enough in advance to receive adequate instruction in use before leaving the hospital?

4. Will he need to be taught how to give himself any medications such as insulin?

5. Do the patient and members of his family need instruction regarding a special diet or other treatments and activities to be continued at home?

6. Is referral to another agency indicated?

PROCESS OF DISMISSAL

Departure procedures are specified by the individual hospital to ensure that the hospital has met its responsibilities to the patient and that the patient receives all of his belongings and is safely on his way, thereby protecting both the patient and the hospital.

Dismissal of a patient from the hospital is a process that involves the cooperation of a number of people. Hospital departments concerned are the business office, the housekeeping department, the dietary department, and perhaps the social service department or others when needed. The social service department may make referral to another agency for further care of the patient. If a patient is unable to obtain needed equipment for home use, the social service worker may make arrangements for obtaining it. The social worker may also assist when the patient's home

conditions are such that basic health needs for rest and nourishment cannot be met. Unsuitable housing situations, poor sanitation, or faulty relationships may nullify even the most satisfactory plan for the restoration of physical and mental well-being.

The nurse may be the first person to recognize that the patient will need additional help after hospitalization, although referrals are usually made by the doctor or social service worker. However, nurses should know what social and health facility services are available in the community for meeting the patient's needs. Referral forms are usually filled out and signed by the physician.

The actual time of departure should be cooperatively planned a few days in ad-

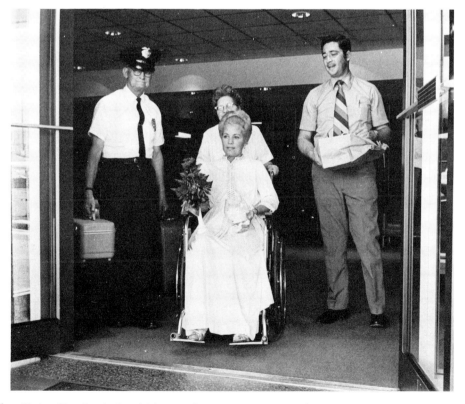

Fig. 14-1. Dismissal should be a pleasant experience for both patient and family. (Courtesy East Tennessee Baptist Hospital, Knoxville, Tenn.)

225

vance by the physician, the nurse, the social service worker, the family, and any other personnel involved in the patient's care. The type of transportation planned for the patient will depend on his condition. A patient usually leaves the hospital by automobile, although ambulance transportation may be arranged if needed. Usually a hospital attendant accompanies the departing patient to the exit, transporting him by wheelchair (Fig. 14-1). Use of a wheelchair is a wise precaution in most instances because the patient may be somewhat weakened by his illness and he may become fatigued or faint with exertion and the excitement of departure from the hospital.

PSYCHOSOCIAL ASPECTS
Dismissal experience

An experience of hospitalization, whether for a brief or a prolonged period, is one that makes a lasting impression on the patient. Just as the events involved in the admission of the patient remain vividly in the mind, so will various factors pertaining to dismissal be important in the remembrance of the total experience.

Disagreeable or unpleasant experiences that may have taken place during hospitalization may soon be forgotten if the patient has a smooth dismissal. Otherwise he may fear future hospitalization and also may make remarks about the agency to other prospective patients. Therefore it is essential that the best nursing care be provided for the patient until the very end of his stay.

Most patients are happy when informed that they can leave the hospital. Dismissal means to them that they can return to their families, friends, and familiar surroundings. However, a few patients may not be happy upon learning that they may leave the hospital because of the realization that they may be returning to a disagreeable job, to the responsibility of a large family, or to unpleasant interpersonal relationships. The patient may think that the time of convalescence will be uninteresting. Visitors might not be so frequent, the physician will not make his daily visit, probably no nurse will be present, and frequent gifts and flowers will no longer be received. Patients become accustomed to these and other daily attentions and may wish them to continue.

Illness brings about a certain amount of regression. Sick persons tend to become dependent and childlike. To return to self-reliance may be a big adjustment to some individuals. The patient usually is pleased with his own progress, anxious to return to his family, friends, and his previous position in the community—yet he is often hesitant to assume the responsibility for his own care and may be fearful that something will happen to retard the progress he is making.

A patient may fear that he has lost his job or that he will not be physically able to return to his former employment. He may fear that his illness will recur. He may wonder how long it will be before he has another acute episode of a chronic condition. Transference of a patient to a hospital for chronic conditions may have a distressing effect upon him, because he may think that there is no hope for his recovery. The nurse may, through encouragement, assurance, and understanding, impart to the patient a desire to live fully and to participate in former activities as much as possible (Fig. 14-2). Many patients with chronic conditions may develop new interests and live happy and useful lives. Understanding the patient's living conditions will aid the nurse in helping the patient make whatever changes may be necessary. With this kind of awareness the nurse will be better able to assist in working out the plan of care realistically with the family, the physician, and at times the social worker.

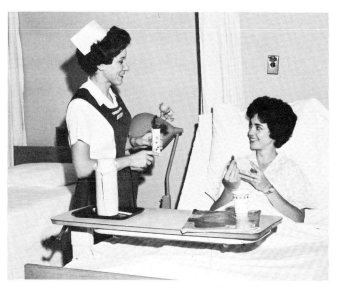

Fig. 14-2. Improvement in physical condition affects the patient's personality.

Postdismissal reaction

Any type of hospitalization limits a person's activity. It was shown in Chapter 6 that this inactivity interferes with normal biologic functioning.

After prolonged illness, muscles are weak and vitality is low. Exertion in any form may be tiring to the patient. This may cause the patient to be nervous, irritable, or demanding. A patient may feel quite well before discharge, but after being home for a few days he may have a relapse or find himself not so well. The probable reason for this may be that while the patient was in the hospital, he did not realize how much service was being provided for him. This is especially true of female patients who upon returning home may have to assume the responsibility of preparing their own meals and also caring for their families. The extra exertion or the sudden awareness on the part of the patient that he cannot yet perform his usual number of activities may produce an emotional response in him. The patient may cry or even become physically sick, yet no organic basis will be evident. This condition is sometimes referred to as "the

blues." It is quite common among surgical patients, stroke patients, and new mothers. The physician usually warns the patient to "take it easy," but with the eagerness to get home, the patient soon forgets his charge. The nurse can often reinforce the doctor's instruction and see that the patient has enough rest immediately before the trip home.

As a person increases in age, so does the time required for the return to normalcy following disease or disability. For the eager patient this can be very discouraging. It is hoped that more home-care programs with home visits by public health nurses or one from the hospital extended care service, will one day be routine for all patients.

FOLLOW-UP PROGRAMS

Medicare legislation has stimulated the rapid development of hospital-extension and home-care programs. Follow-up programs of this type have become popular partly because the link they maintain between the patient and hospital gives a feeling of security to the disabled patient and his family. When the patient's needs

227

are extensive and long-term care is necessary, his home becomes like an annex to the hospital. In this situation services needed by the patient at home may be provided by the hospital. Nonprofessional persons, perhaps family members, may be trained to care for the patient at home. The rising cost of hospital care has also been a stimulus to the development of these programs, since it is far less costly to care for the patient at home, when his condition makes it advisable, than it is in the hospital.

In an increasing number of hospitals a liaison nurse is being employed to provide continuity for necessary care, either at home or, if indicated, in an extended care facility, after the patient leaves the hospital. The liaison nurse, in cooperation with the physician and other members of the health team, helps to determine further care needed by the patient and interprets the plan of care to the family or staff of the extended care facility (Fig. 14-3).

In making a nursing care plan for the family, the nurse must assess the family's strengths and weaknesses as has been done in the hospital setting. The basic pattern is similar but the content will differ in relation to the home environment. In making plans for home care, the same principles of nursing care will apply.

There are certain environmental factors to be considered in each particular situa-

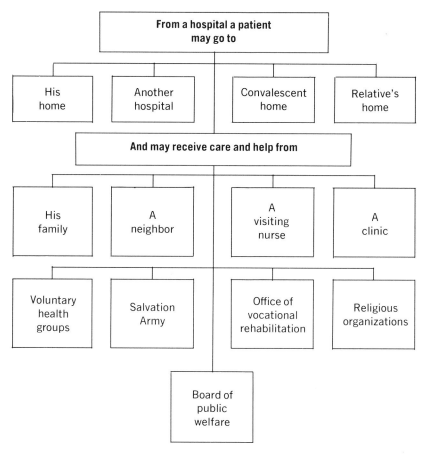

Fig. 14-3. Chart showing where a patient may go and from whom he may receive help.

tion as: (1) location of home in relation to neighbors and relatives, (2) availability of safe water supply and proper sewage disposal (indoor or outdoor toilets), (3) use of gas, electricity, oil, or wood for cooking, heating, and lights, (4) location of doors and windows and whether they are screened, (5) use of double or single beds and number of bedrooms, (6) stairs to be used in entering or leaving home or upon changing levels such as basement or split-level plans, (7) availability of telephone, (8) placement of furniture in relation to traffic through home, and (9) infestation of home with insects or rodents (may or may not be a problem but should be considered in environmental factors, since they seem to increase with other pollution factors).

Socioeconomic factors to be considered are: (1) number in family, (2) age and sex of each member, (3) life style of family, which involves bathing, dressing, eating patterns and food likes and dislikes, sleeping patterns, employment responsibilities of patient, spouse, and children, (4) amount and source of income, (5) general expenses of family, (6) level of education of family members, and (7) family health practices.

Tentative long-range goals are set to aid the patient to return to his life style of activity in the home and community. Short-term goals are set daily, weekly, or monthly, with the patient, family, and neighbors becoming involved. It is an accepted tenet in community health nursing that the nurse helps the patient and family to help themselves. The level of wellness may be one of total dependence on others or full independence with steps of the continuum based on the ability of the family to meet its needs with the help of available resources. These resources may be local, state, or federal (such as Medicare or Medicaid) or they may include friends and neighbors.

When the patient is discharged to an-

other institution, the new agency usually is responsible for the plan of care, but this does not relieve the first nurses from the responsibility of follow-up care. The nursing history and other necessary data should be provided for the new agency so that care may be continued with the fewest number of interruptions or interferences.

LEARNING SITUATIONS FOR THE PATIENT

Instruction, to be of value to the patient, should take place over a period of time and under less exciting conditions than that of departure. Instructions for treatments that the physician desires the patient to continue at home must be fully understood by him or a member of the family. The nurse interprets these directions to the patient and emphasizes the importance of following them. These final instructions may concern diet, treatments, medications, exercises, positioning, and other provisions for the patient's comfort and welfare.

The family may need to be impressed with ways of safeguarding the physical and emotional strength of the patient and with the importance of further care. Sometimes it is necessary to demonstrate a procedure that is to be continued at home. The nurse will demonstrate it to the patient, or to a relative, and assist him to perform it safely and effectively, using the kind of equipment that will be available to him at home.

When the patient is to be referred to another agency, the nurse should be able to explain the functions of that agency to the patient so that he will cooperate and receive the most benefit from the care to be received. If the patient is to return to the outpatient department, the nurse should be sure that he has written instructions including (1) the clinic that he is to attend, (2) the day on which he is to attend, and (3) the hour that he should attend. These instructions should be in written form.

SUMMARY

The important facets of the patient's dismissal from the hospital are handled cooperatively by the various members of the health team according to the policies and procedures established to safeguard both patient and hospital.

The nurse is an active participant in the dismissal process, being concerned with the preplanning necessary for assuring that the patient's departure will be as smooth as possible, with instruction of the patient and his family, and with assisting the patient in the last-minute preparations for leaving the hospital. The nurse's understanding of the psychosocial aspects related to the patient's readjustment following hospitalization will increase effectiveness in working with the patient and his family.

QUESTIONS FOR DISCUSSION

1 Why are dismissal procedures important? When should they be initiated?
2 Why are some patients unhappy upon dismissal?
3 Illness brings about emotional regressions. How is this shown at the time of dismissal?
4 What details of procedure are necessary to refer a patient to another hospital?
5 Where may a patient obtain a wheelchair for home use?
6 What adjustments will a family need to make for a patient who will need to stay in bed at home?
7 How would you explain to a patient the functions of the Visiting Nurse Association?

LIFE SITUATION

Prevention of disease with the promotion of a high level of wellness is the primary focus of the community health nurse in continuity of care. In the case of Mrs. Henry,* who suffered a cerebrovascular accident while visiting her husband in his office, the following information

*Fictitious name, narrative adapted from actual situation.

was of interest to the nurse who participated in her care at home.

History: Mrs. Henry, a 60-year-old white female, lived in a small rural town. While waiting in her husband's real estate office for him to join her for lunch, she became ill. Dr. B., whose office was next door, was called in and he diagnosed a "mild cerebrovascular accident with some slight paralysis of the left side."

He had the patient remain in the office for approximately 1 hour and then removed to her home. A registered nurse was called to accompany the patient home and give care.

Mr. and Mrs. Henry lived in a small five-room house with modern conveniences. Their daughter lived next door and Dr. B.'s house was next to the daughter's. Mrs. Henry's condition appeared to stabilize within a few hours and Dr. B. stated that she could have bathroom privileges, sit up in bed, and be up in a chair for 15 to 20 minutes as she desired. She was to have both passive and active exercises to the affected side.

One week following the initial attack, Mrs. Henry complained of nausea and dizziness and was removed to the nearest hospital, 40 miles away, for further tests and evaluation. Her loss of motion in the affected area had improved upon admission to the hospital, but after 3 days a gradual regression became apparent and she remained under care in the hospital for approximately 3 weeks.

She was discharged with a diagnosis of cerebrovascular accident, left hemiparesis with some ability to use lower extremity, and only a minimal loss of motion in upper extremity. There was some mental confusion but all vital signs were within normal limits. Blood pressure was 130/80 upon discharge.

The community health nurse was notified of Mrs. Henry's discharge and was asked to visit the home to help plan her care. Physician's orders included a full range of motion, rest for 2 hours in the morning and afternoon, a low sodium 1,500-calorie diet, and one Aldomet tablet each morning.

After visiting the home, the community health nurse made a temporary plan of care for Mrs. Henry. Immediate goals were: (1) to find someone to care for Mrs. Henry during the day while her husband worked, (2) to prevent further muscular weakness and contractures, and

(3) to initiate a low sodium, low calorie diet for Mrs. Henry.

Since it was during summer vacation, Mrs. Henry's granddaughters, ages 14 and 12 (children of the daughter who lived next door), agreed to take turns staying with their grandmother during the working hours of their grandfather. Their mother agreed to aid and supervise the children in the care of her mother and also to prepare the meals for the Henry family. The nurse showed the family how to position Mrs. Henry during her rest periods during the day and at night. She also left a printed diet sheet for her to follow. It was agreed that the nurse would return each day for a week or until the granddaughters learned how to help the grandmother with her exercises.

The nurse and the family followed the tentative plan of care (which was composed chiefly of executing the physician's orders) for several weeks, with the nurse revising or adding suggestions as indicated. The nurse noticed that all members of the family tended to "baby" Mrs. Henry, which hindered the long-term goal of returning the patient to her normal daily activities. The nurse therefore made the following suggestions to them: (1) to allow Mrs. Henry to eat meals at the family dining table rather than using a bedside tray, (2) to encourage Mrs. Henry to get things for herself, such as a drink of water, book, and the like, (3) to allow Mrs. Henry to start assuming certain duties as making her bed and helping with the cooking, and (4) to help Mrs. Henry get extra finger exercise by playing the piano, shelling peas, or knitting. Mrs. Henry had previously been the pianist for her Sunday school department.

The granddaughters were very successful in learning how to put their grandmother through a full range of motion, since the nurse had provided them with charts and instructions (similar charts appear in Chapter 19). As a result of their success, each was able to be away for a short camping trip during the summer. A neighbor was kind enough to prepare the Henry meals for the Fourth of July weekend so that the daughter and her entire family could go on an outing.

In the course of events, some weeks were fine and others not so successful. Mrs. Henry did not always stay within her diet. She would forget to take her medicine, so the children had to stick a pin on the calendar and move it each day after she had taken the tablet. Some days the granddaughters would be very helpful, others they would spend most of their time on the telephone. Mr. Henry did not always do the washing exactly right or run the vacuum so that it pleased Mrs. Henry.

Visits to the home became less frequent as the patient assumed more of her household duties. Twelve months from the date of hospital discharge, Mrs. Henry was again able to function as a wife, mother, and community leader. She was again able to drive her car to local stores and meetings; however, she thought it best to let the substitute pianist continue in her old position since she had had to miss so many Sundays at church.

Questions:

1 Had you been the community health nurse, what changes, additions or omissions would you have made in the plan of care?
2 Had Mrs. Henry's daughter not lived so near to her mother, how would you have proceeded to have secured help for the family?
3 Why was it so important for Mrs. Henry to take her medication so regularly since her blood pressure appeared to remain stable?
4 Outline a teaching plan for teaching a relative how to position a patient and to execute a full range of motion.
5 Do you feel that the granddaughters assumed too much responsibility in the care of their grandmother? Give reasons for your answer.
6 What accidents might occur during the care of a stroke patient and how can they be prevented?
7 What are the physiological and therapeutic actions of Aldomet? What are its side effects?
8 How do you suppose Mr. Henry reacted to the situation?
9 How do you suppose the daughter's husband reacted to his wife's spending so much time away from home?

SUGGESTED PERFORMANCE CHECKLIST
Comfort

1 Is assistance given with dressing, if needed?
2 Is clothing suited to the weather?

3 Is assistance given with assembling belongings, if needed?

4 Is the bed patient offered the bedpan before leaving?

5 Are tact and kindness shown?

6 Is the patient reassured regarding his condition?

Therapeutic effectiveness

1 Is the attitude of the patient good?

2 Is excessive excitement prevented?

3 Is provision made for further care, if needed?

4 Does the nurse show courtesy and kindness?

5 Are the physician's orders interpreted?

6 Are the instructions sufficient about future appointments and care?

7 Is the chart completed accurately?

Economy

1 Has the office been notified beforehand?

2 Is a wheelchair or stretcher provided?

3 Are medicines and equipment for home use ready beforehand?

4 Is unused medicine returned to the pharmacy?

5 Has the dietary department been notified?

6 Is equipment returned to proper places?

7 Is the unit stripped at once?

8 Is a record transferred with the patient, if necessary?

9 Is the chart sent to the record room at the appointed time?

Safety

1 Has the physician's dismissal order been checked?

2 Is the proper form filled out for self-release?

3 Was the family properly notified?

4 Are all belongings returned in proper order and signed for?

5 Is the proper conveyance used from the bed to the exit?

6 Does a hospital attendant accompany the patient to the exit?

7 Is the proper conveyance used to take the patient from the hospital to his home?

SUGGESTED READINGS

Canaday, Mary E.: SSPE—helping the family cope, American Journal of Nursing 72:94, January, 1972.

Deakers, Lynn P.: Continuity of family-centered nursing care between the hospital and the home, Nursing Clinics of North America 6:83, March, 1972.

Fielo, Sandra, and Edge, Sylvia C.: Technical nursing of the adult medical surgical and psychological approaches, New York, 1970, The Macmillan Company.

Kinoy, Susan K.: Home health services for the elderly, Nursing Outlook 17:59, September, 1969.

Leaky, Kathleen M., and others: Community health nursing, ed. 2, New York, 1972, McGraw-Hill Book Co.

Mayers, Marlene Glover: A systematic approach to the nursing care plan, New York, 1972, Appleton-Century-Crofts.

Nielsen, Sharon: Home visiting for patients receiving special care, Nursing Clinics of North America 7:383, June, 1972.

Tinkham, Catherine, and Voorhies, Eleanor F.: Community health nursing evolution and process, New York, 1972, Appleton-Century-Crofts.

Tyzenhouse, Phyllis: Care plans for nursing home patients, Nursing Outlook 20:169, March, 1972.

UNIT THREE

Principles related to adaptive response

15 Comfort and rest

CONCEPT OF COMFORT

Comfort is sometimes described as a subjective state in which there is a sense of mental and physical well-being, with freedom from pain, want, or anxiety. It is adversely affected by sensations of physical distress or pain and by dissatisfaction related to the individual's psychologic or physiologic disequilibrium. Conversely, comfort is likely to be achieved by measures alleviating mental or emotional distress as well as by those relieving physical pain or discomfort. The implication in this concept is that the mental and physical elements of the individuals are so integrated that the same causative factor may produce both physiologic and psychologic responses that are experienced as physically uncomfortable sensations.

Merely to achieve the appearance of the "patient being made comfortable," although important, is not of itself a sufficient nursing goal. Morning care of the patient may leave him bathed and clean with fresh linen, with the general appearance of resting, and his unit in order. These hygenic measures may have succeeded in providing for the immediate comfort of the patient. However, for meeting the long-term comfort needs, the underlying causes of discomfort in each instance must first be recognized, and then measures can be provided for reducing the discomfort effectively.

For instance, consider the situation of the patient, Mrs. Lewis, and the nurse, Miss Hunt. Miss Hunt's immediate impression is that Mrs. Lewis has had an uncomfortable night because she presents a generally disheveled appearance with hair and linen rumpled, anxious expression, agitated manner, strained position, labored breathing, and a statement that she is "miserable." If Miss Hunt is exercising common sense she may decide that the giving of routine morning care will restore comfort for Mrs. Lewis, and she may assign this function to a nursing assistant. But if Miss Hunt were to assess the situation, guided by the knowledge necessary to recognize the less obvious causes of physical and psychologic discomfort, and even of possible dangers, she would have identified potential needs that are beyond those satisfied by routine ministrations and that necessitate skillful intervention in order to achieve long-term comfort, rest, and safety for Mrs. Lewis. She would have been able to recognize the possibility of at least these factors: (1) need for thorough measures of positioning and skin care to prevent friction and pressure leading to

235

tissue breakdown and decubitus ulcer formation, (2) bladder distension and constipation resulting from Mrs. Lewis' inability to use a bedpan in the unaccustomed position of bed rest, (3) improper positioning for physiologic body alignment, which, together with the pressure of a distended bladder and colon, produces compression of her chest and results in labored, inadequate respiration, (4) decreased oxygen supply needed for cellular metabolism, (5) muscle tension that could be relieved by full range of motion and proper positioning, and (6) psychologic or social factors contributing to Mrs. Lewis' agitation, which might be alleviated if the causes were recognized.

This hypothetical situation illustrates the point that comfort and safety factors are often interrelated and that the importance of immediate physical comfort may be secondary to the need for preventing long-term serious effects that may endanger the patient. The nurse must be aware of the necessity to provide for both comfort and safety factors, establishing the priority of needs to be met. Thus, in Mrs. Lewis' situation, the implementation of immediate measures to relieve the distension and inadequate respiration would be more important than an immediate bath and change of bed linen. Also, Miss Hunt would be aware of the significance of the communication between herself and the patient and would use her interaction to gain needed information about Mrs. Lewis in assessing the meaning of her response to discomfort and illness. The interaction would then become more purposeful and goal-directed.

The nurse must first recognize the causes of discomfort, identifying the comfort measures indicated, while simultaneously establishing the generally higher priority safety needs of the patient. The next step is to implement appropriate nursing action. The ability to recognize the need for measures to promote comfort, safety, and rest and to initiate nursing intervention is based on knowledge and application of principles drawn from the biologic, physical, and behavioral sciences. Proficiency in the skills of observation and communication, together with knowledge of the underlying principles, serves as a tool that the nurse uses in collecting significant information, identifying existing problems, setting priorities, and implementing appropriate intervention.

SELECTED BIOLOGIC AND BEHAVIORAL PRINCIPLES

Many scientific principles can be identified from the biologic and behavioral sciences that are helpful in understanding, to considerable depth, the relationship of comfort and rest to maintaining or restoring homeostasis. However, this chapter is less concerned with the exploration of contributing scientific facts and theories than it is with describing the role of the nurse in providing for the physical comfort and emotional well-being in the context of meeting the needs of the total person. Therefore, the following statements have been selected for their usefulness in translating concepts into nursing action that is generally applicable in any illness setting.

1. Comfort and well-being of the individual are dependent upon both physical and psychologic factors.

2. Pain and other sensations of physical discomfort may indicate injury, or impending injury, to the body with threat of homeostatic imbalance.

3. An individual may perceive any change or threat of change in normal physiologic or psychologic function as a menace to his life.

4. The sensation of discomfort or pain may be elicited by several stimuli: mechanical (such as pressure against pain receptors), chemical (such as metabolic wastes of cellular activity), and thermal stimuli.

5. Sensations of pain and discomfort may cause restlessness, irritability, insomnia, and emotional tension.

6. Periods of decreased activity, such as sleep, are necessary for cellular restoration.

7. An individual's perception of pain is affected by his emotional attitude toward pain.

8. Discomfort may result from the tension created by the continuation of unmet needs.

9. During illness the primary physiologic needs of the individual (including oxygen, water, food, rest, exercise, elimination) may become a strong motivator of his behavior:

a. These physiologic needs are prerequisite for his continued existence.

b. Priority must be established for meeting these physiologic needs.

c. Individuals vary in their ability to tolerate need deprivation.

10. An individual may be helped to achieve a feeling of comfort and safety in a situation through:

a. Increasing his knowledge about the situation before it occurs

b. Physical care ministrations, which can be used to develop a trusting relationship

c. Supportive relationships with others to whom he may verbalize about the situation

d. The experience of approval and acceptance by the "significant others" in the situation

e. Ability to communicate his needs to a trusted person in the situation

11. Those needs creating the greatest threat to homeostasis should be given priority over those of less import to the welfare of the individual.

COMMON CAUSES OF PHYSICAL DISCOMFORT

The causes of discomfort in illness may be quite simple and easily counteracted or very complex and difficult to explain and relieve. Discomfort and pain may be associated with the existent pathology and the bodily reactions to it and to the psychologic stresses attending hospital admission.

Physical conditions causing discomfort that are commonly encountered by the hospitalized patient include the following.

Nausea. The stimulus for vomiting is usually an irritant in the stomach or duodenum, such as a drug; mechanical stimulation of the pharynx; neurologic or hormonal changes; or changes in carbohydrate metabolism. Such stimuli result in a sensation of nausea that may be followed by vomiting.

Distension. A distended bladder and/or a colon distended by gas and accumulated feces will increase the intra-abdominal pressure, which may be the source of considerable discomfort.

Hunger. The hungry patient is an uncomfortable patient. For example, in hypoglycemia the uncomfortable visceral sensation indicating the body's need for food may be very unpleasant.

Thirst. This uncomfortable sensation is experienced in a marked degree when the oral mucous membranes are dry and the salt concentration of body fluids is increased.

Coughing. The cough reflex is protective in that it keeps the respiratory passages free of obstructive particles. However, it may become exhausting or be self-perpetuating through continued irritation of the trachea and bronchi, or, if paroxysmal, it can cause strain of thoracic and abdominal muscles.

Vertigo. Dizziness, or a feeling of light-headedness that may precede syncope (fainting), occurs in a variety of conditions, including hypotension, hypoglycemia, hypoxia of the brain, or decreased blood level of carbon dioxide.

Headache. Headache is usually perceived by the individual as a painful sensation and is one of the most common of ailments. It may accompany many conditions, including emotional distress.

Muscle tension. Muscle fatigue or spasm may result from improper positioning or emotional tension. This may contribute to restlessness and insomnia.

Pain. Pain is an unpleasant sensation that should always be investigated, evaluated, and reported.

External sources of discomfort can include a great many factors impinging on the patient, although patients may react to these stimuli in a variety of ways and with varying degrees of intensity. Among these factors are the following.

Personal hygiene needs. Dry, coated oral mucous membranes of the mouth not only cause discomfort but may also be a source of possible infective exudate. A weary, restless, perspiring patient with rumpled, soiled bed linens may experience relief from morning care with bath and change of linen skillfully administered.

Improper positioning. An improper position may cause muscle and joint discomfort and may contribute to a variety of other undesirable physiologic effects.

Pressure. Pressure from casts, bandages, and other appliances may be the source of considerable pain and even of actual danger to the patient.

Environmental factors. A great many different environmental factors may be disturbing to a particular patient, such as ventilation, noises, lights, odors, disturbing sights, or behaviors of other patients. These factors may contribute to restlessness, irritability, and emotional tension.

OBSERVATION AND EVALUATION OF DISCOMFORT

Observing for signs of discomfort. An individual may be aware of the source of his discomfort and may be able to communicate with the nurse about it if he receives encouragement to report and discuss his physical needs with the nurse.

When the hospitalized patient is unable to report his needs, he is dependent upon the nurse for observation, evaluation, reporting, and intervention in his behalf. It is particularly important for the nurse to observe the patient for signs and symptoms of physical discomfort when the patient is (1) unconscious, (2) suffering from an illness prone to development of complications, (3) at the extremes of age, or (4) not responsible or having difficulty communicating for any reason.

Nonverbal communication and symptoms that should alert the nurse to the presence of physical discomfort include (1) restlessness, crying, moaning, (2) unusual quietness or withdrawal behavior, (3) unusual position, (4) facial expression, (5) changes in the color and temperature of the skin, (6) respiratory changes such as increased, decreased, or irregular respiration, (7) nausea and vomiting, (8) anorexia, (9) excessive perspiration, (10) rubbing or scratching, (11) insomnia, and (12) behavior changes (for example, depression or irritability).

Evaluating physical discomfort. Complete information about the patient's discomforts should be gathered as accurately as possible and evaluated in relation to such significant factors as the patient's age, his general physical condition, his diagnosis and the commonly associated discomforts and complications, his emotional status, and his attitude toward his illness. Any new, severe, or sudden pain, any discomfort not quickly relieved by nursing measures, or any discomfort related to casts, bandages, or any orthopedic device should be reported promptly.

NURSING MEASURES FOR RESTORING COMFORT

When the nature of the patient's discomfort has been identified and evaluated the nurse may then intervene appropriately to relieve or minimize the discomfort and try to prevent complications.

Whatever is done *for* the patient should be planned *with* the patient when possible, with every effort being made to involve him in the decision-making process. Knowledge of what is to be done and why, with the feeling that he has some control over the situation, will help to restore his feeling of ease and comfort that may have been disrupted by the illness situation and hospitalization.

While listening to the patient will give the nurse many clues as to the dimensions of the patient's problem, it will at the same time help the patient to gain some control over his anxieties and frustrations. When a trusting relationship has been established, the way is open for the nurse to convey an attitude of caring and concern that encourages the patient to express his feelings and also encourages family members and other visitors to gain understanding and comfort through the nurse's explanations and response to their concerns. In a climate of trust and confidence, family members and friends may be of considerable assistance in providing the support needed by the patient in restoring and maintaining physical and emotional comfort.

To be successful in meeting the special needs of individual patients, the nurse's approach will depend among other factors upon the patient's personality, his family background, and his current home and work situation. By listening to and communicating with the patient, information can be learned about his likes and dislikes in regard to food, sleep, personal hygiene, and the like, and this can be used by the nurse in providing a therapeutic environment that promotes comfort and well-being. In this caring, intervening role the nurse is sometimes said to be the patient's advocate, being in a unique position to recognize his needs and assure that the care he receives is in his best interest. In a very real sense the nurse is the patient's go-between within the institution in representing his needs and interests to other personnel.

More specific measures helpful in alleviating common problems of illness and associated discomforts of illness are discussed in the remaining chapters of this unit.

LEARNING SITUATIONS FOR THE PATIENT

In the presence of physical and/or emotional discomfort, the degree to which an individual is ready to learn may be difficult to assess. For the patient who is uncomfortable or in a period of emotional depression, teaching efforts may be quite ineffective or may even have the effect of increasing the patient's fatigue and depression. Consider the example of Mrs. Jones, a young woman recently diagnosed as a diabetic. She is still in a state of depression and anxiety, fearing that she will be an invalid, unable to care for her three small children. Until Mrs. Jones is able to accept the situation, it is probably better to administer care with little emphasis on actual teaching. When Mrs. Jones is emotionally ready, she will be able to adjust to the changes her diagnosis entails and will be able to develop the skill and judgment necessary to assume responsibility for her own diet and insulin regulation and also the remaining facets of her self-care after she goes home.

SUMMARY

In this chapter, the role of the nurse in restoring and maintaining physical comfort has been presented. Content has been selected to emphasize the importance of knowledge of relevant principles in understanding and providing for the comfort needs of the patient.

As with other needs, promotion of comfort is often complex and interrelated with the satisfaction of other physiologic and psychologic requisites of the patient. The importance of providing for both physical comfort and safety needs is emphasized.

The identification and evaluation of the signs and symptoms of discomfort and patient involvement are presented as basic to the decision-making process in nursing intervention.

QUESTIONS FOR DISCUSSION

1 What is the meaning of comfort? of rest?
2 What principles from biologic and behavioral sciences can you identify that are relevant in understanding comfort needs?
3 How is the knowledge of homeostasis useful in providing for the comfort, rest, and safety of the patient?
4 What can you suggest as a significant guiding principle to use in establishing priority of the patient's needs?
5 What behaviors can you suggest for the nurse to employ in creating a trusting relationship with the patient?

LIFE SITUATION

Suppose you are the nurse in our example of Mrs. Lewis. From your initial assessment of her condition, you affirm that she has four major nursing problems. The first is inadequate respiration impeded by improper positioning and increased intra-abdominal pressure; the second is bladder distension and constipation associated with difficulty in using the bedpan; third is the threat of decubitus formation caused by pressure of improper positioning and lack of exercise; and fourth, muscle tension also resulting from improper positioning.

In this situation, what further information is needed in evaluating Mrs. Lewis' condition? What nursing objectives will you define? In planning and organizing your nursing intervention to accomplish these objectives, which of them will likely need your most immediate attention?

Probably you will discover that there is some overlapping among these priorities that necessitates flexibility in making nursing decisions as the plan of care is implemented and the patient's condition changes.

SUGGESTED READINGS

Fass, Grace: Sleep, drugs, and dreams, American Journal of Nursing 71:2316, December, 1971.

Hrobsky, Arthur: The patient on a CircOlectric bed, American Journal of Nursing 71:2352, December, 1971.

Isler, Charlotte: Decubitus/old truths, and some new ideas, RN 35:42, July, 1972.

Williams, Donald H.: Sleep and disease, American Journal of Nursing 71:2321, December, 1971.

16 Hygienic care

PHYSICAL AND PSYCHOLOGIC HOMEOSTASIS

As implied in an earlier chapter, the concept of physiologic homeostasis, involving such processes as blood circulation, fluid balance, and nutrition, may be used in identifying scientific principles applicable to the nursing care of the patient, and it is therefore helpful to direct physical nursing care toward maintaining or restoring homeostasis. However, in maintenance of homeostasis at "high levels of wellness," the critical factors are generally considered to be personal practices related to cleanliness, rest, sleep, exercise, nutrition, elimination, and recreation, as well as emotional equilibrium. Knowledge of these factors and their rational application by any individual are significant in his achieving and maintaining an optimum level of health. When illness or injury occur with associated disequilibrium of homeostasis, certain of these important factors may become even more crucial and at the same time more difficult to practice because of the resulting functional limitations affecting the individual.

In the illness situation the nurse is confronted with the responsibility of assisting the patient to cope with the problems encountered in maintaining his personal hygienic practices in the presence of the limitations imposed by his specific illness or trauma and in relation to the degree of his understanding regarding their importance.

Elements of the nursing process have already been presented, with emphasis on the use of scientific principles in the problem-solving activities of the nurse, regardless of the setting within which one functions. Even though scientific attitudes and techniques are necessary for the solution of a patient's health care problems, to be fully effective as a practitioner, today's nurse must preface the assumption of patient care responsibility by preparation for dealing with the patient's psychologic stresses as well as with his physical needs, if the relevance of the concept of psychologic homeostasis is accepted. The nurse must be cognizant of the role that anxiety plays in the patient's tendency toward regression and dependency in illness, the persistent feelings of discomfort that may be experienced by the patient in response to anxiety, and the resulting patient behavior that confronts the nurse.

Regression is a mechanism through

which the patient unconsciously seeks to cope with the anxiety engendered by the care he may be receiving. When the ill person enters the hospital, he is immediately confronted with the necessity of adjusting to his new role of being a patient, which may mean surrendering some or all of his independence. Even the moderately ill patient soon discovers that he is dependent in some degree upon the hospital staff for the supplying of his physical needs, including the daily ministrations that heretofore he had performed for meeting his own intimate personal hygienic requisites at the time, place, and manner of his own choosing and usually in privacy. Now, he finds he is guided into hospital routines that may or may not be what he would choose for himself, and perhaps this happens without his express wishes having been considered—meals, baths, bedpan, treatments, medications—all of which he may feel he is expected to passively accept in uncomplaining cooperation with the hospital staff. Through regression and increased dependency the patient may be able to tolerate this loss of his adult prerogative in the process of adjusting to his patient role. For the patient who feels he must always be in control, dependency on others represents loss of control, which tends to increase his feeling of discomfort from the resulting psychologic imbalance.

Much is appearing in current nursing literature through which the nurse can increase personal understanding of the psychologic aspects of the care of patients and of the principles underlying interpersonal relationships and the interaction involved; therefore these and related topics are not detailed here. Attention in this chapter is, however, focused on the independent nursing functions available to the nurse in supplying hygienic care and comfort for the patient and on understanding of the scientific basis for these practices.

INDEPENDENT NURSING INTERVENTION

Independent professional nursing responsibilities universally include supervision of the patient and management of his care, based on the exercise of judgment. Again it is emphasized that the nurse bases judgments and intervention in behalf of the patient's welfare on the intelligent assessment of his needs and on knowledge of appropriate underlying principles. In the preceding chapters, techniques have been described that are available to the nurse for (1) assessing the needs of patients and identifying related nursing problems, (2) collecting further information about the patient's identified problems, (3) developing an appropriate nursing care plan in terms of the data collected and relevant nursing principles, (4) implementing the nursing care plan to provide optimum quality of nursing care for individual patients, and (5) evaluating the success of the nursing care plan and adjusting it to meet the patient's changing needs.

This supervision implies that the nurse has a vast amount of ethical and legal responsibility for determining and implementing safe and effective patient care that lies outside the physician's realm of medical diagnosis, prescription, and implementation of therapeutic measures. In most cases the provision of hygienic and comfort measures is a nursing responsibility for which no written medical prescription is needed. So then the nurse independently plans the patient's daily activities to include provision of personal hygienic care and nursing measures for the relief of discomfort, setting priorities and exercising professional judgment in the care of each patient. The nurse also participates in carrying out the physician's therapeutic orders that may have been prescribed for the patient and refers to the physician pertinent observations and information about the patient. Those nursing functions prescribed by the physician are usually termed *dependent* (or restorative) in contrast to the *independent* (supportive, preventive, and rehabilitative) nursing functions that are presented in the various chapters throughout Units One to Three. Very often dependent and independent functions are combined as, for instance, in providing adequate nutrition and elimination. The independent functions are usually performed by the nurse functioning as a member of the health team and of the nursing team.

SUPPORTIVE NURSING MEASURES

Personal practices considered most significant in maintaining homeostasis are usually referred to as supportive nursing measures because their objectives are related to meeting the physiologic and psychologic needs of the patient arising from the stresses imposed by the illness or injury. These practices usually include measures relating to cleanliness, comfort, rest, sleep, exercise, diversional activities, nutrition, elimination, and emotional equilibrium.

The method of carrying out these hygienic practices in the illness situation often requires modification because of the patient's condition, particularly when bed rest has been prescribed, but their significance may be even greater than in health when imbalance in homeostasis caused by the disease process has occurred. The aim of supportive nursing measures is to assist in maintaining or restoring homeostasis.

The following are daily hygienic practices in illness for which the nurse is usually responsible, for either their provision or supervision:

1. Those related to cleanliness and personal appearance:
   a. Bathing and care of the skin
   b. Care of the mouth and teeth
   c. Cleanliness of the eyes
   d. Care of the hair
   e. Care of the nails

2. Those related more directly to body functioning:
   a. Supplying food and fluids
   b. Providing for elimination
3. Those more related to the environment:
   a. Bedmaking
   b. Regulation of sanitation
   c. Safety, atmospheric, and esthetic factors
4. Those related to prevention and rehabilitation, depending on the nature of the individual patient's problems, the medical evaluation, and the prescribed therapy. (Preventive and rehabilitative measures may require both dependent and independent functioning of the nurse. They include measures for comfort, rest, sleep, exercise, diversional activities, and instruction and psychologic support for the patient.)

The following discussion is primarily concerned with those measures affording personal cleanliness, comfort, rest, and exercise.

APPLICATION OF SCIENTIFIC PRINCIPLES

Basic principles can be identified that make promotion of cleanliness and care of the body and its appendages more effective for all patients, although the nurse would need to seek out additional principles pertinent to the specific hygienic and comfort needs of individual patients. The ability to identify and utilize principles pertinent to the specific needs of individual patients is emphasized because understanding of the relationship between the particular problem and relevant scientific concepts enables the nurse to exercise sound judgment for making decisions regarding actions in performing effective nursing intervention. The principles, hypotheses, and facts relating to the situation can be used by the nurse to help the patient either maintain or achieve his health potential in the particular circumstance.

It is intended that these examples of very basic principles will stimulate the student to pursue thoroughly and exhaustively the study of scientific principles and their application to nursing problems in each situation encountered, making this study an integral facet of the whole approach to nursing practice. Surely the techniques of applying scientific principles to the problem-solving process will be a means through which one may develop professional nursing competence, both for today and for the ever-increasing complex and scientific nursing world of tomorrow.

Biologic sciences

The following selected principles are universally applicable in this context:

1. The body's total resistance to stress is enhanced by decreasing the demands placed upon it. Periods of decreased activity allow body cells to restore themselves.

2. An adequate supply of oxygen and nutrients is essential for the normal functioning of all body cells.

3. Substances are transported to and from the body cells in response to changing demands of body tissues. The circulating blood is the transporting agent; therefore a decrease in functioning of any tissue results from a decrease in the volume or pressure of circulating blood.

4. Systemic circulation of the blood can be promoted by massage, by muscle contraction during exercise (passive or active), and by postural changes.

5. A horizontal body position tends to provide the most effective systemic circulation, with the least demand upon the cardiovascular system.

6. The amount of body heat lost through evaporation and convection is affected by the amount of skin exposed, the presence of moisture on the skin, and the surrounding environmental temperature and air currents.

7. Soft, supple skin depends on the presence of a normal amount of sebum, the oily substance produced by the sebaceous glands (Fig. 16-1).

8. Unbroken, healthy skin and mucous membranes present a more or less impassable barrier to microorganisms and other harmful agents. The amount of resistance will vary with different individuals.

9. Some bacteria are found normally on the surface of the skin and are present in body cavities and passages having direct connection with the surface of the body. (Organisms isolated from normal, healthy skin include staphylococci, diphtheroids, gram-positive bacilli, and many varieties of saprophytic fungi. These microorganisms are able to enter the body only through a mechanical or chemical injury.)

10. Soaps and detergents lower the surface tension of water, thereby increasing its wetting capabilities. This wetting aids in the emulsification of fats by the soap; excessive use of these agents for cleansing tends to dry and irritate the skin.

11. Skin and mucous membranes tend to react to the presence of irritants by inflammatory response.

Behavioral sciences

Basic concepts drawn from the behavioral sciences have been selected; such concepts should be helpful to the nurse in developing understanding of the function of human needs as they relate to psychologic homeostasis and to observation of the patient for planning individual patient care. Principles that may be used in planning nursing care are those that:

1. Demonstrate attitudes of acceptance and approval for the patient
2. Increase the patient's feelings of comfort and safety
3. Provide adaptations for the individual patient's particular needs and limitations

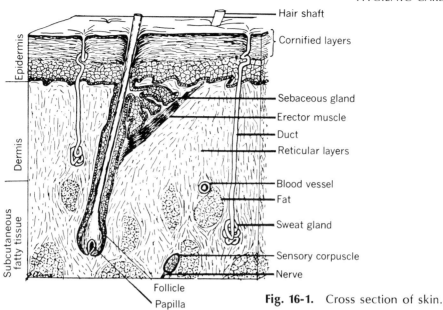

Fig. 16-1. Cross section of skin.

4. Assign priority to those needs that are the most intense

5. Allay the patient's fears, frustrations, and discomforts

6. Motivate the patient to resume independence and responsibility for his own care as his condition permits

Principles applicable are the following:

1. Psychologic homeostasis for the individual is promoted by (a) acceptance of himself and his individual differences by others, (b) the feeling that someone cares about him, and (c) the feeling of interaction with others and the sharing of experiences with them.

2. An individual is likely to respond in a manner similar to the way in which he is approached by others.

3. The individual's needs and response patterns may be altered by illness and hospitalization.

4. In physical illness certain needs may be increased and may also become more difficult to satisfy.

5. A feeling of comfort and safety in any situation promotes the establishment and maintenance of psychologic equilibrium for the individual.

6. Feelings of comfort and safety are engendered for the individual by (a) experiencing a sense of self-identity and self-esteem, (b) knowledge and understanding of the facts about himself and the situation, (c) understanding of the action to be taken in the situation, (d) opportunity to make decisions regarding himself, and (e) opportunity to communicate one's needs with assurance that help is available for satisfaction of the needs.

7. All components of the individual are interrelated, and therefore the individual tends to respond as a whole and with the best response he is able to make at that time.

Regardless of the particular procedure being carried out with the patient, the nurse will have the opportunity to apply the above principles. Often the procedure itself can be used as a vehicle for establishing communication with the patient and initiating meaningful interaction. For instance, the nurse may choose to give a bed bath to a particular patient personally, rather than delegating this responsibility to another team member. The nurse can then interact with the patient according to his individual needs in this situation and apply the principles listed previously or other appropriate principles based on assessment of the patient's needs.

SUGGESTIONS FOR TECHNIQUE

Application of some of the stated principles have been illustrated in earlier paragraphs of this chapter; in the following discussion others may be noted. Many additional applications of principles will be encountered in actual patient care.

Providing for the patient's bath

Several methods of bathing are available to the hospital patient, depending on his condition. They include the cleansing bed bath for the patient confined to bed, the tub bath, and the shower bath.

The bed bath. The cleansing bed bath (sometimes called a sponge bath) can produce several beneficial effects. The following benefits are related to relevant principles that have been stated before.

1. The most obvious effect is cleansing of the skin to remove accumulated perspiration, secretions, microorganisms, and debris from the skin. Removing these accumulations, which can act as culture media for microorgansims, may assist in preventing infection as well as in preserving the healthy, unbroken condition of the skin.

2. The bath can be comforting, refreshing, and relaxing to a tired, restless patient.

3. The stroking motions applied to the skin tend to stimulate circulation, both systemically and locally.

4. The accompanying exercise produces muscle contractions that help to maintain muscle tone and joint motion.

5. Elimination from the skin is promoted.

6. The exercise and change of position tend to alter rate and depth of respiration, which increases the oxygen intake and helps to prevent lung congestion.

7. Assisting the patient to appear well groomed tends to improve his self-esteem; he is then more likely to interact with others in the situation.

The bath should never be thought of as "just another routine" that can be done by anyone. Rather, the nurse should view it as probably the greatest opportunity that any member of the nursing team will have for spending time with the patient. Therefore it is used to evaluate the mental and physical state of the patient. The nurse who is skillful in observing will be able to gather information of value in improving and updating the plan of care for the patient. Time spent with the patient during the bath can be extremely worthwhile, since it gives the nurse an opportunity to listen to the patient, to consider his questions, to communicate with him, and to give him appropriate instructions and emotional support (Fig. 16-2). When patient care assignments are made, the nurse should give careful attention to the level of functioning of the various team members. The patient who is in need of nursing expertise for assistance in coping with the stresses of illness, both psychologically and physiologically, should be assigned to the nurse who is most able to assume this responsibility. Thus the team leader personally might choose to give the bed bath to the patient. Professional judgment and insight are necessary for the nurse making patient care assignments in order to provide the best care available for all patients.

The amount of rest or activity required by the patient, as determined through prescribed medical treatment and nursing assessment, should be used in determining the kind of assistance the patient will need with the bath. For the patient requiring complete bed rest the bath should be administered expeditiously with the minimum amount of exertion. The equipment and procedure will vary with the patient and the hospital; however, the following suggestions for technique may be helpful.

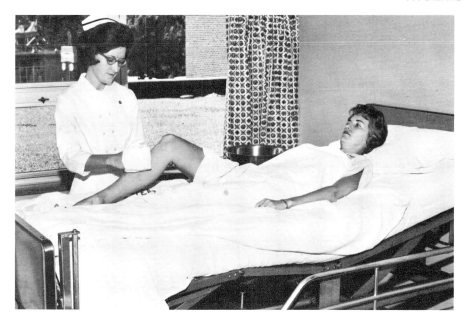

Fig. 16-2. Firm but gentle strokes are necessary to make the bed bath effective. A mitten is used, or a washcloth is palmed to avoid dragging its wet, cold ends over the skin.

The patient's unit should be warm and free from drafts. All needed equipment should be at hand and conveniently placed before beginning the procedure so as to avoid leaving the patient unnecessarily until the entire procedure has been completed. Instructing the patient as the bath progresses will help to conserve his energy by avoiding unnecessary exertion and uncertainty on his part.

The temperature of the bath water should be adjusted for the comfort of the patient, and the water should be changed at intervals to maintain a comfortable temperature and to avoid the drying effect of soapy residue left on the patient's skin. Privacy should be provided by screening and draping the patient to avoid his embarrassment. Only a small area of the body should be exposed and bathed at a time, and use of the bath blanket and towel for draping will also help in keeping the bed linens dry. The washcloth should be held with the corners tucked securely in the palm of the hand to avoid dragging its cold,

wet ends over the skin. Long, smooth strokes with the maximum pressure in the direction of venous return, for example, from the hand toward the shoulder, should be used in washing and drying each part of the body, rather than short, jerking motions. Support should be given to the joints in lifting each arm and leg while washing and drying these parts. Normal range of motion of the joints and muscles can be provided either as passive or active movements during the bathing of the various parts of the body, except when contraindicated.

Placing the patient's hands and feet in the basin is a desirable practice because it is refreshing and promotes more thorough cleansing of the fingernails and toenails, thus minimizing danger from pathogenic microorganisms, which tend to lodge in crevices and under fingernails. Clean, well-rounded fingernails and toenails for both patient and nurse are important. Nails, however, should be trimmed with great care so that the lateral mar-

247

gins lie beyond the distal part of the nailfold to avoid ingrown nails or infections (Fig. 16-3). In some conditions, such as diabetes, the nails should be trimmed only with medical sanction because of the increased susceptibility to trauma and infection.

The patient's entire back should be thoroughly washed and dried and the skin inspected over bony prominences. A nonalcoholic lotion may be used in massaging to avoid excessive drying of the skin. Dusting powder may be used in moderation to absorb moisture and to act as a lubricant between opposing skin surfaces. The powder tends to lessen friction and excoriation. The axillae should be cleansed thoroughly to remove the organisms thought to be most responsible for decomposition of organic material generally regarded as the cause of disagreeable body odors. The patient may wish to use a deodorant in the underarm areas. A deodorant is also an antiperspirant when it contains an astringent, such as aluminum sulfate, that tends to decrease the flow of perspiration.

All skin surfaces should be included in the bathing process, with special care being taken in cleansing and drying creases, folds, and bony prominences, since these parts are most likely to be excoriated by moisture, pressure, friction, and the presence of irritating substances.

The decision about the general order in which the various parts of the body are bathed is based on esthetic concepts as well as on the concept of cleanliness, by proceeding from the area apt to be cleanest to the area that is apt to be least clean. For example, the upper parts of the body would be bathed before the lower parts. If the patient is not able to wash the perineal area, the nurse would wash this area for the patient as the last part of the bath. If surgery has been performed on this area, sterile perineal care may be required and is often carried out at this time.

Pleasant accessories to the bath may have a favorable effect on the patient—cosmetics, a different hair arrangement, and an attractive gown or bed jacket. A desire for cosmetics, attractive pajamas, and, for the male patient, a fresh shave can nearly always be interpreted as an indication that the patient is beginning to think of returning to his place in the community. For the male patient facilities for shaving should be offered as often as needed.

The frequency and time at which a cleansing bath is given should be adjusted for the comfort of the patient as much as possible and upon the physician's orders. For some very critically ill patients the exertion of a complete bath might be too exhausting, but a partial bath might be tolerated. Another patient with very dry skin might prefer a full bath only every other day. Modified daily hygiene usually includes bathing the face and hands, axillae, and back, with massage over any bony prominences. In almost every case, oral care should also be included.

Principles relating to body mechanics that have been described in the preceding chapter should be consciously applied by the nurse in personal position and motions, in the arranging of equipment and the working area, and in positioning of the patient during the procedure.

The self-administered bath. The patient may be encouraged to begin assisting with his bath, or to take a "self-bath" in bed,

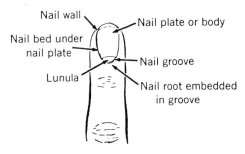

Fig. 16-3. The nail and its surrounding structures.

when he is physically ready for some exercise or when it is not desirable for him to have a tub bath or shower. Care should be taken to prepare the patient emotionally for the self-bath so that he will understand that this is a way of providing needed exercise for him and that it is a desirable step toward resuming his independence. Whether the patient accepts the self-bath on this basis depends on the nurse's attitude and approach, which may avert the unfortunate inference a patient might otherwise think that the nurse is either too busy or just does not want to give the bath. When a self-bath is to be taken, the equipment should be arranged and an explanation given to the patient as to how he can proceed with the bath most conveniently.

The shower or tub bath. A shower bath may provide a more desirable amount of exercise for some patients; a tub bath may be indicated for cleansing or for therapeutic reasons. The shower or tub should be prepared for the patient, with sufficient instruction and supervision to ensure safety and hygienic or therapeutic effectiveness of the bath. The established hospital procedure should be observed for the various types of tub baths, such as the sitz bath or medicated baths. The nurse should always remain with the patient who is likely to become faint; for example, for a postsurgery patient having a first sitz bath, the warmth of the bath could cause fainting by a circulatory reaction in which the supply of blood is decreased in the vital centers of the brain and diverted to the peripheral circulation (Table 16-1).

Providing for oral care

The oral cavity is the entrance to the alimentary tract, respiratory passages, and parotid glands and may therefore be a portal of entry for pathogenic microorganisms. Healthy, clean mouth, gums, and teeth promote the patient's comfort and sense of well-being and tend to promote his self-esteem. In addition to their

Table 16-1 Temperatures for tub baths

Type of bath	Temperature
Excessively cold	40°- 50° F. (4.4°-10.0° C.)
Cold	50°- 60° F. (10.0°-15.5° C.)
Moderately cool	60°- 70° F. (15.5°-21.1° C.)
Slightly cool	70°- 84° F. (21.1°-28.8° C.)
Neutral	84°- 88° F. (28.8°-31.1° C.)
Tepid (lukewarm)	88°- 95° F. (31.1°-35.0° C.)
Warm	95°-105° F. (35.0°-40.5° C.)
Hot	105°-110° F. (40.5°-43.3° C.)

psychologic effect, healthy teeth play a role in proper nutrition since they are necessary for mastication of food.

The patient should have oral care after meals and before retiring. It is also refreshing before breakfast if one has been accustomed to this practice. Equipment that might be used by the bed patient includes toothbrush, dentifrice, mouthwash, curved basin, and towel. The patient is usually able to brush his own teeth if positioned comfortably, with the equipment conveniently arranged for his use. If the patient is unable to brush his teeth, the nurse should give as much assistance as necessary. The toothbrush, or cotton applicator used as a substitute, should be applied gently to avoid abrasion of the gums.

Dentifrices cleanse the mouth through mechanical action by removing food particles and debris from the mouth rather than by chemical action on bacteria. Mouthwashes also have more esthetic than bacteriologic value, because they are neither sufficiently strong nor held in the mouth long enough to kill bacteria. They may help to remove particles loosened by brushing the teeth and are refreshing.

Lack of oral hygiene and insufficient fluids in illness, particularly in the case of mouth breathing, may result in the tongue and gums becoming coated. Frequent and

249

persistent cleansing of the entire mouth is necessary to avoid further accumulation of microorganisms, dried mucus, and food particles, known as *sordes.* This unpleasant condition can be prevented by frequent cleansing of the mouth, perhaps as often as every 2 hours and after meals. Sordes is very much more easily prevented than treated once it has become established. In febrile conditions the lips tend to become dry, cracked, or crusted and also need to be cleansed and lubricated.

Oral care is essential for the patient with artificial dentures. Many patients who wear dentures are sensitive about them, and privacy should be provided while the dentures are being cleansed. Many patients prefer to care for the dentures themselves and can do so if the equipment is provided for them. Otherwise, the nurse should wash them. In cleaning dentures they should be held firmly because water reduces the friction between the teeth and fingers and the dentures are likely to slip and be broken. Care should be taken to avoid applying excessive pressure to any part of dentures, particularly the lower plate. It is safe to clean them over a basin of water. A denture should be dipped in cold water to prevent friction with the mouth and to help it slide easily into place. While the dentures are out of the mouth, a mouthwash should be offered. Dentures should be kept in a safe place when out of the mouth; a small opaque jar makes a good container.

Providing for care of the hair

Care of the hair should be a regular part of the daily hygiene. The purpose of routine care of the hair is to maintain cleanliness, to prevent matting, and to promote comfort. The process of combing and brushing the hair is to remove accumulations of lint, dandruff, and the like and to exercise the scalp.

Equipment needed to care for the hair consists of a clean comb and brush. A comb with both coarse and fine teeth is best, the coarse teeth being used for removing tangles and the fine teeth for removing lint. If the hair is tangled, a little alcohol will aid in loosening the tangles because it tends to dissolve the oily accumulation matting the hair. In case of the acutely ill patient, caring for the hair gives the nurse an opportunity to inspect the scalp and the hair for any condition needing treatment. If the hair is long, it may be combed and braided once a day. If it is short, it may need to be combed more often.

Few women are indifferent to the arrangement of their hair, although they may hesitate to discuss their feelings. The appearance of the patient should always be considered when caring for the hair. A comfortable and becoming hair arrangement gives the patient a sense of being well groomed.

Normal hair and scalp are neither dry nor oily and show little evidence of flaking, and the hair has a natural sheen. The hair normally is kept soft and pliable by the secretion of the sebaceous glands of the scalp, which open into the hair follicles. When the hair and scalp are healthy, there is a constant replacement of falling hair by new growth. The growth of a scalp hair is approximately 1 inch a month, and the average duration of a hair is about 4 years. The general health affects the growth of hair and when the vitality of the body is lowered, the hair suffers in proportion. Illness, especially with fever, worry, and grief, tends to affect the state of the hair. Various endocrine abnormalities and imbalances greatly influence the growth and distribution of hair.

When a person must remain in bed for a long time without a shampoo, the hair becomes sticky and heavy and acquires a sour, unpleasant odor, which may be quite distressing to the patient. A shampoo can be given with almost no exertion on the part of the patient and is usually very satisfying, particularly to the woman patient. Liquid soaps are ordinarily used for shampooing because they are easily rinsed from the hair. Soap emulsifies the oil of the hair and permits it to be washed out easily. A vinegar or lemon rinse softens the water and helps to remove all soap. For a bed shampoo, water and liquid soap, a protector for the bed (such as a shampoo trough), and something for the water to flow into (such as a pail or foot tub) are needed. In combing and shampooing the patient's hair, the nurse should apply the principles related to body mechanics. Positioning the patient close to the edge of the bed will minimize reaching and straining on the part of the nurse. However, the patient should be adequately supported to avoid the danger of falling out of bed. Most hospitals have a specific written procedure that will serve as a guide in carrying out the details of the shampoo.

When the hair is combed evidence possibly indicating the presence of *pediculosis capitis,* which is infestation by the head louse, might be noted. The condition is most apt to occur in children, and its presence is suggested by scratch marks about the scalp, particularly back of the ears, and by nits (eggs) that look like tiny white flakes adherent to the hair shafts. The condition not only is annoying to the individual but also is a hazard because the scratches made by the patient as a result of the local itching may become infected. The existence of this condition may be very embarassing to the patient. His feelings should be spared as much as possible. Many parasiticides that kill the pediculi are available, but some do not affect the nits, which if left will hatch and continue the infestation. For this latter purpose, vinegar (acetic acid) may be used because it dissolves the gummy substance surrounding the nit and attaching it to the hair. When the presence of pediculi is suspected, the condition should be recorded. The physician will prescribe the treatment of choice for the individual patient. There is currently a significant rise in the number of reported cases of pediculosis.

LEARNING SITUATIONS FOR THE PATIENT

A degree of caution should be exercised by the nurse in planning instruction for the patient that will be acceptable to him. It is important to find out first how much the patient already knows about the intended instruction and what his level of understanding is in the matter. Otherwise, the patient may feel that the nurse is "talking down" to him if instruction is attempted on subjects about which he is already knowledgeable.

Some patients may ask questions regarding the value of certain highly advertised products used in personal care. When the nurse is unable to answer questions about specific products or cosmetics, it is appropriate to suggest obtaining further information through such sources as the pharmacy.

The observant nurse will also note whether it is important to explain to the patient that the hands play an important role in the spread of disease and will encourage the patient to use the facilities provided for handwashing and care of the fingernails.

Each patient's instructional needs should be carefully considered and a plan prepared for him based upon his individual needs. The teaching plan should include participation by any other members of the health team who are best qualified to work with the particular patient for an area of teaching content. It is also emphasized that the nurse should be very sure of the validity and relevance of whatever is planned to teach the patient before undertaking the responsibility.

SUMMARY

Basic physical care and emotional support of the patient may be considered in relation to their significance in maintaining or restoring homeostasis. Critical factors in maintenance of homeostasis at "high levels of wellness" are considered to be personal practices associated with cleanliness, rest, sleep, exercise, nutrition, elimination, and emotional equilibrium.

Through independent nursing intervention the nurse seeks to assist the patient in meeting his hygienic, physical, and psychologic needs arising from the stresses imposed by illness or injury. Dependent nursing functions are those prescribed by the physician. Often dependent and independent functions are combined, and they are usually performed by the nurse functioning as a member of the health team and of the nursing team. Examples of basic principles have been selected from the biologic and behavioral sciences to illustrate how understanding of the relationship between the particular nursing problem and relevant scientific concepts enables the nurse to exercise judgment in making decisions for the performance of effective nursing intervention.

A constant commitment of the nurse toward developing sensitivity of perception in recognizing the process and effects of stress in the patient is encouraged. The nurse strengthens such a commitment by keeping it uppermost in mind while planning, implementing, and evaluating the plan of care for the patient.

QUESTIONS FOR DISCUSSION

1 Describe a correct technique for brushing the teeth.
2 Evaluate the advertising claims for popular mouthwashes and toothpastes, indicating whether the claims are well founded for each product. Give supporting evidence for your statements.
3 Identify and illustrate with stick figures the major applications of the principles of body mechanics for the nurse while administering a bed bath. A tub bath.
4 After leaving the bedside, record as accurately as possible your conversation with a patient while you were giving direct patient care. Determine whether you have established and maintained communication with the patient. Discuss your recording and conclusions with your instructor.
5 Identify at least one principle from the biologic sciences and one from the behavioral sciences, not already stated in this chapter, that you consider to be relevant to meeting the daily hygienic needs of your patient.

LIFE SITUATION

Mr. Jones, a 45-year-old man, has been hospitalized for 3 days with a diagnosis of peptic ulcer. He is on bed rest. The nursing assistant reports to you (you are the team leader) that Mr. Jones does not want a bath today because he does not want to be "any trouble." How would you evaluate the patient's needs?

SUGGESTED PERFORMANCE CHECKLIST
Comfort

1 Does the nurse's attitude demonstrate concern for the patient?
2 Is proper attention given to the nurse's own personal hygiene and grooming?
3 Is privacy provided?
4 Is exposure prevented?
5 Are lotions and powder used in back care if indicated and acceptable to the patient?
6 Are the ends of the washcloth held in the hand?
7 Is firm, even pressure used in rubbing?
8 Is drying of the skin thorough?
9 Is soap rinsed off well?
10 Are hands and feet immersed in water?
11 Have extra pillows been removed from under the head during the bath?
12 Is hair well combed and arranged?
13 Is oral care adequate?

Therapeutic effectiveness

1 Is the patient comfortable?
2 Are all parts of the body clean?
3 Is the patient unduly fatigued?
4 Are the nails clean?

5 Does the hair look neat and feel clean?

6 Has the patient's mouth been cleansed?

7 Does the nurse provide an opportunity for the patient to talk?

8 Does the nurse listen and try to interpret the feelings of the patient?

9 Is order maintained during the procedure?

10 Is the unit left in order?

11 Is the nurse skillful?

12 Does the nurse inspire confidence?

13 Is the nurse gentle in touch?

14 Is the patient's call signal within reach?

15 Does the patient look well groomed?

16 Does the patient express a feeling of well-being?

17 Is diversion provided for the patient when indicated?

18 Are unusual symptoms reported?

19 Is charting complete? accurate?

Safety

1 Did the nurse wash her hands before beginning morning care?

2 Are the nurse's fingernails smooth and well rounded?

3 Is the environment warm, with no drafts?

4 Is the nurse continually making pertinent observations?

5 Is the bedding protected from dampening?

6 Is the water changed often enough to ensure a cleansing process?

7 Is the water changed often enough to keep it at a temperature comfortable for the patient?

8 Is support given the extremities?

9 Is the patient kept in good position?

10 Is the back rubbed well?

11 Is care given to the nails?

12 Is the hair handled gently?

13 Is effective care given to the mouth?

14 Is care used in handling dentures?

15 Is special attention given to skin over pressure areas?

16 Is the nurse's posture consistent with principles of body mechanics?

Economy

1 Are all materials assembled before beginning?

2 Is the bedding protected?

3 Is the bedpan offered before beginning?

4 Is there sufficient water in the basin?

5 Is needed equipment replaced?

6 Are materials put away properly?

7 Is linen protected during combing of the hair?

SUGGESTED READINGS

Davis, Ellen D.: Give a bath? American Journal of Nursing 70:2366, November, 1970.

Olson, Edith V.: The hazards of immobility, American Journal of Nursing 67:780, April, 1967.

Peterson, Donald L.: Developing the difficult patient, American Journal of Nursing 67:522, April, 1967.

Robinson, Lisa: Psychological aspects of the care of hospitalized patients, Philadelphia, 1968, F. A. Davis Co., p. 5-25 and 35-52.

Temple, Kathleen D.: The back rub, American Journal of Nursing 67:2102, October, 1967.

Wexler, Louis: Gamma hexachloride in treatment of pediculosis and scabies, American Journal of Nursing 69:565, March, 1969.

17 Nutrients and fluids

The need for food and water is common to all living organisms. Many health agencies employ nutritionists or dietitians to be responsible for planning and organizing food services. The nurse may rely on these health team members for meeting many of the patient's dietary needs. The nurse will, however, need a knowledge of the fundamentals of nutrition and the digestive processes to assist in meeting the patient's health needs as well as personal needs.

Medical or nursing problems of the patient may be directly or indirectly related to nutrition and digestion. A patient with diabetes mellitus, for example, has special dietary needs arising from faulty metabolism of certain food components, whereas a patient with a fracture may have special dietary needs resulting from the inactivity caused by the fracture. But whatever the specific cause, a commonly encountered general nursing problem is to promote adequate nutrition to all body tissues.

The specific purpose of this chapter is to review briefly some aspects of the nutritive process and of fluid and electrolyte balance as a framework for studying the responsibilities of the nurse in dealing with the patient's nutritional needs. However, many details of the complex process of metabolism are omitted here, for it is assumed that related courses in physiology, chemistry, and microbiology will provide greater depth for the study of nutrition.

SCIENTIFIC PRINCIPLES

Nutritional processes are the sum of the physical and chemical activities by which the body uses food for energy, maintenance, and growth. It includes all of the processes necessary for survival of even the simplest living single cell organism—respiration, ingestion, digestion, absorption, circulation, synthesis of new materials, breakdown of materials for energy, response to the environment, excretion, and reproduction. The human being, however, is a complex organism whose multiple cells cannot exist independently

254

but must carry out their complex activities through intricate coordination mechanisms with other cells.

The normal distribution and composition of body nutrients and fluids are necessary for the structure and environment of the cells. All cells require a continuous supply of oxygen, water, and nutrients for maintaining their functions. Oxygen must be supplied moment by moment, whereas in health nutrients are stored to a varying degree within the body so that the cells may be supplied as needed. The kidney functions within limits to regulate the volume and composition of the extracellular fluids. Basic to the nurse anticipating and meeting the nutrient and fluid needs of patients with understanding is some knowledge of the normal mechanisms for maintaining the constancy of the internal environment and the manner in which these mechanisms are altered during illness.

Selected principles from the biologic and social sciences have been included to assist in understanding the significance of nursing responsibilities for determining and meeting the related needs of patients in supplying foods and fluids. Other relevant and useful principles are readily identifiable.

Principles from biologic sciences

Physiology, anatomy, and chemistry are areas from which the following statements have been selected:

1. Normal cellular activity requires a consistent supply of oxygen, nutrients, and other vital chemicals:
   a. As structural materials for all cells of the body
   b. As a source of energy for activity of the body
   c. For synthesis of the regulatory substances, such as hormones and enzymes

2. An optimal nutritional state is maintained by the regular intake of a diet sup-plying the essential nutrients in amounts adequate for the individual.
   a. *Carbohydrates,* as a source of energy
      (1) Small amounts are stored in the body as glycogen.
      (2) An excess beyond the body's immediate need is stored as fat.
      (3) A small fraction of the available carbohydrate is used for synthesis of some regulatory substances.
   b. *Fats,* as the most concentrated source of energy, continuously available from the stores in adipose tissue
      (1) Excess calories from the individual's diet are stored as fat.
      (2) When the diet supplies fewer calories than are needed, adipose tissue will furnish some of the additional needs.
   c. *Protein,* as essential for tissue synthesis and regulation of certain body functions
      (1) Proteins are made up of building units, the amino acids.
      (2) The essential amino acids must be supplied in diet because the body is unable to synthesize them.
      (3) Proteins are not stored in the body to any extent.
      (4) Plasma proteins, albumin and globulin, are essential in maintaining the osmotic pressure of the blood.
   d. *Mineral elements,* as substances that enter into the structure of every cell of the body and that are necessary for efficient cellular functioning
      (1) Some mineral elements are constituents of enzymes, such as iron in cytochromes, and of hormones, such as iodine in thyroxine.
      (2) Some mineral elements are associated with maintenance of osmotic pressure and cell permeability that influence water bal-

255

ance between intracellular and extracellular spaces, maintenance of acid-base balance, ability of cells to respond to stimuli, and contraction of muscles.

(3) A dynamic equilibrium between intake and excretion of an element is maintained provided the supply of nutrients is adequate.

e. *Vitamins*, as organic substances essential for growth and normal metabolism

(1) Each vitamin has specific functions.

(2) Some reactions in the body require several vitamins; one vitamin cannot substitute for another, though lack of one can interfere with the function of another.

(3) When taken in larger amounts than the body needs water-soluble vitamins are excreted in the urine.

3. Water is a medium of all body fluids.

a. In health, homeostatic mechanisms balance water intake against water loss.

b. Definite amounts of water are essential to maintain the fluid balance of the body. Death is likely to follow water deprivation of more than a few days.

c. All the physiochemical changes that occur in the body cells take place in the environment of the body fluids, which normally are regulated within narrow limits.

(1) Water is essential in the hydrolysis that occurs in digestion.

(2) Nutrients and cellular wastes are soluble in water. Nutrients are carried to all cells and wastes are removed to the lungs, intestines, and skin.

(3) Water is the end product in the oxidation of glucose.

(4) Water is a factor in regulating

body temperature by taking up heat produced in cellular activity and distributing it throughout the body.

(5) Water functions as a body lubricant, for example, mucous secretions of the gastrointestinal and respiratory tracts.

4. Precise amounts of certain electrolytes and proteins are required by body cells for efficient functioning and are distributed in all body fluids within the so-called normal range for each.

a. The major cations are sodium, potassium, and magnesium. Sodium is the primary cation in extracellular fluid, potassium is the primary cation in the intracellular fluid.

b. The major anions are chloride, bicarbonate, phosphate, sulfate, and protein. The principal balancing anions in extracellular fluids are chloride and bicarbonate. The principal balancing anions in intracellular fluid are protein and bicarbonate.

c. Precise concentrations of intracellular potassium and extracellular sodium are essential to fluid balance and acid-base balance.

5. The primary function of the kidney is to maintain electrolyte balance by regulating the volume and composition of extracellular fluid through selective reabsorption and elimination of water and electrolytes in the tubules.

a. Deviations either upward or downward from the so-called normal range will have adverse effects on body functions.

b. Sodium chloride may be lost through both urine and excessive perspiration; therefore, diaphoresis can increase the required intake of sodium.

6. When the balance between intake and output of water is disturbed so that more water is lost from the body than is replaced:

a. The extracellular fluid is decreased in

volume and, therefore, is hypertonic in relation to the intracellular fluid.

  b. The resulting increase in osmotic pressure causes intracellular fluid to move from the cell to the extracellular fluid.

  c. The kidney secretes concentrated urine that is decreased in volume.

  d. Circulatory collapse and death will follow if the water deficit continues to the point that failure of the body's adaptive mechanism occurs.

7. When the intake of fluid is greater than the excretion, the concentration of plasma albumins is reduced, with resulting decrease in the osmotic pressure causing fluid retention in the tissue spaces (edema).

8. Hunger is a physiologic state in which the individual is aware of the need to ingest food, feels the unpleasant contractions of an empty stomach, salivates, and displays food-searching behavior. Anorexia is the absence of hunger.

9. Appetite is less related to physiologic activity than is hunger; a psychic desire for food is implied.

10. The extent to which hunger and appetite are affected by hormonal and other biochemical changes in the body or to cultural and social factors is not completely understood.

Principles from behavioral sciences

1. The behavior of an individual is affected by his nutritional state.

2. Most individuals tend to prefer foods they learned to eat as young children and may resist changing their food habits. Established food habits are difficult to alter.

3. The patient may be resistant to necessary changes in his diet when professional staff members display indifference, criticism, or hostility toward him.

4. An individual may eat or not eat to satisfy psychologic needs; he may eat or refuse to eat in order to gain attention or

to gain some measure of control over others.

5. Motivation for eating is based on individual needs, attitudes toward food, and the meaning food has for the individual.

6. Knowledge about a nutritious diet is usually not sufficient by itself to effect change in eating habits of the individual.

Cultural factors play a major part in assessing the patients' nutritional needs and are of importance to both dietitians and nurses in diet planning, preparation, and service. Eating habits usually change during illness. Appetite may range from extreme hunger to complete lack of interest in food. Illness can be a cause or result of malnutrition, and treatment is directed toward alleviating both. Thus with the assistance of the health team a patient may eat better-balanced meals when ill than when well.

The pathway of digestion

Mechanical and chemical processes interact simultaneously during digestion. The digestive canal (Fig. 17-1) is composed of the mouth, esophagus, stomach, small intestines, and large intestines. In the mouth are the tongue, teeth, and salivary glands. Taste buds are found on the tip, edges, and back of the tongue. The tongue is composed of voluntary muscle covered with mucous membrane, and it helps to move the food about in the mouth and in swallowing it. The teeth grind the food, as the lower jaw is moved by muscles that control its action. Saliva contains a starch-splitting enzyme, amylase (ptyalin), which converts starch to sugar.

The mouth connects with the stomach by the pharynx and esophagus. The stomach is a dilated portion of the alimentary tract. Its walls are muscular, and it is capable of distending in order to hold the food that enters it. Food remains in the stomach from 1 to 4 hours, depending on the nature of the food. With the exception of alcohol,

257

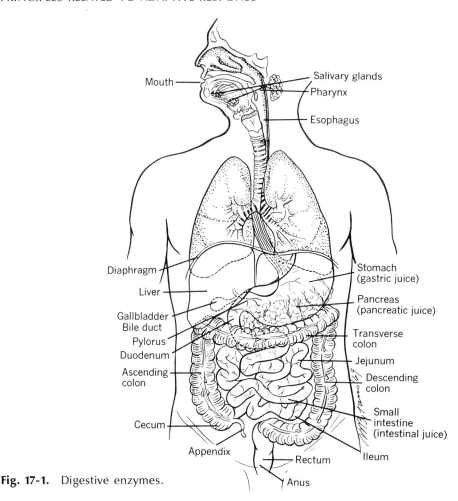

Mouth
Salivary glands
Pharynx
Esophagus
Diaphragm
Liver
Stomach (gastric juice)
Pancreas (pancreatic juice)
Gallbladder
Bile duct
Pylorus
Duodenum
Transverse colon
Jejunum
Ascending colon
Descending colon
Cecum
Small intestine (intestinal juice)
Appendix
Ileum
Rectum
Anus

Fig. 17-1. Digestive enzymes.

food is not absorbed from the stomach. The churning action of the stomach breaks up solid food into smaller particles. Chemical changes take place because of the enzymes in the gastric juice. These enzymes act especially on proteins. Gastric secretions are stimulated by the sight, taste, and odor of food.

The pyloric sphincter guards the passage into the small intestine, which is a long, tubular organ having muscular walls. Further churning in the intestine breaks up the food and mixes it with digestive juices from the small intestine, pancreas, and liver. These secretions act on starches, sugars, proteins, and fats. The end products of digestion are absorbed into the circulation,

and the remaining contents are propelled along to the large intestine.

The large intestine absorbs water from the contents and aids in expelling the undigested and indigestible residue from the body. This residue is composed chiefly of cellulose from carbohydrates, connective tissues from meats, and undigested fats.

The process of absorption of food is by diffusion and selective action of cells. The rate of absorption varies with pressure, the size of the area for absorption, and temperature. Warm fluids will be absorbed from the stomach and intestines faster than cool ones. The enormous area in the intestinal tract permits rapid absorption of food.

Fluid and electrolyte balance

The fluid of the body is composed of water and electrolytes. Electrolytes, often referred to as salts or minerals, develop positive and negative electrical charges (cations and anions respectively) when dissolved in water. These charges balance each other electrically in the fluid compartments of the body. Exchanges of water between these compartments is dependent on the concentration of electrolytes and resulting osmotic pressure regulation. Body fluid is contained in two major compartments, the cellular fluid within the cells and the extracellular fluid. Extracellular fluid is contained in (1) plasma within the blood vessels and (2) interstitial fluid outside the vascular system and the cells.

Physiologic homeostasis within the body requires the presence of an adequate supply of fluids. To maintain homeostasis, the volume and electrolyte composition of fluids must remain balanced. The body normally regulates this balance within a narrow range, even though the fluid intake of a person fluctuates widely. The volume of fluid from food and chemical reactions in the body approximately equals the volume of fluid lost through the skin, lungs, and feces. Therefore, by comparing the amount of fluid taken by mouth with the amount of urine excreted, the general state of fluid balance in the healthy adult can be estimated (Fig. 17-2).

Abnormal differences between gains and losses of electrolytes and water result in body-fluid imbalances. These imbalances may represent a deficient or excessive volume of body fluid as well as a change in the properties of the fluid itself. Ill persons frequently develop water and electrolyte imbalances, resulting in nursing problems common to many patients. Retention of fluid occurs in a variety of medical conditions when the drainage of tissue fluid cannot keep pace with its formation. Excessive loss of fluids often accompanies hyperemesis, prolonged diarrhea, protracted fever, hemorrhage, and burns, which in turn may lead to circulatory and

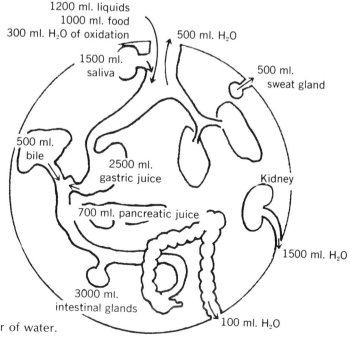

1200 ml. liquids
1000 ml. food
300 ml. H_2O of oxidation

500 ml. H_2O

1500 ml. saliva

500 ml. sweat gland

500 ml. bile

2500 ml. gastric juice

Kidney

700 ml. pancreatic juice

1500 ml. H_2O

3000 ml. intestinal glands

100 ml. H_2O

Fig. 17-2. Normal daily turnover of water.

renal impairment. Accurate records of the patient's weight gains and losses, the amounts and kinds of fluid intake, and the amounts and kinds of fluids excreted by the body are essential in many clinical conditions to help detect or circumvent fluid imbalances. Compensations for water and electrolyte abnormalities may be made through increased or decreased oral intake, tube feedings, or parenteral therapy.

Chemistry of digestion

The chemical changes begin in the mouth with the action of amylase on starch. In the stomach the enzymes protease and rennin act on proteins in the medium of hydrochloric acid, which has a concentration of about 0.5%. Enzymes found in the intestines are lipase, amylase, and protease from the pancreatic juice and the peptidases and the disaccharases from the intestinal juice (Fig. 17-1). Intestinal enzymes act only in an alkaline medium.

Food and body regulators are classed under the headings of carbohydrates, fats, proteins, water, minerals, and vitamins. Carbohydrates and fats contain carbon, hydrogen, and oxygen. They furnish heat and energy, the fats producing twice as much as the carbohydrates. *Carbohydrates* are found in starches, sugars, and cellulose foods. Carbohydrates eventually change to glucose, a form of sugar that the body can use. The amount of glucose in the blood generally is 0.1%. Insulin, an internal secretion from the pancreas, serves to keep the blood sugar at a constant level.

Fats come from the vegetable and animal kingdom. Fats yield fatty acids and glycerol for use in the body. When carbohydrates and fats are burned completely in the presence of oxygen, carbon dioxide and water are formed, which are eliminated from the body through the excretory organs. Fats burn slower than carbohydrates and are digested more slowly, so that they should be given sparingly to ill persons.

In addition to carbon, hydrogen, and oxygen, *proteins* contain nitrogen, usually sulfur, and sometimes phosphorus. Proteins serve as building materials for body tissue, enzymes, and internal secretions. Proteins come from the animal and plant kingdoms, animal proteins being more palatable than vegetable proteins. Proteins are classified as complete or incomplete according to the number of amino acids they contain. The diet should include a variety of protein foods in order to assure a minimum supply of the necessary amino acids. Each person needs 1 Gm. of protein each day for each kilogram (2.2 pounds) of body weight, since proteins cannot be stored in the body. The end products of protein digestion are amino acids.

The minerals most important to the body are calcium, phosphorus, iron, iodine, sulfur, sodium, potassium, magnesium, and chlorine. The most important source of calcium is milk. Calcium and phosphorus are interrelated in that if one is low, the utilization of the other is affected. Phosphorus is found in bone, muscle, and nerve tissue. Important sources of phosphorus are milk, meat, fowl, eggs, vegetables, and fruits. Iron is an essential of hemoglobin. When iron is low, hemoglobin is low and tissue oxidation is below normal. Sources of iron are lean meats, especially liver, egg yolk, dried beans, and molasses. Iodine is normally present in the thyroid gland and must be supplied continually. Fish and other saltwater products have a fairly high content of iodine. Sulfur is a component of the protein molecule. Sulfur plays a part in oxidation in the body. It is a constituent of hair and nails. If protein intake is sufficient, so also will be sulfur.

Sodium and potassium function with calcium in regulating muscular irritability. An imbalance of either mineral disturbs the water balance of the body. Sodium and potassium are seldom lacking in food. Magnesium is present in bones and teeth, in all soft tissues, and in body fluids. It is found in chlorophyll, hence in green vegetables. Chlorine combines with sodium to form sodium chloride, which is present in all secretions, excretions, and body fluids. The chlorides control the osmotic pressure of body fluids.

The chief sources of minerals are milk, vegetables, and fruits. The average balanced diet will furnish adequate minerals that help maintain the acid-base balance in the body, aid in the prevention of certain diseases, help regulate body processes, are necessary for the growth and repair of tissue, and are essential constituents of bone, teeth, blood, muscles, nerves, and glands.

Vitamins are essential for normal nutrition and growth and for resistance to disease. The most important vitamins are A, the B group, C, D, E, and K. The normal vitamin requirements of the body will be found in an adequate, balanced diet.

NURSING RESPONSIBILITIES

The responsibilities of the nurse in dealing with the patient's nutritional needs are many and varied. Several activities typically expected of the nurse are (1) assessing the patient's nutritional requirements, (2) preparing the patient and his environment for food or fluid intake, (3) feeding the patient or assisting him to feed himself, (4) interpreting the patient's diet prescription to him, and (5) observing and recording the patient's food and fluid intake and his reactions to it.

Assessing the patient's nutritional needs

As already stressed in the stated principles, physiologic nutritional requirements are the sum of the processes by which living organisms take in, absorb, and utilize the elements that a body needs to maintain function, to renew its components, and to grow and develop. Human beings need an adequate intake of water, carbohydrates, fats, proteins, minerals,

and vitamins to maintain health. Water is essential for the functioning of every organ of the body. It is the medium in which physiologic changes occur, aiding in digestion, absorption, circulation, and excretion. Carbohydrates and fats yield heat and energy; proteins promote growth and repair of tissues; vitamins act as metabolic catalysts; and minerals act as catalysts, as structural components, and as factors in other vital processes.

In the hospital setting the nurse utilizes knowledge of nutrition in cooperation with the patient's physician and the various members of the dietary service. Awareness of the important effects that nutrition can have in the successful outcome of the patient's total plan of care leads to (1) significant observations of the individual patient's eating problems, for example, difficulties in mastication and swallowing or food preferences or dislikes, the presence of anorexia, or other problems interfering with nutrition that may require positive action, and (2) reporting observations for appropriate action in the team's efforts to provide adequate nutrition for the patient.

Preparing the patient and his environment

The nurse has the ability to influence physical and psychologic conditions surrounding the patient's meals, which should be served regularly and promptly. Before serving a tray, the environment should be made as pleasant as possible. Disturbing physical elements, such as unpleasant sights, should be removed, and disturbing psychologic elements, such as pain and worries, should be reduced to a minimum. Disturbances during the meal may be anticipated and prevented. For instance, the bedpan may be offered before and after mealtime.

Pain, fatigue, and worry inhibit gastric juices and cause tension in the digestive tract, which slows peristalsis. Loneliness

261

and insecurity may decrease or increase the appetite. For most persons, food is associated with things pleasant. When food, as in a special diet, becomes part of medical treatment and there is restriction on types of food or when unaccustomed foods are added to the diet, conflicts may arise. It may be that the only way in which the patient can express himself is through his reaction to food—all his pent-up objections that he has accumulated come to the surface at the sight of his tray (Fig. 17-3). The patient should be placed in a proper and comfortable position, and the atmosphere should be calm and happy. Peace of mind increases the pleasure of eating and stimulates the flow of digestive juices, thereby contributing to health.

Many microorganisms enter the body through the mouth through food and drink. However, the senses of smell and taste reject noxious agents. Harmful organisms that enter the gastrointestinal tract may be engulfed by mucus, destroyed by hydrochloric acid, or rejected quickly by vomiting or diarrhea. The organisms of typhoid, dysentery, and tuberculosis are a few bacteria that may not be affected by hydrochloric acid, and these microorganisms pass on to the intestines and may cause disease. Bacteria normally inhabit the intestines. About fifty different species have been isolated. The lower levels of the small intestine become progressively richer in bacteria, and in the large intestines the number of organisms reaches the maximum. Bacteria cause putrefaction of proteins and fermentation of carbohydrates, disintegrate cellulose to liberate the enclosed food for digestion, and also synthesize vitamins B and K. The kinds of bacteria depend on diet. Fluids dilute bacterial

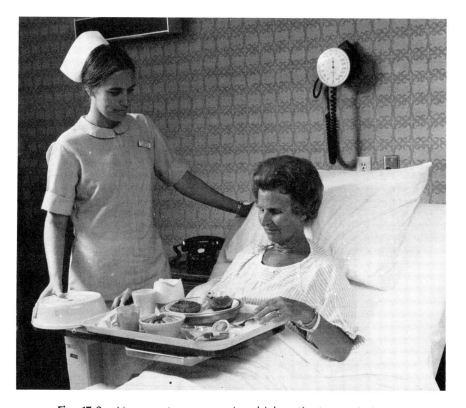

Fig. 17-3. Nurse notes manner in which patient accepts tray.

toxins and aid in their removal from the body.

In preventing food-producing disease, the first essential is cleanliness, which includes keeping the food uncontaminated, preparing it carefully, and having clean hands for preparation, serving, and eating. Handwashing facilities are provided for patients before their meals. Some hospitals place on the food trays packaged skin cleansers that may be used before or after eating.

Bacteria may be passed from one to another by unclean eating utensils, so all silverware and dishes should be thoroughly washed and sterilized before being used again. At home, dishes may be cleansed adequately by washing with water and a detergent, scalding, and then air drying. This method is advocated by health departments.

Sanitary regulations regarding handling, storing, and preparing food, as well as regulations regarding dishwashing and the disposal of waste food, are observed in a hospital. Food handlers in most hospitals have physical examinations to be sure that they are not carriers of disease. In some cities the board of health certifies a person to be a food handler.

In its proper function of protecting citizens from frauds, adulteration, and deterioration of food supply, the federal government passed two food laws in 1906 that were carried out originally be the Department of Agriculture. The Pure Food and Drug Act, the original name, prevents adulteration and misbranding of food and drugs. A second law provides for inspection of meats. State and city laws also govern the distribution of foodstuffs.

Prescribed diets

Hospitals usually provide modifications of daily diets that may be classed as general, light, soft, liquid, or clear liquid. The *general* (or regular) diet is comparable to a normal, adequate daily diet. A *light* diet is similar but excludes highly seasoned, fried, and fatty foods and foods high in roughage. A *soft* diet is made up of pureed foods or those with a fine texture and less cellulose content and may exclude meat. A *liquid* diet is composed of all liquid foods, including gelatin and ice cream, whereas a *clear liquid* diet includes broth, tea, coffee, strained fruit juices, and gelatin.

The diet ordered by the physician is well cooked and served as attractively as possible. An adequate explanation is given to the patient about the kind of food that has been prescribed. If the food prescribed is limited, there is all the more reason for ingenuity on the part of the dietitian and the nurse for variety. For liquid diet, for instance, different kinds and colors of liquids should be considered. The patient's likes and dislikes are considered. Food habits of the patient should be learned soon after admission so that he will not need to be questioned before each meal.

FEEDING OR ASSISTING THE PATIENT
Serving food

Some patients need to be helped at mealtime. It is necessary to make the food more easily accessible for some and to actually put each bite into the mouth for others.

Many patients need some assistance in cutting meat, buttering bread, or having a dish placed within reach (Fig. 17-4). After serving the tray, the nurse should not leave the patient until it is certain that he feels secure and comfortable about eating. When it is necessary to feed a patient, the tray should be placed where the patient can see it, and he may suggest the rotation of food. If the nurse sits down, the patient is more likely to feel at ease. The food should be served slowly, in small quantities, and in proper sequence, and the desire for fluids should be anticipated. The patient may feel embarrassment at having to be fed. The nurse can help pre-

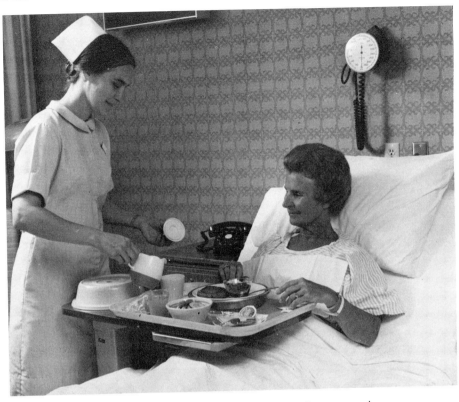

Fig. 17-4. Assisting the patient according to needs.

vent this feeling of dependency by a quiet attitude and a willingness to be helpful.

A cup of coffee frequently represents more than just a cup of coffee. It has become a symbol of sociability and adulthood. Patients appreciate the coffee that is offered before breakfast or between meals. A head nurse may wish to contact her patients on a friendly and informal basis by refilling the breakfast-tray coffee as she makes her morning rounds.

Food too has a socializing value. When trays are served to ward patients in their beds, their curtains and screens can be removed so that they may converse with each other. Or they may eat at a small table in their rooms. Some hospitals have dining rooms for ambulatory patients, and these facilities resemble normal community life.

In illness the patient is usually dependent on others for bringing him food and drink, for feeding him perhaps, and for satisfying his appetite. The diet department prepares the menu and may distribute a list of food to be selected by the patient. A dietitian may visit the patient to discuss his wishes for particular food. The professional nurse, the practical nurse, the nurse's aide, or sometimes a volunteer may feed the patient.

Gavage

A few patients are fed through a tube placed into the stomach. This is called *tube feeding* or *gavage* if the tube is introduced into the stomach through the mouth or the nose. If the tube is put through an incision into the stomach, the method is termed *gastrogavage*. The patient's cooperation should be obtained, if possible, and an explanation of the procedure given. Tube feedings may be administered by gravity flow or by a mechanical pump and should provide essential fluids and nutrients.

Before use, the tube is chilled by being placed on ice or in the refrigerator because cold hardens the rubber and makes it easier to control. The end of the tube is wet before insertion, since the wet surfaces will offer less friction to the mucous membrane than will dry surfaces. While liquid food is being poured into the tube, the speed of flow is controlled by the height of the funnel and the diameter of the tube. Pouring the fluid against the side of the funnel tends to lessen the amount of air introduced into the patient's stomach. The mixture should be given slowly in small amounts to prevent distension, nausea, and excessive peristalsis.

Cultural influences

Some of the deepest emotional experiences are concerned directly or indirectly with food. Racial and religious influences play an important role in eating habits. Folkways include foodways that must be taken into consideration with patients, and where at all possible the desires of the patient should be satisfied. What is served and how and where it is served may be of signal importance to the welfare of sick persons. A dietary situation that fits both the patient's physiologic needs and his emotional and cultural expectations can be one of the strongest bonds that the hospital is capable of forging with him.

Food preferences and customs vary among social classes and among ethnic groups even in the same community. Among factors to be considered in food customs are the manner in which certain foods are prepared, foods that are particularly liked or disliked, foods that are taboo or thought to be harmful in some way, foods that are used for festive occasions, and foods that are especially helpful to the sick.

Nutritional diseases constitute the greatest medical problem from the point of view of disability and economic loss. Barriers to good nutrition are economic conditions, lack of appreciation of the right food, poor health habits, and resistance to changing eating habits. About one fourth of the people in the United States are ill fed because of inadequate income. More than one half of the earth's population does not have enough of the right kind of food. The Food and Agriculture Organization (FAO) of the United Nations is a supranational organization formed to help alleviate this problem by attempting to match the world's food supply more nearly with the world's food needs.

Free or low-cost school-lunch programs have been established in many communities in an attempt to increase the quality and amount of food for children. Some social and welfare agencies furnish food, cash, or food tickets to families that cannot provide sufficiently. Carbohydrate foods are found in excess of others in food orders supplied by relief organizations. A large number of families whose self-respect would be affected by public assistance do not receive adequate diets.

In health, food habits and tastes are influenced by early training, nationality, the part of the country, mental attitudes, religious customs, and the family budget. Food tells much about people: whether they like others, whether they are friendly in extending another an invitation to eat with them, whether they wish to share words and thoughts during a meal, and whether they accept others and wish to continue the relationship.

INTERPRETING DIET PRESCRIPTIONS TO THE PATIENT

If the nurse and the patient have identified a learning need regarding food that will be useful to the patient, the nurse has an excellent opportunity for initiating planned learning activities with the patient. The nurse answers questions regarding food and may furnish pertinent literature for the patient to read. Why the prescribed diet is of therapeutic value and why it is just as necessary as any other treatment must be understood by the patient. The nurse encourages the patient to take the proper amounts of food unhurriedly and to masticate thoroughly. Instruction may be needed in the preparation of food, and these suggestions should be made in relation to the facilities available for cooking at home.

The nurse explains how water is necessary in the body as an aid to elimination and to the regulation of body processes. She also provides sufficient fluids for the patient between meals, thus enabling him to carry out instructions.

The patient who is on a special diet in the hospital may have to continue it at home. He will need instruction from the nurse or the dietitian in regard to the selection of food for the diet. A member of the family may need to be taught how to prepare food and feed a patient at home.

Sometimes a patient may be encouraged to eat foods that are good for him but that he has not been accustomed to eating.

A balanced diet may be discussed. The patient is made aware of foods contained in the four basic groups: (1) milk group—milk and milk products; (2) meat group—meat, poultry, fish, eggs, and legumes; (3) vegetable-fruit group—fruits (including citrus), vegetables (including green leafy); and (4) bread and cereal group—whole grain or enriched bread and cereals and potatoes. The patient is told that a balanced diet may be obtained by including the designated servings from the four groups into each day's menu (Fig.

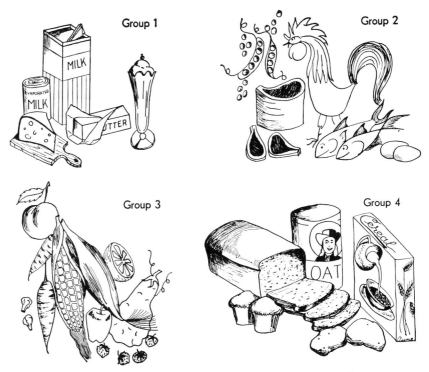

Fig. 17-5. The basic four groups of protective foods.

17-5). The following servings have been recommended.*

Group 1—milk group: 3 to 4 cups of milk for children; 2 cups of milk for adults; 4 cups of milk or equivalent during pregnancy; and 6 cups of milk or equivalent while nursing a baby

Group 2—meat group: 2 or more servings daily; 1 ounce portions of lean meat, poultry, and fish are approximately equal in protein value; substitutes include 1 egg, 1 slice of yellow cheese, 2 tablespoons of creamed cottage cheese or peanut butter, or $\frac{1}{2}$ cup cooked dried beans or peas

Group 3—vegetable-fruit group: 2 fruits and 2 vegetables; 1 serving of a dark green or yellow vegetable at least every other day and 1 serving of a citrus fruit or its equivalent each day; substitutes include tomatoes, raw cabbage, cantaloupe, and strawberries

Group 4—bread and cereal group: 4 or more servings daily; a serving includes 1 slice of bread or $\frac{1}{2}$ to $\frac{3}{4}$ cup of cereal (including rice, grits, cornmeal, and macaroni)

If possible, menus should be planned a week in advance. Minor changes may sometimes be necessary. In planning the menu, the basic four (protective) foods should be chosen first and then other foods added to make the meal palatable and attractive.

The nurse helps the patient to know that it is not always how much but rather what food is important and may guide him in selecting foods of relatively low price but of good nutritional value.

The patient may have questions regarding highly advertised vitamins and other concentrates. The nurse advises that these should be used under the prescription of a physician and that it is better to eat the proper foods than to depend on "pills." The patient may also ask about reducing diets, and the nurse will advise the patient who wishes to reduce to do so under the counsel and supervision of his physician.

A definite relationship exists between family education and the selection of food. The nurse, knowing that the smaller the expenditure for food, the more careful must be the planning for an adequate diet, may help the family select proper foods

*Dairy Council of St. Louis, Mo., 1961.

for an adequate diet and assist parents in establishing in their children good eating habits and attitudes toward food. The nurse may promote community understanding of, and an interest in, good nutrition for everyone.

EVALUATING PATIENT'S FOOD AND FLUID INTAKE

Observing and recording the patient's food and fluid intake are as important as other nursing activities carried out to meet the patient's basic nutritional needs. The food and fluid intake of all patients are evaluated, reported, and, if necessary, changed in order to supply adequate nutrition to all body tissues.

A nurse's general estimate of the patient's reaction to prescribed food and fluid intake and output may be sufficient. A record that the patient is eating, drinking, and retaining most of the food and fluids served to him would indicate that his needs for nutritional intake had been assessed and were being met as prescribed. On the other hand, an exact record of all food and fluid intake and output might be needed in order to help make the judgment or evaluation. A patient may have specific problems in which there is continued loss of nutrients from the body through vomiting and diarrhea, for example, or in which there is inadequate utilization of food because of liver disease or endocrine disorders. In such cases, the nurse should maintain a concise written record of all food and fluid intake (and usually output) so that the patient's nutritional deficiencies can be investigated, evaluated, and treated. Health agencies adopt or adapt appropriate forms for the purpose of recording patient's accurate food and fluid intake (and output) records, often showing totals for 8-hour and 24-hour periods.

SUMMARY

The principles of nutrition require the assessing and meeting of the individual's

267

nutritional needs so that adequate nutrition will be supplied for all body tissues whenever possible. Illness may change a patient's eating habits and his reactions to food and fluids, and a nurse may have the opportunity to improve the patient's nutritional status by providing a balanced or therapeutic diet, interpreting needed information to him regarding his prescribed diet, and keeping a record of his reactions. Cultural practices and specific health problems affect the utilization of food and fluid components, and the patient may need help in planning balanced daily diets and in understanding that adequate diet not only prevents disease but also helps to give a margin of vigor and reserve that makes for buoyant health.

QUESTIONS FOR DISCUSSION

1 List five foods under each of the basic four.
2 What scientific principles do you observe when you eat a meal?
3 Describe the role of the dietitian and of the physician in food and its service.
4 Describe how you would prepare a patient for his food tray in bed; in a chair.
5 What is the FAO?
6 The original food law was called the Pure Food and Drug Act. What is it now called?
7 Discuss some folkways in regard to food.
8 Discuss some religious customs in regard to food.

LIFE SITUATION

Bert Brown, 16 years of age, has been hospitalized with a broken leg. With each meal he is served milk. The second day he asked for coffee and did not drink his milk. When the nurse questioned him, he said he did not like milk. How would you help him to understand that he needed milk? In what other ways could his need for calcium and other nutrients be met?

SUGGESTED PERFORMANCE CHECKLIST
Comfort

1 Is the bedpan offered before the meal?
2 Is the tray placed within convenient reach?
3 Is the food attractively served?
4 Is the patient's posture good and position comfortable while eating?
5 Are the patient's likes and dislikes considered?
6 Is treatment equipment out of sight?
7 Is a fresh glass of water provided?
8 Are the patient's needs anticipated?
9 Are ambulatory patients encouraged to be up for their meals?
10 Is the bed neat and comfortable?

Therapeutic effectiveness

1 Is an adequate amount of food eaten?
2 Are trays served as soon as possible after hot foods are placed on them?
3 Is the environment pleasant?
4 Is food served in an appetizing manner?
5 Is tact used in feeding?
6 Is plenty of time allowed for feeding the patient?
7 Does the patient understand the importance of balanced food and fluid intake?
8 Are significant observations made and recorded?
9 Is recording adequate and accurate?
10 Are strong emotions and excessive fatigue avoided?
11 Do foods correspond to the patient's religious and national preferences?

Economy

1 Is the tray complete?
2 Is the bedside prepared before the tray is served?
3 Is the tray inspected before serving?
4 Are servings in the proper amount for the individual patient?
5 Is the bedding protected adequately?
6 Is the energy of the patient on bed rest conserved according to the patient's needs?

Safety

1 Are the patient's hands washed before the meal?
2 Are the nurse's hands clean?
3 Is the prescribed food served?
4 Is the tray service in good condition?
5 Is the tray marked with the patient's name?
6 Is a disposable drinking tube used if needed?
7 Is the tray well supported in carrying?

SUGGESTED READINGS

Burke, Shirley: Composition and function of body fluids, St. Louis, 1972, The C. V. Mosby Co.

Callahan, Catherine L.: The White House Conference on Food, Nutrition and Health, Nursing Outlook 70:58, January, 1970.

Chappelle, Mary Lou: The language of food, American Journal of Nursing 72:1294, July, 1972.

Crim, Sarah R.: Nutritional problems of the poor, Nursing Outlook 17:65, September, 1969.

Fenton, Mary: What to do about thirst, American Journal of Nursing 69:1014, May, 1969.

Grant, Jo Ann, and others: Parenteral hyperalimentation, American Journal of Nursing 69:2392, November, 1969.

Metheny, Norma Milligan, and Snively, William D.: Nurses' handbook of fluid balance, Philadelphia, 1967, J. B. Lippincott Co.

Nelson, Alice H.: Self-recorded diet histories, American Journal of Nursing 72:1601, September, 1972.

Pasquali, Elaine Ann: Learning about a poverty budget, American Journal of Nursing 72:1419, August, 1972.

Robinson, Corinne H.: Normal and therapeutic nutrition, New York, 1972, The Macmillian Company.

Snively, W. D., and Beshear, Donna R.: Textbook of pathophysiology, Philadelphia, 1972, J. B. Lippincott Co., chaps. 8 and 9.

Weldy, Norma Jean: Body fluids and electrolytes—a programmed presentation, St. Louis, 1972, The C. V. Mosby Co.

Williams, Sue Rodwell: Nutrition and diet therapy, ed. 2, St. Louis, 1973, The C. V. Mosby Co.

18 Maintaining excretory function

AVENUES OF ELIMINATION

In the preceding chapter nutritional intake and the significance of fluid and electrolyte balance were discussed. Closely related to and of equal importance in preserving the body's homeostatic condition is the excretion of waste products and toxic substances formed in the body. The focus in this chapter is on maintaining the relatively narrow range between intake and output that is essential for the continuance of life. Efficient body functioning is dependent upon the complex physiologic machinery necessary for maintaining the fine adjustments that hold in balance the body's temperature, chemical composition, and osmotic pressure. Elimination, or output, is accomplished mainly through four channels: the integumentary, respiratory, and urinary systems and the gastrointestinal tract.

Water and certain mineral salts, such as sodium chloride, are excreted in perspiration by way of the sudorific glands in the skin. The significance of this process is

mentioned in the preceding chapter. Perspiration becomes a problem factor in skin care, as noted in Chapter 16. However, another important function of perspiration is the cooling of the body by the evaporation of water in the maintenance of normal body temperature.

A second avenue of elimination is that of the lungs. The elimination of carbon dioxide and water are important in maintaining the acid-base balance of the body, as described in other chapters.

The third avenue is that of the large intestine. Residue from digested food, indigestible objects, mucus, and other products secreted during digestion are expelled by this channel. Because the gastrointestinal tract is highly influenced by conditions of stress, this route of elimination is also an important factor in maintaining physiologic homeostasis in and during illness.

A fourth avenue of elimination is by way of the urinary system. The kidneys are designed for a dual purpose: (1) waste

270

disposal and (2) regulatory functioning, primarily in achieving the constant composition and volume of the blood that result in homeostasis in the extracellular and intracellular compartments of the body. The functioning also involves regulation of the osmotic pressure, the electrolyte and water balance, and the acid-base balance. In the process of the kidneys producing urine, excess water, solutes such as sodium, chloride, and other substances including metabolic by-products (for example, urea), and ingested toxic substances are eliminated. Urine is transported to the bladder by way of the ureters and stored in the bladder until the amount is sufficient to produce a reflex mechanism that causes it to empty itself.

In this chapter, relevant principles and nursing problems dealing with elimination form the urinary system and the intestinal tract will be considered.

ELIMINATION FROM THE URINARY SYSTEM

The content of this section will be limited primarily to normal elimination. It is assumed that management of patients with acute or chronic renal failure will be dealt with in other contexts. Some of the related principles appear in Chapters 16, 17, 19, and 29 and are not repeated here.

Principles from biologic sciences

A balance is maintained between intake and output via the kidneys through certain mechanisms that preserve a constancy in volume and chemical composition of body fluids.

1. The kidneys function to preserve the homeostasis of body fluids and electrolytes by screening waste products from the blood plasma.

2. Certain factors extraneous to the kidneys influence them in the amount of fluid and electrolytes they should reabsorb or eliminate in the urine to preserve homeostasis.

a. The antidiuretic hormone (ADH) governs the amount of water reabsorbed by the renal tubules in response to fluctuations in the osmotic pressure.

b. Aldosterone, a hormone secreted by the adrenal cortex, stimulates the renal tubules to reabsorb sodium and excrete potassium. Since sodium is retained, the resulting increase in osmotic pressure is followed by release of ADH, which produces a decrease in water loss. A reverse situation increases the water loss.

c. The load of solid wastes to be eliminated by the kidneys also affects the water loss. In diabetes mellitus a greater volume of water is required to eliminate the excess sugar, which accounts for the increased urinary output and excessive thirst occurring in this condition.

3. Solids must be in solution in order to be removed via the kidneys.

a. Excess inorganic salts are removed.

b. Most of the nitrogenous wastes from protein metabolism are removed, including urea, uric acid, and creatinine. Normally blood urea nitrogen level is held between 8 and 28 mg. per 100 ml.

4. The cystic bladder is a hollow, muscular organ of considerable elasticity.

a. It serves as a reservoir for urine.

b. The musculature of the bladder is capable of great distension.

c. Urine is retained in the bladder by an internal sphincter, the sphincter vesicae, which is located at the opening of the bladder into the urethra.

d. The bladder is emptied by contraction of its muscles. The desire to urinate results from sensory stimulation in the bladder caused by the pressure of urine, the chemical composition of urine, or reflex stimulation. In a healthy adult urination is a voluntary act.

e. Accumulation of 300 to 500 ml. of urine in the adult will normally cause awareness of the need to void. The urge to void may be increased by bladder or urethral irritation.

f. Normally, the urinary system is free from bacteria except at the urethral meatus.

In considering the body's fluid balance, the ability to withstand water loss is sometimes referred to as the individual's water reserve. In the event of fluid deficit, the question of how good the individual's water reserve is becomes significant. The one with the greatest percentage of body water has the greatest reserve. Normally water content is about 50% for women and 60% for men. Adipose tissue water content is low. Therefore, obesity is one of the commonest causes of decreased body water. While infants have a relatively high percentage of body water in comparison with adults, they have poor reserve because their fluid loss via urinary output each 24 hours is high. Infants and the obese develop severe dehydration easily in the stressful situations of illness.

Principles from behavioral sciences

Normally, voiding is under complete control of the individual and does not usually present any problems. However, the hospitalized patient may suddenly become dependent on the assistance of others to perform this function. The dependency and resulting embarrassment can cause problems.

1. Psychic states of fear, excitement, and embarrassment increase the tonicity of the muscles of the bladder.

2. The volume of urine produced is influenced by emotional stress because stress affects the blood pressure.

Terms and definitions

The act by which urine is expelled from the bladder is called *micturition, urination,* or *voiding.* The terms to *urinate,* to *void,* and to *pass water* (used by patients) are also used in reference to the act. When urine cannot be expelled from the bladder, the condition is called *retention,* which is relieved by catheterization. *Retention with overflow* means that the patient voids small amounts but does not empty the bladder, and the bladder eventually becomes distended. When there is no urine secreted by the kidneys, the condition is called *suppression.* Suppression may be known as *anuria* or lack of urine. *Hematuria* means blood in the urine. *Pyuria* means pus in the urine. *Polyuria* means an abnormally large amount of urine. *Oliguria* means a reduced daily output of urine. *Dysuria* means painful urination. *Albuminuria* means albumin in the urine. *Glycosuria* means sugar (glucose) in the urine. *Incontinence* is uncontrolled urination (also applies to uncontrolled defecation). *Frequency* means the patient urinates often, whereas *urgency* refers to the immediacy of urination.

Normal urine

Urine is a complex watery solution of organic and inorganic substances, most of which are waste products from metabolism of body cells and food. Urine contains about 95% water and 3.7% organic and 1.3% inorganic wastes. Specific substances found in urine are wastes, mineral salts, toxins, pigments, sex hormones, and sometimes abnormal constituents The color of urine varies from light yellow if dilute to a dark brown if concentrated. The color is derived from several pigments, the most abundant of which is urochrome. Urochrome is a constant product of metabolism but may vary in amount under abnormal conditions.

Substances normally in the urine are mainly inorganic salts and compounds of nitrogen. Inorganic salts include the sulfates, chlorides, and phosphates and the bicarbonates of sodium, calcium, magnesium, potassium, and ammonium. The most abundant of these is sodium chloride, which makes up about 20% of the solid matter of urine or about 10 to 15 Gm. a day.

Of the organic matter in urine, urea is the most important and abundant, forming about 50% of the solids. Urea is excreted to the extent of 20 to 30 Gm. a day, the amount depending on the amount of protein in the diet.

Creatinine is a product found in the normal urine of adults. Uric acid, usually in the form or urates, represents a small but important constituent of normal urine. Normal urine will contain a few white blood cells and a small number of epithelial cells. Some drugs may be excreted by the kidneys and be found in the urine.

The specific gravity of urine varies, according to the amount of solids in it, from 1.010 to 1.030. Specific gravity of urine is the weight of a given volume of urine as compared with the weight of an equal volume of pure water and is measured by a urinometer.

Urine ordinarily is slightly acid, the pH being between 5.5 and 7. The acidity is attributed to the presence of acid phosphates, particularly sodium acid phosphate. When urine stands for some time, its reaction may become alkaline because of the production of ammonia. Some types of bacteria that cause disease in the urinary tract may influence the reaction. The reaction of urine varies also with the diet. Meats tend to make the urine acid, whereas vegetables and fruits cause an alkaline reaction. Certain drugs change the reaction of urine.

The odor of freshly voided urine is faintly aromatic as a result of the presence of a substance called urinod. As urine stands, fermentative bacteria change urea to ammonium carbonate and then to ammonia, giving an odor of ammonia to the urine. The odor of urine may be changed by the ingestion of certain drugs and vegetables.

Abnormal urine may be red from fresh blood or dark brown from old blood. A brown color may result from an excess of bilirubin. Various drugs and foods may color urine.

Constituents of abnormal urine are albumin, sugar, acetone bodies, casts, calculi, and pus.

ELIMINATION THROUGH THE GASTROINTESTINAL TRACT

Many problems may arise from improper functioning of the intestine. These usually result from poor hygiene, prolonged bed rest, surgery, or other disease entities. Because the digestive system is controlled by the autonomic nervous system, it is influenced by emotions and also by many drugs given for other therapeutic purposes. To understand the problems of elimination, one should be familiar with the normal process.

Principles from biologic sciences

Significant activities of the large bowel include movement, secretion, and absorption, which are essential in the process of eliminating food residues and gases via the gastrointestinal tract. The large intestine is a thin-walled musculomembranous tube similar in basic structure to the rest of the intestine, but wider in diameter and more distensible, with greater capacity for retention of its contents.

1. Peristaltic movement propels the intestinal content toward the anus:
   a. Innervation is by fibers from both divisions of the autonomic nervous system: craniosacral stimulation increases peristalsis, thoracolumbar stimulation decreases it.
   b. Peristaltic movements are reflexly stimulated (gastrocolic reflex) by the entrance of food into the stomach, especially in the morning when the stomach has been without food overnight.
   c. The external aperture of the colon,

the anus, is guarded by the internal and external sphincters, which keep the orifice closed except during defecation.

2. Practically all the processes of food digestion and absorption are completed in the small intestine. Only the indigestible components pass through the ileocecal valve into the large intestine.

3. The important function of the colon is reabsorption of water and electrolytes and the storing of the dehydrated contents to form feces.

   a. The amount of water absorbed into the capillaries of the large intestine is affected by the body's state of hydration.

   b. Prolonged retention of feces results in increased water absorption and hardened fecal mass. Rapid passage of contents through the intestine decreases water absorption, resulting in soft or liquid feces.

   c. Fecal material normally is composed of food residue, bacteria, epithelial cells, mucus, bile pigments, and some inorganic salts.

4. The sudden propulsion of feces into the rectum initiates the defecatory reflex.

   a. The reflex stimulates the internal sphincter to relax.

   b. The external sphincter is relaxed voluntarily; it must be relaxed for evacuation of the rectum.

   c. Voluntary contraction of abdominal muscles and the diaphragm against the abdominal organs assists in defecation.

   d. Repeated ignoring of the defecation reflex causes loss of the normal stimulation by distension and pressure, through sensory adaptation, allowing fecal accumulation and constipation to develop.

5. A viscous, alkaline mucus is secreted by the large intestine.

   a. Mucus lubricates feces, facilitating evacuation.

   b. Mucosa is protected from mechanical and chemical injury by the mucus secretion.

   c. Bacterial acids are neutralized in the alkaline secretion, permitting constant putrefaction of whatever proteins were not digested and absorbed in the small intestine.

   d. Irritation of the mucosa from bacterial action, foodstuffs, or excessive craniosacral stimulation in stress situations results in increased output of mucus and an attempt to dilute and remove the irritant. Frequent liquid stools (diarrhea) is the result.

6. Reflex stimulation originating with emotion will initiate movement of feces into the rectum.

Principles from behavioral sciences

1. An individual patient may experience difficulty using a bedpan for defecation because it is a new experience in an unnatural position and under unusual circumstances.

2. The individual's feeling of safety and confidence in using the bedpan may be increased by receiving appropriate instructions before attempting the use of the pan.

3. Prompt response to the request for a bedpan may lessen the patient's feeling of frustration in this experience.

4. A feeling of comfort and safety is apt to be enhanced by providing privacy during use of the bedpan.

Healthy individuals tend to have a bowel movement at approximately the same time each day. Others who are equally healthy have two or more a day or one every other day with no appreciable ill effects.

Illness often results in irregularities in intestinal elimination, with a loss of independence. This loss then in itself also becomes a problem. A few social scientists and some psychologists agree that the adult personality is profoundly influenced by early toilet tranining and other experiences connected with elimination. Elimination habits are also influenced by cultural patterns, the chief one being that of privacy.

Terms and definitions

The intestine is referred to as the *bowel.* The content of the large bowel is called *feces. Defecation* is the process of expelling fecal material from the rectum. *Stool* means the fecal discharge from the bowel. A stool may be called a bowel movement. *Incontinence* means inability to control the sphincter that guards the rectum (also inability to control urination). *Constipation* is infrequent or difficult evacuation of hard feces. *Diarrhea* is abnormal frequency and liquidity of the feces. *Flatus* means gas in the intestines. *Flatulence,* tympanites, or meteorism is the condition of having flatus. *Tenesmus* is unsuccessful straining. *Melena* refers to stools that are very dark or black because of the presence of blood.

The process of elimination from the bowel

The large intestine is made up of the cecum, colon, and rectum and is about 5 feet long in the adult. Separating the small intestine from the large intestine is the ileocecal valve, which opens in one direction, preventing the passage of material in the opposite direction. Fluid injected in a treatment cannot go beyond the ileocecal valve. The cecum is a large, blind pouch at the beginning of the large intestine. The colon, or the section of the large intestine between the cecum and the rectum, is divided into the ascending colon, which goes up on the right side; the transverse colon, which crosses the abdomen; the descending colon, which comes down on the left side, and the sigmoid flexure, which ends at the rectum. The rectum is 5 to 6 inches long and terminates at the anus. (See Fig. 18-1.) The anal canal is an aperture about 1 inch long leading to the exterior. It is guarded by an internal and an external sphincter. These sphincters are controlled by nerves from the central nervous system.

The walls of the large intestine are made up of longitudinal and circular muscles. Involuntary muscle tissue relaxing and contracting produces peristalsis, which moves the contents of the intestine in a downward direction. The reaction of muscle tissue to irritation is contraction. Intestinal muscle may be irriated by food bulk or by gas formed by chemical reaction.

Action in the intestine is controlled by the autonomic nervous system. When a certain amount of fecal matter has arrived

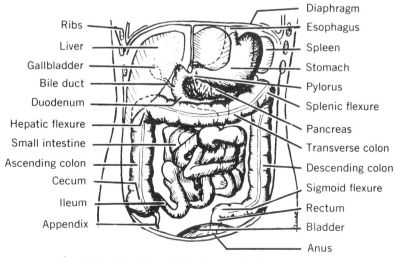

Fig. 18-1. The large intestine and other structures.

in the descending colon or rectum, sensory nerve endings are stimulated and induce a desire for evacuation. Defecation is, in part, a voluntary process, being largely caused by powerful contractions of the abdominal muscles. If the desire for evacuation is not heeded, water is absorbed from the feces, which become hard, and constipation may result. Sometimes the intestinal contents pass too rapidly so that water is not absorbed. They may be eliminated too frequently and give rise to diarrhea. The frequency of evacuation depends largely on the nature of food eaten. A diet with much cellulose produces more frequent and more watery stools than a bland diet does. Cellulose acts as a mechanical stimulus to peristalsis. Other aids to proper elimination are exercise by which the muscles of the abdomen are massaged and stimulated and also proper position of the body in walking, standing, and sitting. Good posture gives room for the abdominal organs to function and increases muscle tone.

About one third of the weight of feces is bacteria, most of which are dead. More than fifty species of bacteria have been found in the intestinal canal. They are classified as those that are regarded as normal inhabitants and those that are pathogenic. The group of organisms referred to as the colon bacilli normally constitute about three fourths of all living bacteria in feces. As a rule, the colon group do not have much initial pathogenic power and attack the intestinal wall only after it has been made more vulnerable by obstruction ischemia (local anemia), malignancy, and so on. Among other organisms are staphylococci, sarcinae, and yeasts. These organisms do no harm unless they escape to wounds on the skin or to other organs of the body. They may contaminate the urinary tract and the vaginal tract because of the improper use of toilet tissue. Common pathogenic bacteria causing intestinal disease are typhoid and dysentery organisms. Injurious substances of endogenous origin may be excreted from the blood directly or indirectly into the intestines.

Parasites that may be found in the intestinal tract are roundworms, hookworms, pinworms, and tapeworms (Fig. 18-2). These may be killed or removed by drugs taken orally or injected rectally.

If a fresh wound that provides a channel for the entrance of bacteria is present, such as after a hemorrhoidectomy or a perineorrhaphy, or if the tissues have been stretched widely, thus lessening resistance to infection, such as in childbirth or in instrumental dilation, it is necessary to cleanse the area well after a bowel movement. Cleansing this area is called perineal care. In administering this care, an antiseptic may be used to wash or flush the vulva, or soap and water used with a clean cloth may be employed. Drying may be done with cotton, a clean towel, or soft tissue, and it is done gently in order not to injure the tissues further.

Because of the prevalence of bacteria in the intestinal excretions, it is important that the nurse's hands be washed well after caring for the bedpan or after giving a rectal treatment, since the commonest method of germ transfer is contaminated hands. It is also necessary to provide the patient with handwashing facilities after he has used the bedpan. The skin of incontinent patients should be well cared for to prevent irritation caused by excretions on the skin.

The nurse should form the habit of keeping the hands away from the face and mouth, since the channel of infection for bacteria that produce intestinal infection is the mouth.

Bedpans are made of materials that can withstand frequent sterilization by heat. Individual bedpans prevent infection. The usual cleaning of a bedpan, where bedpan sterilizers are not available, consists of rinsing with cold water and then a thor-

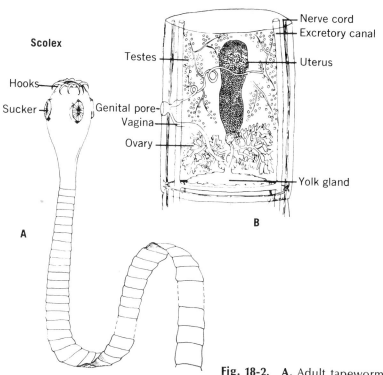

Scolex

Hooks

Sucker

Genital pore

Vagina

Ovary

Testes

Nerve cord

Excretory canal

Uterus

Yolk gland

A

B

Fig. 18-2. **A,** Adult tapeworm. **B,** Proglottid.

ough washing with warm water and a disinfectant. The disinfectant is not in contact with the material of the bedpan long enough to kill bacteria. They are removed by flushing and rubbing action. The disinfectant in most cases is also a deodorant.

When pathogenic bacteria are present in the feces, it is sometimes necessary to disinfect the stool before emptying it into the waste pipes. A proper chemical, such as chlorinated lime, is mixed with the stool, which stands for a period of at least 1 hour.

The character of the bowel contents is a result of chemical and mechanical action. Besides digested and indigestible material and bacteria, the feces contain intestinal secretions, products of bacterial decomposition, some purine bases, pigment, and inorganic salts. A quantitiy of gas may be present. Swallowed air contains 70% nitrogen, which is a heavy gas and diffuses slowly from the intestines and so produces

gas pains. Inorganic salts in feces are salts of sodium, potassium, phosphorus, calcium, magnesium, and iron. A group of bacteria form lactic acid and acetic acid from carbohydrates. Protein putrefaction is a constant and normal activity in the large intestine. In these processes gases are produced. Acids and gases stimulate the intestinal musculature. Methane, carbon dioxide, hydrogen, nitrogen, and hydrogen sulfide have been found in the large intestine.

The normal color of feces results from digested food or metallic compounds and from a normally present pigment, stercobilin or urobilin, which is derived from the bilirubin of the bile. Abnormal colors may be caused by disease or drugs. Bismuth and iron cause stools to be black.

The odor of feces is mainly the result of skatole and indole, two substances produced by bacterial action on amino acids.

Hot water coagulates protein. All body

excretions contain some protein. Cleansing the bedpan consists of first rinsing it with cold water to dissolve the protein and thus aid in its removal.

NURSING RESPONSIBILITIES IN MAINTAINING NORMAL ELIMINATION
Observation

A very necessary nursing responsibility for all patients is the recognition of optimal patterns of elimination, while being alert to detect any indication of impending or existing problems with this important bodily function. Evaluation regarding the efficiency of elimination for every patient is important in order that any interference with the normal mechanisms of elimination that requires intervention will be detected promptly.

Observation and reporting about the act of voiding and the characteristics of urine should include at least the following:

1. Character of the urine. Amount, color, clarity, odor, cloudiness, sweetish odor, or smell of ammonia in freshly voided urine or other unusual odor or appearance should be noted.
2. Frequent voiding of small amounts. This may indicate urinary retention with overflow (a distended bladder can usually be felt above the symphysis pubis).
3. Anuria or scanty urine. This may indicate suppression.
4. Discomfort, pain, or burning associated with the act of voiding
5. Urgency in the need to void

When unusual characteristics of either the act of voiding or of the urine itself are noted, the excretory functions of the skin and respiratory tract should also be observed for changes that may indicate related systemic problems. Significant observations might include changes in the rate and character of respiration and the odor of expired air (as a "fruity" odor in diabetic acidosis or fecal odor in intestinal ob-

struction), or uremic "frost" (white, powdery urea crystals appearing on the skin areas, such as the forehead, indicating renal failure in the normal process of excreting this substance) or diaphoresis causing further loss in fluid and electrolytes. There is a direct relationship between water lost through the kidneys and the skin; usually when large amounts of water are lost via the skin, the volume of urine is decreased.

Observation and reporting about the act of defecation, the characteristics of the feces, and the bowel habits that would be most significant in early detection of problems of elimination from the gastrointestinal tract would include at least the following points:

1. Character of the feces
   a. *Consistency and form.* The stool should be soft and formed to the shape of the colon (not liquid, loose, hard, or of unusual shape, such as pencil-like, possibly indicating a change in the bowel, for example a mass or tumor).
   b. *Color.* The stool is usually dark brown, not clay colored, indicating absence of bile, or black and tarry resulting from bleeding in the intestine. It should not show the presence of fresh blood, mucus, or other unusual constituent, such as visible parasites.
   c. *Odor.* A foul odor should be reported.
2. Act of defecation
   a. *Frequency.* Normalcy for an individual means regular evacuation daily or according to the individual's own usual bowel habits, which may be a stool every day or every second or third day (constipation is indicated by infrequent, difficult stools and diarrhea by frequent liquid stools; fecal impaction with frequent, small liquid stools is a possibility to be considered).

b. *Discomfort and tenesmus* (ineffective straining to evacuate)
c. *Flatus* (gas in the intestine). Flatulence and tympanites are terms indicating the presence of excessive gas in the stomach or intestine.

Pain may be an indication that problems of elimination have developed and should therefore be carefully observed, described, and reported. For example, cramping abdominal pain with distension might be associated with intestinal obstruction or fecal impaction; severe pain in the abdomen or flank that may radiate to the thigh or genitalia is suggestive of renal calculi passing through the ureter; pain and burning experienced with voiding often indicate urinary tract infection.

Recording fluid intake and output

Evaluation of fluid intake and output relationships is very important in the total evaluation of the patient's excretory functioning and in determination of the need for restorative measures. A discussion of the significance of fluid and electrolyte balance in maintaining the body's homeostasis was given in the preceding chapter. Accurate records of all fluid intake and excretory output must be kept throughout the 24 hours if the intake and output balance is to be correctly interpreted. A deficit in fluid intake and output is a guide in assessing the need for intervention.

Intake measurement includes all fluids taken orally, by tube feeding, or by intravenous infusion. All internal irrigation fluids should also be considered in the total fluid intake estimate.

Normally, fluid output is directly related to fluid intake. Output measurements include fluids lost by urine, voided or collected by catheter, vomitus, and drainage. Insensible losses of fluid through perspiration, rapid respiratory rate, and diarrhea should be noted. Normally, water loss per 24-hour period can be estimated as follows: (1) urine, from 1,000 to 1,500 ml.;

(2) feces, from 100 to 150 ml.; (3) insensible perspiration, 450 to 800 ml.; and (4) lungs, 250 to 350 ml. A balanced intake/output record based on these figures might possibly, for example, be as follows:

INTAKE

Fluid intake (oral and intravenous)	1,200 ml.
Water content of ingested food	1,000 ml.
Water of oxidation	250 ml.
Total	2,450 ml.

OUTPUT

Urine	1,200 ml.
Feces	150 ml.
Via lungs	300 ml.
Insensible loss	800 ml.
Total	2,450 ml.

Excessive loss of fluid by diarrhea, vomiting, persiration, or hemorrhage, loss through the kidneys, or loss from burns causes decrease in the plasma and interstitial compartments. Failure to ingest sufficient quantities of fluid may further deplete the fluid balance.

Failure to correct the fluid deficit eventually leads to depletion of the intravascular volume, falling blood pressure, electrolyte imbalance, and appearance of shock. If this situation is allowed to continue, anuria will develop with retention of metabolic wastes; coma and death may follow.

In each hospital situation a specific routine for measuring and recording intake and output is established for the use of all personnel.

Measures for assisting the patient to maintain optimal excretory function

When the patient has bathroom privileges, the nurse has responsibility for instructing him regarding such matters as location of the bathroom and, if intake and output recording is indicated, how the urine is to be measured and recorded and either discarded or saved as a specimen, in order that the patient will be spared confusion with these matters.

Whenever possible the patient should go to the bathroom or use a commode for both bowel and bladder evacuation because dependency on use of the bedpan creates many problems for the patient. Just the necessity of having to request the bedpan from strangers is a source of embarrassment, and he may not ask for this service when he feels the urge, especially for defecation. Or he may delay in following the urge to evacuate because the staff members seem busy and he hesitates to make his needs known. The delay in responding may contribute to occurrence of constipation and to difficulty in voiding. Other problems the patient may experience with the bedpan include difficulty in either voiding or defecating in the unusualness of the situation; using a receptacle in bed; trying to relax the sphincters sufficiently in a recumbent position to permit voiding and defecation; using a cold bedpan (cold tends to cause muscle contraction); and embarrassment from using the pan in the same room with others.

Measures that can be employed in assisting the bedfast patient to cope with these problems include reassuring him so that he will ask for the pan or urinal when needed; prompt response to the patient's request; warming a cold bedpan for the woman patient; assisting the patient to assume the most natural position on the pan that is possible for the individual and instructing him in its use to help in allaying his tension in the experience; screening him and placing toilet tissue and signal cord in convenient location. Such measures will help to reduce some of the anxiety experienced, thus making evacuation on the pan easier for the bed patient.

The nurse should endeavor to learn about the patient's normal pattern of elimination so that the bedpan can be offered according to this pattern, thus helping the patient to continue in his normal elimination habits with the least amount of tension.

LEARNING SITUATIONS FOR THE PATIENT

The patient should be encouraged to develop regular dietary and elimination habits if he has previously neglected these health measures. These matters may be discussed sufficiently with the patient to assess his degree of knowledge before attempting to instruct him. The medical therapy plan should also be ascertained.

If the patient needs more information of this nature, it is usually appropriate to discuss the essentials of a balanced diet, explaining the need for including some roughage, six to eight glasses of fluid daily, good posture, daily exercise, necessary amounts of rest, and relaxation. The value of setting a regular time for defecation can be emphasized by offering the bedpan at certain stated times. This may help the patient to establish regular habit patterns or to return to desirable habits that have been interrupted by illness. It is well also to encourage the patient to understand and use correct terminology in referring to elimination.

The problems associated with dependence upon the use of laxatives and enemas may be mentioned, explaining that these measures give only temporary relief, that they can be habit forming, and that their continued use decreases the ability of the intestine to respond to normal stimulation, thus tending to aggravate constipation. The patient may ask about drugs that are widely advertised to relieve constipation. He should be advised to consult the physician if constipation persists after being discharged from the hospital.

Handwashing after use of the bedpan can be encouraged by providing handwashing facilities for the bed patient and giving instructions according to the level of the individual patient's knowledge. It may also be advisable for some patients to explain the proper method of using toilet tissue when the tissue is placed within reach.

SUMMARY

Elimination has been discussed as an essential activity of the body closely related to preserving the body's homeostatic condition. It is dependent upon complex physiologic machinery necessary for maintaining the fine adjustments that hold in balance the body's temperature, chemical composition, and osmotic pressure. Output is accomplished mainly through four channels: the integumentary, respiratory, and urinary systems and the gastrointestinal tract. The focus of the chapter is on maintaining a balance between intake and output as affected by the functioning of the urinary system and the gastrointestinal tract.

Principles selected from the biologic and behavioral sciences are related in the discussion to nursing responsibilities in assisting the patient to maintain normal elimination. Stress is placed on the need for nursing intervention to be individualized and coordinated throughout each 24-hour period, with emphasis on opportunities for the patient to develop or reestablish regular bowel and bladder habits that were interrupted by illness.

QUESTIONS FOR DISCUSSION

1 What is the function of the glomerulus and renal tubule in relation to volume and composition of urine?
2 Why do some patients have difficulty in voiding?
3 Discuss the responsibilities of the nurse for the patient on intake and output.
4 An adult, Mr. S., is admitted to the hospital, undiagnosed but with a history of vomiting

for 2 days and scant output of urine. The physician's orders include: (1) nothing by mouth, (2) 3,000 ml. of physiologic saline with 5% glucose to be given intravenously during the first 18 hours, and (3) measurement of intake and output.
   a. Why is the urinary output decreased in amount?
   b. What is a physiologic saline solution?
   c. Why would the saline and glucose solution be ordered?
   d. What electrolytes are being lost by vomiting?
   e. If Mr. S. is perspiring profusely (as in diaphoresis with fever), how will the total body fluids be kept within normal limits?
   f. Discuss the responsibilities of the nurse for the patient on intake and output.
5 What can observation of the patient's feces reveal?
6 Why do some hospitalized patients have problems with constipation?
7 How would you account for the fact that constipated stools are hardened?
8 How may the nurse assist the patient to maintain adequate bowel function?
9 Mrs. N. is a new patient who has been admitted for observation. She requests an enema right away, saying to the nurse, "I always take an enema every day." How might the nurse respond to Mrs. N.'s request?

LIFE SITUATION

Mrs. S. was placed on measured intake and output following surgery. After the indwelling catheter was removed she began early ambulation, which included bathroom privileges. Her understanding of managing output consisted only of the fact that she was to void in a certain container placed on the toilet seat. She followed these instructions accurately according to her understanding, but each time the other patient sharing the room with Mrs. S. needed to void, she was confronted with how to use the toilet because the collection receptacle for Mrs. S. was still in place and the output measurement had not been made.

How could the nurse have avoided the frustration in this situation for both patients? What further instructions might Mrs. S. have been given?

SUGGESTED PERFORMANCE CHECKLIST

Comfort

1 Is the pan offered as soon as needed?
2 Is the pan removed as soon as possible?
3 Is the pan placed comfortably?
4 Is privacy provided?
5 Is necessary explanation given to the patient?
6 Is aftercare of bed and room adequate?
7 Is the backrest raised for use of the pan?

Good workmanship

1 Is assistance given as needed?
2 Is tact used to prevent embarrassment?
3 Is the patient covered as much as possible?
4 Is knowledge of principles evidenced?
5 Is observation good?
6 Is the charting pertinent and adequate?

Safety

1 Is the bedpan placed securely?
2 Is the bedpan clean and dry?
3 Is the bedpan in good condition?
4 Is the bedpan padded if necessary?

5 Is the bedpan warm if necessary?
6 Is the bedpan cleaned thoroughly?
7 Is the patient handled gently?
8 Are handwashing facilities provided for the patient?
9 Did the nurse use the handwashing facilities after assisting the patient with elimination?

SUGGESTED READINGS

Barnes, Mauvine R.: Clean colons without enemas American Journal of Nursing 69:2128, October 1969.

Birum, Linda, and Zimmerman, Donna S.: Catheter plugs as a source of infection, American Journal of Nursing 71:2150, November, 1971.

Delehanty, Lorraine, and Stravino, Vincent: Achieving bladder control, American Journal of Nursing 70:312, February, 1970.

Dison, Norma G.: An atlas of nursing techniques, St. Louis, 1971, The C. V. Mosby Co.

Dobbins, Janet, and Gleit, Carol: Experience with the lateral position for catheterization, Nursing Clinics of North America 6:373, June, 1971.

Rowson, Lorraine: The lateral position in catheterization, Nursing Clinics of North America 5:175, March, 1970.

19 Daily rehabilitative processes

CONCEPT OF REHABILITATION
Overview

The five broad categories within which complete health service can be most effectively provided have already been introduced. (The reader is referred to Chapter 1, p. 5.) The fifth stage of these recommended categories of health service is considered to be that of rehabilitation. This stage merges with the preceding, more acute clinical stage but is also considered to be sequential to it. The significance of this overlapping of clinical and rehabilitative stages is that the preventive aspects of rehabilitation are most effective when begun during the acute phase of the patient's illness.

During the onset and early stages of a physical illness, secondary complications and physiologic damage may be associated with the inactivity of prolonged bed rest. The deteriorative effects may be more disabling or handicapping to the patient than his initial acute disease entity or injury. These preventable secondary conditions leading to chronic disability and invalidism are often described by the term "disuse phenomena." Common examples are cited in the following brief outline of causes and resulting phenomena:

CAUSES	DISUSE PHENOMENA (deteriorative effects of disuse)
1. Inactivity	Muscle atrophy and weakness Contractures and ankylosis with limitation of joint movement and resulting deformity
2. Prolonged pressure with decreased circulation	Decubitus ulcers
3. Recumbent and/or poor position with lack of chest expansion	Hypostatic pneumonia Venous stasis resulting in circulatory thrombosis Edema contributing to development of decubitus ulcers Constipation Distention Anorexia
4. Lack of weight bearing and muscle pull	Chemical imbalance contributing to osteoporosis, urinary lithiasis, and/or infection
5. Excessive stress	Psychologic responses: depression, dependency, withdrawal, anger, confusion

An undesirable cycle of causes and resulting phenomena tends to develop, leading to further inactivity, aggravation, and extension of disuse effects. Unchecked, the results of the cycle may be a chronically ill, confused patient with weakness, decubitus ulcers, contractures, osteoporosis, and other phenomena in which deterioration of otherwise healthy parts of the body may also occur.

Consider the situation of a patient who has suffered a cerebral vascular accident. The nurse's active part in rehabilitation begins almost immediately by providing proper support to affected limbs in such a way as to maintain physiologic positioning of all parts of the body. This will assist in preventing damage to affected body members that may result when flaccid muscles are left unsupported or spastic muscles are allowed to develop contractures. To preserve the range of joint motion for such a patient, the nurse may put his passive limbs through the complete range of joint motion while administering daily nursing care. By preventing contracture deformities from developing, the long-range rehabilitation potential of the patient will be much greater than if correction of deformities must first be attempted before further rehabilitation measures can be instituted.

From the foregoing illustration it can be seen that during the acute phase of illness the nurse utilizes many rehabilitative techniques to help the patient prevent disuse effects. The patient should become a most active participant in his own rehabilitation as soon as the acute phase of his illness has subsided. In the case of the cerebral vascular accident patient just cited, this will probably be from the third day of illness or as soon as the patient is conscious, the objective being to prevent deformities and helplessness while assisting the patient to care for himself. Helplessness in this context means the inability of the patient to perform such basic tasks as feeding, dressing, bathing, using the toilet, walking, and changing his body position. The acutely ill patient's condition may be such that it is necessary for him to receive the help of the nurse for those functions when complete bed rest is prescribed.

In each patient's situation it is important to understand both the therapeutic purpose and the adverse effects of complete bed rest in order to reduce the hazards of restricted motion. Common purposes of bed rest include: (1) immobilization of a wound, such as a fracture, (2) restricted motion following certain types of operations and to promote healing, rest, and comfort in the acute course of disease process, (3) increased cardiac output and venous return in case of shock, and (4) reducing the effect of gravity in such conditions as edema, varicosities, and protruding hernia. The patient may have enforced limitation of motion as a result of brain or spinal cord injury. When the specific purpose of the bed rest is understood, it is often possible to limit the prescribed restriction of motion to the involved body part or system in order that the rest of the body need not remain totally inactive.

Thus it becomes important to evaluate the patient's total situation and to determine what action can be taken to minimize the physiologic and psychologic effects of inactivity, since many of the preventive measures are nursing activities and can be independently initiated by the nurse. There is growing evidence that prevention of disuse phenomena depends in a large measure on nursing care that is based on a plan for maintaining a balance between rest and activity.

Definition

From the foregoing discussion it can be seen that rehabilitation may be defined as a process of assisting a disabled, acutely or chronically ill, or convalescent person to realize his particular goals in living and working to the utmost of his potential. This process involves various aspects of the individual's physiologic, psychologic, social, economic, and vocational functioning, and it includes almost all of those persons receiving health care.

The individual patient's goal in rehabilitation may vary all the way from achieving ability to give his own daily care to becoming gainfully employed. The word "rehabilitation" itself means "retraining" or "restoring" in contrast to the word "habilitation," which refers to the initial capacity for learning. For example, when a baby first learns to walk, the process is habilitation, but when an individual learns to walk again, it is rehabilitation. The degree of the patient's own motivation to undertake the retraining process is of special significance when illness or injury results in disability.

A patient's need for rehabilitation may or may not be obvious, for not all patients who need rehabilitation have visible handicaps. A patient with heart disease may need as much rehabilitation as does the patient who has lost a limb. Therefore, an evaluation is necessary to determine the individual patient's rehabilitation needs. His needs may be minimal or extensive, depending on his total physical, emotional, social, and economic state, including the degree of effectiveness of previous measures for the prevention of deformities and helplessness.

Rehabilitative process

During the *acute phase* of illness, therapy and nursing care are directed toward assisting the patient to recover from his disabling disease or injury with a minimum of superimposed impairment, social, psychologic, and physical. The prevention of secondary disabilities and the provision of emotional security are equally important. Since the preventive aspects of care relative to the patient's ability to assume

285

activities of daily living are important functions of nursing, the nurse's goal in the acute stage is to pilot the patient safely through to the restorative phase with a minimum of secondary disability, emotional as well as physical.

The *restorative* and *retraining phase* of rehabilitation follows when the patient's immediate lifesaving needs have been met. Long-term considerations must then be examined as early as possible so that appropriate actions geared toward realistic goals for the patient may be instituted. This phase usually includes evaluation of the patient's functional status, potentials, and existing deficits; the determining of realistic goals; and the setting up of a rehabilitation program to enable the patient to achieve self-sufficiency within the level of his capabilities and motivation. This program may require measures to improve his general physical condition, correction of deformities when indicated, passive and active exercises, teaching the patient how to resume self-care, measures to maintain or restore psychosocial equilibrium, therapy for specific disabilities such as speech therapy, training in the use of mechanical devices such as braces, crutches, or prostheses, vocational retraining and employment, teaching the family members how they may accept and help the patient, and providing for appropriate social and recreational activities.

The basic aims of rehabilitation are generally considered to be (1) prevention of further limitation of body function, (2) maintenance of existing abilities, and (3) restoration of as much function as possible.

Team approach to rehabilitation

Rehabilitation usually encompasses a number of special health services that may be made available to the individual patient on the basis of his particular need. Personnel representing these special services include the physician and the nurse and may also include a physical therapist, occupational therapist, psychiatrist, speech therapist, social worker, vocational counselor, or other professional personnel when indicated. Because rehabilitation is a complex process involving the patient and a number of professional personnel, a team relationship usually provides the structure through which each member can make his special knowledge and skills available for the greatest benefit to the patient. The team evaluates the patient's need for rehabilitation and develops a plan whereby he may receive maximum assistance in achieving his rehabilitation goals. However, the success of the plan partially depends on the patient's attitude; therefore, the nurse should be guided by the consideration that the patient is a key member of the team and that the degree of his determination to be rehabilitated may be the deciding factor in the success of the plan.

The nurse's role as a member of the rehabilitation team

The nurse can make a valuable contribution to the effectiveness of the rehabilitation team. The nurse may stimulate development of motivation through an attitude of respect for the patient and confidence in his ability to return to the highest level of independence possible for him. Through a supportive relationship with the patient the nurse observes, listens, and evaluates and so may be able to contribute pertinent information about the patient's condition and progress that might not otherwise be available to the team. The longer contact that the nurse has with the patient often provides the opportunity to act as a coordinator in planning the patient's day, thus enabling other team members to schedule their special rehabilitation services more effectively for the welfare of the patient. The nurse may also work with the other team members in assisting the patient; for example, the physical therapist may enlist the help of the nurse in maintaining correct body alignment and in carrying out some of the frequently repeated exercises to achieve the best therapeutic results.

SCIENTIFIC PRINCIPLES
Concept of activity

Maintenance of the patient's equilibrium, with resulting prevention or counteraction of the physiologic effects of immobility, are often dependent upon knowledge and application of basic scientific principles in dealing with the deteriorating effects of prolonged bed rest. In this context it is a fundamental and useful concept that *the functional ability of the body and its various systems is based on activity*, that body systems tend to function abnormally during prolonged inactivity, and that the resulting adverse effects of inactivity can have drastic physical and emotional consequences more disabling than the initial illness or injury.

Some examples of the more pertinent principles have been selected from the biologic and behavioral sciences. To be all inclusive of principles related to rehabilitation is not possible in this presentation because the exact principles applicable in a particular patient's situation will vary, depending on the nature of his illness or injury, the body structures affected, and his psychologic and emotional state. It should also be remembered that a true principle may not be identifiable as a basis for every nursing action since scientific knowledge is incomplete in many areas, but the nursing action may be continued on empirical grounds if it is known to be effective.

Principles from biologic sciences

The concept of physiologic homeostasis has served as a basis for identifying scientific principles selected from anatomy and physiology that are applicable to the nursing care of a patient with rehabilitation needs, regardless of the specific illness.

1. Normal cellular activity requires:
    a. A consistent supply of oxygen, nutrients, and other vital chemicals
    b. A continuing process for the removal of metabolic by-products
    c. Circulating blood as a means of transportation of oxygen, nutrients for cellular utilization, and elimination of metabolic by-products
    d. Maintenance of the volume and pressure of the circulating blood within certain limits to provide for the changing demands of cellular activity

2. A decrease in the volume and pressure of the circulating blood in a tissue causes a decreased functioning of the tissue.

3. Movement of voluntary muscles assists venous return of blood to the heart by exerting pressure on the veins of the body. Backflow is prevented by the presence of venous valves.

4. Under normal conditions, contraction of skeletal muscles during exercise causes an increase in the blood supply to the muscles involved.

5. Movements of the body are brought about by muscle contraction, through shortening and lengthening of the fibers under nervous control. This produces a full range of body motion.

6. The energy for muscle contraction is produced through complex oxidation-reduction reactions requiring a constant supply of oxygen to the muscle cells.

7. Bone is living tissue requiring a balance between the catabolic and anabolic processes for normal function.
    a. In the process of maintaining a state of equilibrium in the bone, osteoblastic cells are responsible for bone absorption. Osteoclastic cells have an opposing function, which is adsorption of substances back into the bloodstream.
    b. The stresses and strains of mobility

and weight bearing stimulate the osteoblastic cells in their function of building up calcium in the bone matrix.

  c. Some decalcification of bone occurs in the absence of the process of locomotion for a prolonged period of time.

8. Damage to a blood vessel acts as the stimulus to clotting. Thrombocytes are stimulated to release thromboplastin, a vital chemical in the clotting reaction.

  a. The presence of calcium ions is essential for the formation of a blood clot.

  b. Blood calcium and thromboplastin secreted from thrombocytes activate prothrombin to form thrombin.

  c. Thrombin in turn is the catalytic agent to transform the blood-clotting protein, fibrinogen, into fibrin, which forms the network of the clot.

9. The kidneys function to preserve the homeostasis of body fluids and electrolytes by screening waste products from blood plasma.

10. The relative concentration of carbon dioxide and oxygen in the body fluids are principal chemical regulators of the respiratory rate.

11. Continued strong stimulation of tissue eventually leads to fatigue and to depression of normal function.

Principles from behavioral sciences

Selection of principles derived from the behavioral sciences has been based on factors that influence the person's psychosocial equilibrium while he is in a situation requiring nursing care.

1. Perception, influenced by the individual's current physiologic and psychologic states and past experiences, affects his behavior.

2. The individual reacts to a situation as he perceives it, regardless of the reality of the situation or of how others see the situation, and therefore he may be suscep-

tible to errors or distortion in his perception.

3. Psychologic equilibrium is affected by strong emotion that may interfere with rational thinking and behavior.

4. Psychologic factors may cause either subjective physiologic symptoms or changes in physiologic functioning. These psychologic factors may or may not be within the individual's awareness.

5. The individual's body image contributes to his own total self-concept.

6. The threat of change in an individual's self-concept is almost always accompanied by anxiety.

7. Motivation is a requirement for behavior change.

  a. Behavior change is more likely to occur when an individual sees the relationship between the behavior and his personal needs and problems.

  b. Motivation of behavior change in the desired direction is facilitated by anticipation of desirable conditions that will result from the behavior.

APPLICATION TO PLANNING NURSING CARE

The nurse approaches specific responsibilities in providing nursing care by utilizing the framework of the nursing process as presented in the preceding chapters. In utilizing this framework the reader has thus far been introduced to (1) methods of assessing the needs of patients and identifying related nursing problems, (2) methods of collecting further information about the patient's identified problems, and (3) methods in developing an appropriate nursing care plan in terms of the data collected and relevant scientific and nursing principles.

The task at this point is to apply these concepts (1) to begin developing methods for implementing the nursing care plan to provide optimum quality of nursing care to assist the individual patient in maintenance or restoration of homeostatic equilibrium, and (2) to begin developing methods of evaluating the success of the nursing care plan and adjusting it to meet the patient's changing needs.

USING RELATED PRINCIPLES IN SOLVING NURSING PROBLEMS

Continuing with the rehabilitation needs of the immobile patient, some of the common problems most likely to be found in the care of a long-term bed patient have been selected as examples to demonstrate how the related principles become meaningful to the nurse in solving the problems encountered while planning and administering direct patient care.

Problems in maintaining integrity of movement

The necessity of motion, tonicity, and intermittent work load of the skeletal muscles in maintenance of the structural stability and metabolism of the musculoskeletal system has been well documented. From the biologic principles inferences can be made that normal daily activity (1) contributes to cell nutrition through efficient blood circulation, (2) maintains muscle integrity, (3) is a complex, integrated activity coordinated through the nervous and endocrine functions, and (4) is a factor in maintaining calcium and other ionic equilibria within the body.

Adverse effects on motor function develop rapidly when the immobility of bed rest is allowed to continue. Early symptoms often are noticeable within 2 to 3 days and progress rapidly with continued immobility. Problems of musculoskeletal deterioration commonly seen by the nurse are muscle weakness and atrophy, contractures, decubitus ulcers, and proneness to fracture from the loss of bone matrix and calcium characteristic of osteoporosis. Injury occurs to cells when they are deprived of oxygen, essential nutrients, and the stimulation of activity. In the condition of immobility, cells decrease in size as the nutrient and functional demands decrease, which is a means of maintaining a degree of homeostasis. *Disuse atrophy* is the term used to denote this loss of substance in a cell or tissue that develops in response to inactivity. It is an adaptive mechanism that permits cells to survive unfavorable conditions. However, if the amount of deprivation is too severe, the cells will die such as in a decubitus ulcer.

Atrophy and contractures occur when muscles do not have the activity necessary to maintain the integrity of their function, which is shortening and lengthening of their fibers to produce a full range of motion. Regardless of the factors causing contractures of the involved muscles, weakness and atrophy result in a limited range of motion of the associated joint. Fixed deformities, such as "clawhand," develop when there is an imbalance in the pull of opposing muscles, that is, one muscle is weaker than its antagonist. Additional effects of gravity, muscle spasm, and edema may also further limit muscle activity and joint motion. Once a contracture has developed, the process may often be reversed through rehabilitative exercises and stretching. If allowed to progress the process will involve tendons, ligaments, and the joint capsule. The condition may eventually become irreversible, with joint motion being impossible even if the original disease or injury would allow it. Surgical intervention may, in selected cases, be successful in restoring some function to the disabled part; however, it is better to prevent contractures that to treat them.

Problems in maintaining integrity of cardiovascular function

The major hazards of immobility to cardiovascular functioning have been identified in current literature as thrombus formation and increased work load of the heart.

While the exact etiologic role of immobility in thrombus formation has not been

289

entirely explained, the findings of related studies seem to support the statement that venous stasis and other identifiable effects of immobility can be contributing factors to venous thrombus formation. The most obvious cause of venous stasis during bed rest is the lack of muscular contraction promoting venous return, which normally occurs as a result of exercise.

Other factors possibly contributing to venous thrombus formation include dehydration leading to increased coagulability of the blood by increasing the concentration of formed elements in the blood, which in turn results in greater viscosity and a greater tendency for clotting. Increased levels of blood calcium occur in the process of bone decalcification, which may result in further hypercoagulability of the blood. Another predisposing factor, the effect of external pressure on the blood vessels, is common knowledge in nursing. Any situation restricting circulation with resulting damage to the blood vessel intima may lead to clot formation because the blood thrombocytes deposited on the damaged area form predisposing plaques. Examples of such situations include a lateral recumbent position with the upper leg lying on the calf of the lower leg or pressure on the popliteal vein from pillows or bent knee gatch.

There is some disagreement in literature regarding the work load of the heart when the patient is in the resting supine position as compared to the resting sitting position. The more recent studies indicate that the heart works 30% harder when a person is supine than when in the sitting position because of the altered distribution of blood in the body, which occurs with the release of gravity pressure in the supine position. Part of the blood is redistributed from the lower extremities to other parts of the body. This increase in the volume of the circulating blood adds to the work load of the heart. The studies also show that the heart rate increases with the added work

load and that there tends to be a progressive decrease of ability in cardiovascular function as the patient remains bedfast. A prolonged period of reconditioning is necessary for the heart to return to its capacity prior to the period of bed rest.

Problems in maintaining integrity of urinary function

The effects of prolonged bed rest on urinary function are primarily related to metabolic changes that cause the kidneys to excrete larger amounts of calcium and other minerals that contribute to the formation of renal calculi, sometimes called "stones of recumbency." As a consequence of bone decalcification, an excess of calcium occurs in the extracellular fluid, which is excreted by way of the kidneys. The high content of urinary calcium may lead to the formation of kidney or bladder stones. This condition occurs when factors predisposing to precipitation of salts are present, such as urinary stasis, infection, alkalinity, decreased volume of urine, insufficient citric acid, and increased concentration of phosphates. According to one theory, salts in the urinary tract are held in suspension in combination with citric acid. Therefore, the stone-forming salts are more apt to precipitate when the urine becomes alkaline. The decreased muscle activity of the immobilized patient contributes to alkalinity of the urine because the acid end products to be excreted are also decreased. Medications taken by the patient may contribute to these changes. Urine alkalinity may also be increased through bacterial activity.

Urinary stasis, a common development when the patient is immobilized, may occur within a few days if the patient is supine because in this position urine formed must be passed from the kidney pelvis into the ureter against gravity.

An implication of the foregoing statements for nursing is that the urinary tract complications may often be prevented or minimized through appropriate nursing measures directed toward reducing the effects of bed rest when the reasons for the adverse effects are understood.

Problems in maintaining integrity of respiratory function

A constant flow of oxygen in amounts necessary to maintain oxidative reactions in the cells and the elimination of carbon dioxide from the tissues are processes necessary for maintenance of life. The movement of air in and out of the lungs during respiration provides the supply of oxygen necessary for survival. The gaseous exchange occurs through the thin moist membrane of the alveolar and capillary walls, which are essential parts of lung tissue. Oxygen is essential to cellular metabolism. Deprivation of oxygen for more than a few minutes, even for as brief a period as 4 or 5 minutes, will result in irreparable damage or cellular death in tissues most sensitive to hypoxia such as cerebral cortex, myocardium, and kidney.

In spite of great differences in the level of tissue activity at various times, homeostatic mechanisms operate to maintain the amount of oxygen available to the body cells within quite narrow limits:

Activity →Increased cellular metabolism
↓
Increased carbon dioxide formation
↓
Vasodilation
↓
Increased blood flow
↓
Increased oxygen demand
↓
Increased respiratory rate and depth
↓
Increased gaseous exchange in tissues and alveoli (oxygen supply increased, carbon dioxide eliminated)

The effect of exercise is to bring fresh blood to the tissues via the capillaries. This action changes the local pressure as well as the fluid environment of all the cells, which aids the body in maintaining homeostasis. The effect of immobility, however, is decreased cell metabolism, diminished metabolite production, and less oxygen need. The first response to immobility is adaptive in that the balance in concentration between carbon dioxide and oxygen is maintained temporarily through decreased cell metabolism and decreased oxygen need. As immobility is prolonged, decreased respiratory movement and oxygen–carbon dioxide imbalance will develop.

Some of the common factors limiting respiratory movement and thus interfering with expansion and effective ventilation of the lungs include:

1. Any position of the patient that limits chest cage expansion, that is maintained over too long a time, that compresses the thorax, or in which pressure against the bed limits respiratory movement
2. Muscle weakness limiting movement of the chest wall, as in the case of a paralyzed, debilitated, or otherwise inactive patient
3. Pharmacologic agents such as anesthetics, narcotics, and sedatives, which act on the central nervous system and may depress the rate and depth of respiratory movement
4. Anything creating intra-abdominal pressure and limiting action of the diaphragm during respiratory movement, such as abdominal distension from pressure of accumulated feces, gas, fluid, or tight abdominal binder

The adverse effects of limited respiratory movement are manifested as stasis and pooling of secretions in the tracheobronchial passages, because coughing and movements that normally aid in moving secretions from the respiratory passages are not used by the patient. Coughing may be further inhibited by medications that depress the cough reflex. Inadequate fluid intake and medications may contribute to mucus secretions becoming thick and tenacious and more difficult to move, thereby tending to fill the alveoli with fluid and obstructing the airway. As aeration is further decreased, hypostatic pneumonia may intervene. Collections of static secretions serve as likely medium for pneumococci, staphylocci, and other common pathogenic organisms, increasing the possibility of respiratory tract infections and filling of the alveoli with inflammatory exudate.

As the act of breathing becomes more difficult in the presence of these inhibiting factors, the efficiency of ventilation is decreased, causing the patient to increase the effort needed for breathing. The greater effort requires a greater oxygen supply, with more carbon dioxide produced but with increasingly limited diffusion of oxygen and carbon dioxide in the alveoli. The result is a buildup of carbon dioxide in the blood and progressive tissue hypoxia as the imbalance becomes greater.

Initially, the increased carbon dioxide concentration in the blood acts as a respiratory stimulant. In time, however, the respiratory center will become depressed, and eventually carbon dioxide narcosis will result. Respiratory acidosis follows when the retention of carbon dioxide reaches a concentration sufficient to cause interference with the bicarbonate buffer system. The body attempts to compensate by producing metabolic alkalosis. If the condition is unrelieved, respiratory failure will lead to death of the patient.

$$\text{Buffer system}$$
$$H_2CO_3 \leftrightarrows H^+ + HCO_3^-$$
$$\Updownarrow$$
$$H_2O + CO_2$$

Problems in maintaining integrity of gastrointestinal function

Just as all cells of the body require an adequate amount of oxygen to maintain optimum function, so also do they need adequate nutrition. Normal cellular activity requires a constant supply of nutrients maintained by the regular intake of a properly balanced diet that supplies all of the essential nutrients in adequate amounts. Within limits, the individual is able to adapt to variations in supply of nutrients, as with other homeostatic mechanisms. However, the individual consigned to bed rest encounters complex physiologic effects in relation to gastrointestinal function. Depending on the nature of the original disease process and the general physical condition, this may require astute nursing intervention for maintenance of homeostatic equilibrium.

The major functions most usually involved are those associated with food intake and with elimination. These problems are discussed briefly here but are more fully developed in Chapters 17 and 18.

The healthy individual in a normal state of nutrition is in nitrogen balance since the nitrogen intake and excretion are equal. Positive nitrogen balance, a state in which the intake of nitrogen is greater than the output (meaning that the anabolic processes exceed the catabolic processes), occurs during periods of growth or convalescence from injury or debilitating illness. When nitrogen is being lost more rapidly than it is being supplied by the diet, a state of negative balance exists. This is an unfavorable state because it means that the body is oxidizing its own protein.

Although there may be many reasons for a negative nitrogen balance, it is well documented that with continued bed rest, even for healthy individuals, a negative balance will occur initially. But for the ill patient the catabolic activity is apt to accelerate, producing breakdown of tissues and resulting in protein deficiency. The rate of tissue repair is diminished, synthesis of plasma proteins and hemoglobin is interrupted, and resistance to infection is sharply decreased. Over a period of time a state of malnutrition will develop, with loss of weight and strength and loss of resistance of the tissues to pressure. This contributes to the occurrence of decubiti that may not respond to treatment unless the nutritional deficiencies are corrected. Diminished ability to respond to stress together with anorexia frequently occurs in the presence of protein deficiency. The effect on the individual will vary, depending on such factors as the condition responsible for the bed rest, the rapidity with which the condition developed, and the time element involved.

The nutritional problem is made more difficult when anorexia is accompanied by psychologic problems and other factors leading to failure of the patient to eat. Even though the desire to eat may be lacking and energy requirements are reduced, the nutrients necessary for maintenance of basal cell metabolism and restoration of nitrogen balance are needed by the immobilized patient.

Some of the predisposing factors to the development of problems with elimination from the intestine include lack of muscular exercise, malnutrition, limited food and fluid intake, unfamiliar diet, medications such as barium used in x-ray of the colon, weakness and debility, and difficulties the patient may experience in using a bedpan. The abnormal posture assumed in using a bedpan and the psychologic effects resulting from embarrassment and anxiety add to the difficulties.

Failure to defecate, for any reason, will eventually cause the colon to lose muscular tone and become increasingly unresponsive to the normal stimuli for defecation. The rectal mucosa and musculature become insensitive to the presence of a fecal mass, and sooner or later constipation will have developed. Prolonged retention of feces may lead to fecal impaction, an accumulation of hardened fecal material. Stool retained in the colon tends to become hard and dry because water is absorbed, and it

is then extremely difficult or impossible for the hardened mass to be expelled in a normal process of evacuation. The pressure of a large impaction will create a mechanical obstruction of the bowel with the following symptoms characteristic of blockage: distension aggravated by accumulating fluid and gas, impaired circulation resulting from pressure on the blood vessels of the area, depressed intestinal function leading to failure of absorption and to fluid and electrolyte imbalance, and, as the intra-abdominal pressure increases, labored breathing, pain, and discomfort.

An early fecal impaction may not be easily recognized because the irritation of the intestinal mucosa by the hard fecal particles may cause liquid stool to seep around the impaction, thereby simulating diarrhea. Frequent liquid seepage without passage of normal stool should always be investigated as a possible indication of fecal impaction. Since the effects of immobilization on gastrointestinal function can be so extensive and difficult to relieve, it is obviously imperative to prevent them from occurring if it is at all possible. Continuous, well-planned nursing management can in most cases prevent these drastic physiologic effects.

Problems in maintaining integrity of the skin

When the patient is unable to move about freely in bed, the pressure on skin and underlying tissues, particularly over a bony prominence, will cause a decreased blood supply, threatening the structural integrity of the skin. Referring to the principles selected for their relevance to this problem, pressure from the weight of the patient's body resting against the bed will impair the volume of circulating blood in the area, with resulting decrease in the supply of oxygen and other nutrients necessary for cellular metabolism in the skin and underlying tissues. This produces a situation in which there is an inadequate supply of oxygen to maintain homeostasis.

Any break in the continuity of the skin is a potential source of infection, and decubiti are no exception. They are difficult to manage because the circulation to the tissues has been allowed to fail. The integrity of the skin may be further endangered by the presence of urine and feces when the patient is incontinent. Too often those responsible for patient care may not be aware of the possibility of decubitus formation until it occurs, overlooking the fact that decubiti can develop withing 24 hours. Therefore, preventive measures should begin at the time of admission for any patient who for any reason has limited motion, particularly if he is debilitated and undernourished.

Problems in maintaining psychologic integrity

Emotional support is as significant as physical care, because illness and hospitalization are almost always disruptive for the patient and are accompanied by feelings of fear and anxiety that may threaten his powers of emotional adaptation. The need to understand and deal with the cultural aspect of the hospitalized patient's illness was introduced in Chapter 7. At this point attention is directed toward maintaining the psychosocial equilibrium of the patient consigned to bed rest.

In reference to the stated principles, it is suggested that in the acute stages of illness the immobilized patient will experience feelings of helplessness, inadequacy, and dependency on those around him and, most likely, problems related to the loss of role activity. His behavior will be influenced by the responses from the nurse, family members, and other significant persons in the situation. When a sudden, long-term, or permanent disability has been sustained, the more disruptive effect on the patient is that of profound emotional shock. His immediate reaction is

usually that of denial, because it is difficult for him to believe that this has really happened to him. He may express denial in a variety of different ways, such as by apathy and by refusing care and rehabilitative measures. As the full impact of the disability can no longer be denied, a period of depression and anxiety will usually follow while the patient seeks to deal with his altered perception of himself and with the significance of the disability in terms of the effect on his former way of life, family situation, and vocational and financial problems to which he may see no acceptable solution. He may express these feelings by continuing to reject care, food, and fluids or sometimes by withdrawal. He may even become abusive, expressing frustration and anger.

The value of assisting the patient to work through these agonizing stages to the point of eventually accepting the disability should be understood by the nurse. If these behaviors are understood and managed properly, the patient may come to recognize his abilities and potentials as well as the limitations. As he regains emotional equilibrium the patient is ready to join the team and take an active part in his own rehabilitation.

NURSING MEASURES

Preventive and maintenance measures undertaken during acute care shorten and enhance restorative care, and they are often continued as an integral part of the restorative care of the disabled. Since these aspects of care are so often overlooked in the acute phase when preventive measures are most crucial, they are presented as nursing measures appropriate for the beginning stages of bed rest, unless specifically contraindicated for individual patients. They are discussed here in relation to isolated body systems, but it is well to recognize that the various body systems are interdependent and that they are all involved in the complex interactions through which restoration and maintenance of homeostasis is achieved.

Maintaining integrity of the skin

The nurse is applying knowledge of the principles related to integrity of the skin when selecting nursing measures designed to facilitate the supply of blood to the tissues affected. Appropriate nursing action based on the principles used in solving the problem of maintaining the integrity of the skin and underlying tissues would include these steps:

1. *Observing* the patient's limitation of motion and recognizing its significance in relation to maintaining the health of local tissues
2. *Inspecting* the skin for signs of pressure, especially over the bony prominences of the coccyx, trochanters, shoulder blades, heels, and elbows (significant effects of blood stasis would be recognized by redness, or mottled appearance of the skin, that does not disappear quickly with change of position or with rubbing)
3. *Concluding* that continued pressure on the area would cause death of the tissues affected (decubitus ulcer)
4. *Selecting* appropriate nursing measures to restore and maintain adequate circulation in the area (these measures might include frequent changes of the patient's position, passive range of motion while giving hygienic care, and gentle massage of the reddened skin areas to stimulate circulation)
5. *Reporting* beginning skin changes so that other more effective therapeutic measures may be instituted to prevent further damage to the tissues

Similar effects resulting from impaired circulation may occur when there is pressure from casts, splints, braces, or other mechanical devices with which the patient may be fitted during the course of rehabilitation.

Prevention of decubiti is, of course, a primary aim in patient care. This objective is usually achieved through such nursing measures as the following:

1. Definite schedules for assisting and/or encouraging the patient to shift the body weight off the bony prominences should be maintained. Principles of body mechanics and positioning are included in Chapter 4. In some instances oscillating beds, turning frames, and the like may be helpful, but they cannot substitute for meticulous skin care. To be avoided are rubber rings and doughnuts, which are less than helpful because they create pressure around the bony prominence, thereby tending to restrict circulation in the threatened tissues.

2. The patient's skin should be clean and dry and the bed linen dry and wrinkle-free. Any massage lotion containing alcohol should be avoided because the drying effect on skin oils tends to contribute to the breakdown of the tissues in vulnerable areas.

3. Close inspection of vulnerable areas when giving skin care and changing the patient's position to note the first warning indications of impending decubitus formation, such as a reddened or mottled area or a break in the integrity of the skin, is a nursing responsibility.

4. Regular bowel and bladder toilet schedules will aid in controlling incontinence, which predisposes to tissue breakdown and ulcer formation.

5. Prompt therapy to encourage healing should be instituted if a pressure area does develop.

Coping with musculoskeletal deterioration

Disuse atrophy of bone and muscle tissue can often be limited or averted through the prompt application of nursing measures that have as their objectives (1) prevention of atrophy by assisting the patient to carry out a planned program of appro-

Text continued on p. 307.

295

Fig. 19-1.   Shoulder flexion and extension.

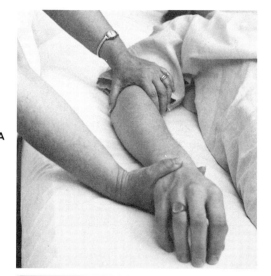

Begin by placing one hand above the patient's elbow. Hold the patient's hand with the other hand.

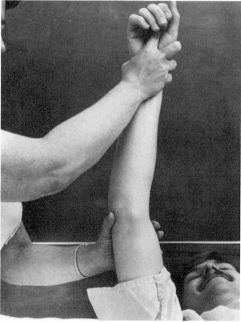

Raise the arm upward from the side of his body.

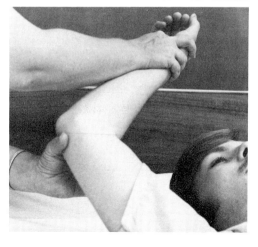

Next, in one flowing movement, carry the arm slowly and gently toward the patient's head as far as possible without causing pain. *Repeat motion.* (Should the headboard interfere, the arm may be bent at the elbow.)

Fig. 19-2. Shoulder abduction and adduction.

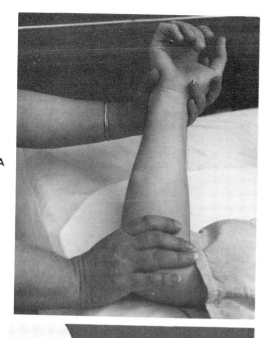

While supporting the patient's wrist and elbow,

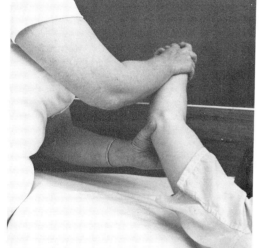

slowly move the arm straight over the patient's head.

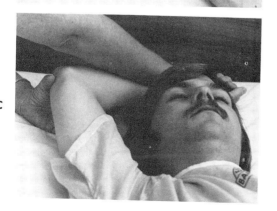

Next, bend the elbow and push the arm gently toward the top of the patient's head, then lower the arm to the starting position (Fig. 19-1, *A*) and *repeat motion.*

297

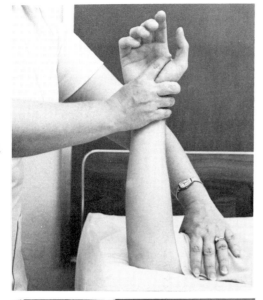

A

Fig. 19-3. Shoulder internal and external rotation.

Begin with the arm even with the shoulder, the elbow bent, and the wrist supported.

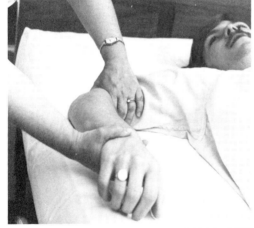

B

While keeping the upper arm even with the shoulder, move the hand and forearm toward the bed, touching the mattress with the patient's hand (palm down).

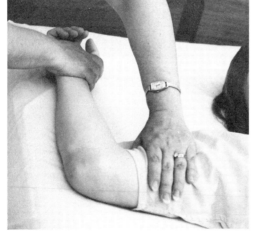

C

Move the arm toward the patient's head, again touching the mattress with the patient's hand (palm up). *Repeat motion.*

Fig. 19-4. Shoulder cross adduction.

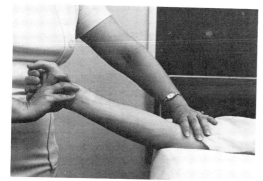

Begin by holding the patient's arm away from his body and supporting the wrist.

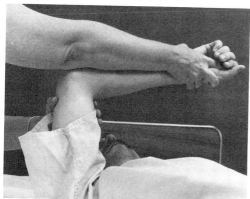

Lift the arm while bending it at the elbow.

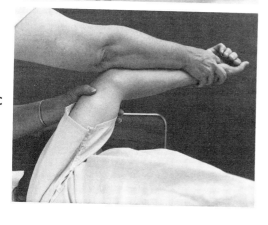

Gently carry the arm across the chest, then return to the starting position (**A**) and *repeat motion.*

299

Fig. 19-5. Forearm supination and pronation.

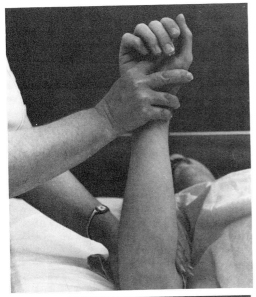

A

With the elbow bent and wrist supported, twist the wrist toward the patient's face,

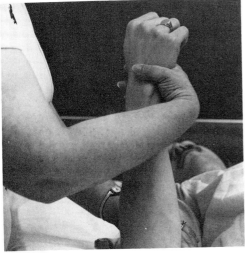

B

then twist the palm toward the patient's feet. *Repeat motion.*

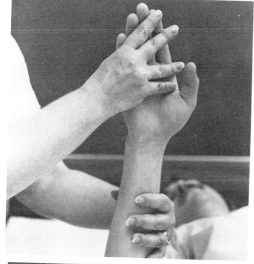

Fig. 19-6. Wrist flexion and extension.

Bend the patient's wrist forward,

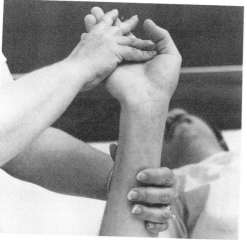

then bend it backward, keeping the fingers straight. *Repeat motion.*

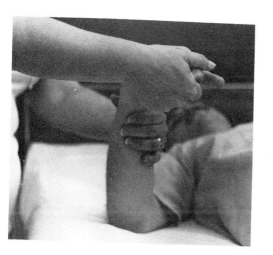

Fig. 19-7. Finger extension and flexion.

Bend the fingers forward while closing them to make a fist, then open. *Repeat motion.*

301

Fig. 19-8. Thumb flexion and extension.

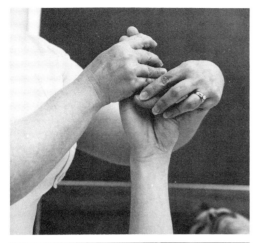

A

Begin by holding the patient's fingers straight, then bend the thumb into the palm.

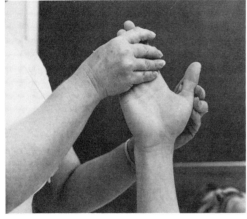

B

Next, pull the thumb away from the palm. *Repeat motion.*

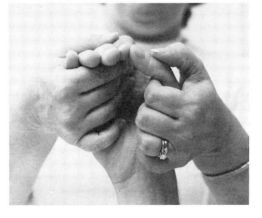

C

Then move the thumb toward the index finger so as to form a circle.

Fig. 19-9. Knee and hip flexion.

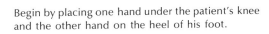

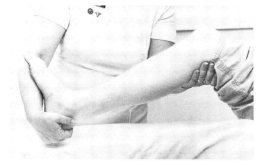

Begin by placing one hand under the patient's knee and the other hand on the heel of his foot.

Lift the leg while bending it at the knee.

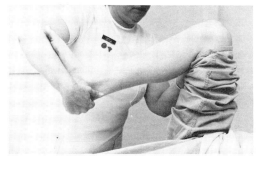

Next, move the leg upward toward the patient's head as far as possible without causing pain. *Repeat motion.*

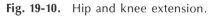

Fig. 19-10. Hip and knee extension.

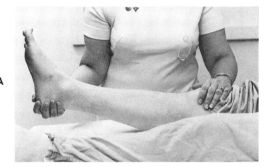

A

Place one hand under the patient's heel and the other hand under the knee.

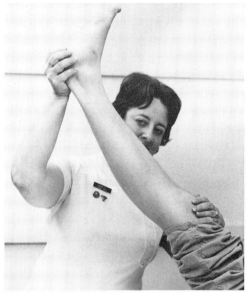

B

Lift the leg while keeping the knee straight, pushing gently to stretch the back of the leg. *Repeat motion.*

Fig. 19-11. Hip abduction and adduction.

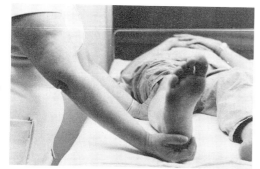

Begin by placing one hand under the patient's knee and the other hand under the heel. Then, while holding the leg straight, lift it approximately 2 inches above the mattress.

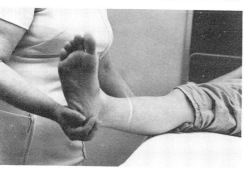

Next, pull the leg toward you,

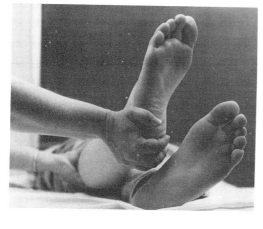

then push the leg back toward the patient's midline. *Repeat motion.*

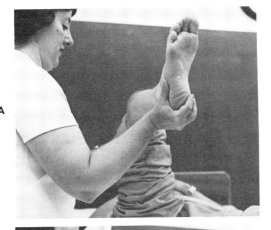

Fig. 19-12. Hip internal and external rotation.

Begin by placing one hand under the patient's knee and the other hand under the heel. Then lift the leg while bending it to form a right angle at the knee.

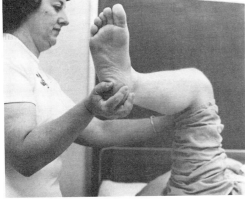

Pull the foot toward you while holding the knee in place.

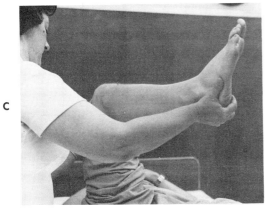

Push the foot away, then back to the starting position **(A).** *Repeat motion.*

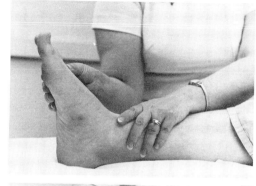

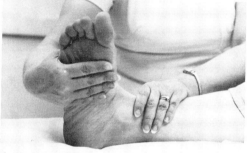

Fig. 19-13. Foot inversion and eversion.

Begin by turning the foot outward,

then turn the foot inward. *Repeat motion.*

priate exercises, (2) maximizing maintenance of the patient's functional capacities, (3) prevention and relief of pressure on any body part or tissues, (4) assistance to the patient in maintaining the principles of body positioning and alignment, and (5) assistance to the patient in maintaining adequate nutrition. The focus in this section is primarily on the first two objectives, because the remaining ones are discussed in other sections.

A program of therapeutic exercises is prescribed by the physician and carried out under the guidance of the physical therapist, often with the assistance of the nurse. On the basis of the concept of activity and the related principles already presented, it can be assumed that the exercises will stimulate circulation, assist in maintaining muscle strength and joint function, prevent deformity, and assist in the return to physiologic functioning of the respiratory, gastrointestinal, and nervous systems.

There are four types of exercises, but all have a common goal, which is the restoration and/or maintenance of function. The exercises can be arranged in progressive steps, depending on the condition of the patient.

1. *Passive exercises* are performed for the patient by the therapist or nurse, without the patient's assistance, either because of the patient's inability to move the parts or when it is undesirable for him to move the part or parts himself. The recommended method is to stabilize the proximal joint and, while supporting the distal part, move the joint smoothly, slowly, and gently. The usual procedure is to move the joint through its *full range of motion*, which is the *extent that it is normally capable of being moved* without pain or undue force.

2. *Assistive active exercise* is the second step in which the exercise is carried out by the patient with the assistance of the therapist or nurse. This may be for the purpose

307

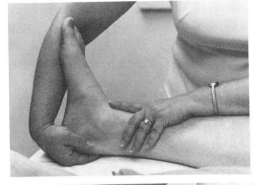

A

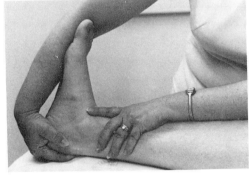

B

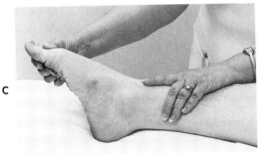

C

Fig. 19-14. Ankle dorsiflexion and plantar flexion.

Begin by holding the heel, allowing your arm to rest against the sole of the patient's foot.

Press the arm against the sole moving it toward the shin.

Then move the hand to the top of the patient's foot just below the toes and push downward so as to point the toes. *Repeat motion.*

of encouraging the patient to resume active voluntary movements and to build muscle strength. The therapist or nurse supports the distal part while the patient is encouraged to take the joint through its range of motion with as little assistance as possible, avoiding excessive fatigue or pain.

3. *Active exercise* is that which is accomplished by the patient without assistance to further increase muscle strength. The movement is initiated and produced by the patient and should be slow, smooth, and rhythmic. The exercise should be stopped when there are signs of fatigue.

4. *Resistive exercise* is the final step. This is performed by the patient against some force, mechanical or manual, for the purpose of increasing muscle power.

Another type of exercise that may be performed by the patient is *muscle setting,* which is used to maintain muscle strength when a joint is immobilized. The patient is taught to tighten the muscle as much as possible without moving the joint, hold for several seconds, and then relax.

The range of motion program should be planned to meet the individual needs of the patient, the objective being to maintain

Fig. 19-15. Toe flexion and extension.

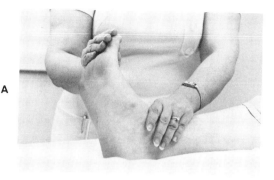

Begin by pulling upward on the toes,

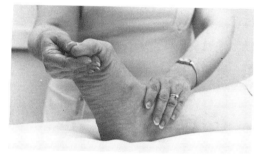

then pull downward. *Repeat motion.*

and/or achieve the amount of motion necessary for him to perform the activities of daily living. However, it should not be assumed that performance of the personal self-care activities by the patient will alone be sufficient to prevent contractures and to maintain joint integrity and mobility, because the performance of these activities does not necessarily require a full range of motion. Therefore, the nurse should be alert to the need for other preventive measures, including change of position, proper body alignment, and support of the various body parts, and a planned program of therapeutic exercises based on the patient's individual needs and capabilities and arranged to be performed within his daily schedule.

During the acute phase of illness the passive range of motion exercises can be carried out by the nurse while giving physical care, in order to minimize disabilities of inactivity, except when contraindicated for specific patients. In most cases the passive range of motion exercises can be utilized by the nurse until a planned

rehabilitative program of therapeutic exercises can be instituted. During the range of motion exercises the patient should be comfortable in the supine position with proper support of the various body parts maintained during the exercises. Utilization of correct body mechanics is important for both the patient and the nurse. Figs. 19-1 to 19-15 demonstrate an acceptable method of carrying out passive range of motion exercises for the various body joints.

Personal self-care activities (a term sometimes used synonymously with activities of daily living) include three areas: (1) performance of personal hygiene activities, such as bathing, oral hygiene, nail care, hair care, and other grooming tasks, (2) ability to care for bowel and bladder toilet needs, and (3) eating. The nurse can do much to prepare the patient for beginning self-care activities when he is ready, physically and psychologically, to begin to move toward independence by assuming some responsibility for his own care. When it is time for the patient to realize

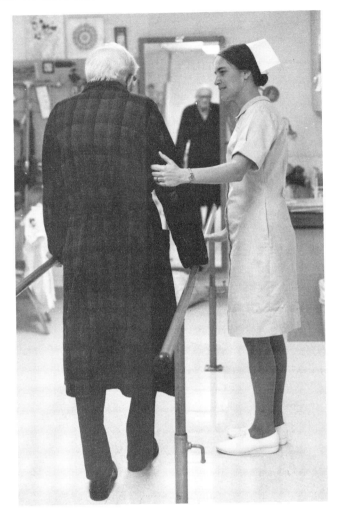

Fig. 19-16. Daily accomplishment brings self-confidence to the patient. (Courtesy Hoag Memorial Hospital, Newport Beach, Calif.)

that he can do things for himself, it is important that his activities be within his developing muscle strength and that the nurse assume responsibility for teaching him how to perform these activities safely. Maintaining or regaining independence will help him to progress from illness toward physical and emotional health. Often, judgment on the part of the nurse is required to decide when and how much the patient should be assisted in order to avoid taxing the patient beyond his capacity or, by assisting him unnecessarily, delaying his progress from dependency and self-centered attention toward independence. More specific information on personal self-care activities is included in Chapter 4. Assistive devices and techniques designed for use by patients with various types of disabilities are described in the suggested reference readings at the end of this chapter.

Preventing respiratory complications

Vigilance on the part of the nurse will often lead to the recognition of variations

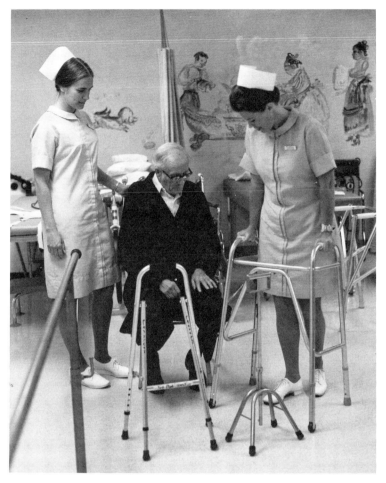

Fig. 19-17. Reassuring the patient learning to use an assistive device. (Courtesy Hoag Memorial Hospital, Newport Beach, Calif.)

in the patient's condition that suggest the need to alter the plan of care in order to meet his changing needs. This is true, for instance, of the patient lying passively in bed who does not maintain proper position and who may therefore not expand his lungs adequately, thus increasing the danger of hypostatic pneumonia. Respiratory depression from any cause predisposes to the pooling of bronchial secretions. Regularly turning the patient helps to avoid the pooling of secretions on one side. The possibility of early pulmonary complications might be suspected by changes in the respirations, such as slow, shallow, labored breathing, and by restlessness.

Active preventive measures at this early point may be effective in helping to halt the changes in the normal physiologic functions of the respiratory system. By the time late signs of hypoxia have developed—including dyspnea, cyanosis, anxiety, use of neck muscles to aid in respiration, productive cough—a complication such as hypostatic pneumonia may already have developed.

Nursing measures that are essential in counteracting ill effects of immobility on the respiratory system are based on the

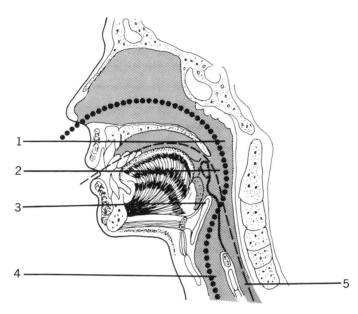

Fig. 19-18. The problem of aspiration may occur because the pathways for inspired air and ingested food cross at the epiglottis. *1,* Nasopharynx; *2,* pharynx; *3,* epiglottis; *4,* trachea; *5,* esophagus.

understanding and meeting of the patient's need to breathe efficiently. A definite schedule to assist the patient to turn, cough, and breathe deeply should be included early in the plan of care. Since coughing and breathing deeply may be painful, it is usually necessary to help the patient to understand the benefit of breathing deeply and coughing to loosen secretions and clear them from the respiratory passages. The patient may find that sitting up in a chair, whenever possible, results in easier breathing and stimulates greater depth of respiration. Arranging regular periods for activity and rest is usually beneficial in facilitating adequate oxygen–carbon dioxide exchange, which is significant in preventing respiratory complications in vulnerable patients.

Maintaining nutrition

An adequate food intake serves an important role in maintaining homeostatic balance. Cellular nutrition will therefore suffer when for any reason the food intake is deficient or there is interference with the integrity of the gastrointestinal tract. Nursing measures should be directed toward assisting the patient in solving problems related to the ingestion of food and to maintaining the function of the gastrointestinal tract.

Problems encountered with ingestion may include at least some of the following factors:

1. Failure of the patient to eat, either because he does not feel like eating, such as in the presence of anorexia of nitrogen imbalance, does not like the food served, or has some contributing condition in the mouth, such as ill-fitting dentures; or he may be too weak and ill to feed himself.
2. Failure of the swallowing mechanism to function, resulting in aspiration of food or fluids.

The problem of aspiration may arise because the pharynx serves as a common passageway for both food and air. (See Fig. 19-18.) As inspired air is drawn downward

312

it passes through the larynx and onward to the lungs. A bolus of food passing through the pharynx, however, must be diverted away from the larynx and pass via the esophagus into the stomach. This is accomplished during the act of swallowing by reflex action causing elevation of the larynx, pressing it upward against the epiglottis to block the passage of swallowed material into the larynx. Gravity and peristaltic waves then assist the passage of food along the esophagus and into the stomach. The danger of failure of the mechanism with resulting aspiration of food or fluids into the respiratory passages is greatly increased for the very weak or paralyzed patient or for the patient in a prone position. Aspirated material endangers the patient because it may block the airway or may be the cause of an inflammatory process in the lungs of an already ill patient.

In dealing with problems of ingestion, an important nursing responsibility is to note when the patient is failing to eat adequately and then to determine the nature of the problem. When the causes are known, it is often possible to discover ways of assisting the patient with the process of eating. By confering with the physician and dietary staff, balanced meals supplying nutrients necessary for cell metabolism may be served that will have more appeal to the patient or be easier to masticate when there are denture problems or when the patient is edentulous. Attention to reducing stress factors whenever possible may also help to improve the appetite.

Assisting the patient during mealtime either by positioning for greatest ease in feeding himself or by feeding him when necessary, and by adjusting the rate and size of bites to the patient's ability to eat, are all nursing responsibilities.

Measures to prevent aspiration include positioning the patient with head elevated to aid gravity in the swallowing process, observing that the swallowing reflex is present before attempting to feed the patient, and testing the patient's ability to swallow food with a small amount of semisoft nourishment first because it is less apt to be aspirated than liquids. Caution should always be exercised in feeding a patient to avoid the dangers of aspiration. If vomiting occurs the patient's head may be turned to the side to lessen the possibility of aspirating vomitus.

Preventing bowel problems

For every immobilized patient prevention of constipation, with its threat of more serious complications, is always a possibility to be considered in the plan of nursing care.

A plan for bowel hygiene management is based on the information obtained from the patient about his normal routine and pattern of elimination. Habits of elimination are learned and therefore vary from individual to individual and also among age groups. Information that may be obtained from the patient, or family members, before planning care would include such data as:

1. What is the patient's normal time of day for a movement?
2. What is his usual frequency of movements?
3. When was the last movement?
4. Is there any difficulty or discomfort associated with the process of elimination?
5. Does he use laxatives or other means to stimulate bowel movement?
6. What is his usual diet?
7. How much fluid does he usually take?

With the pertinent information gathered the nurse can proceed with the planning of care.

Success of the plan of care often depends on the patient's understanding and participation in measures that take his regular pattern into consideration. Whenever possible the patient should help to regulate his own diet and daily schedule. Since peristalsis is apt to be strongest following meals, particularly breakfast, regularity is encouraged by providing time in the schedule at that point for the patient to respond to the urge to defecate. Some patients may already be accustomed to an evening schedule at daily, or perhaps every other day, intervals. The significant features of the schedule are that a specific time of day be selected at no longer than 3-day intervals and that the patient be encouraged to respond when the urge to defecate occurs. A prolonged schedule of more than 2- to 3-day intervals is usually unsatisfactory because fluid is absorbed, increasing the difficulty of evacuating the hardened fecal mass.

Consistency of the stool is an important factor in the success of bowel hygiene management. A soft, formed stool is most easily evacuated and should be promoted by regulating fluid and diet intake. A high fluid intake (2,000 to 3,000 ml. per day), with perhaps a hot drink before breakfast, may be recommended to stimulate peristalsis. A diet that adds bulk and cellulose from vegetables and certain foods that tend to increase bowel activity, such as lemon juice, prunes, oranges, figs, and other fresh fruits, should be individualized according to the natural laxative effect of these foods on each patient. Through dietary adjustments the need for medications may be reduced. With some patients stool softeners may be necessary. Generally speaking, the frequent use of laxatives and enemas should be discouraged because they tend to interrupt the pattern of colonic action and may lead to cathartic habituation.

Other measures that may encourage bowel response and that are often used temporarily during the establishment of a management program include suppositories, laxatives, enemas, and gentle stimulation of the anal sphincter with a gloved finger. Exercises designed to strengthen weak abdominal muscles may also be helpful in preventing bowel problems. Impaction should rarely occur if the nurse accurately observes, interprets, and reports the frequency, color, amount, and consistency of the stools and uses the information in adapting nursing measures to prevent the physiologic effects of immobility on the gastrointestinal system. In the event an impaction does form in spite of a well-planned bowel management program, the hardened fecal mass is usually removed manually. These measures for encouraging normal bowel action are discussed further in Chapter 17.

In summary, the steps in planning of nursing care for the prevention of bowel problems usually follow this sequence:

1. Gather relevant data about the patient's elimination habits.
2. Begin developing a plan of care with the patient as an active participant whenever possible.
3. Assist the patient according to his capacity to increase his understanding of the physiology of bowel function and the purpose of the proposed measures.
4. Assess the effects of various foods, stool softeners, or other measures attempted and the degree of success in maintaining bowel function.
5. Adjust planning accordingly.
6. Incorporate the plan for bowel hygiene management into the total nursing care plan.

Preventing problems related to the urinary tract

As previously stated, the common urinary tract problems of patients on prolonged bed rest are usually responsive to preventive nursing measures based on understanding of the related physiologic principles. Common problems that are either preventable or amenable in some degree to nursing care include urinary stasis, infection, retention with the incontinence of overflow, and calculi.

In order for the plan of nursing care to be effective, appropriate measures adapted to the needs of the individual patient must be conscientiously carried out on a 24-hour basis. The measures most apt to be indicated include the following:

1. Adequate fluid intake. Fluid intake up to 3,000 ml. daily will maintain hydration. Urinary stasis, precipitation of calcium particles, and infection are less apt to occur when the urine is dilute.

2. Measurement of fluid intake and urinary output. This will help to identify the need for fluids and for voiding.

3. Periodic observation for bladder distension. A distended bladder with overflow should be suspected when the patient is frequently incontinent of small amounts of urine. The mass of a distended bladder can usually be identified above the symphysis pubis.

4. Scrupulous skin care. When the patient is incontinent, one of the major nursing responsibilities is prevention of decubiti by keeping the patient clean and dry.

5. Nursing measures to aid in initiating normal micturition. Every effort should be made to assist the patient to void when there is no mechanical obstruction to the normal passage of urine, in order that the patient may remain catheter free. There is always danger of infection associated with the use of a catheter whether introduced for temporary or extended use. The prolonged use of a catheter will often result in infection and ultimately in kidney damage.

6. Prevention of urinary tract infection. Exacting aseptic technique is always indicated when a catheter is used.

7. Promotion of mobility in prevention of urinary stasis. The patient usually needs encouragement and assistance with passive and active exercises, ambulation, and positioning. Nursing intervention in this aspect needs to be individualized.

8. Participation in dietary measures. A diet that is acid-ash and low in calcium is usually recommended to decrease the likelihood of calculi formation. The nurse can be of assistance in observing the patient's likes and dislikes and in noting individual reactions to various foods and fluids.

9. Bladder training program. The aim of a bladder training program is to enable the individual patient to gain bladder control without the prolonged use of the catheter whenever possible.

Dealing with the psychologic impact

The initial reaction to the temporary or permanent loss of a function has already been presented from the standpoint of understanding the psychologic reaction to physical disability. Although the basic problem may be physical, the situation is often multifaceted, including such requirements at various times as financial, vocational, housing, and transportation factors. At times the psychosocial adjustment may be the priority need.

The possibility of motivation toward rehabilitation usually increases when the patient gains a measure of acceptance of his disability that enables him to view the potential for some restoration of function through rehabilitation as a way of beginning to move toward achieving satisfaction in dealing with his personal needs and problems. As he is able to work through the initial impact of shock, denial, depression, fear, dependency, and anger, the patient gradually reaches some measure of acceptance of the physical problem. In some instances a residual disability means that the patient will be faced with reorganization of his entire life, whereas in others he may be able to return to his former routine with some modifications, or perhaps even with no modification. However, the patient must be given time to recover from the initial period of disorganization and anxiety before the process of adaptation begins and before he can respond to the goals of rehabilitation for promoting ego integrity and the feeling of self-worth.

In seeking to understand and work with the patient's behavior, it is helpful to remember that the *disability* is the degree of impairment that exists, while *handicap* is generally used to imply the individual's total adjustment to the disability. Two individuals may have similar disabilities but varying degrees of handicap. For example, each may have the right leg amputated at the knee; one is independent, managing his own business and supporting his family, while the other one remains at home in a wheelchair, continuing in the dependency stage. Disparity between the degree of impairment and the individual's total adjustment to the disability may be an indication for psychotherapy.

Nurses should be alert to the behavior and signs and symptoms through which the patient's physical and emotional progress and readiness for participation in the rehabilitation process may be assessed. Flexibility on the part of the nurse is essential in order to vary the approach according to the individual patient's state.

Application of the behavioral principle that the individual reacts to a situation as he perceives it, regardless of reality or of how others see the situation, and that he is therefore susceptible to errors and distortions in his perceptions will assist the nurse in trying to understand the patient's behavior in working with him.

Goals that are set with the patient should be realistic and planned with progressive steps so that the patient can gain some satisfaction with accomplishments, regardless of how slow the progress. Sincere recognition of accomplishments may be a source of encouragement for most patients. However, an approach that is too cheery is usually inappropriate.

An important point in nursing care for the patient undergoing rehabilitation is to encourage him to do all that he can for himself. Allowing sufficient time for his slow movements will avoid the impression that he is imposing on the nurse or that he is inadequate merely because he cannot do something quickly. When the patient cannot perform acts for himself, he then should be allowed to make as many decisions as possible. He should be encouraged to start planning his care in such a way that the routine will be continued at home. If he is accustomed to an evening bath, then this should be planned in the hospital so that the adjustment to home will be minimized.

Hostility expressed by the patient should not be taken personally by the nurse but should be considered to be an expression of his need for help. If the nurse is unable to meet a patient's psychologic needs at any time, members of the rehabilitation team should be consulted to assist the patient in meeting these needs. Aiding him in either establishing or reestablishing his identity may require the efforts of the entire rehabilitation team.

A patient should not be told to forget his handicap, thus denying it; rather, he should be supported in developing his ability to accept the reality of his situation. To help maintain a patient's sense of wholeness, many hospitals provide recreational, occupational, and vocational therapy. As the patient's condition improves, it may be beneficial for the patient to take outings from the hospital before discharge so that he will have a chance to adjust and to realize what problems he may face.

When the patient goes home, he should immediately start doing things for himself. Although it may be quicker and neater for the family to perform these tasks, they will be robbing him of his identity, his feeling of usefulness, and, most of all, his hope of independence.

Both nurses and family need to understand the emotional aspects of the patient's condition. Fear itself is a large factor. The patient often has fears of not being accepted by his family, his friends, or society and also has fears concerning his new limitations and of the future in general. A patient who is worried and afraid may express his feelings in a multitude of ways. However, he may not be able to express these feelings as fear or anxiety. If they are not expressed as fear and worry, they may appear as irritability, frustration, hostility, depression, embarrassment, or shame.

When the husband is removed from his role, either temporarily or permanently, the wife can help him to maintain his feeling of usefulness by consulting with him as she formerly did before the disability occurred. Although plans may be long range, the patient gradually resumes his place in the family and in society. If a wife or mother is taken from her role, she can be sustained as a functioning member of her family by helping with the planning of family activities and meals.

Working with a patient who is undergoing rehabilitation requires that the nurse be a teacher and offer support, not only to the patient but also to his family. The nurse should help convince the family and others that it is natural for the person with a handicap to resent offers of help on the basis of his disability; instead he wants to be accepted as would another individual.

In order for the patient to make plans for the future, he may need to talk with the nurse to clarify his own ideas and to be reassured that his plans are realistic, that is, if they are realistic. The family, too, may need assistance in recognizing, accepting, and solving future problems.

SUMMARY

This chapter deals with the concept of rehabilitation in relation to the associated ill effects of bed rest and inactivity. The secondary physiologic damage and complications of immobility may result in deteriorative effects that can be more disabling or handicapping to the patient than his initial disease entity or injury. These effects are referred to as disuse phenomena.

In each patient's situation it is therefore important to understand both the therapeutic purpose and the adverse effects of the imposed complete bed rest in order to reduce the hazards of restricted motion. Many of the preventive measures taken to minimize the physiologic and psychologic effects of immobility are nursing measures that must begin during the onset and early stages of a physical illness in order to interrupt or diminish the undesirable cycle of causes and resulting phenomena, which if allowed to develop lead to further extension of the disuse phenomena.

Rehabilitation is defined as a process of assisting a disabled, acutely or chronically ill, or convalescent person to realize his particular goals in living and working to the utmost of his potential. It is presented as a process dealing with the physical, psychologic, social, economic, and vocational aspects of the patient's life.

During the acute phase of illness, the rehabilitative process is directed largely toward the prevention of secondary disabilities and the provision of emotional security. The restorative and retraining phase of rehabilitation follows, in which a long-term program geared toward the realistic goals of the patient may be instituted.

The basic aims of rehabilitation are usually approached through the efforts of the rehabilitation team, of which both the patient and nurse are participating members.

The concept of activity and relevant principles from the biologic and behavioral sciences are discussed with examples of application to the solving of nursing problems. Nursing measures to counteract the ill effects of bed rest, while seemingly infinite, must be adapted to the individual patient's situation to help him identify and fulfill his needs.

QUESTIONS FOR DISCUSSION

1 Define rehabilitation and habilitation.
2 What is meant by the statement: "Rehabilitation is a philosophy"?
3 List some types of handicaps that are appar-

ent to the observer. List some types that are not apparent.

4 List the members of the rehabilitation team and give the function of each.

5 What resources are available in your community to help a patient with a rehabilitative need?

6 How may the patient react to his disability?

7 Why is an adequate diet important in rehabilitation?

8 Identify the effects of passive exercises.

9 Discuss correct methods of crutch walking with the physical therapist:
   a. List the important points to use in teaching crutch walking.
   b. Identify the advantages and disadvantages of the different types of walking aids.

LIFE SITUATION

Mr. Micheals, 48 years of age, is admitted to the hospital with a diagnosis of cerebral vascular accident and symptoms of right hemiplegia and aphasia of a mixed type. Mr. Micheals has a master's degree in political science and is a professor at a university. He is married and has three children, 20, 18, and 16 years of age. His wife has never worked, and the children are all in school. Identify the factors that could interfere with Mr. Micheals' return to his teaching position. How could the rehabilitation team assist him to compensate for these aspects of his illness?

SUGGESTED READINGS

Beavers, Stacie V.: Music therapy, American Journal of Nursing 69:89, January, 1969.

Brower, Phyllis, and Hicks, Dorothy: Maintaining muscle function in patients on bedrest, American Journal of Nursing 72:1250, July, 1969.

Brunner, Lillian S., and others: Textbook of medical-surgical nursing, ed. 2, Philadelphia, 1970, J. B. Lippincott Co.

Burt, Margaret M.: Perceptual deficits in hemiplegia, American Journal of Nursing 70:1026, May, 1970.

Carnevali, Doris, and Brueckner, Susan: Immobilization—reassessment of a concept, American Journal of Nursing 70:1502, July, 1970.

Drury, John H., Jr.: Handbook of range of motion exercises, Nursing '72 2:19, April, 1972.

Eyre, Mary K.: Total hip replacement, American Journal of Nursing 71:1384, July, 1971.

Foss, Georgia: The how to's of bed positioning, Nursing '72 72:14, August, 1972.

Fox, Madeline J.: Talking with patients who can't answer, American Journal of Nursing 71:1146, June, 1971.

Grey, Howard A.: The aphasic patient, RN 33:46, July, 1970.

Goldstrom, Deborah Kuttin: Cardiac rest: bed or chair? American Journal of Nursing 72:1812, October, 1972.

Griffin, Winnie, and others: Group exercise for patients with limited motion, American Journal of Nursing 71:1742, September, 1971.

Kamenetz, Herman L.: Selecting a wheelchair, American Journal of Nursing 72:100, January, 1972.

Kamenetz, Herman L.: Exercises for the elderly, American Journal of Nursing 67:780, August, 1972.

Martin, Nancy and others: the nurse therapist in a rehabilitation setting, American Journal of Nursing 70:1694, August, 1970.

Morris, Victoria, and Traber, Wilma: After the battle, American Journal of Nursing 72:97, January, 1972.

Olson, Edith V., and others: The hazards of immobility, American Journal of Nursing 67:780, April, 1967.

Ranalls, John: Crutches and walkers, Nursing '72 2:21, December, 1972.

Rusk, Howard A.: Rehabilitation medicine, ed. 3, St. Louis, 1971, The C. V. Mosby Co.

Shaw, Bernice L.: Revolution in stroke care, RN 33:56, January, 1970.

Stryker, Ruth Perin: Every nurse a rehabilitation nurse, Nursing '72 2:13, January, 1972.

Stryker, Ruth Perin: Rehabilitative aspects of acute and chronic nursing care, ed. 1, Philadelphia, 1972, W. B. Saunders Co.

West, Wilma L.: Occupational therapy—philosophy and perspective, American Journal of Nursing 68:1708, August, 1968.

20 Adaptation and the dying patient

CHANGING CULTURAL ATTITUDES

During the first half of the ninteenth century, western civilization lived and died within the Christian faith. Prior to our drug era, there was little relief from pain. Success in coping with death was based on faith that one was rewarded in the hereafter. A related philosophy was also reflected in childbirth when the mother was rewarded for her pain and suffering when she held her living child within her arms.

In the days before the control of most common childhood communicable diseases, a mother could expect to lose at least half of her children before they reached age 12. Death was a reality and a common part of everyday living.

Today, we live in an aspirin age. Death is considered to be something morbid. It is a traitor to the physician, for he is expected to conquer it. It is a threat to the pharmacist who seeks to relieve its pain. Actually, death is very "un-American,"

for it robs one of his inalienable rights, "life, liberty, and the pursuit of happiness." In the obituary column, the word "death" is usually removed from all notices. The stark realities of death are hidden from us through rituals and amenities that cast a veil between it and those who are left to mourn. Afterward death once more becomes a reality.

Death is most real to the dying patient. The cardiac monitor tells him that time is running out. His loved ones are only permitted to see him for 5 minutes every hour or so. The patient is shrouded in bottles and tubes. His life is dependent upon machines. Human hands are no longer useful. Modern man is also tongue-tied. Even with all the advances in science, man is still destined to die. Yet man continues to fight his enemy either by accepting a transplanted organ or, when the battle is lost, by giving his organs to the living so that he may yet still live in part.

Sigmund Freud considered death to be

319

a part of growth. The infant becomes a child; the child, a youth; the youth, a young man; the young man, an adult; the adult, a middle aged person; the middle aged person, an elder; and the elder, the dying. Normal growth takes place within a family environment, in a society with friends and communication. However, modern urbanization reduces the circle of social communicants for the elderly. The children go to school, the parents to work. There is no place in the modern home or society for the elderly. They must either live alone or join others in institutions who share similar burdens. Although many of these institutions do excellent jobs in providing physical care and comfort, the person is still deprived of the most contributing factor of growth—the family.

It is within this framework that today's nurse practitioner must seek to meet the needs of the terminally ill or dying patient and his surviving relatives and others who care.

THE NURSE'S PERCEPTION OF DEATH

In spite of the fact that each of us expects to die and expects all others to die, an element of uncertainty and helplessness is almost always present when death does occur. Few patients are wholly prepared for their own deaths and less often are nurses prepared for the death of their patients. No matter how seasoned in the care of the living, a nurse typically approaches a dying patient with at least some feeling of uncertainty, helplessness, and anxiety—uncertainty that all is being done to make the patient as comfortable as possible, to postpone dying, or to prevent death altogether; helplessness in being unable to perform tasks that will keep the patient alive; and anxiety about how to communicate effectively with the patient and his family. All these factors severely tax the nurse who attempts to help those who experience the process of dying. The usual goals in nursing are to attain or maintain health. Here the nurse has no hope of attaining these goals and must therefore seek other objectives in the care of the patient. The nurse often responds to these feelings by dissociating from the patient and from death itself. The nurse then may unconsciously or consciously focus on nursing tasks, equipment, the patient's disease process, superficial conversation designed to inhibit expressions of fear and death, and the like.

Sometimes the nurse may avoid contact with the patient altogether. Observations made in hospitals where nurses were involved in caring for both curative and terminally ill patients have shown that the nurses took significantly longer time in answering the signals of the patients who were suspected of dying. By withholding themselves from the patient through these kinds of activities, nurses shield themselves from feelings about death that cause them discomfort. If nurses understand their own behavior together with the realization that each can do much to determine how the patient will live through his last days, it will give impetus to their dealing rationally with the "here and now" when encountering delicate and difficult problems among patients.

During the last decade, many studies have been made regarding the behavior of dying patients, those by Dr. Elisabeth Kubler-Ross and the Reverend Carl Nighswonger being the most noted. Basic principles of some of their findings plus our own are presented in this chapter so that the nurse may better understand the psychology of dying and the sociologic impact on both the patient and his social environment (Fig. 20-1). With this understanding, the nurse should be able to build a plan of care that will be meaningful for the patient and realistic in the nurse's own goals.

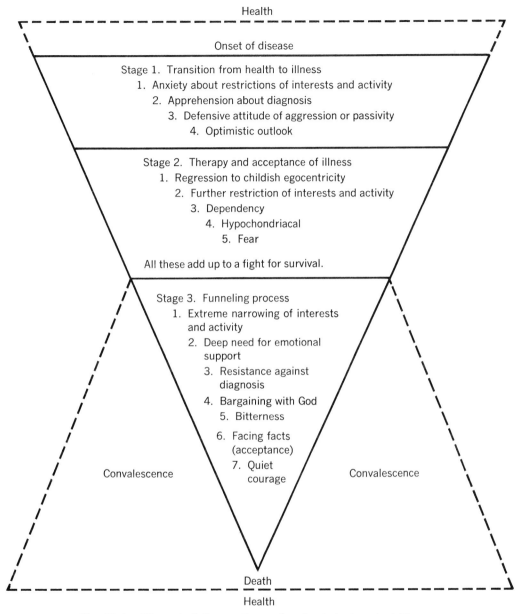

Fig. 20-1. Characteristic reactions of patients to terminal illness.

THE PATIENT'S PERCEPTION OF DEATH

The dying patient deserves the most perceptive, individualized, and carefully planned medical and nursing care that can be achieved, for here lies his only hope for understanding in the face of doubt and for comfort in the midst of pain and suffering. Nursing had its beginning as a profession among the dying during the Crimean war, when more lives were being lost by the lack of respect and love than by the war itself.

In addition to his physiologic needs, the

321

personal, moral, religious, legal, and economic issues associated with death will invariably influence the patient who encounters it, whether it comes gradually or suddenly without warning. Everyone is ready to agree that death is something that happens to someone else. Therefore, there are a series of defenses and attitudes that are highly unique and specific to death. The ability to help both the patient and his family greatly depends upon the knowledge of normal psychology as well as the physiology of death and dying.

Probably the most common question that the practitioner familiar with the terminally ill patient is asked is, "Should the patient be told the truth about his condition?" The proponents of informing the patient maintain that such is not only morally right but that silence condemns the patient to dying alone with a reality of which he is probably aware. Silence deprives him of his best resource, namely, the empathetic communication with his physician, nurses, friends, and family at a time when he needs it most.

Those who support the opposite view—that it is inappropriate to tell a patient of his impending death—are also able to marshal very convincing arguments. They maintain that the fear of death is unique among human fears and, as such, is normally defended by a degree of denial. They also agree that no man can envision his own death, and to force him in view of such a powerful universal fear is to do him great harm. Studies show that both positions have merit. Patients have been driven to the brink of madness by well-meaning physicians who have bludgeoned them with the naked truth about their condition. Patients have also been condemned to the pain of facing death alone because of a conspiracy of silence formed by a well-meaning physician and relatives. Both extremes should be avoided and can probably best be done by becoming fully acquainted with the broad spectrum of the patient's history and the type of personality that he has become. It has been said that one cannot be expected to die a Socratic death if he has not lived a Socratic life.

The patient's personal perception of death will affect his moral and religious attitudes toward it. He may be prepared to die and look forward to it as a deserved rest, relief from pain, or spiritual renewal. He may deny that he is dying to himself or to others. Or he may feel or accept the fact that death is imminent, yet feel the need to deny that he is not aware of it, perhaps to "protect" himself and his family from expressing grief. The patient may want to talk, be silent, or cry, or he may demonstrate feelings of fear, anger, guilt, or stoicism. He may wish to be alone or he may fear being alone above all else. No set rules can be applied as to how the terminally ill patient will react; however, studies show that patients do more or less follow a general pattern. If nurses and other workers are aware of this pattern, they will be more able to understand the patient's behavior and therefore more able to meet his needs. This pattern of behavior is described in the following paragraphs.

THE PSYCHOLOGY OF DYING

When a patient is told that he has a fatal or terminal illness, it is usually a shocking experience. Denial is the emotional shock absorber that allows one to pretend that he did not hear that which he cannot emotionally accept. Denial functions as a buffer after unexpected shocking news, allows the patient to collect himself, and in time permits him to mobilize a less radical defense. Denial is usually a temporary defense and will soon be replaced by partial acceptance. Studies show that continual denial to the end is rare except in a few instances. In summary, then, the patient's first reaction may be a temporary state of shock from which he recuperates gradually. As he begins to collect himself, again his usual response is, "No, it cannot be me."

Denial appears to be accompanied by isolation, which may be physical because of efforts by the family and medical personnel to also evade the presence of death. Studies indicate that most patients will eventually talk about their problem and will at least partially accept the inevitable if there is someone who will listen and share their loneliness. Here the minister, chaplain, friend, or one special family member becomes the support upon which the patient leans. For a husband or wife, it may be the surviving spouse; for the elderly widow, her minister or priest.

When the patient is no longer able to maintain denial, it is usually replaced by feelings of anger, envy, or resentment. This is one of the most difficult stages for the nurse to accept because this anger is often projected onto the environment and in all directions with nurses and physicians bearing the brunt of it. "The doctors are no good," "The hospital regulations are too severe," "All nurses do is to bother you, they wake you up to give you a sleeping pill. . ." are common expressions. This anger is also often exhibited spontaneously and at random. One patient, a 35-year-old banker, was very courteous during admission and joked about his illness, saying he was just in for tests at the insistence of his physician. An hour later he was yelling at the nurse and saying, "Get me something for this pain." It was later learned that this patient exhibited symptoms similar to those of his father, who had died of a brain tumor, and the patient feared that the same thing was happening to him.

The stage of anger may not remain very long, for like a misbehaving child, the patient soon learns that he may gain favors by being good or asking for just one more chance. This bargaining is often made with God. The patient may make all types of promises of a changed life or to be willing to die if only he can live to attend a certain event as a daughter's graduation or the birth of a grandson. This bargaining is really an attempt to postpone reality. A patient may have guilt feelings about the way he has lived and therefore promises to attend church or dedicate his future life to God. These guilt feelings may first be picked up by the chaplain, who should be a member of the health team for all patients. The function of the chaplain here is not so much "to save the patient's soul" as it is to be a support for other team members as well as for the family.

When the patient can no longer bargain and must finally face reality, as in the case of a cancer patient requiring extensive surgery, for example, a total laryngectomy, depression usually ensues. Two types of depression may occur. The first may be reactive and accompany the loss of the vital organ. A second type is that which is associated with impending loss—that of the patient's own life, his loved ones, his everything. For the nurse to try to cheer up the patient at this point would be again to deny the inevitable. Studies show that if the patient is allowed to express his grief, final acceptance seems much easier. The patient will be grateful for those who stay by him and remain loyal.

NURSING CARE OF THE TERMINALLY ILL PATIENT

The major objective in the care of the terminally ill patient is to give care through keeping the patient physically comfortable and offering "realistic" hope. The hope is not a cure for himself but that a cure might be found for others who follow in the same path, hope in fact that his life has been well spent.

To be more able to meet these objectives, the nurse must be aware of the different emotional stages through which a patient may pass. All dying patients will not move through these stages, and the nurse should be able to recognize what is happening. Also, any of the stages may be interrupted by sudden death caused by hemorrhage, embolism, or sudden failure of any of the vital systems. In an accident case, it is quite possible that a patient might pass through all stages in just a few hours.

Some problems that the nurse might expect to encounter are the following.

Panic. Rather than denying the fact of one's illness, the shock may be so great as to cause the patient to panic and resort to impulsive, uncontrolled, and unrealistic behavior. Fright and terror may bring about a situation so fluid that the patient sees no way out except to escape reality through magic (or faith healing), suicide, or psychosis. The competent nurse is aware of these possibilities and watches for symptoms that help to precipitate the patient's behavior. Sometimes it is the nurse who panics and flees the patient.

Emotion. As reality sets in, it brings with it the second drama or emotion that either finds expression in catharsis or is turned inward against the self in depression. This is the period that the nurse will find the most trying because much of the patient's anger may be directed against hospital personnel, family, and friends. All too often, the patient is not allowed to experience the catharsis so essential at this time. Nurses are prone to stifle this behavior, since it is much more pleasant to care for the more cooperative patient. Some patients by virtue of their philosophy find it against their superego to express their negative feelings. For them it is wrong to be angry, it is un-Christian and maybe it is a sin. When feelings are kept inward rather than being expressed, realistic guilt and shame may reach neurotic proportions. Thus the patient's life ends in the depressive state and the patient becomes resigned to this state, which ends in forlornness. Here the nurse can be most helpful by letting the patient know that the reason for his anger is understood and that even God understands situations of this nature. Dr. Ross so uniquely expressed it when she said in one of her workshops, "God is a big man, He can take it."

Negotiation. During the stage of negotiation, the patient may resolve the conflict by "selling out" instead of living through the bargaining stage, or he may just say, "What's the use." In either case, the drama ends in spiritual bankruptcy. The danger for the nurse in this stage is in being prone to reinforce the negotiation rather than remaining realistic.

Commitment. It is sometimes difficult to distinguish just when realistic hope moves into acceptance, just as it is difficult to recognize when despair ends in resignation. Essentially there is a shift from intellectual assent to emotional response. Hope is confirmed in the assurance that everything will be all right, whereas in resignation, the patient accepts the inevitable.

Completion. As death finally approaches, the patient completes his life with either a sense of fulfillment or forlornness. The forlorn patient tolerates each pain and welcomes death as an end to suffering. In contrast, the patient who reaches the stage of fulfillment not only dies in dignity but often enriches the lives of those around him. Here, the nurse should not be disturbed if emotionally involved. Involvement is often essential in giving the needed care. Sometimes it is helpful if the nurse takes time to discuss this with the chaplain, minister, or priest.

When the patient has made his final commitment and has found some peace, his circle of interest may diminish. He wishes to be left alone. Problems of the outside world are left for someone else to solve. As an example, a particularly avid baseball fan refused to have the television turned on during an entire World Series. Prior to the day of his death, he had remarked to his minister that it was all over. Some observers thought that he was referring to the winning team, but his minister knew differently.

This is the time when it is unwise to force diversion on the patient. Communications are more nonverbal than verbal. Visitors are limited to close friends and relatives. The patient may wish to make a will or express gratitude to those most dear to him, as one patient who said to his wife, "Honey, I knew you were good when I married you, but I never dreamed that you would be the jewel that you are." The patient was referring to her loyalty through the previous years of his illness. In contrast, an elderly cardiac patient on the evening prior to his death completely rejected his wife. Previously, his whole life had been centered around her. The rejection began during the evening when she served dinner. This continued throughout the night. During the early morning hours she went to his bed to check on him. He apologized for his previous behavior and apparently rose from his bed because of severe chest pain and fell to the floor. The wife gently picked him up and he died 15 minutes later in her arms.

PHYSIOLOGIC PROCESS OF DYING

Just as it was essential to understand the psychology of death in order to meet the patient's emotional needs, so it is necessary to understand the physiology of death to meet the physical discomforts of it, since many of the unpleasant characteristic symptoms result from the cessation of normal body functions.

Usually there is a series of changes that make the appearance of death known. The process of dying is a progressive failure of the vital functions. Organs absolutely essential to the maintenance of life are known as vital organs. The sovereign three vital systems are the central nervous system, the circulatory system, and the respiratory system.

The approach of death is shown by various physical signs: fast, irregular pulse, irregular and maybe noisy respirations, restless moving about, relaxation of muscles, excessive sweating, great thirst, pale cold skin with mottling the dependent portions, gradual disappearance of reflexes, and glazed and half-closed eyes.

Changes in pulse, respiration, and temperature result mainly from circulatory changes. The general slowing of the circulation from the lower extremities upward is evidenced by coldness, which is caused by failure of peripheral circulation. As a rule the heart continues to pulsate after respirations have ceased. The radial pulse gradually fails, and only an apical heart rate can be counted. As the peripheral circulation fails, there usually is a drenching sweat and the body surface cools. However, the patient feels warm, and his restlessness may be the result of his sensation of heat.

Respirations may be rapid and shallow or abnormally slow. Many times Cheyne-Stokes respirations (cycles of dyspneic respirations) are present. The breathing may be of the alae nasi type. That is, the sides of the nose may be drawn in with each inspiration. In order to make breathing easier, the head and shoulders may be elevated. Fresh circulating air should be provided to furnish the much-needed oxygen. The sagging jaw may move, and the flaccid cheeks may be drawn in and out with each breath.

Mental alertness varies from absolute unconsciousness to perfect consciousness.

As sight begins to fail, the dying patient turns instinctively toward the light and sees only what is near. Speech is made with an effort and is usually mumbled and confused.

Because of excessive sweating (diaphoresis) there is a great thirst. Discomfort of a dry mouth may be relieved by sips of water or other fluids given by teaspoon or by applying lubricants to the lips and mouth. Swallowing gradually becomes more difficult, and finally the patient cannot swallow at all. Because of aphagia (inability to swallow) mucus may collect in the mouth and throat. Air passing through the secretions may give rise to a gurgling sound referred to as the death rattle. Turning the patient on his side will allow gravity drainage of the secretions from the mouth.

Hearing is supposed to be the last sense to leave the dying person. He may be able to hear and be disturbed by noises long after he is unable to respond. There is no way of knowing when hearing ceases. Words spoken to the dying should be pronounced distinctly and close to their ears. Nothing should be said that would be distressing to him in the event he hears the conversation.

Because the muscles are becoming flaccid, the body assumes a supine position. The patient is not able to change his position or to make known his needs. The alert nurse will turn the patient often and will fluff his pillows to support varying parts of his body. Peristalsis may cease, the anal sphincters may relax, and the stomach simply distends with what is swallowed. The bladder sphincters may also relax. Incontinence of the bladder or rectum may occur, and protection should be provided for the bed. Placing the bedpan under the patient at intervals may help to keep the bed dry and clean. In case of urine retention, the physician will order catheterization.

As a result of anemia and loss of muscular tone, the face in long-continued illness may take on the expression called facies hippocratica, characteristics of which are ashy, pale skin, sunken and glazed eyes, sharp, pinched nose, and prominent chin and cheeks.

Physical nursing care for the dying patient consists chiefly of compensating for the loss of physiologic function.

PREPARATION OF A WILL

If the patient wishes to make a will or change an existing will, the policy of the health agency should be followed. A hospital may appoint someone from the business office to witness and handle necessary legal documents. Rarely would a nurse need to act as a witness for such procedures, but the nurse may contact the family or those designated by the health agency policy to see that the patient's wishes are carried out.

RELATIVES AND FRIENDS

In the care of the dying patient, relatives and friends are an integral factor, for they are a part of the social environment and must also cope with their own grief process (Fig. 20-2).

As has been previously stated, death is a family matter, and to separate the patient from his family at this time would be very unkind. Many problems could be solved or prevented entirely if the nurse would only take time to consider the total situation.

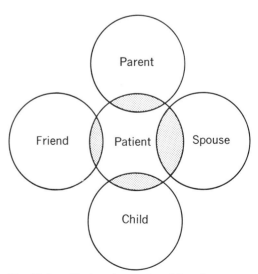

Fig. 20-2. Circle of emotional involvement.

In taking a history for the new patient, one is quite careful to inquire as to what one's parents or other relatives died of in order to try to diagnose a physical ailment. But rarely does one inquire as to how recently a patient lost a relative in order to diagnose his emotional problem.

In general practice the nurse will have many patients who in addition to their physical ailments will be in a period of grief and must work this out in order to cope with the ordeal.

Relatives of dying patients also sometimes pass through emotional stages similar to those of the patient. The nurse should remember this when their behavior is demanding and brusque.

Accepting their behavior often helps them to work through their grief, which in turn aids in more supportive care for the patient. The younger the patient, the more involved will the family be, especially if it is an adolescent or young child. The stillborn child presents little problem in himself but leaves a grieving mother for whom care must be continued.

Whether death occurs suddenly or gradually, the family is never ready and typical behavior can never be anticipated. Since thirst usually accompanies shock, a refreshing drink (nonalcoholic) offered to them at this time will be very much appreciated and physically comforting.

RELIGIOUS CUSTOMS

The observance of certain religious practices often brings comfort to the dying patient and his family.

Long prayers, sermons, and other such practices are inappropriate at this time and often tiring to the patient or his family. An expressive handshake and the mere

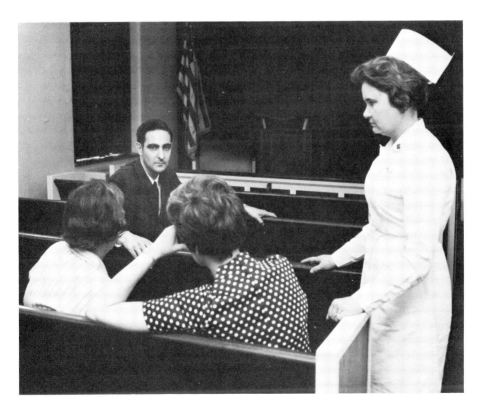

Fig. 20-3. The hospital chaplain is a friend to all in time of need.

presence of a familiar face seem to be all that is necessary.

Most agencies have set up routine practices for the major faiths so that priests are automatically called for the Catholic patient, and the administration of last rites is recorded on the chart. At the time of death the chaplain should be notified regardless of the patient's faith. Most hospital chaplains now have special preparation in this area and know the proper thing to do (Fig. 20-3).

If a clergyman is not available, the nurse may baptize a patient, pray, or read from the Bible. Nurses should not allow their own faith to prevent them from performing any spiritual procedure needed by the patient, since acts done at this time would probably be classified as nursing duties rather than religious practices.

GUIDING PRINCIPLES IN PLANNING NURSING CARE

Maintaining psychologic equilibrium at the time of approaching death is one of the dying patient's most urgent needs. Nursing problems arising from these needs frequently include promoting effective communication between the patient, his family, and the persons responsible for his care. Ideally, all members of the health team as well as others in contact with the patient should be cognizant of the planned regimen.

In collecting data prior to formulating a trial plan, the nurse should typically try to assess the meaning of death to the patient, his acceptance or denial of it, his awareness or lack of awareness of it, and the physician's plan for informing the patient of his prognosis.

To resolve the nursing problem of communicating effectively with the dying patient, the nursing care plan could call for a variety of approaches and a variety of principles on which to base these approaches. The following generalizations and examples of applications in nursing

are among the many from the behavioral sciences that could be used as a guide in planning meaningful communication with the dying:

1. Death has psychologic, spiritual, and social meanings that vary with each individual. Assessing the patient's perception of death as well as personal ideas makes the nurse better prepared to meet the dying patient's needs.

2. The dying patient's behavior is a function of his interactions with significant persons around him. If the experience of dying is to be made as satisfying as possible for the patient, hospital social systems need to provide a climate in which this can be achieved.

3. Culturally sanctioned roles require specific social behaviors. In death, for example, the patient may be expected to show peaceful acceptance; the bereaved, grief; the nurse, compassion; the doctor, omnipotence. The nurse must be prepared to understand and accept behavior that is to the contrary. The patient may demonstrate denial; the bereaved, relief; the nurse, hostility; and the physician, helplessness.

4. The protective mechanisms of dissociation or denial serve to control or suppress emotional reaction. Entering into active discussion about death usually carries a high emotional risk for the patient as well as the nurse; nevertheless, it can provide strength and comfort to both. If the patient wants to discuss his death, he should; if he does not, his defenses to avoid discussion should be supported for as long as he seems to need them.

5. The need for man's belief in a meaning to existence is universal, and every human culture has some form of organized religious behavior. During periods of stress and uncertainty, spiritual needs tend to increase in intensity. When a need for spiritual help exists, a nurse alert to cues communicated by the patient can assist the patient in being willing and able

to discuss his concerns with the spiritual leader of his religion.

These general principles and nursing measures are representative of those that a nurse might use in planning for optimum communication and human contact with the patient at a time when the patient's opportunities for open communication and human contact are limited. Principles related to the physiologic needs of the patient are not less important and, in general, these needs are somewhat dependent on the patient's physical condition. Reference to previous chapters will provide the reader with principles applicable to meeting unique physical needs of the patient, as well as additional principles relating to psychologic needs.

ASSESSING THE TIME OF DEATH

Cessation of breathing and of the heartbeat is considered evidence that death has occurred. Nursing personnel note the time the patient's heartbeat and breathing stop and record it on the medical report. A physician pronounces the patient dead. Lifesaving measures may be instituted following cardiac arrest, however, and the patient who has apparently died may be restored to life.

The contrast between life and death is not always clear-cut. Legally, the physician pronounces the patient dead. The time of death is estimated to occur when the patient's heartbeat and breathing have ceased. At times, estimating the time of death may be an ethical question as well as a legal one and may be reflected in nursing practice. Whether to initiate or continue heroic measures to delay death when it is "known" to be imminent may be a controversial decision. Determination of the exact time of death may be crucial when the dying patient's organs are to be used for transplantation to the living.

The physician or nurse may also bear the less critical but nonetheless important responsibility for estimating the expected time of death so that family members who wish to be present when the patient dies can be notified in time. When death is sudden, notification may not be possible, but when life lingers for days or weeks, families who come from great distances may be particularly affected by being notified either too soon or too late.

POSTMORTEM CARE

Preparation of the patient's body for transfer to the undertaker is carried out by the nurse or assistant. The patient is placed in a supine position with the head slightly elevated. He should be clean and appear comfortable. Drains are removed, unless contrary to the physician's order; dressings may be applied to prevent the drainage of fluids from the body orifices, such as the rectum and vagina. If the jaw, ankles, or wrists are tied, this should be done with soft gauze and sufficient padding so that bruising is minimal. Dentures may be put in place or labeled and sent with the patient when he leaves the hospital unit. The patient's identification should be carefully checked and labels added if required.

There are important changes that follow death. Cooling of the body is rapid for a short time and then proceeds more slowly until about 24 hours after death, when the temperature of the environment is reached.

Rigor mortis, a stiffening of the body after death, is caused by the fixation of muscles. Rigor mortis generally appears in the course of a few hours, but the time varies considerably. It first involves the muscles of the jaw and passes successively down the neck, arms, trunk, and legs. The arms and legs cannot be bent while rigor mortis is present unless the tendons are torn. It disappears in 1 to 6 days, and the muscles resume their soft consistency but will never contract again. Postmortem hypostasis is a dark red or bluish discoloration caused by the settling of the blood.

Since gravity affects the level and distribution of fluids, raising the head and shoulders on pillows or with the backrest prevents the blood from settling in the face and discoloring it. As far as possible, good posture of the patient is maintained, although loss of muscle tone renders the patient incapable of maintaining his position. Hence, supports such as pillows and rests are needed.

Embalming fluids are germicidal and permeate all the tissues of the body. However, in cases of communicable disease, state laws may provide that added precautions be taken to prevent the spread of disease.

The death certificate is signed by the physician and sent to the local health department. It must be filed before a burial permit can be issued. The physician secures permission for an autopsy in writing, except in coroner's cases, from the nearest relative. Coroner's cases include those in which death occurred after a brief period in the hospital and those in which there may be an element of crime. An autopsy will show why the patient died, the extent of the condition, and the effectiveness of treatment. The entire procedure is similar to an extensive surgical operation, and there is no mutilation of the body. The mortician prepares the body so that there is no visible evidence that a postmortem examination has been conducted.

SUMMARY

Patients view death from individual and cultural value systems. Assessing and respecting these systems is of key importance in planning nursing care of the dying.

Doctors and nurses are committed to saving lives and promoting health and well-being. When the limits of the healing professions dictate that the patient will surely die, this conflicts with the primary purpose of care, and feelings of frustration and failure are almost certain to occur. These feelings are frequently manifested by the development of hospital social systems that support a collective professional attitude of withdrawal from death. Avoidance of discussion with the dying patient about death prevents him from facing or preparing for the fact of his own death by isolating him from meaningful interactions with others. Active interaction is avoided and the patient is depersonalized at a time when his feeling of loneliness and abandonment may be at its peak. An active encounter can provide added strength and help the patient feel safe and better able to face dying with courage and dignity.

Physiologically, death is a gradual process that is complete when breathing and heartbeat cease. Care of the patient after death is directed toward preserving a natural, comfortable-appearing person who is asleep and toward providing comfort for the patient's family.

QUESTIONS FOR DISCUSSION

1 How is the dying patient supported psychologically?
2 Describe a patient's reaction to dying as shown by his behavior. Describe your own feelings.
3 What is meant by apparent death?
4 What are the physical signs of death?
5 How is the dying patient made physically comfortable?

LIFE SITUATION

The following terminally ill patient was visited by a nurse instructor on several occasions. The information gained through observation and interviews was later used by the instructor and her students to formulate a plan of care for the patient. Name, nationality, and place changed to conceal identity of patient and family.

Mrs. Lueke, a 47-year-old nurse supervisor, was admitted to Blank Hospital for palliative therapy for metastatic carcinoma. Her medical history revealed that 9 years previously she had sought medical care for a back injury. During the routine physical examination, a lump was discovered in her right breast. Diagnostic studies were done immediately and revealed a malignant tumor. Mrs. Leuke did not immediately accept the reality of her diagnosis. She signed a release and left the hospital. However, a few days later she returned for radical surgery. The patient then remained symptom free for $4^1/_2$ years, at which time lymph node enlargements occurred in the left axillary area. These were surgically removed. Other enlargments have been excised on discovery.

Mrs. Lueke's social history indicates that she has been married twice. Her first husband simply vanished about 6 years ago. She had one daughter as a result of this marriage. The daughter is enrolled in a local university and is majoring in sociology. Her present husband is a mechanic.

Mrs. Lueke is a very meticulous person. This was observed in her personal appearance during the first contact with her. The first interview was geared to health history, course of disease, and medical therapy. There was little discussion about the prognosis, but she admitted that she had accepted her illness and had previously been through the stages of denial and anger. A neighbor was visiting at the time of the first interview. The purpose of the interview was explained and Mrs. Lueke requested that her guest remain. The guest consented but remained silent throughout the period except for a couple of comments on the whereabouts of the patient's present husband.

Mr. Lueke drinks heavily and, according to the patient, denies that she is ill. After threatening her life, they separated 3 weeks before this hospitalization. He had visited her once during this admission. The patient stated, "I am better off without him because he is self-centered. My daughter is happy over the separation." During the early part of the marriage, Mrs. Lueke also drank heavily and her husband considered her a good drinking partner.

Since the separation the patient has been living with her parents. Her mother is a retired school teacher and is presently employed as a teacher's aide. Her father has Buerger's disease and one extremity has been amputated. Both parents visit twice a day. She is a member of a Protestant church. Various ministers visit her frequently; however, her own minister only started visiting her recently. The multiplicity of ministerial visitation sometimes irritates Mrs. Lueke. She has not been a strong church goer, but the daughter stated that she had become more religious recently.

Observations of the patient revealed a well-built frame that did not appear acutely ill. Her present admission was primarily caused by nausea and vomiting. Her abdomen appeared slightly distended, and there were periods of dyspnea and intermittent tremors of the upper extremities. Bed clothing did not permit extensive observation of the physical aspects. She complained of constant constipation. Attempts to aid bowel integrity included enemas and cathartics. She denied any difficulty with bladder integrity although a Foley catheter had been inserted and removed a few days before.

Gastrointestinal integrity was related to eating. Nausea and vomiting were aided by the use of dexpanthenol (Ilopan), hydroxyzine (Vistaril), and prochlorperazine (Compazine). Hydromorphone (Dilaudid) had been used for pain, but the patient developed an allergy to the drug. Meperidine (Demerol) was being received for pain, which was located in the abdomen. She denied pain in any other part of the body. Because of nausea and vomiting, she had been receiving intravenous therapy. However, she had a selected menu and the Dietary Department allowed her to have what she wanted at any time. Independent action for bowel integrity such as prune juice had been ineffective. She had been eating cracked ice for episodes of nausea and vomiting and occasionally applied a cold washcloth to her throat.

During the second interview, the patient's mother was present. The mother was assessed to be overanxious and overprotective. When Mrs. Lueke became nauseated and requested the cold cloth, the mother reached for the cracked ice and stated, "I should have refilled this." Realizing her error, she stated, "I want to do things right but I act on impulse and do the wrong thing." She complained about the overloaded bedside table and stated, "You won't be able to hide a mouse in it." She expressed desire for her daughter to be at home, but not before the physician felt it advisable. Throughout the remaining portion of the interview, the mother talked about her work as a teacher's aide and invited the nurse to visit the family at home. Mrs. Lueke passively ate ice and held the cool washcloth to her throat.

Observation of the patient revealed increased tremors that involved most of her body and more frequent and severe episodes of dyspnea and nausea. The room was warm, thus more of her body was exposed, which revealed edema of the upper extremities that tapered off near the shoulders and across the scapula. Her face also appeared edematous. The body had a grayish jaundice color. The sclera of the eyes were definitely jaundiced. The right eye protruded outward more than the left. The patient stated she had received cobalt therapy because of "lumps" above the eyelids. Her entire body appeared edematous but at the same time adipose loss was obvious. A sore on the anterior portion of the right thigh had a sanguineous discharge that the patient immediately covered with a cloth. Enlarged nodes were noted on various parts of the body.

During the next contact with the patient she had an episode of nausea and did not feel like talking. Her daughter was home for spring vacation. Time was spent interviewing the daughter, who was a highly intelligent and attractive young lady. Tears came in her eyes as her mother's physical condition was discussed. She stated, "At first I could not believe it, but now I have accepted what is happening because she has." Information obtained from the daughter indicated that the mother was now living each day as it came. Mrs. Lueke was discharged the next day because she wanted to go home.

The first day home, Mrs. Lueke ate some onions and lettuce. Abdominal distension became extensive and she became severely dyspneic. She complained of difficulty in moving her right leg because of severe pain.

Two days later Mrs. Lueke was readmitted because of inability to control the pain, lack of use of the lower extremity, generalized abdominal distension, and severe dyspnea. She talked about plans for summer cookouts and visiting the beach because she would have her daughter home for summer vacation. She had changed the beneficiary on her insurance policy from her husband to her daughter. This was her last major objective.

Throughout her illness, she had administered her own intramuscular medications, made decisions about which drugs were more effective, rejected drugs that she felt were "no good," and always made sure she had sufficient drugs on hand.

She eventually became comatose and died a few days later.

Questions:

1 Some of the objectives and nursing actions that were included in Mrs. Lueke's plan of care were as follows:
  a. Keep patient as comfortable as possible by relieving nausea, vomiting, and distension.*
  b. Control pain insofar as possible without undue suppression of respiration and in accordance with physician's directions.
  c. Allow parents and daughter to visit whenever they desire.
  d. Endeavor to exclude all ministers and religious workers except Mrs. Lueke's own minister.
  e. Continue to allow Mrs. Lueke to make decisions in relation to her care as seem feasible.
  f. Encourage family members to express their feeling of grief by accepting their behavior.
  g. Allow time to answer questions asked by family and time to just listen to them.
2 If you had been the nurse caring for Mrs. Lueke, would you have included the above? If so, why? What other objectives might have been included?
3 Why was Mrs. Lueke's mother concerned over the untidy bedside table and her inability to do things "right"?
4 Identify the various emotional stages through which Mrs. Lueke passed.
5 Discuss the basis for Mrs. Lueke's second marriage.
6 What coping mechanisms did Mrs. Lueke use?
7 In what stage did Mrs. Lueke die—acceptance or forlorness?
8 What coping strategy was Mrs. Lueke using when she planned summer cookouts with her daughter? If you had been Mrs. Lueke's nurse, would you have shared in these plans? Give reasons for your answer.
9 Review the principles of communication as presented in Chapter 5 and decide what methods are most appropriate in caring for the terminally ill patient and his family.

*Detailed measures for executing this objective can be found in Chapter 28, Gastrointestinal Disorders.

SUGGESTED READINGS

Blewett, Laura J.: To die at home, American Journal of Nursing 70:2603, December, 1970.

Brimigion, Jeanne: Living with dying, Nursing '72 2:23, June, 1972.

Browning, Mary, and others: The dying patient—a nursing perspective, New York, 1972, The American Journal of Nursing Company.

Burnside, Irene M.: You will cope, of course, American Journal of Nursing 71:2354, December, 1971.

Craven, Ruth, F.: Anaphylactic shock, American Journal of Nursing 72:718, April, 1972.

Craytor, Josephine, K.: Talking with persons who have cancer, American Journal of Nursing 69:774, April, 1969.

Death in the first person, American Journal of Nursing 70:336, February, 1970.

Eisman, Roberta: Why did Joc die? American Journal of Nursing 71:501, March, 1971.

Faber, Heije: Pastoral care in the modern hospital, Philadelphia, 1971, The Westminster Press.

Fond, Karen Ikuno: Dealing with death and dying through family-centered care, Nursing Clinics of North America 6:53, March, 1972.

French, Jean, and Schwartz, Doris R.: Home care of the dying in two cultures, American Journal of Nursing 73:502, March, 1973.

Gage, Frances B.: Suicide in the aged, American Journal of Nursing 71:2153, November, 1971.

Goldfogel, Linda: Working with the parent of a dying child, American Journal of Nursing 70:1674, August, 1970.

Gordon, David C.: Overcoming the fear of death, New York, 1970, The Macmillan Co.

Hershey, Nathan: On the question of prolonging life, American Journal of Nursing 71:521, March, 1971.

Hoffman, Esther: Don't give up on me! American Journal of Nursing 71:60, January, 1971.

Johnson, Joan M.: Stillbirth—a personal experience, American Journal of Nursing 72:1595, September, 1972.

Kneisl, Carol R.: Thoughtful care for the dying, American Journal of Nursing 68:550, March, 1968.

Krienke, Chris: Death and me, RN 32:51, September, 1969.

Kubler-Ross, Elisabeth: Anger before death, Nursing '71 1:12, December, 1971.

Laney, M. Louise: Hope as a healer, Nursing Outlook 17:45, January, 1969.

Maxwell, Sister Marie B.: A terminally ill adolescent and her family, American Journal of Nursing 72:925, May, 1972.

Mervyn, Frances: The plight of dying patients in hospitals, American Journal of Nursing 71:1988, October, 1971.

Mitchell, Kenneth R.: Hospital chaplain, Philadelphia, 1972, The Westminster Press.

Murdaugh, Jessica: Mr. Jones, your wife has cancer, RN 44: March, 1969.

Nighswonger, Carl A.: Ministry to the dying as a learning encounter, Journal of Pastoral Care 26:86, June, 1972.

Oerlemans, Marguerite: Eli, American Journal of Nursing 72:1440, August, 1972.

Pacyna, Dorothy A.: Response to a dying child, Nursing Clinics of North America 5:421, September, 1971.

Poi, Kathleen M.: Who cared about Tony? American Journal of Nursing 72:1848, October, 1972.

Prattes, Ora: Helping the family face an impending death, Nursing '73 3:16, February, 1973.

Robinson, Lisa: The demanding patient, Nursing '73 3:20, January, 1973.

Roglieri, John L.: What you should know about autopsy, RN 33:51, March, 1970.

Ross, Elisabeth K.: What is it like to be dying? American Journal of Nursing 71:54, January, 1971.

Ross, Elisabeth K.: Learning about death and dying, American Journal of Nursing 71:56, January, 1971.

Vaillot, Sister Madeleine C.: Living and dying, American Journal of Nursing 70:268, February, 1970.

Waechter, Eugenia H.: Children's awareness of fatal illness, American Journal of Nursing 71:1169, June, 1971.

Wells, Ronald V.: Dignity and integrity in dying (insights from early 19th Century Protestantism), Journal of Pastoral Care 26:99, June, 1972.

When does a patient die, RN, 34:23, July, 1971. (RN Notes and Quotes).

Wilkinson, Laura: Death is a family matter, RN 33:50, September, 1970.

Yates, Susan A.: Stillbirth—what staff can do, American Journal of Nursing 72:1592, September, 1972.

Principles related to administration of medications and therapeutic agents

21 Preparation and administration of therapeutic agents

VARYING ROLES OF THE NURSE
Dependent versus independent functioning

In the preceding chapters, the nursing roles have been presented as (1) independent, (2) dependent (assistive), and (3) health team member (collaborative). The focus of discussion has been mostly upon those activities that lie primarily within the province of nursing, those that may usually be initiated without specific direction. These activities have included providing comfort and support through nursing ministrations, skillful observation, listening and responding purposefully, assessment, and planning and implementing of appropriate nursing care. These activities are a part of the independent role of the nurse and are based on principles applied from the various sciences. As they are performed, the nurse relies on the powers of observation, perception, and judgment, which are developed through learning and experience.

The nurse has also been presented as an actively participating member of a health team in which each team member has a definite role in the coordinated effort toward accomplishment of comprehensive patient care. The role of the nurse in this context is multi-faceted. Essentially, however, it is the application of nursing measures in assisting the patient, or "doing for him," to accomplish those things that help him to maintain his capabilities while preventing further disabilities, in the joint effort toward his restoration to home and community (insofar as these goals are possible). The nursing process, as described, is the framework within which the nurse functions in the delivery of health care service. In the collaborative role as a team member, the nurse both gives and receives assistance in relation to the other health team members in the care of the patient. This implies elements of both dependent and independent functioning, the establishing and maintaining

337

of open channels of communication, and the responsibility for coordinating the patient's activities in the total plan of care.

The nurse functions in the assistive (dependent) role when carrying out specific therapeutic orders of the physician, thus participating in his plan for achieving the goal, which is the patient's recovery. There are both dependent and independent aspects of this nursing role. The dependent elements are those in which the nurse waits for the specific order to be given and then either assists the physician in administering the treatment or procedure or carries out the order in its entirety, for example, administering a medication prescribed by a written order. The independent elements in this are discernible as the nurse uses judgment in carrying out the order—for example, seeking clarification regarding any questions as to dosage, method of administration, or patient reaction—instructing the patient, and observing changes in the patient's condition. These observations are shared with the physician to help him determine the effectiveness of the therapy.

Even though there is a great deal of overlapping in these roles a review of them is useful to the nursing student to enable the individual to more clearly recognize those competencies over which there is decision-making command and those that are predominately assistance functions, particularly when there is much overlapping, as illustrated by looking at both the dependent and independent aspects of medication administration. Such clarification is also useful to the nurse in being able to respond appropriately and quickly in assuming different roles that may be performed in quick succession or almost simultaneously.

Legal aspects related to nursing roles

The law attempts to distinguish between nursing practice and the practice of medicine. However, in some situations the line of demarcation between medical and nursing practice may not be entirely clear. The increasing pressures for nurses to assume responsibilities for activities formerly considered to be solely the practice of medicine seem to have made delineation more difficult. Therefore, in order to avoid the charge of practicing medicine without a license, it is essential that the individual nurse exercise care in identifying both dependent and independent functions and keep informed regarding policies in these matters in the geographic region as well as in the local agency.

From the legal standpoint, the difference between independent and dependent nursing functions is determined on the basis of whether or not a physician's order is needed for the nurse to perform the function.

Negligence in nursing practice is usually defined as performance that does not meet the standards of safe practice as established by law for the protection of the patient against harm resulting from incompetence or carelessness. The conduct is compared with the performance expected of a reasonably prudent nurse in similar circumstances. The intent of the law is to assure that when giving care, the nurse, student or graduate, will exercise the professional knowledge acquired through specialized education. Failure to exercise due care may result in a charge of malpractice and imposed liability.

The nurse is expected to understand the purpose and effect of treatments and procedures performed, whether they are in the area of dependent or independent functioning, and should not undertake responsibilities without adequate preparation. In exercising due care the nurse is also expected to question the physician's orders if they are not clear or if the order seems contrary to usual procedure, in awareness of the individual responsibility for competent performance in both assistive and independent functioning.

The major emphasis of Unit four is on the area of assistive functioning in the administration of common therapeutic agents and measures.

ADMINISTERING THERAPEUTIC AGENTS

The physician's order

The first consideration before administering a therapeutic agent or measure is to ascertain that the physician's order has been correctly written in all of its parts. A written order is better than one given orally because there is less chance for error. The order is written on a particular form specified by the agency and is usually attached to the patient's chart. The patient's name should always appear on the order sheet.

The order is examined by the nurse, who checks it for at least the following information:

Date and time the order was written. This is significant for a variety of reasons; for example, narcotic orders are by law valid only for a period of 24 to 48 hours.

Name of the therapeutic agent or measure to be administered. Official nomenclature is usually encouraged. The nurse is responsible for correctly identifying the exact therapeutic agent, to avoid any type of error and to be able to judge the effect on the patient.

Dosage of medication and concentration to be administered. The metric system is coming into common usage. However, both the metric and apothecaries' systems may be used in the same agency. The nurse needs to be familiar with both systems and to be able to use common equivalents. Any uncertainty regarding dosage should be clarified before preparing and administering the agent.

Time and frequency of administration. These directions are usually given in standard abbreviations. Common abbreviations are listed in the Appendix.

Route of administration. The route by which a medication is to be administered should be clearly understood. In some agencies it is generally accepted that the oral route is intended unless otherwise stated. When a preparation can be administered by more than one route, the nurse must be certain that the intended method of administration is employed.

The physician's signature. An unsigned order should always be questioned by the nurse.

Basis for questioning an order

It is possible for an error to be made in writing any part of the order, or it may be that the nurse does not understand it or perhaps cannot be sure what the order requires because it is illegible. In such an instance the nurse should find out from the physician what the order intends and, when in doubt, how it relates to the plan of care.

Failure to detect an error that results in harm to the patient may have serious implications for the nurse, who can be legally charged with negligence in the situation even though the physician is responsible for the order he has written.

SUMMARY

The roles and functions of nursing are basic to its practice, and independent, assistive, and collaborative types have been identified. While these roles overlap, distinguishing between them is useful. It assists in recognizing those responsibilities over which the nurse has decision-making command and in clarifying nursing responsibility in functions that are predominately assistive in type but that have independent elements.

The intent of the law is to delineate between the practice of medicine and the practice of nursing and to provide protection for the patient against harm resulting from negligent nursing care. While the physician is responsible for the order he writes, the nurse, by reason of her specialized education and experience, is expected to note any errors in the order and seek clarification from the physician.

SUGGESTED READINGS

Budd, Ruth: We changed to unit-dose system, Nursing Outlook 19:116, February, 1971.

Conway, Barbara, and others: The seventh right, American Journal of Nursing 70:1040, May, 1970.

Foreman, Nancy J., and Zerwekh, Joyce: Drug abuse jargon, American Journal of Nursing 71:1736, September, 1971.

Hecht, Amy B.: Self-medication, inaccuracy and what can be done, Nursing Outlook 18:30, April, 1970.

22 Oral medications

GENERAL CONSIDERATIONS

Drugs produce their therapeutic effects within the body by altering or modifying body functions or cell metabolism in some way. All drugs, though tested and assayed, are capable of producing not only the therapeutically desired effects but also effects that are potentially harmful. Therefore, it is essential that the actions of both well-established drugs and newer preparations be known. It is equally important to be able to apply this pharmacologic knowledge together with the other aspects of nursing care. In order to integrate drug administration into the total plan of care, the nurse needs some understanding of the patient's pathophysiology and how the drug being administered is expected to favorably alter body functioning toward restoration of homeostasis. The nurse needs to know the expected action of the drug together with nursing measures that will tend to enhance the desired results and decrease the possible adverse effects.

In recent years, the number of different medications has been tremendously increased. When drugs are dispensed under their trade names, one drug may appear under several names and in different colors, sizes, and shapes. Since this contributes to the occurrence of errors in drug administration, the current trend is to require the use of official names and preparations.

In the process of preparing and administering medicines, the nurse must assume responsibilities that are subject to human error, such as reading and interpreting the physician's orders, transferring the order to the Kardex or medicine card (depending on the established procedure in the agency), and identifying the correct preparation of the drug ordered. Thus the nurse is obligated to be informed about the legal, ethical, and procedural practices in the giving of drugs that are essential for their safe administration and for consulting resources through which one may keep abreast of the continuing advances in drug therapy.

There are several possible routes of drug administration, depending upon the nature of the preparation, effect desired, rate

341

Table 22-1   Routes of drug administration

Route of drug administration	Method of administration	Type of effect
Oral:	Patient swallows medication (most desirable route when practical)	Local (may have local effects in gastrointestinal mucosa) Systemic (if absorbed into bloodstream)
Nonoral: Parenteral (via any route other than gastrointestinal tract; in practical usage refers to injection of a drug beneath the skin)	Injection of a drug into the tissues when oral route is not desirable	
	Subcutaneous, hypodermic, or hypodermoclysis: injection of drug into subcutaneous tissues	Systemic
	Intramuscular: injection of drug deeper between layers of muscle tissue	Systemic
	Intravenous: introduction of drug directly into bloodstream, by-passing all barriers to absorption	Systemic
	Intradermal (intracutaneous): injection of a small amount just below surface of skin, producing a wheal	Local
	Intrathecal: spinal injection by physician	Local (high concentration of anesthetic or other drug in subarachnoid space)
	Intrasynovial or intra-articular injection by physician	Local (high concentration of drug in inflamed joint)
Skin or mucous membranes:		Both systemic and local
Mouth, nose, throat, mucosa	Sublingual: tablet placed under tongue	Systemic
	Buccal: tablet placed between tongue and cheek	Systemic
	Local applications of anesthetic, astringent, or antiseptic solution in form of sprays, drops, lozenges, tampons, and so on	Local
	Snuffing	Systemic
Mucosa of deeper respiratory passages	Inhalation	Systemic and local

342

Table 22-1 Routes of drug administration, cont'd

Route of drug administration	Method of administration	Type of effect
Rectal mucosa	Irrigation: enema or Harris flush	Local effect usually intended
	Suppository or drug in retention enema	Systemic or local
Genitourinary mucosa	Irrigation: douche, bladder irrigation Instillations, suppositories	Local effect usually intended
Skin	Application of lotions, liniments, ointments	Local (ordinarily the skin acts as a barrier to most drugs applied to it)
	Inunction: dermal application with friction. A few substances, such as mercury ointment or methyl salicylate (oil of wintergreen) may be absorbed by way of the sebaceous glands to attain therapeutic blood levels.	Systemic
	Moist dressings	Local

of absorption, and condition of the patient. When a local effect is to be achieved, the drug preparation is applied directly to the tissues in which the action is desired—for example, application of benzalkonium chloride (Zephiran Chloride) or similar solution directly to a wound for cleansing and antiseptic action or topical ointment applied to control itching in skin lesions.

A systemic effect occurs when the medication is absorbed into and transported by the bloodstream to affected tissues remote from the site of application, as, for instance, when insulin is injected into the local tissues but it affects the body's metabolic processes. Routes of administration are outlined in Table 22-1.

The path by which the drug is introduced into the body is one of the most important factors influencing its action, because it affects the rate and completeness of the drug's absorption into the bloodstream and the speed, intensity, and duration of its action. The physician determines the most desirable route of administration for the particular drug for the individual patient, and the nurse must be absolutely certain that there is no misunderstanding regarding this point.

SCIENTIFIC PRINCIPLES
Selected biologic concepts

Selected concepts have been drawn from the biologic sciences that are useful in explaining the basis for some of the things nurses do in the process of preparing and administering oral medications and for accepting the fact that every medicinal agent, even in minute doses, is potentially able to produce an effect when taken into the body. The reader should give thought to identifying other physiologic chemical, and psychosocial principles

343

that will account for specific effects of various therapeutic agents as they are encountered in patient care.

1. The skin and mucous membrane in different parts of the body have varying absorptive powers.
2. The rate of absorption, distribution, and excretion of a drug depends upon its composition and concentration and upon the volume of the circulating blood supply.
3. A drug must be in solution in order to be absorbed into the circulating blood.
4. A drug is a foreign material in the body. When absorbed and distributed to the tissues by the circulating blood, a drug modifies cell metabolism and may thus modify or alter body functions.

Application of principles

The oral route, as already indicated, is usually the most desirable method of drug administration because of convenience, relative safety, and economy. It is the simplest method of introducing the drug into the body in such a way that it can be absorbed into the bloodstream. Also, the effects produced by oral administration of the drug are more easily controlled than when it is given parenterally. Another reason for making drugs available in oral forms whenever possible is that they are less expensive than injectable preparations, which must be sterile and which are intended for administration by qualified personnel.

Oral dosage forms include solid preparations, primarily tablets, capsules, and, to a lesser extent, pills, and liquid dosage forms in a variety of pleasantly flavored liquids, which may be water, alcoholic, or hydroalcoholic.

Tablets are a compressed, dry form of the drug that is readily swallowed and then disintegrates and dissolves in the stomach. Water ingested with the tablet aids in the process of the tablet being dissolved and the drug absorbed. Tablets may be coated with soluble substances to make them more palatable.

Certain drugs in tablet or capsule form have *enteric coating* to delay the release of a stomach-irritating drug until it reaches the alkaline intestinal secretions, where the coating will be readily dissolved. Irritating drugs are less apt to cause stomach upsets if given following a meal when the gastric mucosa is somewhat protected by the presence of food.

Some coated tablets and capsules are prepared as *prolonged action* or delayed action forms of the drug, such as Spansules or Graduments. The purpose of the coating in this case is to produce a sustained effect, since small amounts of the drug are gradually released and absorbed over a period of time. The action begins immediately as some of the drug is released in the stomach, but it extends over a 10- to 12-hour period as small amounts are gradually dissolved out while the tablet passes through the gastrointestinal tract. This is often desirable because it reduces the number of doses the patient must take in order to produce the therapeutic effect of the drug.

An important point in administering time-disintegration products, and to a certain extent with any other preparation, is that *to alter the dosage form in any way will probably alter the dosage.* For example, to crush a sustained-action tablet or empty this type of capsule for administration is to release the entire amount of the drug for immediate absorption and action, thus producing overdosage with possible serious effects for the patient. It is usually acceptable, however, to obtain an ordered dosage by dividing a single dose tablet scored for this purpose or to crush a single dose tablet for the patient who thinks he can swallow it better that way.

The mouth is lined with mucous membrane, which absorbs some substances.

Drugs, however, are so quickly swallowed that little absorption takes place in the mouth. Occasionally a drug is placed under the tongue, where it dissolves and is absorbed, as in the case of sublingual nitroglycerin used by the patient with anginal attacks.

The taste buds are located on the sides, tip, and back of the tongue. The most unpalatable flavors of drugs are the bitter and the salty tastes. Liquid preparations with these disagreeable tastes may be disguised in order to avoid nausea and vomiting. While for some adults it might be helpful to disguise the taste of such drugs as potassium iodide by adding milk or fruit juice, some individuals may learn to dislike the food because of this unpleasant association. Generally, the taste buds are stimulated least by cold fluids. Whenever possible, pharmaceutical companies try to make liquid drugs available in pleasantly flavored vehicles, such as syrups, aromatic waters, emulsions, and similar substances.

Some drugs in watery solutions are suspensions, which should be well shaken before use to evenly distribute the particles in order that dosage of the mixture will be accurate. Many of these drugs can be readily diluted with water if so desired, just before the dose is administered. The elixirs, on the other hand, should be administered undiluted because in some instances the addition of water may cause the drug to precipitate. A common example of an elixir is elixir of terpin hydrate with codeine.

The administration of drugs is often timed in relation to meals. Irritating drugs are usually given with or following food while other drugs are best given between meals, so that the absorption is not delayed by the presence of food in the stomach. When nausea and vomiting interfere with the ingestion of a prescribed oral medication, the physician should be consulted concerning the giving of the medication in a dosage form suitable for another route of administration.

Drug absorption is most rapid from the small intestine. Bile in the intestinal secretions saponifies oils and renders them soluble so that they may be absorbed.

The digestive processes are controlled by the nervous system. If the nervous system is not functioning properly, the rate of absorption of the drug may be changed. The rate of absorption also depends on the blood supply to the digestive organs. Shock causes inadequate circulation and hence slows absorption.

Conditions under which a drug may not be given by mouth are as follows: when absorption is slow, when coma renders the patient incapable of taking a drug by mouth, and when the patient is unable to swallow. Oral preparations are frequently witheld preoperatively.

Most drugs are given during the waking hours of the day. However, for some drugs such as the antibiotics, certain blood levels must be constantly maintained for therapeutic action. In order to maintain the desired level, as determined by laboratory blood tests, the medication must be administered at regular intervals during day and night.

Some radioactive isotopes are given by mouth. A very commonly used one is radioactive iodine in the diagnosis or treatment of thyroid conditions. Drugs are made radioactive by bombardment with deuterons in the cyclotron. The dose of the drug is measured in millicuries, which is a measure of disintegration per second. The path taken by an extremely small amount of a radioactive drug may be easily followed during the course of its metabolism by a scanner. Radioactive drugs are hazardous to the patient, the nurse, and the physician. They are very carefully controlled and are prepared and administered by especially trained technicians.

PREPARING AND ADMINISTERING MEDICATIONS

Every agency has its own equipment and detailed procedures by which medications are to be prepared and administered. These must be followed explicitly by the nurse in each situation. For example, in recent years various commerical systems, such as the Brewer system, have been introduced and rather widely used. These often include an elaborate portable medicine storage cart in which the patient's supply of ordered drugs is kept and from which dosages are prepared and administered as the cart is moved through the corridors (Fig. 22-1).

Innovative practices in handling drugs are also beginning to appear that could have major effects on the nurse's responsibility for the actual preparation of dosage to be administered to the individual patient. The use of pharmacy technicians and pharmacists is an illustration of this type of innovation. These workers may

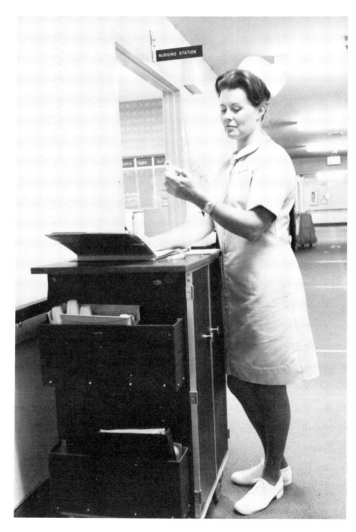

Fig. 22-1. Transportable medicine storage cart from which dosages are prepared and administered as the cart is moved through the corridors.

346

appear under different titles and with varying responsibilities, but in general, they are persons who transcribe the physician's orders onto the Kardex and stocks the medicine cart with a 24-hour supply of unit doses of each patient's medications. These unit doses are then administered by the nurse as ordered. This type of procedure is said to reduce the number of medication errors.

Although there may be marked variations in equipment and technique employed, some considerations remain quite constant and are therefore suitable for inclusion in this context.

Accuracy of dosage

Every dose of medicine is potentially dangerous. Accuracy of measurement is essential for both solid and liquid preparations and can be assured through meticulous attention to established procedural details and safety measures. The smaller the effective dose of the drug, the greater the need for exactness in calculating and measuring the dose. In the newer medication systems the nurse seldom finds it necessary to calculate and prepare divided dosages. However, every nurse needs to understand the basic principles of calculation should the necessity to use them arise, and in any event the nurse must be able to recognize errors on the part of technicians or perhaps inconsistencies in the physician's orders, should these occur. A misplaced decimal point or number may have serious consequences for the patient.

It is also important that there be adequate lighting and freedom from distractions and interruptions wherever the nurse is preparing and administering drugs. Deliberate, informed concentration on the task at hand is necessary to avoid errors. Errors are apt to occur when the nurse is distracted or proceeds automatically from habit without thoughtful attention to carrying out each step of the procedure.

In the event that a medication error does occur, the patient's welfare is the matter for first concern, and this is best served by immediate notification of the physician. Most agencies have a policy governing the handling of medication errors.

Purposeful action by the nurse in promoted through application of the "five rights to safety" in giving drugs.

The five rights to ensure safety in giving drugs

It is expected that the nurse will recognize certain critical factors in the preparation and administration of medications that need special emphasis for patient safety. They are often referred to as the "five rights":

Right patient:
1. Read the physician's orders.
2. Read the patient's name on the chart, Kardex, nursing care sheet or card, medicine card, bed, or wrist tag.
3. Ask the patient his name.
4. Be very careful if the patient is deaf or otherwise does not understand.

Right drug:
1. Read the physician's orders.
2. Be sure the drug is copied correctly on the Kardex or order sheet, on the nursing care sheet, and on the medicine card, if a card is to be used.
3. Select the right drug from the cupboard or elsewhere.
4. Say the patient's name.
5. Read the label three times: (a) before taking the drug from the shelf, (b) before measuring it, and compare with the medicine card or Kardex, and (c) when returning it to the shelf before removing the hand from the container.
6. Look at the appearance of the drug and note its odor.
7. Have clean labels on the containers. Labels are replaced only in the pharmacy.

347

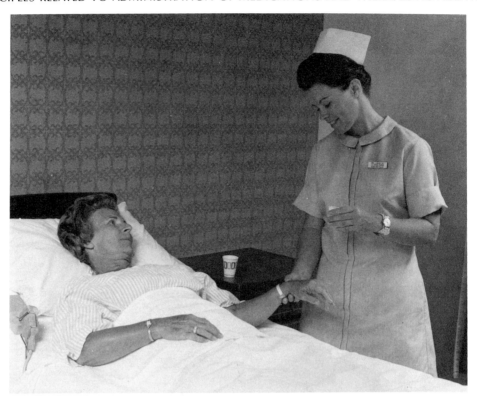

Fig. 22-2. Nurse identifies patient by checking wrist tag before administering the medication.

8. Become familiar with the trade names.

9. Be careful of drugs whose names sound alike, as Pyramidon and Pyridium.

10. Know abbreviations of drugs, such as M.S., Scop, A.S.A., E.T.H.cC., and so on. (See appendix for list of other abbreviations of drugs, physician's instructions, and hours of administrations.)

Right dose:

1. Read the physician's orders.

2. Consider the age of the patient, especially of a child or an elderly patient.

3. Measure liquids accurately: thumb on medicine cup; minims or drops as ordered.

4. Look at the dose on the label.

5. Consider how many tablets or capsules for the dose.

6. Know abbreviations and symbols of amounts, such as ss (viiss), Gm., gr., gtt., m.

7. Be sure of metric and apothecaries' equivalents.

8. Known maximum and minimum doses.

9. Help weak or helpless patients to get all of the drug.

Right time:

1. Read the physician's orders.

2. Know the hospital routines for intervals.

3. Give near the time ordered—within 15 minutes before or after the designated time.

4. Give at stated intervals for blood levels, such as every 8 hours.

5. Know abbreviations for times, such as a.c., p.c., b.i.d., t.i.d., q.i.d., o.d., B.T., or H.S.

348

Right method:

1. Read the physician's orders.

2. Dilute in milk, fruit juice, or water if indicated.

3. Give orally if no method is stated or indicated.

4. Know that certain drugs are given by certain methods.

5. Know the methods for giving drugs: orally, hypodermically, intradermally, subcutaneously, intramuscularly, intravenously, inhalation, aerosol, rectally, topically, and insufflation.

6. Know abbreviations for methods, as O., H., I.M., I.V.

7. Keep the drug and the card together if a card is to be used.

8. Think. Keep your mind on your work.

9. Give only drug dosages that you have prepared.

10. Ask if not sure as to the correct method.

11. Pour drug directly into medicine glass. Once a drug has been removed from the container, do not return it.

12. Pour tablet, pill, or capsule into inverted lid of container and then into medicine cup to avoid touching the drug with the fingers.

13. Record after drug is given.

Exercising judgment in drug administration

Even though innovative systems and equipment have been devised in an attempt to relieve nurses of the mechanical aspects of drug administration, the crucial responsibilities involved in translation of the physician's order into the individualized administration of the drug are still vested in the nurse. Regardless of the system in use, there is a great deal of nursing judgment required in carrying out the following nursing responsibilities:

1. Assuring that the patient is actually given the drug as it was prescribed and in a way that is most beneficial

and safe for the patient (Fig. 22-3)

2. Administering the drug dosage to the patient, except when the patient has permission to take his own medications

3. Observing the patient's reaction to the drug therapy

4. Recording the administration of the medication

5. Reporting untoward patient reaction promptly to the physician

6. Instructing the patient who has permission to take his own medication

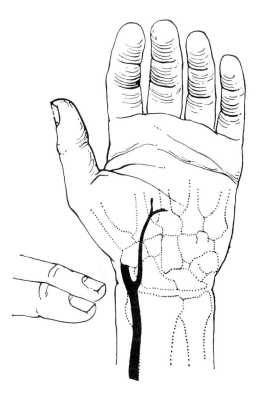

Fig. 22-3. Counting the pulse. This is done as a precautionary measure by the nurse when administering drugs that are likely to slow the action of the heart, such as members of the digitalis group. Radial artery is shown in relation to the bones of the hand and radius and ulna. (From Bergersen, B. S.: Pharmacology in nursing, ed. 12, St. Louis, 1973, The C. V. Mosby Co.)

in such matters as dose, time interval, method, and so on

7. Instructing the patient's family regarding the medication regimen if use of the drug is to be continued at home

8. Exercising judgment in giving p.r.n. medications

9. Integrating the drug administration into the total plan of patient care

The crucial element of nursing judgment in the preceding list of responsibilities inherent in the administration of medications is illustrated by the situation of Mrs. Dillon, a patient who has a new cast on her foot and leg. She tells the nurse, Miss Hunt, that she needs "something" for the burning pain in her foot. As she continues to complain of pain, Miss Hunt, knowing that Mrs. Dillon has a p.r.n. order intended for the control of pain, gives the medication immediately without further action. The patient still continues to call the nurse at frequent intervals to complain that the pain is not getting any better. Miss Hunt is extremely busy and responds that Mrs. Dillon should try to sleep and "everything will be okay," promising to repeat the p.r.n. pain medication when it can be given again in 4 hours. She keeps her promise.

Nevertheless, the patient is still crying with pain as Miss Hunt goes off duty. She reports to the on-coming nurse, Miss Wise, that Mrs. Dillon will probably need another administration of the p.r.n. order as soon as it can be repeated.

Miss Wise immediately visits the patient to assess the situation. She listens to Mrs. Dillon's tearful complaints, then looks for indications as to the condition of her toes which extend out of the cast. She notes that the toes are swollen, discolored, and cold and that the cast obviously fits too tightly around the toes. Recognizing the seriousness of these observations, Miss Wise promptly reports the situation to the physician. A window is quickly cut in the cast and it is found that an extensive area of tissue damage has already developed, resulting from inadequate blood supply to the tissues in the presence of swelling against an unyielding cast. Much costly treatment and time will be required to correct the problem, which could probably have been prevented through the prompt exercise of nursing judgment when the first p.r.n. medication was given.

If Miss Hunt had consulted all available sources of information before deciding to give the first p.r.n. medication for pain, she would have been reminded that the patient's toes were to be regularly checked for possible swelling and that complaint of unusual pain coupled with indications of impaired circulation should be reported at once. Also, she might have realized that failure of the first p.r.n. drug administration to bring significant relief from pain was an alarm signal calling for further investigation, even if she had missed the first cue.

This illustration supports the statement made earlier that the administration of medications is to be integrated into the total plan of care for the patient, that nursing is more than an accumulation of technical skills. It is the exercise of concerned judgment based upon knowledge and informed observation, as well as technical skill combined with experience, that makes nursing uniquely more than a series of tasks performed.

Recording of medications administered

It is necessary, of course, that all drug administration be recorded according to the established policies in the agency. Essential information to record usually includes (1) amount of each dose, (2) time administered, (3) reason for administration (for p.r.n. medications), (4) who gave it, (5) response of the patient to the medication, and (6) statement of the reason when a dose is omitted.

Prompt recording of drugs administered

is always important, but it is particularly so when p.r.n. orders are given, to avoid possible duplication of administration.

Provision for narcotics and other special drugs

In the interest of safety and efficiency in storing and handling drugs, each patient care unit has a facility designed for this purpose that is not accessible to the patient or the public. It may be a special room or, more likely, a cabinet or dispenser devised to facilitate the administration of various types of medicinal preparations, for which a nurse carries the keys.

Invariably, there is a special locked compartment in this facility for the storage of narcotics. Originally, the Harrison Narcotic Act of 1914 was devised to control the traffic in narcotic drugs, in this context, to control the distribution of opium and coca and their derivatives and certain synthetic drugs that are considered to be capable of causing and sustaining addiction. Only physicians registered under the Harrison Narcotic Act were authorized to order these drugs, and any prescription that the physician wrote containing any of these drugs had to bear his narcotic registration number.

In 1952, the federal Food and Drug Administration was empowered to determine which medications could be dispensed only upon a physician's prescription. This was an attempt to deal with rules for the refilling of prescriptions and was aimed at unsupervised self-medication and the abuse of barbiturates that were not controlled by the Harrison Narcotic Act. In 1965 another amendment added more stringent controls over a long list of central nervous system depressants and stimulants.

These regulations have since been replaced by the Federal Controlled Substances Act of 1970 and new regulations issued by the Director of the Federal Bureau of Narcotics and Dangerous Drugs. These became effective May 1, 1971. The drugs controlled by the new act are in five general categories:

Schedule I. Hallucinogenic substances and some opiates for which there is no accepted medical use

Schedule II. Drugs of high abuse potential such as most narcotics, amphetamines, and some closely related compounds (former Class A)

Schedule III. Depressants such as barbiturates, straight paregoric, certain amphetamine combination drugs, and narcotics formerly of the Class B group

Schedule IV. Chloral hydrate, meprobamate, paraldehyde, and some long-acting barbiturates

Schedule V. Paregoric combination preparations and other drugs and compounds of lower abuse potential than those listed in Schedule IV

All prescriptions for controlled drugs (Schedules II to V) must contain the full name and address of the patient, the full name and address of the physician, the signature of the prescribing physician, and the BNDD (Bureau of Narcotics and Dangerous Drugs) number of the prescribing physician.

In addition to the federal laws there are not only many state and municipal regulations for handling of narcotics and other special drugs, but local hospitals have also established their own policies and procedures for the handling and accounting of these drugs. Health agencies are required to provide record forms for use in recording the dosage of each narcotic that is administered, the record usually including such information as (1) name of the patient receiving the narcotic, (2) dosage (or amount of narcotic removed from the supply on hand), (3) time of the administration, (4) name of the physician ordering

351

the narcotic, and (5) name of the nurse administering the narcotic. Each nurse administering a narcotic is responsible for accuracy of this record and for carrying out the letter of the law, which is aimed at controlling the misuse of drugs.

Each agency has a system for ensuring accuracy of the narcotic record, which commonly requires a narcotic count with each of the three changes of shift. When the narcotic count cannot be made to check exactly with the record, the discrepancy must be reported immediately.

It is common practice in most hospitals that emergency carts be kept at strategic locations ready for immediate use. Such carts are checked daily and after each use to make certain that they are equipped at all times with the drugs commonly employed in emergency situations, together with the equipment necessary for their use.

Medications given by rectum

When it is not advisable to administer a medication orally, it is sometimes given per rectum. Since rectal medications are absorbed by way of the gastrointestinal tract, they are usually included along with oral medication.

The same safety precautions previously applied to oral medications are also applicable to rectal medication; however, the dosage is usually increased because of slower and less adequate absorption. Preferably, they should be given before or between meals, since food intake often stimulates peristalsis, which could result in expulsion of the drug.

Medications given per rectum are usually in suppository or liquid form and may be given to produce systemic effects, local effects upon the rectum, or both. Capsules and tablets are also sometimes inserted into the rectum; however, it is better to dissolve them in a little warm water (or in oil in some instances) and give them by retention enema. A catheter and bulb syringe make a good vehicle for administering medications per rectum. When administering a liquid medication per rectum, it is well to limit the total amount (drug plus diluent) to 150 ml. to avoid expulsion of the solution. Saline cathartics and lubricating oils are often given by this method to relieve constipation.

Suppositories are usually made of glycerin, lanolin, or a wax that melts at body temperature. They may be used entirely for their mechanical effects or may contain a medication. For insertion of a suppository, a glove or finger cot will be needed. The addition of a lubricant also adds to the ease of insertion. For insertion of a suppository, the buttocks are usually separated, with one hand exposing the anus. The suppository is then inserted with the thumb and forefinger of the gloved hand, followed by the forefinger to see that it has passed the sphincter muscle. The anal canal is about 1 inch in length, so an insertion of about 2 inches is sufficient. Suppositories are usually kept in a refrigerator and should be allowed to warm to near room temperature before insertion.

Other preparations often administered per rectum are disposable-unit enema preparations. They are available in both cleansing and oil-retention forms. The Fleet enema is an example of a disposable-unit cleansing enema and comes in both adult and children's dosage. Instructions for insertion are included with the product.

Medication per rectum is usually contraindicated in cases of rectal surgery or disease unless given for that specific condition as suppositories for painful hemorrhoids.

Psychosocial aspects of drug administration

In the past it was generally accepted that the patient should know little or nothing about the medications or treatments prescribed for him. This philosophy, however, is being generally questioned. The question of how much information any patient should be given about his illness, medications, and other aspects of his therapy must be determined on an individual basis and in reference to the judgment of the physician. Many physicians now request the pharmacist to include the name of the drug on the prescription label

This change of attitude in the direction of more open communication with the patient seems to be based on experience indicating that patients benefit in many ways from having the opportunity for active participation in their own plan of care rather than being expected to merely follow instructions without question. It is important to listen to the patient's questions or his comments regarding medications that he could not tolerate in the past or, if he questions the accuracy of a medication or a dosage, to take the time to evaluate his concerns, because this may be the means for averting an error in administration or a serious drug reaction on the part of the patient.

Listening to the patient and giving him the opportunity to express his fears and anxieties—perhaps about the value of the medication, or maybe about his resistance to what he believes to be drug-induced discomforts, or possibly about his cultural or religious beliefs—may give the nurse an opportunity to assist the patient with these negative feelings.

Positive suggestions that the nurse is concerned about the patient's welfare and wants him to get well may help the patient be emotionally prepared to expect the medication to be effective. Taking the time to interact with the patient, explaining what to expect, particularly when giving a drug by injection, is more effective than hurrying through the procedure without recognizing the patient as a person and with no explanation to him.

On the other hand, some patients may think they are not receiving adequate care unless they have some medicine and are not content until they do receive something. On rare occasions a placebo, an inactive substance usually in the form of a tablet, may be ordered to satisfy a patient's demand for medicine. However, the emotional support provided for the patient sensing the nurse's sincere attitude of caring and of concern for his welfare is more apt to be effective in the patient's positive response to his therapy. The nurse can sometimes communicate these positive suggestions quietly and wordlessly by the very manner of proceeding with patient care activities.

The nurse should stay with the patient until the drug is taken. If the drug is a sedative or a hypnotic, the environment should be prepared before the drug is given so that the patient will not be disturbed after the drug is given. The light should be dimmed, maybe the back rubbed or extra warmth added, and ventilation provided because these things are conducive to rest for most patients.

The patient's emotional reaction should be considered. For example, a patient may feel embarrassed when having a medication administered per rectum. The provision for privacy and composure of the nurse may contribute greatly to ease the patient.

The senses of the sick person are often very acute. Stimulation of the senses that would mean nothing to the well person may be very irritating to one who is ill. The sight, odor, and taste of drugs may be very distasteful to the patient. Most persons prefer a colored medicine, perhaps because it looks as though it contains something of efficacy. Although not of great importance from the therapeutic standpoint, proper flavoring and coloring are psychologically significant. The flavoring is more important than the coloring, although sometimes the flavoring agent serves as a coloring agent also. The most pleasing colors are red and brown: a red color may be syrup of cherry and a brown color may be chocolate. The use of attractive equipment helps to make the taking of medicine more agreeable for the patient.

LEARNING SITUATIONS FOR THE PATIENT

If the patient is to give himself medications upon his return home, he should be taught how and be allowed to prepare and give himself his medication several days before he leaves the hospital. Instructions to the patient about his medication should be clear, concise, correct, and, if necessary, written. The label on the bottle or box should be interpreted to the patient. The name of the drug or the number of it is found on the box, as well as the amount to take in each dose and the times for taking it. The nurse should be sure the patient understands each item exactly.

Proper instructions regarding the use of measuring devices, whether teaspoon, tablespoon, or medicine dropper, should be given. The patient should be instructed to shake certain liquids before measuring the required dose and warned about exceeding the prescribed dose, since many drugs are toxic in large doses. Other drugs become habit forming if taken over a long period of time.

The nurse has the opportunity to encourage the patient to seek prescriptions from a competent physician. In many instances the patient may save money when the prescription is written by the physician, for he uses the scientific name of the drug, whereas the same drug under a patented name costs more.

The nurse may warn the patient of the grave danger of taking drugs not prescribed by a physician. Self-medication provides inadequate medication at best. Vitamins and minerals are drugs, and as such they need to be prescribed. Sometimes one vitamin or mineral in excess causes imbalance in another vitamin or mineral. The patient may not be aware of these imbalances.

The patient may be reminded that drugs prescribed for him are for him and should not be passed on to another member of the family or to anyone else. Portions of drugs left over after recovery from an illness should be properly destroyed since the nature of some drugs changes with age.

The opportunity might arise for telling a mother to place drugs in a medicine cabinet out of the reach of young children and to keep poisons away from drugs taken internally.

SUMMARY

Material presented in this chapter is intended to be helpful in motivating the nurse toward broadening and deepening a growing personal understanding of how drugs achieve their therapeutic effects and how they may be administered to enhance their therapeutic effectiveness.

The integration of pharmacologic knowledge with the plan of care will enable the nurse to provide better patient care when pharmacotherapeutic agents are being administered. Examples of scientific principles have been included in this context with some application to the nurse's role in drug administration.

Details of the various techniques that may be employed in the preparation and administration of medications have not been included, but the discussion has been centered on the more generally constant factors pertinent to the nursing role.

QUESTIONS FOR DISCUSSION

1 What are the chief advantages of administering a drug orally?
2 How should the nurse deal with the patient's questions about his medications?
3 What is meant by absorption of an administered drug?
4 What is meant by the term "drug idiosyncrasy"?

5 When is the rectal route of administration preferred to the oral route? What are suppositories? What is the proper method of inserting a suppository?

6 List measures applied routinely to avoid making medication errors.

7 What basic knowledge should the nurse have about each drug administered in order to fulfill the ethical and legal responsibilities for drug administration?

8 How may the nurse enhance the effectiveness of drugs administered to produce sleep or relieve pain?

LIFE SITUATION

The nurse was giving Mr. Tone his medicine. He said, "You should see my medicine cabinet at home. You know, every time I hear of a drug on television for aches and pains, I go to the drugstore and buy it. I think I must have about twenty different headache remedies. Then I come to the hospital and get one dose of something the doctor ordered and all my pains are gone. Why?" How would you respond to Mr. Tone?

SUGGESTED PERFORMANCE CHECKLIST
Safety

1 Is the physician's order read before preparing the drug?
2 Is the dose prepared without distraction?
3 Is the dosage the usual amount ordered?
4 Is the medicine given on time?
5 Is the equipment clean? Are the nurses' hands clean?
6 Is the label read three times?
7 Is the door to medicines kept locked?
8 Is the calculation accurate?
9 Is the label on the bottle or box clear?
10 Is light by the medicine cabinet adequate?
11 Is an identifying card carried with the drug?
12 Is the nurse who gives the drug the same one who prepared the drug?
13 Is the patient identified at the bedside before the drug is administered?

14 Are symptoms of overdosage noted before giving a drug with a cumulative action?

Therapeutic effectiveness

1 Is the ordered dose of drug given?
2 Is the drug given on time?
3 Does the nurse stay with the patient until the drug is taken?
4 If the dose seems unusual, is the order questioned through proper channels?
5 Are factors in the environment that are conducive to sedation utilized before a sedative drug is given?

Comfort

1 Is the dose as palatable as possible?
2 Is water given with the drug when indicated?
3 Is a sense of hurry avoided?
4 Are suppositories warmed and lubricated?
5 Is the patient assisted as indicated?

Economy

1 Is the equipment returned clean to its proper place?
2 Is equipment sufficient?
3 Are drugs kept clean?
4 Is the supply of drugs adequate?
5 Are paper containers used for isolated patients?
6 Are liquid medicines poured on the side of the bottle opposite the label?

Good workmanship

1 Is the patient observed carefully?
2 Does the nurse show skill in giving medications?
3 Is the equipment removed from the bedside at once?
4 Is the charting concise and adequate?

SUGGESTED READINGS

Bergersen, Betty S.: Pharmacology in nursing, ed. 12, St. Louis, 1973, The C. V. Mosby Co.

Johns, Marjorie P.: Pharmacodynamics and patient care, St. Louis, 1973, The C. V. Mosby Co.

Levine, Myra E.: Breaking through the medication mystique, American Journal of Nursing **70:**799, April, 1970.

23 Parenteral medications

GENERAL CONSIDERATIONS
Nonoral routes of medication administration

As indicated in the preceding chapter, there may be a number of existing factors that require the selection of a nonoral route of administration for a therapeutic agent. Common factors include (1) condition of the patient that renders the oral route unsafe or impractical, such as unconsciousness, difficulty in swallowing, immediate preoperative situation, or nausea and vomiting; (2) irritating properties of the drug that make it necessary to bypass the oral route; (3) failure of drug, for a variety of reasons, to attain a therapeutic plasma concentration when given by mouth, for example, certain antibiotics such as streptomycin; and (4) impaired circulation in the gastrointestinal tract, as in shock.

Parenteral administration

Literally, the term "parenteral" means any route outside of the gastrointestinal tract. However, in general usage the term is applied to any of the ways by which suitable liquid preparations of drugs are injected by needle into the tissues or directly into the bloodstream. Commonly included with the parenteral routes are subcutaneous (hypodermic), intramuscular, intradermal, and intravenous injections.

Parenteral injections are sometimes more advantagous than oral medications because of the greater rapidity and efficiency of absorption from the injection site when systemic action is desired, and the simplicity of administration to unconscious or critically ill patients.

Parenteral medications are not without some disadvantages, which should be kept in mind when administering any needle injection:

1. Aseptic technique must be maintained during the preparation and administration of the drug.

2. The injection may be painful and the tissue damage at the injection site may be a predisposing factor to infection.

3. It is possible for the needle to break off in the tissues.

4. An irritating or slowly absorbed drug may cause tissue necrosis, skin slough, abscesses, and persistent pain.

5. Injury to a nerve may occur if the site of injection is incorrectly located.

356

6. Inadvertent intravenous injection of a solution not suitable for that route can happen.

7. Once the drug has been injected, it is difficult (or impossible if given intravenously) to recall it or to prevent it from being fully absorbed in the event of an adverse reaction developing to it.

Equipment

The administration of medications by parenteral routes requires equipment that is sterile, accurate in measuring dosage, and convenient for use, that will produce as little discomfort and/or hazard for the patient as possible, and that will be acceptable in appearance for the psychologic effect on the patient, should it come within his line of vision, regardless of the method of administration.

Needles are made of steel or other metal and are either reusable or disposable. They vary in length from $3/8$ inch to 5 inches. The outside diameter is measured by Stubs gauge, which is an English wire measure, standard throughout the United States (Fig. 23-1). The diameter sizes of needles are indicated by numbers 14 to 27, with decimal equivalents in thousandths of an inch. However, the higher the gauge number, the smaller the diameter of the needle. The gauge number is usually found on the hub. (See Table 23-1.)

A needle has two parts, the hub and the cannula. (See Fig. 23-2.) The point of bending and breaking is most often where the cannula and the hub join. The slanting tip of the needle containing the opening is called the bevel. A short bevel is used for intravenous injections in order that the entire opening will be within the vein. A long bevel has a sharper point and is used for all injections except intravenous. Needles should be sharp and shiny in order to penetrate the tissues quickly and safely.

Syringes may be made from glass only or glass reinforced at the ends with metal. Syringes may also be made of plastic, and these are disposable. The most usual sizes are 2, 5, 10, 20, 30, and 50 ml. (cc.). (See Fig. 23-2.) Beyond the 10 ml. (cc.) size the syringe becomes unwieldy.

The 2 to 5 ml. (cc.) sizes of syringes are used most frequently because larger quantities of solution are seldom injected into the muscles. Usually, less than 2 ml. would be injected subcutaneously (Fig. 23-2). The insulin and tuberculin syringes are designed and calibrated for specialized use. The scale on the insulin syringe is

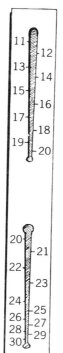

Fig. 23-1. Stubs gauge is used for measuring the diameter of hypodermic needles.

Table 23-1 Usual size of needles for various purposes

Use	Size
Intradermal	26 gauge, $3/8$-$1/2$ inch long
Intramuscular	20 gauge, 1-2 inches long
Subcutaneous	25-26 gauge, $5/8$ inch long
Hypodermoclysis	21-22 gauge, 3 inches long
Intravenous	20-22 gauge, 1 $1/2$ inches long

357

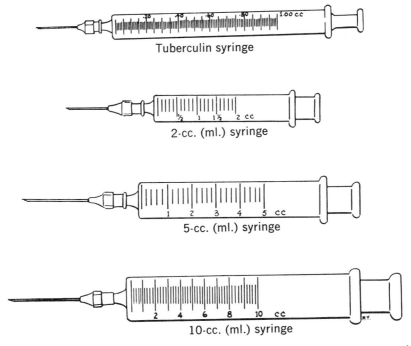

Fig. 23-2. These syringes are used to accurately measure varying amounts of liquids and liquid medications. The tuberculin syringe is graduated in 0.01 ml. (cc.). It is a syringe of choice for administration of very small amounts. The 2-ml. (cc.) syringe is the one commonly used to give a drug subcutaneously. It is graduated in 0.1 ml. (cc.). The larger syringes are used when a large amount of drug is to be administered. (From Bergersen, Betty S.: Pharmacology in nursing, ed. 12, St. Louis, 1973, The C. V. Mosby Co.)

marked off in units according to the concentration of insulin being used, such as U40 or U80 (Fig. 23-3). The tuberculin syringe is a long, narrow syringe calibrated in tenths and hundredths of a milliliter (cubic centimeter). It is used when great accuracy is required for measuring a minute amount of a drug (Fig. 23-2).

The syringe is made in two parts: the barrel and the plunger. Now these parts are generally being made interchangeable with other syringes of the same capacity, although there are still some syringes available for which the barrel and plunger have been specially fitted and marked with identical numbers. These are not interchangeable with other syringes. On the barrel of all standard syringes is a scale indicating milliliters (cubic centimeters). On

small syringes—2 ml. (cc.) size and less—a scale for measurements in minims is added.

Disposable syringes with needles are available in various sizes. A needle protector keeps the needle sterile. The agency's policy for discarding disposables should be followed.

A one-dose discardable hypodermic syringe with needle has been perfected. The dose of drug or serum already in the syringe is separated from a compartment that holds the needle by a rubber diaphragm. An opening on one end of the compartment is set against the point of injection, and pressure is applied to the plunger. This pressure causes the near end of the needle to pierce the diaphragm and release the drug, while the other end

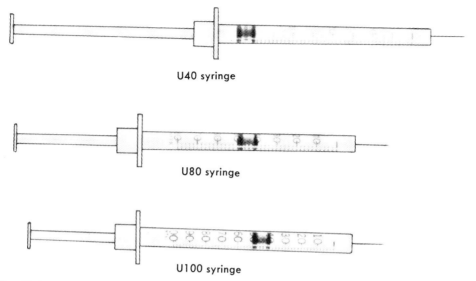

U40 syringe

U80 syringe

U100 syringe

Fig. 23-3. Insulin syringes calibrated in units. (Courtesy Eli Lilly & Co., Indianapolis, Ind.)

of the needle is injected into the patient. Many antibiotics are dispensed in syringes of this kind.

Physicians, visiting nurses, and patients who must have a hypodermic syringe for instant use carry disposable equipment or a kit that permits keeping the syringe sterile and safe.

Ampules and vials

Drugs for hypodermic or intramuscular use are most frequently in ampules and vials and occasionally are supplied in tablet form for drugs that deteriorate in solution. Tablets must be dissolved before use, usually in sterile distilled water or physiologic saline solution.

Glass ampules are designed as single-dose containers because once an ampule has been opened, there is no way to preserve sterility of the contents for future use, as there is with the vial. Some ampules have a constriction in the stem at which it may be scored and then broken off. It may be necessary to tap it to bring the drug down out of the stem, if it is an ampule with a constriction. The fingers are protected with sterile cotton or gauze

when snapping off the stem. The drug may then be drawn up into the syringe as illustrated in Fig. 23-4. Ampules that are prescored are usually marked with a colored line at the constriction and need not be filed before being opened.

After breaking off the stem of the ampule, the nurse can withdraw the medication from its container by inserting the needle through the opening made in the stem and aspirating the solution into the syringe. In so doing, it is important to avoid contaminating the needle by touching the edge of the opening with it and to avoid possible damage to the sharp point of the needle by jabbing or scraping it against the bottom of the ampule while withdrawing the solution. However, withdrawal of the solution is facilitated by keeping the tip of the needle immersed while aspirating the solution.

The vial can be either a single-dose or a multiple-dose dispensing container because the rubber seal, which is the route of entrance into the vial, remains intact to protect the sterility of succeeding doses, providing principles of aseptic technique are used in withdrawing each dose. Using

359

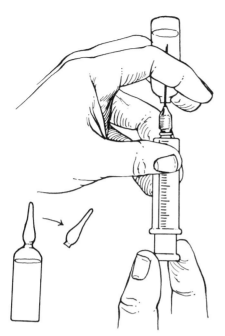

Fig. 23-4. Withdrawing medication from an ampule. An ampule may be made like the one in the lower left part of this illustration—it will break easily when pressure is exerted at the constriction portion—or the ampule may be made so that a metal file must be used at the neck to secure a clean break. (From Bergersen, Betty S.: Pharmacology in nursing, ed. 12, St. Louis, 1973, The C. V. Mosby Co.)

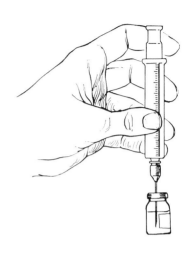

Fig. 23-5. Inserting hypodermic needle into a stoppered vial. When a hypodermic needle is inserted into a vial of this type, it is important that air be injected first to facilitate withdrawal of the liquid medication. Note that the plunger has been withdrawn and is supported by the index finger. After the plunger has been pushed down to the end of the barrel, the vial can be turned and held much like an ampule. The desired amount is then drawn into the syringe. (From Bergersen, Betty S.: Pharmacology in nursing, ed. 12, St. Louis, 1973, The C. V. Mosby Co.)

friction when cleansing the rubber seal with an antiseptic sponge before inserting the needle each time will aid in preventing contamination of the vial's contents.

To remove a dose of medication from the vial, one first draws an amount of air into the syringe equal to the desired dose. The needle is inserted through the center of the cleansed rubber seal and the air is injected into the vial (Fig. 23-5). The increased air pressure in the vial will facilitate removal of the desired dose.

Pressure is a factor of concern in all needle injections. When a solution is drawn from an ampule into a syringe, the needle is put into the fluid and the plunger

is pulled back, thus lowering the pressure in the syringe. Fluids tend to flow to an area of low pressure, so that the solution comes into the syringe. When a solution is drawn from a rubber-capped vial, the plunger is pulled back to admit as much air as the amount of fluid desired. The needle is then introduced into the vial, and the air is pushed from the syringe into the vial (Fig. 23-6). In this way the air pressure within the vial is raised, and when pressure on the plunger is released, the compressed air in the vial pushes the solution into the syringe.

Pressure exerted against the plunger of a hypodermic syringe is transferred to the solution, and the solution is deposited in

360

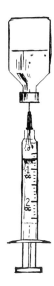

Fig. 23-6. Compressed air in the vial forces the plunger of the hypodermic syringe out.

the tissue. Pressure in the tissue is greater than in the capillaries, so that the fluid is forced into the capillaries.

SCIENTIFIC PRINCIPLES

Most of the principles included in Chapter 22 regarding oral medications are also useful in explaining the basis for nursing activities in preparing and administering parenteral medications. They are restated here together with additional principles that are related more specifically to parenteral medications.

1. The rate of absorption, distribution, and excretion of a drug depends upon its composition and concentration and upon the volume of the circulating blood supply.

2. A drug must be in solution in order to be absorbed into the circulating blood.

3. A drug is a foreign material in the body. When it is absorbed and distributed to the tissues by the circulating blood, it modifies cell metabolism and may thus modify or alter body functions.

4. Fluids tend to flow to an area of lower pressure.

5. When the integrity of skin or mucous membrane is broken, a possible route of entry is opened for invading microorganisms.

6. Microorganisms are always present on the surfaces of the body.
   a. Application of bacteriostatic agents decreases the number of organisms present but does not sterilize skin.
   b. The use of friction when applying the cleansing agent on the skin decreases the transfer of contaminants.

7. More sensory fibers for pain are found in the skin than in any other place in the body.

8. An individual's sensitivity to pain is affected by:
   a. The way he perceives the pain
   b. His emotional attitude toward pain
   c. His personal reaction to the pain as he perceives it

9. Efficiency of the cardiovascular system is promoted by maintaining unobstructed normal blood flow. This implies that:
   a. Immiscible substances will not be injected intravenously.
   b. Blood transfusion must be preceded by blood typing and cross-matching.
   c. Air must be removed from equipment preceding intravenous injection so that air will not be allowed to enter the bloodstream.

10. The osmotic pressure of body fluids is normally about 0.9% sodium chloride.
   a. Physiologic saline solution (normal saline) is isotonic with body fluids, which is approximately a 0.9% aqueous solution of sodium chloride.
   b. Change in this osmotic pressure can result in damage to cells (such as red blood cells) by overhydration or dehydration of the cells.

11. The filtration of water from the capillaries to the interstitial fluids varies in relation to a number of factors including:
   a. The higher the concentration of sodium ions in the interstitial fluid, the greater the filtration.
   b. The lower the osmotic pressure of

the blood caused by loss of plasma proteins, the greater the filtration. Therefore, blood volume replacement by intravenous administration of isotonic saline brings quick relief to dehydration of tissues but does not maintain the normal circulating volume of the blood. Osmotic balance is restored by transfusion of whole blood or blood plasma, which increases the osmotic pressure of the circulating blood and hence decreases the filtration rate of water from the capillaries into the interstitial fluid.

12. A constant cellular environment with a pH value of about 7.4 is required for normal cellular functioning.

   a. Blood pH is of great importance because this determines the pH of the cellular environment.

   b. The proper pH is maintained partly by the buffering action of phosphate, bicarbonate, and protein.

   c. All fluids injected into the bloodstream should conform as closely as possible to the reaction of normal blood.

APPLICATION OF PRINCIPLES
Prevention of infection

Since microorganisms are always present on the skin, the area of injection and the hands of the nurse in each situation should be conscientiously cleansed in such a way as to reduce to a minimum the number of bacteria present. The skin of the patient is usually cleansed with alcohol wipes (70% alcohol) or other suitable bacteriostatic agent.

The moistened pledget is placed directly over the site selected for giving the injection. Beginning at this point, a circular motion is used, cleansing outward in ever widening circles, extending at least 2 inches beyond the point of injection. This is a more effective routine in preparing the injection site than is an unpatterned back

and forth motion that may simply redistribute organisms over the area rather than wash them outward and away from the central point. It may even be advisable to cleanse the skin first with soap and water when the skin is grossly contaminated, as may be in the case with certain types of laborers admited to the hospital directly from work or perhaps with an incontinent patient.

The site selected for an injection should be an area free from skin lesions, abrasions, bruises, or scar tissues.

Handwashing for the nurse should precede preparation of the injection. In assembling and preparing materials, careful handling will avoid contamination of the sterile parts and also avoid injury to the nurse's hands, for instance, in breaking off the stem of a glass ampule.

Sometimes the drug needs to be drawn into the syringe or a dry drug may need to be mixed with fluid either in a vial or in the syringe. The various steps are performed carefully to prevent contamination of the needle, parts of the syringe, and the drug. A protector covers the needle during transportation to the patient's unit. Wet gauze over the needle is an inadequate barrier against the penetration of bacteria.

Capillary attraction involves a liquid. When a sterile needle is put in or on a wet sponge, whether held in the fingers or laid on an unsterile surface, bacteria may rise in the sponge by capillary attraction and may contaminate the needle and also any drug in the syringe.

Depth and angle of injection

Drugs are injected at various angles and depths beneath the surface of the skin. A subcutaneous or hypodermic injection permits the introduction of fluid into the loose tissue under the skin (Fig. 23-7, *A*). Drugs are given subcutaneously in order to secure more rapid absorption of a drug or to prevent its destruction by the action of digestive secretions. The intradermal or intra-

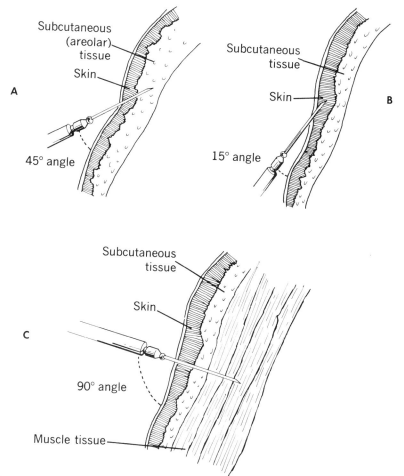

Fig. 23-7. **A,** Subcutaneous injection; **B,** intracutaneous injection; **C,** intramuscular injection.

cutaneous method is used chiefly for diagnostic purposes (such as the Schick test), for sensitivity tests (introduction of allergens), and for local anesthesia. They are also given subcutaneously when the patient is unable to take them by mouth. In an intramuscular injection the material is injected between layers of muscle (Fig. 23-7, *C*). An intracutaneous or intradermal injection is the introduction of material into the skin (Fig. 23-7, *B*).

The skin contains numerous blood vessels, lymph vessels, and nerves. More sensory fibers for pain are found in the skin than in any other place in the body,

and the nearer the surface of the skin a needle is injected and the fluid is placed, the more pain is connected with the treatment. The fluid is taken up quickly by the lymph vessels and is carried to the bloodstream. Intradermal injections are made in areas in which the skin is soft and yielding, such as the flexor surface of the forearm. Directly under the skin is found loose areolar tissue, which contains a good blood supply, lymph vessels, and nerves. To minimize the pain of a subcutaneous injection, areas poorly supplied with sensory nerves, such as the outer side of the arm or the thigh, are chosen if possible. Since complete circulation time is near 20 seconds, the effect of a subcutaneous or intramuscular injection appears within a brief time.

Muscles are well supplied with blood vessels that are larger than those in the skin, but muscles are not so well supplied with sensory nerves as is the skin, hence, deep injections are not so painful as the more superficial ones. One danger in giving an intramuscular injection is that of entering a blood vessel. This danger may be avoided by pulling back on the plunger after the needle is inserted but before the drug is injected.

Site of injection

Intradermal injections are made in areas in which the skin is soft and yielding, such as the flexor surface of the forearm. Very small amounts of fluid are injected intradermally, usually for a local effect. Often the tuberculin syringe is the only one with fine enough calibrations to measure the minute dose to be used. A 26-gauge needle $^3/_8$ to $^1/_2$ inch in length is usually selected and is inserted with the bevel up to make a small bleb just under the surface of the skin and between its layers.

The *subcutaneous* (hypodermic) injection is introduced into the loose areolar tissue just beneath the layers of skin, where there are fewer sensory pain receptors than in the skin and where the drug will cause less pain than if given intracutaneously. Also, a larger amount may be injected hypodermically, although the amount should not exceed 2 ml. to avoid pressure on surrounding tissues. When the drug is in an isotonic solution, it generally produces very minimal or no stinging sensation. It is well to avoid injecting the drug into adipose tissue because there is a less abundant blood supply and the drug will be poorly absorbed. A suitable size of needle to select is 25- or 26-gauge and $^5/_8$ to 1 inch in length, depending upon the state of obesity and hydration of the in-

dividual patient. A 45- or 90-degree angle may be used, depending on needle length.

Almost any area of the body with abundant soft tissue and distant from large nerves and blood vessels may be selected for the hypodermic injection, but the most common sites of injection are the outer aspects of the upper arm, the anterior aspects of the thigh, and the loose abdominal tissue. When the patient is to administer his own injections, the abdomen and thighs would, of course, be the most convenient areas. If the injections are to be continued over a period of time, the sites of injection should be alternated regularly to be sure that there is complete absorption of the drug. Otherwise, induration and itching from unabsorbed drug may occur when repeated injections are permitted in the same site. A definite schedule for rotating the sites may be included in the patient's plan of care.

The *intramuscular* route seems to be increasingly more popular, even for some drugs formerly given by hypodermic injection. Perhaps this is for a combination of such reasons as drugs too irritating for use subcutaneously can be given intramuscularly, and larger quantities can be given per dose. The maximum amount to be injected at one site is usually considered to be 5 ml. A dose requiring more than this would be divided between two different sites. Other characteristics of the intramuscular injection are that the medicine is deposited in muscle tissue where it is more gradually absorbed into the bloodstream to produce a longer and more sustained effect than if given intravenously. It is thought to be the safest, easiest, and best tolerated of the injection routes when it is given properly.

For the intramuscular injection, a 2- or 5-ml. syringe and a 21- or 22-gauge needle 1 to $1^1/_2$ inches in length would be selected. The length of the needle should be sufficient to place the drug deep within the muscle. A larger gauge needle might be needed for thick or oily drug preparations. A common practice is to draw a small air bubble of 0.1 to 0.2 ml. into the syringe so that all of the drug will be forced from the needle into the muscle. Otherwise, the drug left in the needle at the end of the injection may "track" into the subcutaneous tissues from the needle as it is withdrawn. An irritating drug is more readily injurious to fatty tissue than to the muscle. For the same reason some authorities recommend using the Z track method of inserting the needle when injecting some of the very irritating drugs to prevent leaking of the solution along the needle track from the muscle into the subcutaneous tissue. Usually instructions are provided with such preparations by the pharmaceutical companies that give the details for using the Z track technique.

The use of presterilized disposable syringes and needles is recommended, not only for greater convenience but primarily to avoid transmission of infection in the tissues at the injection site and the transference of systemic disease, such as hepatitis.

Choice of the proper site for injection of the intramuscular medication is most crucial in preventing tissue damage at the injection site. Identification of a suitable site is based on the use of definite anatomic landmarks, located by palpation. Four injection sites are usually recommended for adults:

1. Dorsogluteal site. In this area, injection is made into the gluteus maximus muscle, which is not to be confused with the area designated as the buttocks (Figs. 23-8 and 23-9).
2. Ventrogluteal site (von Hochstetter's site). Injection in this area is made into the gluteus minimus and the gluteus medius muscles (Figs. 23-10 and 23-11).
3. Vastus lateralis site. This site is located on the lateral aspect of the thigh

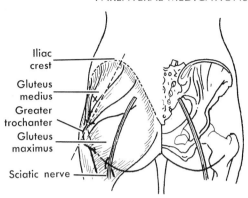

Fig. 23-8. Anatomic landmarks used in locating the dorsogluteal site for intramuscular injection. Draw a line from the posterior superior iliac spine to the greater trochanter of the femur. Select an injection site lateral and superior to this line and 2 to 3 inches below the crest of the ileum.

and uses the vastus lateralis muscle (Fig. 23-12).
4. Deltoid site. This is an easily available but generally less useful shoulder site around the deltoid muscle.

The *dorsogluteal site* seems currently to be the most generally used intramuscular injection site. The recommended method of locating a safe point for insertion of the needle is to draw a line from the posterior superior iliac spine to the greater trochanter of the femur. This line would be lateral to and somewhat parallel with the sciatic nerve. Selecting a point lateral and superior to this line and 2 to 3 inches below the crest of the ilium would place the injection within the gluteal muscle and at a safe distance from the sciatic nerve, large blood vessels, and bone.

The more traditional method of dividing the buttock into quadrants as a means of locating the dorsogluteal site requires the drawing of an imaginary perpendicular line intersected by a horizontal line and placing the injection in the upper outer quadrant. This is not as safe as the preceding method because the landmarks are not as definite.

365

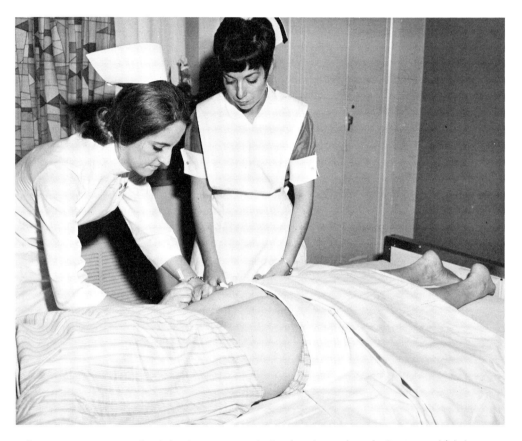

Fig. 23-9. Intramuscular injections are made in the dorsogluteal site to avoid injury to the sciatic nerve.

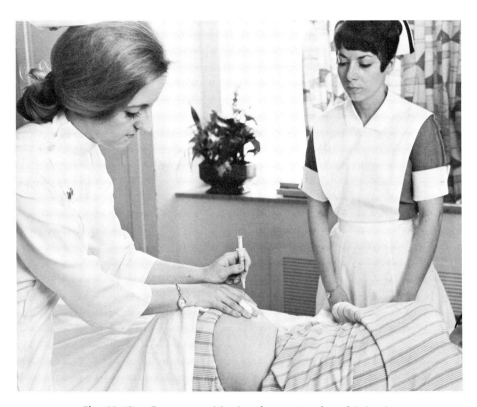

Fig. 23-10. Correct positioning for ventrogluteal injection.

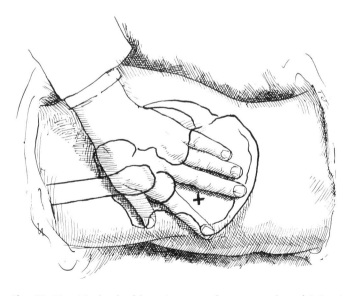

Fig. 23-11. Method of locating area for ventrogluteal injection.

367

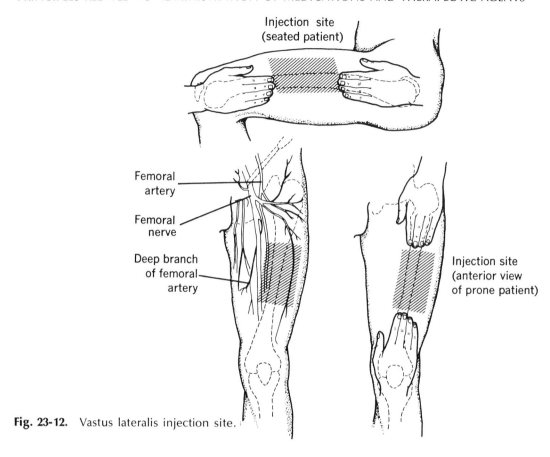

Fig. 23-12. Vastus lateralis injection site.

For this reason there is greater danger of locating the injection too close to the sciatic nerve with this method.

Ideally, the patient should be lying in the prone position, with the toes turned in and the muscles relaxed, although a comfortable side-lying position may be more reasonable for the patient to assume. There should be sufficient exposure to clearly locate the anatomic landmarks. (See Fig. 23-9.)

Assuming that the medication has been prepared following the "five rights" and that the injection site has been identified, the nurse should cleanse the area as previously described. The skin is drawn taut with the fingers of one hand and with the other hand controlling the syringe, the injection is made smoothly and firmly with a quick thrust, the needle penetrating per-

pendicularly (90-degree angle). Holding the skin taut facilitates the needle passing through the skin layers with the least amount of discomfort.

When the needle is in place, the pressure on the tissues is released and the fingers used to steady the syringe, thus preventing the needle from moving once it is in proper position. The nurse aspirates the syringe gently by pulling back on the plunger. Should blood appear in the syringe, indicating that the needle has penetrated a blood vessel, the policy in most agencies indicates that the needle should be withdrawn and a fresh dosage prepared, using another syringe and needle. Suitable explanation should be given to the patient for the second injection.

If upon aspiration, however, no blood appears in the syringe, the solution, and

368

the air bubble are slowly injected, allowing the tissues to distend and accommodate to the medication as it is being deposited. Then, as the needle is quickly withdrawn, the nurse applies light pressure over the puncture site to encourage hemostasis. Since massage of the area appears to be somewhat controversial, it is probably best to refrain from rubbing the area unless the instructions usually supplied with parenteral preparations specifically recommend massaging the puncture site.

A specific schedule for rotating injection sites may be included in the plan of care for the patient, using the different recommended muscle groups. This becomes important for the patient receiving repeated intramuscular doses.

A more recent trend is to use the *ventrogluteal* area. This site has been recommended for children and frail or emaciated adults because it is free of large nerves, blood vessels, and fat. The area is also more accessible than the gluteal site. The site is located by placing the tip of the index finger on the anterior superior iliac spine and the third finger on the crest of the ilium. The middle finger is lowered slightly below the crest, with the palm of the hand resting on the thigh. The triangular area formed by positioning the fingers as designated forms the point of injection (Fig. 26-11).

The *vastus lateralis muscle* is a favorable injection site that is becoming more popular because the muscle is thick and free from major nerves and blood vessels. The injection can be given with the patient lying on his back or in the sitting position. The recommended injection area is about 2 to 3 inches wide between the midanterior and the midlateral thigh. It extends a hand's breadth below the greater trochanter at the proximal end and another hand's breadth above the knee at the distal end. This is a relatively large area and can usually tolerate many injections. The same general technique would be used as for

injections given in the dorsogluteal site. (See Fig. 23-12.)

The deltoid muscle, although easily accessible, is used infrequently because of the proximity of major bones, blood vessels, and especially the radial nerve, which may be injured unless the injection site is selected with care. The injection site is located approximately $1\frac{1}{2}$ to 2 inches below the acromion process. Since the area is small, it is suitable only for injections of no more than 2 ml. of nonirritating drugs. Repeated doses in this area may cause more discomfort for the patient than in the other recommended injection sites.

Psychosocial aspects

Fear of pain seems to be a universal trait of mankind. When a needle injection is given, pain is induced by the needle going through the skin or by the pressure of the fluid in the tissues, and discomfort may be caused by muscular tension during the injection. Some patients are more sensitive to pain than others. An explanation to the patient about what is to be done and what to expect will help the patient to relax his muscles and to accept the injection. Children especially are afraid of a needle injection. The fears of adults may result from the memories of a past painful procedure. Pain may be prevented or alleviated by distracting the patient's attention by conversation or by creating interest in another subject. For some apprehensive patients the physician may prescribe the use of a cold and volatile spray to numb the sensory pain receptors.

Before a procedure, the bedpan should be offered; if it is needed the patient should be put in as comfortable a position as possible.

Sometimes suggesting the effect of the treatment, especially if it is sedative in nature, will produce better relaxation because of mental comfort.

Cooperation is necessary when a physician administers the treatment. In such a situation the nurse may prepare the syringe and place the container of drug by it, and a resident physician or intern draws the drug into the syringe and administers it. Or if the nurse draws the medication into the syringe, the container should be placed with the syringe so that the physician may check the label. In most institutions nurses give subcutaneous, intramuscular, intravenous, and intracutaneous injections. In others there may be some variation in policy regarding this matter. In any case, cooperation is needed between the patient, the nurse, and the physician. The nurse observes and records the proper notations on the chart to provide pertinent information to the physician and other nurses. A visiting nurse may call at a patient's home to give a hypodermic injection.

The patient is dependent on his physician for the prescription for the drug. Many drugs are controlled by federal and state laws and can be obtained only by prescription.

Intravenous route of administration

The intravenous injection is the introduction of a small quantity of drug or the infusion of a large quantity of fluid into a vein. Drugs are given intravenously (1) to obtain a rapid action, (2) to test circulation time, and (3) to administer a drug that is irritating to the subcutaneous or muscle tissue. When a large quantity is given by gravity, the method is called infusion or venoclysis. Intravenous infusions are injected to supply the body with (1) fluids when the patient is unable to take adequate amounts by mouth, (2) the salts of tissue fluids in order to restore or maintain electrolyte balance, (3) food in the form of glucose when the patient is unable to take enough food, (4) vitamins, and (5) whole blood or blood plasma.

Drugs and fluids are given by vein to produce an immediate effect (Fig. 23-13). The walls of veins are elastic and movable,

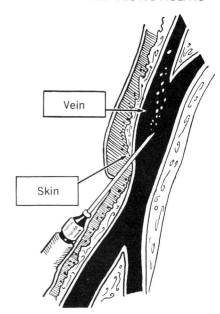

Fig. 23-13. Intravenous injection.

and they may move away or dilate or contract when touched by the needle. Hence, mastery of correct technique for introducing a needle into the vein is needed to avoid undue trauma to the vein wall. Veins contain sensory nerves, and a little pain is experienced as the needle pierces the blood vessel wall. Convenient superficial veins used for injection are the basilic or the median cubitus veins inside the elbow. Other veins that might be used are those of the back of the hand or on the dorsum of the foot (Fig. 23-14). Since the fluid is deposited within a blood vessel, time for absorption is eliminated. The blood can utilize fluids given at the average rate of 30 to 60 drops a minute. With rapid infusion, reactions caused by overloading may appear.

Infusion solutions in large amounts immediately increase the heart rate, blood pressure, and secretion of urine and relieve thirst. If glucose has been used, hunger also is relieved. The cells of the body can utilize glucose as it is given in infusions.

The hydrogen-ion concentration of the

370

blood is of much clinical importance. The average pH value of the blood is approximately 7.4, showing that the blood is slightly alkaline. If the pH rises above 7.8 or falls below 7, life is endangered. Coma usually occurs when the pH of the blood falls slightly below pH 7, whereas tetany is generally present when blood alkalinity rises to a pH of 7.7 or 7.8 Buffer salts, such as sodium bicarbonate and disodium phosphate, constantly present in the blood keep it within normal pH limits. A buffer substance is one that prevents changes in hydrogen-ion concentration when small amounts of acids or bases are added. The most important buffers in the blood are in the bicarbonate–carbonic acid system. The phosphate and protein buffers are of less importance. The kidneys and the lungs also play a large part in maintaining the normal acid-base balance. All fluids given into the bloodstream should conform as closely as possible to the reaction of normal blood.

Solutions for subcutaneous injection should be clear, sterile, nearly neutral in reaction, isotonic if possible, and non-hemolytic, and only those substances that are soluble in water may be used.

The selective flow of certain components of a solution through a semipermeable membrane is called osmosis, and the resulting pressure is called osmotic pressure. Osmotic pressure is unbalanced pressure causing the phenomena of osmosis and diffusion. Osmosis is the passage of water molecules across a membrane. Diffusion is the process brought about by the movement of the molecules of water, gases, and dissolved substances. All soluble inorganic salts, being electrolytes, possess the property of exerting osmotic pressure. Solutions developing the same osmotic pressure as the blood are called isotonic with

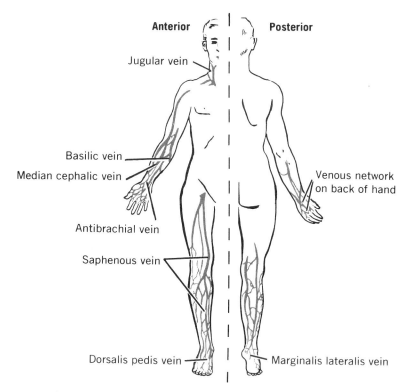

Fig. 23-14. Veins most frequently used for intravenous injections.

the blood. Those producing less osmotic pressure than the blood are called hypotonic. Those producing more osmotic pressure are called hypertonic. The blood contains 0.9% salts of calcium, sodium, potassium, and magnesium.

Physiologic salt solution is 0.9% sodium chloride, which combines with the blood very well. It resembles most of the body fluids in action, density, and osmotic pressure. Markedly hypotonic solutions are not injected because they destroy red blood cells. Hypertonic glucose solutions are occasionally used to reduce edema. Concentrated plasma or serum, administered intravenously, raises the osmotic pressure of the blood and thereby draws fluid from tissues into the vascular system. The kidneys are important in regulating the osmotic pressure of the blood.

Blood transfusions are given to increase the blood volume and to increase the number of red blood cells. The amount of blood given depends on the condition of the patient, the purpose for which it is given, and the amount available. Blood is preferred to plasma, but certain types of patients benefit as much from plasma as from whole blood. However, plasma may be given intravenously with less fear of reaction than whole blood.

Solutions of saline and glucose are lost rapidly from the circulation because they lack colloidal osmotic pressure. A substitute for plasma that contains a high osmotic pressure and has a colloidal particle size large enough to be retained in the circulation for several days is a preparation of gelatin. It is administered in a 6% solution in normal saline.

The *equipment* used for intravenous administration is, for the most part, disposable, which has greatly reduced the incidence of toxic reactions in patients caused by contamination with pyrogenic organisms.

Fluid leaves an inverted hanging flask by the force of gravity. If a clamp is used on tubing, it should be applied as near as possible to the needle to prevent the development of negative pressure within the tubing.

Pressure is used in applying the tourniquet to cut off the flow of blood in the veins. Blood, not being able to escape from the arm, pushes outward on the elastic blood vessel walls and distends them.

The operation of a vacuum bottle for the collection of blood depends on differences in pressure. Air has been removed from the bottle, thus lowering the pressure within it. When it is connected to a vein, blood runs into it because pressure of blood in the veins is greater than in the bottle.

Factors influencing the rate of flow of an intravenous solution are the size of the needle, the height of the flask, and the viscosity of the fluid. Solutions flow less voluminously through a needle of a small bore than through a needle of a large bore. The higher the container, the faster the flow of fluid. Usually the rate of flow is regulated partially by the size of the needle. Blood flows slower than an aqueous solution because the tubing offers more resistance to viscous substances. A larger needle is used with transfusions of blood. The rate of flow should be regulated carefully according to the tolerance of the patient.

Tubing with a small lumen facilitates expulsion of air from it, since the fluid runs through it as a solid column and does not trickle down the side. Tubing should be smooth inside to reduce friction as well as to prevent pits and wrinkles wherein bacteria and blood may lodge.

Increasingly, policies are being developed that permit the nurse to assume responsibility for intravenous administration. It is becoming common practice for joint statements to be prepared and approved by the medical, nursing, and hospital associations within an individual state that establish the criteria whereby registered nurses may qualify for this responsibility. Such criteria usually provide that a specific plan be set up in each agency for additional preparation for the registered nurse in the technique of intravenous administration, to assist the nurse in mastering the necessary skills in the technique of intravenous administration. Therefore, details of the technique are not presented here, but attention is directed to the responsibilities that the nurse is expected to assume for the patient who is receiving an intravenous infusion.

Nursing responsibilities for patient care include the following:

Comfort of the patient. The patient should be as comfortable as possible before the infusion is begun, since several hours are usually required for it to be completed. The bedpan should be offered if the patient is on bed rest. The patient's position should be arranged as comfortably and conveniently as possible and changed frequently if he is to remain in bed. If an arm is being used for this injection, the call signal and personal belongings should be left within reach of the unrestrained arm.

Position of the patient's arm. When the injection is administered in a vein of the patient's arm, the arm is often placed on a padded arm board, with the forearm pronated and the fingers grasping the edge of the board in as nearly normal a position as possible. It is important to check the hand and forearm to be sure that the bandages or ties securing the arm to the board are not interfering with circulation.

Rate of flow. The physician usually indicates the rate of flow at which the solution is to enter the vein. The usual rate of flow is 30 to 40 drops of solution per minute. The nurse is responsible for maintaining the rate of flow as ordered (Fig. 23-15).

Development of infiltration. If the needle should slip out of the vein, the nurse will be able to recognize it because the solution will flow out into the subcutaneous tissues around the needle, causing tissue swelling, whiteness, and a cold feeling to the touch. This is referred to as *infiltration.* When this happens, the clamp on the tubing should be fastened immediately. A test to determine whether or not the needle is still in the vein is to lower the container of solution below the level of the vein. If blood appears in the tubing, the needle is still in position in the vein. If no blood appears, the needle is not in the vein, and the usual procedure is to remove the needle.

Observation for signs of reaction. The injection site and areas along the course of the vein should be observed for signs of inflammation, such as redness, tenderness, and pain, which may indicate developing thrombophlebitis. Generalized complications for which the nurse should be on the alert during the therapy include pyrogenic reactions and circulatory overload.

A pyrogenic reaction usually begins to appear about a half hour after starting the infusion and include an abrupt temperature elevation, chills, backache, headache, general malaise, nausea, and vomiting. When these symptoms occur the infusion should be stopped immediately and the physician notified.

The excessive administration of intravenous fluids may overload the circulatory system. Symptoms that should cause the nurse to suspect circulatory overload include coughing, shortness of breath, increased respiratory rate, increased blood pressure, venous distension, and cyanosis. The infusion should be stopped and the physician notified. Assisting the patient to a sitting position will help the patient to breathe more easily.

Ambulation of the patient. If the patient is to be ambulatory during the infusion, the nurse assists the patient by ei-

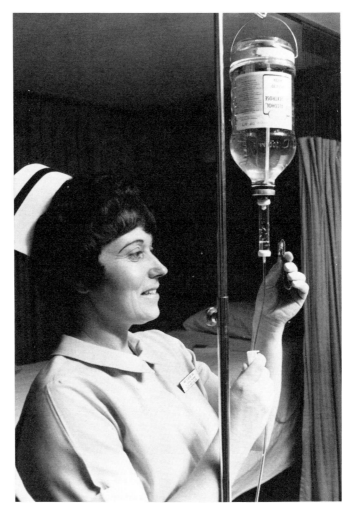

Fig. 23-15. Maintaining an even rate of flow at which the solution is to enter the vein.

ther supporting the infusion container or hanging it on a portable intravenous standard that can be easily moved along with the patient. The patient may also need assistance in handling the tubing so that the needle is not dislodged from its position in the vein.

Addition of more solution. It should be known whether or not another container of solution is to be added before the current one is completely empty. If so, it is usually a nursing responsibility to attach the additional container. However, extreme caution is necessary to ensure that

no serious error occurs. In each agency there is usually an established procedure for managing infusions so that everyone concerned with the patient will know exactly what has been given and what is yet to be given.

Discontinuation of the infusion. When the ordered amount of solution has been administered, the nurse assumes the responsibility for discontinuing the infusion. This is accomplished by removing the arm board, if one is in use, and removing the tape holding the needle. The needle is withdrawn quickly and digital pressure applied immediately over the injection site with an alcohol wipe to encourage hemostasis and sealing of the puncture wound.

The patient will appreciate assistance in moving the arm (or leg) involved after the hours of immobilization. Passive range of motion is usually acceptable.

Record of the administration. Each agency has specific charting procedures, but the information that the nurse would usually expect to record includes date and time the infusion was started, kind and amount of solution injected, name and amount of any drug added to the infusion, time discontinued, and reaction of the patient.

In addition, any symptoms of adverse reactions of the patient should be charted, together with any measures to relieve the symptoms.

Hypodermoclysis

Interstitial infusion and subcutaneous infusion are other terms that mean the administration of large amounts of fluid into subcutaneous tissue. The purpose is to supply the patient with fluids and electrolytes when fluids cannot be taken orally or intravenously by the patient. This type of infusion is used much less frequently now than before.

The equipment is similar to that required for intravenous therapy, except that two 20- to 22-gauge needles 3 inches long are used. The needles are inserted at a 20-degree angle into the subcutaneous tissue and taped in place. The usual sites for administration are the anterior aspect of the thighs and the abdominal wall above the crest of the ilium. The rate of flow ordered is usually between 60 and 120 drops per minute.

In some agencies, the hypodermoclysis needles are inserted by the nurse, in others by the physician. During the infusion the nursing responsibilities are similar to those for intravenous injection.

LEARNING SITUATIONS FOR THE PATIENT

In the process of administering medications to the patient, there may be opportunities to assist the patient to an understanding of why he is taking these particular drugs and what he may or may not do to help achieve the desired effects. There may also be openings in the conversation to answer questions regarding self-medication or perhaps about the current drug problem.

Other patients may need to acquire specific skills and knowledge in order to continue medicinal therapy at home. In this case, definite patient teaching plans may be formulated and included in the patient's total plan of care. This is usually considered to be a nursing responsibility. An example of this kind of learning situation is the patient who needs to become competent in managing his own insulin administration and associated diabetic diet, together with the other details of his life that must be modified because of his diagnosis.

SUMMARY

The reasons for selecting nonoral drug administration routes are discussed, together with their advantages and disadvantages. Pertinent information about equipment used in giving parenteral drugs is reviewed.

Relevant scientific principles have been included that give a basis for understanding nursing responsibilities in administering or assisting with the administration of parenteral drugs and fluids. Examples of the application of these principles to administration of drugs and fluids by the various parenteral routes are explored.

Concepts have been the central focus rather than procedural steps, although many practical applications of principles to each technique have been included.

QUESTIONS FOR DISCUSSION

1 List all of the medications ordered for your patient.
   a. For what purpose is each ordered?
   b. By what route is each being given?
   c. What is the safe dosage range for each?
   d. Do any of these medications require precautionary measures?
   e. What learning needs does the patient have regarding these drugs?
   f. What adverse symptoms might be observed with each?
2 Which needle has the larger lumen, the 25 gauge or the 18 gauge?
3 Why is physiologic saline a frequent solvent for parenteral medications?
4 What observations would you make regarding a patient's intravenous infusion?
5 Identify the parts of a syringe that should be kept sterile until after the injection.
6 For each of the four recommended intramuscular sites, identify the particular structures to be avoided during injection of needle.
7 What are the anatomic boundaries for each of the four recommended intramuscular injection sites?
8 When administering an intramuscular or subcutaneous medication, why should you aspirate before injecting the drug?

LIFE SITUATION

Mrs. McPherson's physician told her he was ordering some penicillin for her. When the nurse brought in the intramuscular preparation of penicillin, Mrs. McPherson said, "I don't like needles. When my little boy needed penicillin, the doctor gave him some liquid medicine. Why can't I have mine by mouth too?" How would you answer Mrs. McPherson's question?

SUGGESTED PERFORMANCE CHECKLIST

Safety

1 Is the equipment sterile?
2 Are the inside of the barrel, the outside of the plunger, and the needle shaft kept sterile until the injection?
3 Is the skin properly prepared?
4 Is the needle sharp?
5 Does the nurse wash her hands before preparing the materials?

6 Is the arm immobilized for an intravenous injection?
7 Is air expelled from the apparatus before injection of the needle for an intravenous administration?
8 Is the physician's order checked?
9 Is the needle securely fastened in place?
10 Is the plunger pulled back after insertion of the needle (if not an intravenous injection) to be sure the needle is not in a vein?
11 Is the label on the preparation checked before using?
12 Is the rate of flow as ordered?
13 Is the injection (unless intravenous) made in an area to avoid large blood vessels and nerves?
14 Is the patient helped to relax?
15 Is an explanation given during the steps of the procedure?
16 Is discardable material disposed of safely?

Therapeutic effectiveness

1 Is the injection made at a proper angle?
2 Is pressure made at the site of injection after the needle is withdrawn?
3 Is the ordered amount of drug given?
4 Does the nurse know why the medication or fluid is being given?

Comfort

1 Is the insertion of the needle quick?
2 Is the withdrawal quick?
3 Is the arm in a relaxed position for an intravenous injection?
4 Are the signal light and personal belongings within reach?
5 Is the patient kept as comfortable as possible during the treatment?
6 Is the bedpan offered before beginning a prolonged treatment?
7 If the treatment is prolonged, is the patient's position changed within safe limits?

Economy

1 Are materials returned to their proper places after the treatment?
2 Are materials effectively used?
3 If a physician is required, does the nurse save his time by preparing equipment beforehand and anticipating his needs?
4 Is the equipment cleaned or disposed of immediately after use?

5 If reusable, are the plunger and the barrel separated immediately after use?

Good workmanship

1 Is the patient positioned for adequate identification of the injection site?
2 Is the patient's condition noted before, during, and immediately after the treatment?
3 Is the equipment checked frequently during a prolonged treatment?
4 Are untoward symptoms reported at once?
5 Is charting pertinent and accurate?

SUGGESTED READINGS

Bergersen, Betty S.: Pharmacology in nursing, ed. 12, St. Louis, 1973, The C. V. Mosby Co.

Brandt, Patricia, and others: Intramuscular injections in children, American Journal of Nursing 72:1402, August, 1972.

DiPalma, Joseph R.: Precautions with the anticoagulants, RN 34:57, October, 1971.

Dison, Norma Greenler: An atlas of nursing techniques, ed. 2, St. Louis, 1971, The C. V. Mosby Co.

Donn, Richard: Intravenous admixture incompatibility, American Journal of Nursing 71:325, February, 1971.

Durr, Eleanor E., and Fierro, Louis: I.V. therapy as a nursing responsibility, RN 33:38, September, 1970.

Gahart, Betty L.: Intravenous medications—a handbook for nurses and other allied health personnel, St. Louis, 1973, The C. V. Mosby Co.

24 Oxygen and medications for inhalation

ADMINISTRATION OF THERAPEUTIC AGENTS BY INHALATION

The importance of normal respiratory functioning is discussed in Chapters 11 and 19, together with examples of related principles. Application of these principles is useful in this context also with the administration of drugs and oxygen by inhalation.

Pharmacology of respiration

It is possible to administer gases and drugs in vapor form for systemic effects because absorption into the bloodstream occurs very rapidly via the large vascular surfaces of the alveoli and other areas of the respiratory tract. Medications given by inhalation may have either a systemic or local effect on mucous membranes of the respiratory tract.

In order to administer a drug by inhalation it must be in a vapor form. Very few drugs are of a volatile nature and must therefore be added to a vaporizing or nebulizing agent. Steam, either hot or condensed, is one of the chief agents used. Steam in itself is also soothing. In addition to providing moisture, some of the new commercial humidifiers also provide "airconditioning."

Nonvolatile drugs may be administered by nebulization. By this method a mistlike spray is produced, breaking the drug into minute particles for inhalation. A gas such as oxygen is used.

The nebulizer depends on Bernoulli's effect, which is that a moving stream of air reduces the air pressure about it. The air pressure being lower than the upward pressure of the fluid in the nebulizer, the fluid is forced up into the area of less pressure, is broken up into a fine spray by the force of the air, and is carried into the respiratory tract with the oxygen (Figs. 24-1 and 24-2).

Many bronchodilators and detergents are administered in the preceding manner (Fig. 24-3). In most institutions all drugs given by inhalation are under the supervision of the inhalation department and are administered by the therapist or inhalation technicians. However, the nurse is often responsible for preparing the medication.

Drugs that act upon the respiratory system may be classified as (1) respiratory stimulants and depressants, (2) those that act on the mucous membrane, and (3) those that change the size of the bronchioles.

The most important respiratory stimulants are carbon dioxide, caffeine, nikethamide (Coramine), atropine, and ammonia. Spirits of ammonia and amyl nitrite are used as emergency stimulants. Carbon dioxide is used therapeutically to stimulate respiration in carbon monoxide poisoning. The opiates depress the respiratory center and slow the respirations. Drugs that act on the mucous membrane include demulcents, antiseptics, and expectorants. These may be administered in the form of sprays, in water vapor, or in cough syrups. The warmth of water vapor relaxes the involuntary muscles of the bronchi. Drugs that change the size of the arterioles include the nitrites and adrenergic agents.

Oxygen is prescribed to supply a deficiency of oxygen in the body, which occurs in pneumonia, in carbon monoxide poisoning, and in heart disease with cyanosis, and it is used following surgery. The usual flow of oxygen for an adult varies from 6 to 14 liters a minute.

Water vapor therapy is sometimes ordered for the treatment of conditions in which secretions accumulate in the bronchial tubes and in the larynx. The high humidity of inspired air reduces the evaporation of water from the mucous membrane, and the thinner secretions may be more easily expectorated. If a tent is used with steam, a blanket should serve as a foundation of the canopy since the porous blanket will absorb, by capillary attraction, the condensed water and the drug vapor, thereby preventing accumulation of the vapor.

Physiology and mechanics of oxygen therapy

Since many patients who have respiratory problems receive oxygen, it is essen-

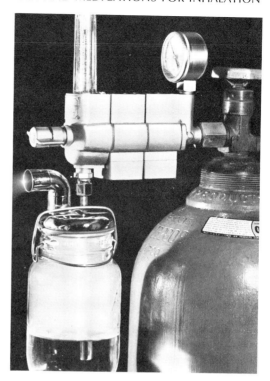

Fig. 24-1. Jet humidifiers produce aerosols that can be used for high humidity and the administration of drug solutions. (Courtesy Union Carbide Corporation, Linde Division, New York, N.Y.)

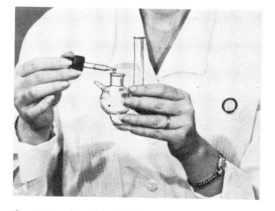

Fig. 24-2. Small nebulizers can be used for the administration of antibiotics and bronchodilators. (Courtesy Union Carbide Corporation, Linde Division, New York, N.Y.)

379

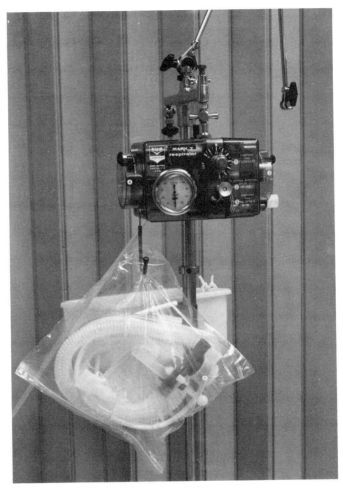

Fig. 24-3. Bird machine. This may act as a mechanical bronchodilator through intermittent positive pressure breathing (IPPB).

tial that the nurse have an understanding of the basic principles on which its administration and effectiveness is based. Below are listed some of the more common facts and principles related to oxygen therapy.

The purpose of oxygen therapy is to supply oxygen in conditions in which there is some interference with the normal oxygenation of the blood.

Oxygen therapy raises the concentration of percentage of oxygen in the lungs and therefore the partial pressure of oxygen, forcing it into the blood more readily, since the rate of diffusion of gases is proportional to the pressure. In anoxia the

oxygen in the tissues is reduced below normal. This loss does not cause signs of distress until the amount is below 14%. If the percentage of oxygen in the inspired air is increased from 20% to 40%, the oxygen pressure in the tissues is increased by about 25% above normal. However, in some conditions part of one lung or both lungs may not be functioning, and the oxygen that is diffused more rapidly because of increased pressure through the functioning part of the lungs may be just sufficient to maintain a normal supply of oxygen to the tissues.

Oxygen can be administered by many

380

different types of equipment. It may be given by nasal catheter (Figs. 24-4 and 24-5) or inhaler, by face mask, or by tent. The choice of apparatus can have an important bearing on the effectiveness of the treatment. Face masks can deliver oxygen throughout the therapeutic range, up to concentrations approaching 100%. Oropharyngeal catheters deliver oxygen directly into the oropharynx in moderate concentrations (35% to 50%), and they are considered to be the most economical methods. Tents are suitable for the administration of moderate oxygen concentrations, up to 55%. In addition, their air-conditioning features add greatly to the patient's comfort (Fig. 24-6). A plastic hood is a closed apparatus capable of deli-

vering oxygen throughout the therapeutic range up to 100%. Hoods are available in sizes suitable for infants, children, and adults, but they are used most often for children. Oxygen chambers, formerly in use, are now considered too expensive. Many hospitals now have oxygen banks from which oxygen is piped throughout the hospital. This method is very convenient and eliminates the necessity for bringing tanks to the bedside. A few hospitals have installed hyperbaric chambers for giving oxygen under pressure.

When piped oxygen is not available, oxygen is supplied for therapeutic purposes in cylinders that contain 244 cubic feet of oxygen under 2,200 pounds of pressure per square inch. Before a high-pressure

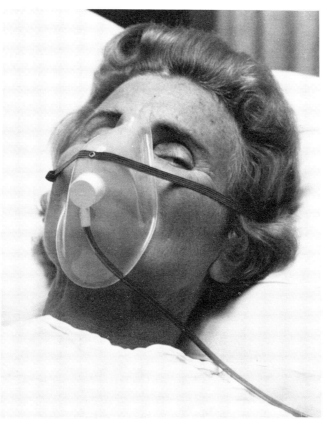

Fig. 24-4. Oxygen administered through face mask. (Courtesy Hoag Memorial Hospital, Newport Beach, Calif.)

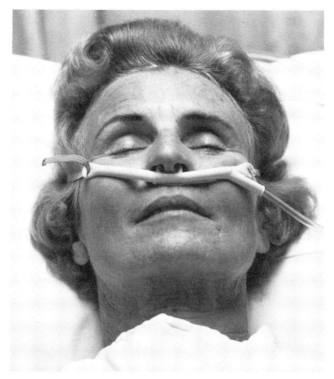

Fig. 24-5. The nasal route is the most economical means of delivering moderate concentrations of oxygen. (Courtesy Hoag Memorial Hospital, Newport Beach, Calif.)

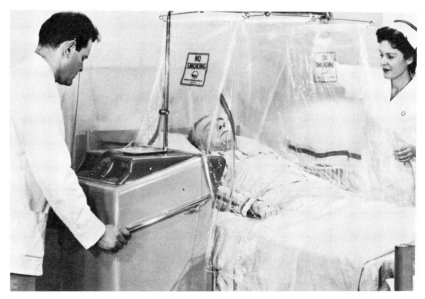

Fig. 24-6. An oxygen tent is a closed-circuit apparatus in which temperature, humidity, and oxygen concentration of the circulating atmosphere are closely controlled. (Courtesy Union Carbide Corporation, Linde Division, New York, N.Y.)

cylinder can be used safely, a pressure-reducing regulator must be attached to the cylinder valve outlet. The regulator reduces the high pressure of the oxygen coming from the cylinder and enables the nurse to control the rate of flow to the patient. Most regulators are of the two-stage type. In the first stage, oxygen pressure is reduced before it enters the second stage, where flow is regulated. A regulator has two gauges. One indicates pressure in pounds per square inch the amount of oxygen in the cylinder, and the other registers flow to the patient in liters per minute (Fig. 24-7).

The flow rate is not a sure indication of oxygen concentration. The only way to be sure of oxygen concentration is to use an oxygen analyzer. Some analyzers measure oxygen concentration using the principle of chemical absorption. A known volume of gas from the tent is injected into a chamber and the oxygen is absorbed. The decrease in volume is measured on a scale giving the reading of the concentration.

Another type of analyzer uses the principle of magnetism to determine the concentration. A sample of gas from the tent is pumped by a bulb into a section of the analyzer, which has a magnetic field. Oxygen, unlike other gases, is capable of being attracted by a magnet. The action is registered on a cailbrated scale. The higher the concentration, the greater the deflection on the scale.

When a hospital is piped for oxygen, a flowmeter must be attached to the wall outlet to control flow to the patient (Fig. 24-8).

The purpose of a gauge is to reduce the higher pressure, which would destroy lung tissue, to a pressure of 20 pounds, which the patient can safely bear. A pressure of 20 pounds is above that of the atmosphere, which is 14.7 pounds per square inch.

Since oxygen flows into the lungs under pressure higher than that of the atmosphere, rapid evaporation of the surface fluids on the mucous membranes takes

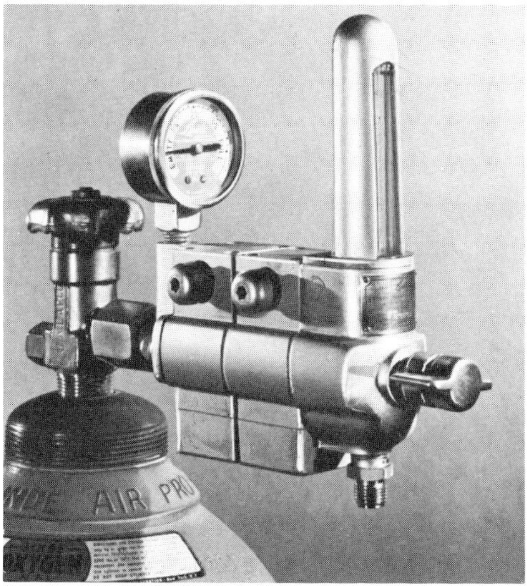

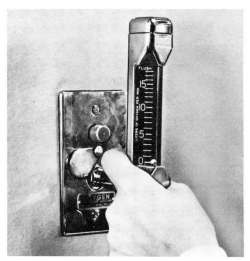

Fig. 24-7. A pressure-reducing regulator must be attached to a cylinder before oxygen can be withdrawn for therapy. (Courtesy Union Carbide Corporation, Linde Division, New York, N.Y.)

Fig. 24-8. An oxygen outlet at the bedside allows therapy to be begun without delay. The nurse has only to attach a flowmeter and connect the administering apparatus. (Courtesy Union Carbide Corporation, Linde Division, New York, N.Y.)

place. To overcome this drying action, some moisture is added to the oxygen. Two methods of humidifying oxygen are employed. One is the attachment of a bottle of water to the cylinder through which the oxygen bubbling on its way from the cylinder picks up some moisture (Fig. 24-1). The other is the passage of oxygen over ice on its way from the cylinder to the patient, thus picking up some of the water from the surface of the ice.

Hyperbaric oxygenation is the administration of oxygen in an environment of increased atmospheric pressure. This permits more oxygen to be dissolved in the body fluids. Pressure of a gas will increase or decrease inversely to the volume or space in which it is contained. If the space is constant, addition of an increased amount of gas increases the pressure of the gas. The amount of gas that dissolves in a liquid depends on the partial pressure of that gas. As the atmospheric pressure increases, more gas dissolves in the blood and eventually in the tissues. The amount of gases dissolved will depend on the composition of gases inspired, the degree of increased pressure, the time one stays in the environment, and the degree of circulatory efficiency. As the total atmospheric pressure increases in the hyperbaric chamber, the individual partial pressures of the gases being breathed increase proportionately.

The oximeter is an instrument for measuring the amount of oxygen in the blood. It depends on the fact that oxyhemoglobin transmits more red light than does reduced hemoglobin. The color can be measured and interpreted in terms of amount of oxygen in the hemoglobin.

Oxygen-helium therapy

The inspired air contains about 78% nitrogen, which has a molecular weight of 28. The breathing of this heavy gas produces fatigue and dyspnea in certain respiratory conditions. A substitute is made for it with helium, which has a molecular weight of 4. A mixture of 75% helium and 25% oxygen can be inhaled with less effort than nitrogen. Helium-oxygen mixtures are also used in conditions involving obstructions in the larynx or the trachea. This treatment is based on the fact that helium is one seventh as dense as nitrogen, so that mixtures are used in which the atmospheric nitrogen is replaced by the helium. Helium is used in some hyperbaric chambers in place of nitrogen. Much less effort is required to get the life-giving oxygen past the laryngotracheal obstructions and through constricted bronchioles. Helium is noninflammable, tasteless, odorless, and colorless.

PSYCHOSOCIAL ASPECTS

Oxygen deprivation caused by anoxia in the brain brings apprehension. The patient must be reassured and made as comfortable as possible. If oxygen is to be used, the patient should be given an explanation of its purpose and method of use before the equipment is brought to the bedside. As little noise and disturbance as possible should take place while the equipment is being set up. If a cylinder of oxygen is used, the regulator should be attached to the cylinder outside the patient's room.

The nurse should know how to put the equipment together and how to adjust it in order to maintain patient confidence. Transparent canopies help the patient to see what is going on about him. Since they are not soundproof, the patient can hear and talk and feel less confined than in canopies that are not transparent. When oxygen therapy is begun, the nurse should visit the patient often to reassure him and to note his progress.

Oxygen equipment is supplied to homes through the home service division of oxygen supply companies. Contact with the home service division is made by the physician. Resuscitators used by the fire departments contain oxygen and carbon dioxide and are used in emergencies.

Visitors may be limited for patients who are receiving medicated inhalations or oxygen. The patient who requires these treatments is usually either acutely ill or very uncomfortable.

LEARNING SITUATIONS FOR THE PATIENT

The nurse may explain to the patient the need for inhalations of medications or steam. The nurse may also suggest some devices that may be used at home for an inhalation, when these are needed after the patient leaves the hospital.

Many patients have a fear of oxygen therapy. A careful explanation of the reason for its use should be made to the patient and also to his relatives. The family should know the hazards presented by the use of oxygen. They should be told why smoking is not allowed. The patient can be reminded that an emergency oxygen supply may be obtained from the nearest welding shop or industrial plant.

The services of a visiting nurse may be discussed. The patient may be told that these services are available to all and that a nurse may be called to aid in mechanical adjustment of equipment, to carry out a treatment, or to aid the family in carrying out the physician's directions.

SUMMARY

Respiration is a vital function of life. Observation of the respirations provides a measure of how well the respiratory system is functioning. Respiration is a physical and chemical process. Breathing is the mechanical side of respiration. Respiration depends on the partial pressure of gases in the air and in the bloodstream. Breathing depends on pressures of the atmosphere, of the alveolar air, and in the intrapleural space. Oxygen therapy is treatment by supplying added oxygen to the alveolar air to relieve anoxia or lack of oxygen in the tissues. During treatments on the respiratory tract the patient needs to be reassured, and careful explanation should be given.

QUESTIONS FOR DISCUSSION

1 Why is oxygen used therapeutically?
2 Why is helium used therapeutically?
3 How does oxygen get into the bloodstream?
4 How is oxygen pressure in a tank reduced to a safe pressure for breathing?
5 What is an oximeter? How does it work?
6 Explain how an oxygen analyzer works.
7 What fears does a patient who is receiving oxygen have and what can you do about them?
8 What explanation would you give to the relatives of a patient who is in an oxygen tent?
9 What is the difference between industrial oxygen and medical oxygen?

LIFE SITUATION

Mrs. Zelinski, a Polish Catholic patient, was dying. She was in an oxygen tent. Her husband approached the chart desk and asked for a match. When the nurse asked why, he said that during his wife's lifetime she had always hoped that a candle would be lighted for her when the time came for her to go and that he wanted to grant this last request. What would you do about it?

SUGGESTED PERFORMANCE CHECKLIST
Administering oxygen and helium
Comfort

1 Is an adequate explanation of the treatment given?
2 Is the position of the patient comfortable?
3 Is the patient warm?
4 Is noise around the tent prevented?

Therapeutic effectiveness

1 Is proper concentration maintained?
2 Is the patient relieved of distress in breathing?
3 Is the pulse rate reduced after oxygen is started?
4 Is the oxygen discontinued gradually?
5 Is the patient observed frequently?
6 Is skill shown in handling equipment?

7 Is an explanation given to relatives?

8 Are immediate reports made of change of condition?

9 Is recording pertinent and accurate?

Economy

1 Is waste of oxygen prevented by the following:

  a Tucking in the tent well?

  b Not loosening the skirt of the tent more than necessary?

  c Keeping the tent tucked about the neck while bathing?

  d Inspecting the canopy for breaks and tears?

2 If helium is used, is extra care taken to prevent its loss?

Safety

1 Is the order checked?

2 Is chilling prevented?

3 Is sufficient oxygen on hand?

4 Are warning signs against smoking displayed?

5 Is a hand bell provided instead of the electric button?

6 Is the patient observed carefully?

7 Is humidity provided?

8 Is overheating prevented?

9 Is oxygen turned off if candles are to be lighted?

10 Is rubbing avoided?

SUGGESTED READINGS

DiPalma, Joseph R.: Oxygen as drug therapy, RN **34**:49, August, 1971.

Flatter, Patricia A.: Hazards of oxygen therapy, American Journal of Nursing **68**:80, January, 1968.

Gaul, Alice, and others: Hyperbaric oxygen therapy, American Journal of Nursing **72**:892, May, 1972.

Shaw, Bernice L.: Whatever happened to hyperbaric medicine? RN **32**:50, November, 1969.

Wade, Jacqueline F.: Respiratory nursing care—physiology and techniques, St. Louis, 1973, The C. V. Mosby Co.

25 Physical agents

HEAT, COLD, AND RADIATION

PHYSICAL AGENTS

Physical agents appear on the earth in countless forms, and many of them have profound effects on man. Some physical agents, such as heat, cold, light, and radiation, may have therapeutic effects when used properly. Otherwise, they become causative agents for disability and even death.

For a long time physical agents have been used therapeutically. References to the use of sunlight, water, heat, and massage for curing and relieving disease can be found in the early writings of Greek and Roman scholars. In modern times the therapeutic use of certain physical agents such as x-ray and radioisotopes has been developed.

The purpose of this chapter is to focus on the nursing responsibilities that are frequently encountered in the care of patients receiving diagnostic or therapeutic treatment with common physical agents.

HEAT AND COLD
Agents for application and withdrawal of heat

In recent years, great strides have been made in the rehabilitation of patients through the use of heat, cold, and motion. Because of the newer and more technical equipment, most treatments are administered in physical therapy departments by therapists. However, the nurse of today may still have occasion to perform some of these treatments and should therefore understand the principles on which therapy is based.

The application of heat means the use of an agent warmer than the skin, which may be applied in either a moist or a dry form. In an application of moist heat, the body, or a part of it, is wet. In dry applications, no moisture is on the skin.

Many of the forms of hot applications so popular in the past are seldom used in current hospital practice, but they are listed here for the sake of the occasional need to clarify the terms for treatments that may be in use in some areas.

Hot wet applications have traditionally included baths, packs, soaks, saturations, compresses, stupes, fomentations, and poultices. A bath implies putting the entire body or a part of it in water. Pack, saturation, fomentation, and compress usually mean applying a wet cloth (or gauze) to a part. Stupe may mean the same as fomentation, or sometimes the term is used in referring to hot wet material put over an application of an irritant drug. A poultice is an application of a hot moist mass of some substance that is light and holds the heat well, such as flaxseed meal. Poultices as well as the compresses, stupes, and fomentations are seldom used today. A soak usually refers to the immersion of a part of the body, such as a foot or a hand, or it may refer to wrapping the part in gauze and saturating it with a fluid. Hot dry applications include the hot-water bag, the electric heating pad or blanket, and packs.

The withdrawal of heat means putting an agent on the skin that is cooler than the skin—in other words, cold materials. Cold applications are also either moist or dry. Moist applications include cold compresses, sponge baths, and packs. A dry application would be an ice bag. Moist applications of either heat or cold are more penetrating than dry ones.

Heat is applied to increase suppuration, to soften exudates, to bring more blood to the part and thus hasten healing, to warm a chilled part, to relax tissue, and to increase temperature. Materials used for applying moist heat include flannel, Turkish toweling, woolen blankets, or gauze. The manner of wetting these materials varies with the method used. The material may be wrung out of hot water in a basin, or hot water may be poured over the material and then the material wrung out, or the material may be steamed. Another method is to apply the material dry and then wet it with a syringe or a small pitcher. Therefore, the nurse takes precautions to avoid burning the patient by testing an unsterile application on the back of the hand and then putting it on the patient slowly.

Cold is applied to reduce inflammation in a part, to slow metabolism, or to reduce temperature. Materials used for applying cold include gauze and sheets. Since cold applications are seldom sterile, the materials are wrung out of cold water. Seldom is cold applied continuously. It may deplete the blood supply so much that nutrition to the part is impaired.

Heat and cold may be used intermittently to stimulate circulation in a part. For this purpose, ice bags may be alternated with hot-water bags, or local hot baths may be alternated with local cold baths. These may be called contrast baths.

Scientific principles

Relevant statements have been selected —primarily from anatomy and physiology, microbiology, chemistry, pharmacology, and physics—that help to explain the physiologic effects produced by hot and/or cold applications. Through blood vessels and nerves of the skin and underlying tissues and the connections they make with the nerves and blood vessels in distant parts of the body, other portions of the body may be influenced by applications of heat and cold to the skin.

1. Application of heat may cause local vasodilation.

2. The local response to cold applications depends on length of time.

   a. Short application may cause vasodilation.

   b. Prolonged application may cause vasoconstriction.

3. The increased blood supply resulting from vasodilation tends to increase the exchange of cellular nutrients and waste products in the tissues.

4. The effects of hot and cold applications result from stimulation of the temperature receptors in the skin.
   a. Impulses are carried via the somatic afferent fibers to the hypothalamus and the cerebral cortex.
   b. Impulses conveyed to the cerebral cortex arouse the conscious sensation of temperature.
   c. Impulses conveyed to the hypothalamus affect the caliber of blood vessels.
   d. The temperature receptors adjust quickly to mild stimulation, so that the sensation of either warmth or coolness decreases.
5. Tissue tolerance to temperature varies:
   a. In different skin areas of the same individual
   b. In different individuals according to such factors as age and condition of the vascular and nervous systems
   c. With the length of exposure time
   d. With the size of skin area involved
6. Tissue injury occurs with extremes of temperature, but the exact point at which injury begins varies with the individual.
7. Water is a more efficient conductor of heat than is air.
8. Cold applications conduct heat from the tissues.
9. Heat increases the speed of chemical reactions.
10. Low surface tension tends to increase the penetration ability of a solution.

Application of principles

Anatomy and physiology. End organs of sensory nerves in the skin convey the sensations of cold, heat, pain, and pressure. Sensations are interpreted in the brain. If the nerve pathway or brain is impaired, impulses may not be conveyed over the nerves and thus the skin may be injured by hot or cold applications. This principle is of great importance in the care of patients receiving paraffin baths. The paraffin bath (a mixture of paraffin and mineral oil at 126° F.) is one of the newer and very effective methods of applying moist heat. Moisture is brought about by a reflex action of the sweat glands in the skin. The treatment brings temporary relief of pain and helps to increase joint range. The patient *must* be neurologically sound, in that he should be able to feel heat and to perspire. If not, the blood vessels will not dilate as rapidly and the patient will stand a strong possibility of being burned (Fig. 25-1).

The skin is plentifully supplied with blood vessels and lymph vessels. The capillaries of the skin are so numerous that when distended they can hold one half to two thirds of the blood in the body. Heat applied to one area is carried by the blood to other areas. The intensity of the effect of heat or cold depends on the difference in the temperature of the application and the temperature of the skin and the length of the application. Moderate heat applied to the skin provides general warmth. It dilates superficial blood vessels, bringing more blood to the area. Prolonged application of heat is undesirable because it weakens the cutaneous cells, and the skin is then more vulnerable to injury.

The local vasodilation resulting from the application of heat lasts for approximately 1 hour. Then, it is thought, homeostatic mechanisms will bring about reflex vasoconstriction through the autonomic nervous system. The effect of vasodilation will return if the hot application is removed for a period of time. This explains why hot applications are usually alternated with periods of rest rather than being applied continuously.

The *sitz bath* is used to apply moist heat to the pelvic area, usually following rectal or pelvic surgery. The preferred method is to use a special sitz bathtub so constructed that the patient's buttocks are submerged in water to about the level of the crest of

389

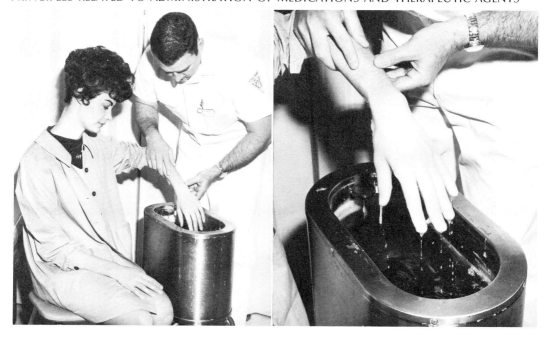

Fig. 25-1. Paraffin bath.

the ilium but that permits the feet and legs to remain out of the water. A bath blanket or gown may be draped over the shoulders to avoid unnecessary exposure and chilling. The temperature of the water will vary from 100° to 115° F., depending on the specific purpose for the patient, and is usually continued for 10 to 20 minutes at a time. Since the patient may recently have had surgery, his tolerance to heat may be reduced. Therefore, the pulse should be checked and the patient observed closely for signs of fainting. He should be supported in as comfortable a position as possible and without pressure on the legs if his feet do not reach to the floor. Following the sitz bath the patient is usually returned to bed until circulatory readjustment has occurred. In recording this treatment the appearance of the wound, amount and character of discharge, and any untoward reaction of the patient should be charted.

Because of the vasodilation the area covered by a hot application becomes hyperemic. This increased blood supply makes better nutrition of the cells possible, which is important in tissue repair, increases the number of leukocytes, and promotes the process of supperation when present. The increased exchange of oxygen and waste products hastens absorption of exudates and softens fibrous tissue. Heat tends to draw blood to the surface from a deep congested area, promotes muscle relaxation, and thus tends to relieve stiffness and fatigue. These effects of heat may be summarized as being antispasmodic, analgesic, decongestant, or sedative in its action on tissue.

Different degrees of heat and cold produce different effects. Temperatures to the skin above 120° F. (48.8° C.) contract involuntary muscles and superficial blood vessels and produce pain. Cold has the same action, although, if not renewed after an hour, the cold application becomes warm and the effects of heat become manifest. The vasoconstricting effect of cold may be used to check bleeding. Extreme heat and cold may destroy tissue if their application is continued over a sufficient period of time. The therapeutic effect desired from brief applications of extremes of temperature to the skin is contraction, which is followed by relaxation upon removal of the application. This tonic effect is stimulating to tissue.

The relief of deep congestion by application of warmth to the skin, either by hot applications or by chemicals, is spoken of as the counterirritant effect. A large quantity of blood is brought to the skin because the blood vessels in the skin are dilated. The blood tends to be redistributed from the deeper congested parts and in this way may bring relief from the pressure there.

Heat and cold serve as irritants, and the vasomotor center responds by producing reflex and local changes, owing to irritation of cutaneous sensory nerve endings. Heat and cold applied by baths, compresses, stupes, or dry appliances penetrate no more than 2 mm. The effect on the deep structures is usually explained by the possibility that the skin surface over each organ is reflexly associated with that organ. Sensation from the application is carried to the spinal cord by sensory nerves. The impulses pass over nerves that enter the chain of sympathetic ganglia and so pass with the sympathetic nerves to the internal organs. The same effect, in a measure, may then be produced on the internal organ as is produced on the skin by the application. All reactions to heat and cold are modified by mode and duration of application, the degree of heat or cold applied, the condition of the tissue, and the surface of the body covered by the application.

The local effect of heat is the same regardless of the method employed. Heat produces peripheral vasodilation, raises capillary blood pressure, and, by relaxing the capillaries, increases the area of the capillary wall available for fluid exchange.

Microbiology. The application of heat or cold to open wounds or to lesions that may rupture demands a sterile technique.

The compresses and instruments are sterile, and the insulating material and the solution are sterile. Hot compresses for the eye are sterile because they are used in conditions that make the conjunctiva very susceptible to infection. Sterilization of materials is accomplished by steam under pressure. Solutions used in a sterile technique are tested by a sterile thermometer or by pouring some solution into an unsterile container and testing that with an unsterile thermometer. In some instances the nurse tests the temperature of the solution by pouring some of it on the inside of the wrist.

If the application is for its thermal effect and there is no wound, the materials and solution must be clean but not sterile. The nurses hands are carefully washed before the application to reduce transfer of bacteria by this route.

To avoid transferring infection, hot-water bottles and ice caps are washed with soap and water and dried well after each patient's use. Soap and water mechanically remove bacteria, and drying kills some kinds of pathogens.

Cold diminishes the formation and absorption of bacterial poisons. A cold application may conduct so much heat from the tissues that the growth of organisms causing infection may be checked.

If a sterile technique is used with cold applications, the container of sterile solution is set in a bowl of ice.

Chemistry. Heat generally increases the speed of a chemical reaction. Since metabolism is largely caused by chemical reactions, the application of heat speeds metabolism, either local or general.

The solvent action of water may be increased by adding other substances, such as soap or magnesium sulfate, to water used for soaks or baths. Crusts and scaly skin will be penetrated by solutions of low surface tension and will be removed more readily.

Chemical heating bottles may make use

of sodium salts and other chemicals that produce heat through the action of crystallization. "Medi-Cold," a disposable first-aid ice pack, likewise produces instant cold by a reverse action in which heat is lost in the process of dissolution.

Pharmacology. The addition of a drug reinforces the effect desired from the hot application. Irritant drugs that have been used more in the past than at present are turpentine and mustard. Turpentine, used in the turpentine stupe, is diluted with oil and painted on the skin. Mustard may be used in the form of plasters, pastes, and local baths. Mustard contains an enzyme, myrosin, that acts on the sinigrin in mustard in the presence of warm water and changes it to dextrose and a volatile oil, which is the active ingredient. Since the volatile oil is destroyed by hot water, lukewarm water is used.

Turpentine and mustard are used for their irritant effects. If left on too long or if the solutions are too strong, these drugs may blister. These drugs are seldom used in the hospital but often appear in the home in the form of commercially prepared plasters.

Flaxseed meal may be used for hot moist poultices because of its mucilaginous and oily ingredients.

Hot compresses are used to apply heat and sometimes to apply a mild antiseptic as well. Drugs used for solutions for hot compresses may be magnesium sulfate (Epsom salt), witch hazel, or salt. Witch hazel is an astringent used over draining areas. A salt solution (1 teaspoon of salt to 1 pint of water) may be used because it is nonirritating.

Physics. Applications of heat and cold employ physical agents: water, heat, light, and electricity (Fig. 25-2). Heat is the most valuable and most versatile physical force for treatment. Water is often employed to convey heat to tissue. Water has a great heat capacity and undergoes change more slowly than does any other substance. It also gives off more heat than any other substance when cooling. Water is a flexible agent and is used in three states. It can be converted into a gas or into a solid by varying its temperature. It absorbs twenty-seven times as much heat as air does. The effect of a hydrotherapeutic procedure is modified by the difference

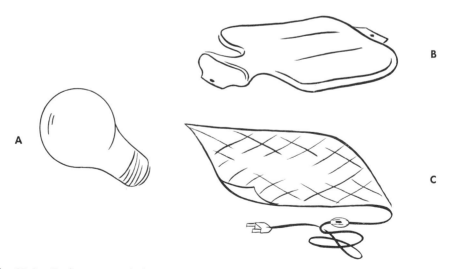

Fig. 25-2. Both water and electric wiring are good conductors of heat and are therefore dangerous. Heat may be supplied by radiation (light bulbs, **A**), water (hot-water bottle, **B**), or electrical energy (heating pad, **C**).

between the temperature of the water and the temperature of the skin, called the temperature gradient.

The immediate effect of an application of heat is purely physical—a rise in temperature in the tissues. The degree and extent of this effect will vary according to the source of the heat, its intensity, and its length of application.

Heat may be transferred from one place to another by conduction, convection, or radiation. Heat is applied by conduction when a heated object, such as a hot-water bottle, heating pad, blanket, or poultice, is put in contact with the skin. Conduction implies contact. In conduction, transference of heat takes place by molecular collision. Conduction varies with differences in temperature and differences in tissue. It is the chief method by which effects at a depth are obtained.

The difference in conduction between water and air explains the difference in temperature of application between hot moist packs and dry heat, such as a hot-water bottle. A substance that is a poor conductor is often used as an *insulator.* This partially explains why hot-water bottles are made of rubber or plastic rather than of metal, which would be more apt to produce a burn. It also explains why the hot-water bottle should always be used with a flannel cover or why the skin is usually covered with a layer of petrolatum before a hot pack is applied.

Convection, characterized by the word circulation, is transfer of heat by actual motion of the heated fluid, whether liquid or gas. It is employed in baths—in the tub bath with the water running, in the sitz bath with the water running, or in the whirlpool bath.

Radiation is the transfer of heat through space. It is employed with heating lamps, bed lamp, infrared lamp, or ultraviolet lamp.

The good effects of a poultice are brought about by the heat that is held in the soft spongy mass. Flannel is used for stupes because its loose weave holds large amounts of warm water. Gauze, used in sterile procedures, does not hold heat as well as wool does. Therefore gauze compresses need to be renewed more often than flannel ones do.

Pressure is not exerted on a hot application because reducing the air layers increases the risk of burning. Also, as a wet dressing dries, it shrinks and becomes tighter.

Because water conducts heat well, the materials should be wrung as dry as possible. The patient's bedding and clothing should be protected from the wet dressing by waterproof material. Rubber or plastic sheeting or waterproof pads make good protectors and insulators of heat as well. Damp bedding may conduct heat from the body.

Electric pads need to be insulated well because water is a good conductor of electricity and so a short circuit may occur from wetting open wires. The dampness may come from a wet dressing or perspiration on the patient's skin. The nurse should not handle electric devices with wet hands. Insulating material is chiefly rubber since rubber is a poor conductor of electricity.

A convenient method of applying a hot compress is by use of the Aquamatic K Pack. Its effectiveness is based on the principle of maintaining even temperature through continuous circulation of water. The temperature is controlled by a thermostat. The device is time saving in that frequent changing of compresses is unnecessary and the bed and surroundings are kept neat and comfortable (Fig. 25-3).

Water for a hot-water bag is tested with a thermometer. The degree varies from 120° to 135° F. (48.8° to 57.2° C.), depending on the thickness of the cover, the area to which the application is made, the condition of patient, the condition of the area,

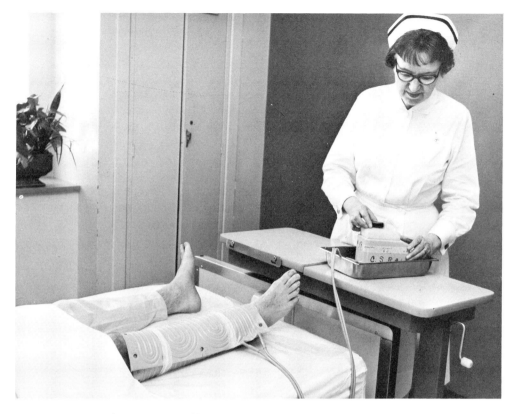

Fig. 25-3. An effective method of applying moist heat.

and the physician's orders. The thicker the cover is, the more heat will be absorbed by it. Some skin areas are thinner and more sensitive than others and will burn more quickly.

If an application is very hot, a layer of oil on the skin will keep it from burning, since oil prevents or delays both evaporation of moisture and conduction of heat of the compress.

The weight of the bed covers on an ice bag causes ice to melt. Iced water stays at a uniform temperature until all the ice is melted. Then the temperature of the water takes on the temperature of the environment. The application is no longer a cold one, and so ice bags need to be refilled or renewed often.

In melting, ice uses up heat that must come from whatever source is near. In the case of an ice bag applied to the body, the heat comes from the body, thus reducing local temperature. Ice bags become wet on the outside because the bag, being colder than the atmosphere, condenses the moisture from the air. The ice bag cover needs to be changed often enough to keep it dry and thus comfortable. When an ice bag is filled, air must be expelled from it because air melts ice rapidly.

In the *sponge bath,* given to *reduce temperature,* the treatment depends on the fact that evaporation is a cooling process. To evaporate, a liquid must draw heat from some source nearby. The temperature of the skin is lowered because it gives up heat in the process of vaporization of the water from the skin. Large areas of the body are wet at one time with water or alcohol. Alcohol, 50% to 75%, is used because it evaporates faster than water, and, because of this fact, the cooling of the skin will be more rapid.

The rate of vaporization depends on the temperature of the skin, the temperature, humidity, and movement of the air, and the size of the area exposed. The warmer the skin and the environment are, the drier and the more moving the atmosphere is, and the more movement in it, the more rapid will be evaporation. Evaporation is faster on a large surface than on a small one.

Evaporation of 30 ml. of water lowers the temperature of 76.5 kg. (168 pounds) of water, or of flesh that is largely water, by about 0.2° C. (nearly 0.4° F.).

Friction produces heat, so little or no friction is used during a bath that has reduction of the temperature of the body as its purpose.

Psychosocial aspects

In treatments involving heat or cold, patients may be afraid of pain. The nurse should test the temperature of warm solutions carefully before bringing the solution to the bedside and put on the application slowly in order to prepare the patient for a difference in temperature, at the same time explaining the purpose of the treatment. The nurse watches the patient carefully during hot or cold applications so that he will not be injured and will obtain the most benefits possible from the treatment.

A patient may prepare and administer a hot or cold application to himself. In many cases he does not. He is dependent on a nurse in a hospital, a private or a visiting nurse in his home, or a member of his family for the treatment. He needs to cooperate with his physician and with the person who carries out the treatment in order for it to be effective and to aid in his early recovery.

The nurse who administers the hot or cold treatment observes the effects and charts the treatment and its results for the information of the physician and other nurses. Adverse effects should be reported to the physician immediately.

The patient's plan of care should include the prescribed application as often as necessary to produce the desired results. The hospital administrator expects the nurse to carry out the ordered treatments efficiently and with safety to the patient. A great number of legal suits against hospitals have arisen because of burns caused through negligence in applying heat by means of a hot-water bottle, heating lamp, or electric heating pad.

Learning situations for the patient

The nurse should explain the purpose and the nature of an application of heat or cold. If the treatment is to be continued at home, the nurse may explain to the patient how the application is prepared, which solutions may be used, how they are prepared, and what to substitute for hospital equipment. Although many devices may be purchased in a drugstore, some household articles may be used just as well. Warm, dry blankets will convey heat to the body. A sieve or double boiler may be used for heating wet flannel for stupes. The patient should be told to use a cover on a hot-water bottle, to test it for leakage, to pull the sides apart before closing it when putting it away, and to watch the skin carefully when it is in use. The temperature may be tested by holding the bag against the inside of the wrist. The patient should be warned against the indiscriminate use of heat over the abdomen for the relief of pain.

The patient may be told about the services of the visiting nurse who may be called to help him with a treatment. He may also be told that the Red Cross home nursing course, available to anyone who wishes to take it, teaches proper methods of applying heat and cold treatments.

RADIATION
Radiotherapy

Radio waves, heat waves, light waves, and x-rays are all manifestations of the same phenomenon. Frequencies in the billions and trillions per second and wavelengths that are so short as to be measured in angstrom units make up infrared heat waves and visible light and, as they increase still further in frequency, become ultraviolet rays and then x-rays. Radiation is the process by which energy is propagated through space. Radiant energy may be used therapeutically for diagnosis and for treatment of various disease conditions. Treatments dependent on radiation that the nurse may carry out or assist with in some way include the use of infrared rays, ultraviolet rays, and medical diathermy and treatments with x-rays, radium, and radioactive drugs. Electromagnetic waves are measured in angstrom units (called after a Swedish physicist of that name). An angstrom unit (Å) is one ten-millionth of a millimeter. Each type of ray has its own wavelength (Table 25-1).

Rays on the violet end of the spectrum

Table 25-1 Electromagnetic spectrum

Wavelength			Wave	Source	Effect
In Angstrom units 3×10^{17}	miles	1,000 100 10 1	Electric	Alternating currents in circuits	More penetrating than infrared; can be sent over long distances
	feet	1,000 100 10 1	Radio (Hertzian)		
	inches	1			
		0.1 0.01 0.001	Infrared	Sun and other hot substances	Penetrates opaque matter; used in heat therapy
		0.0001 0.00001	Visible	Incandescent matter	Affects human eye; gives discrimination of color
		millionth	Ultraviolet	Sun, electron tube	Produces chemical and biologic effect (bactericidal)
		ten-millionth hundred-millionth	X-ray	High-voltage tubes	Less penetrating than gamma rays
3×10^{-7}		billionth ten-billionth hundred-billionth	Gamma	Radioactivity (radium and other nuclear processes)	Penetrates several inches of metal

are essentially light rays. Rays on the red end of the spectrum are essentially heat rays. Any object hotter than its surroundings will radiate infrared rays. The human body itself emits a long-wave infrared radiation of about 9,400,000 Å. However, these rays are not sufficiently powerful for use as treatment.

Treatment with infrared radiation is the exposure of the body to an electrically heated unit capable of producing sufficient infrared rays so that they can be used to produce a physiologic change. The apparatus used to produce infrared radiation consists of a generator and a reflector. The reflector should be kept polished bright so that it will reflect the rays downward.

The advantages of using infrared over some other forms of heat application are that the dosage can be regulated easily, the application has no weight, and the patient can be made comfortable and left undisturbed through the treatment. The duration of the treatment is from 30 to 45 minutes. The length of time will depend on the amount of erythema produced during the treatment. The treatment may be ordered once or twice a day.

The lamp is placed 18 to 24 inches above the skin area to be treated. The rays should strike the skin at a right angle. If too much heat is produced, the distance may be increased.

Infrared treatment is used with caution over areas in which nerve or circulatory impairment exists. It finds its chief usefulness for conditions in which heat without contact is desirable.

Ultraviolet treatment is the exposure of the body to the ultraviolet portion of the light spectrum. Ultraviolet rays are obtained from the sun, but the sun varies in intensity according to the season, the climate, the time of day, and cloudiness. For therapeutic purposes, a mercury vapor lamp or cold quartz lamp is used for producing ultraviolet rays. Dosage with a lamp can be regulated easily. The time of exposure for the first treatment is usually 1 minute. With each succeeding dose the time is increased by 1 or $1^1/_2$ minutes until a maximum time is reached. Treatment may be given once a day or once every other day. The timing is very important, for reaction to ultraviolet rays is not manifest for about 24 hours. The skin will be reddened. It may blister and peel as with sunburn.

The lamp is placed at a distance of 30 to 36 inches from the skin. Since ultraviolet rays cause conjunctivitis, the eyes should be protected during treatments. Ultraviolet radiation is ordered for a great number of skin conditions. A physiotherapist usually applies ultraviolet rays. The operator and the patient wear dark goggles to protect the eyes.

Medical diathermy means the production of conversive heat in the tissues when a special type of high frequency current is used. A high frequency current is an alternating current consisting of a million or more oscillations per second. The heat produced in medical diathermy has insufficient local intensity to produce destruction of tissues or to impair their vitality.

Cables on the machines are heavily insulated. Pads or coils are applied to the patient, although with some types of apparatus no part of the equipment touches the patient. Heat in medical diathermy penetrates all tissues. Diathermy is applied by a physiotherapist.

Surgical diathermy or electrosurgery denotes the application of electricity for the destruction of new growths and diseased tissue and for cutting through normal tissue with minimal bleeding.

X-ray therapy is treatment of a part of the body by means of x-rays. The method of producing x-rays is by accelerating electrons to a high velocity in an electrostatic field and then suddenly stopping them with a solid body, the so-called target (Fig. 25-4). The application of x-ray thera-

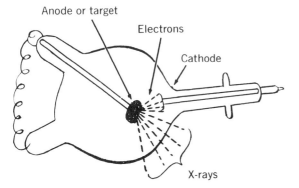

Fig. 25-4. X-rays are formed when electrons hit a target.

py is painless. It is a treatment often prescribed for cancer. X-rays also cause certain substances to fluoresce. This makes fluoroscopy possible, by which the size, shape, and movements of various organs such as the heart, stomach, and intestines can be observed. The operation of x-ray machines is carried out by specially trained persons.

Radium therapy is treatment by means of radium or radon. Radium is obtained from pitchblende or carnotite. It is not used in pure form but is combined with bromine to form a salt of radium. It is put into seeds, needles, and tubes for insertion into parts of the body. The patient is usually hospitalized during treatment with radium, since observation is needed while it is in place to ensure the correct position of the radium applicator. Radium therapy is often used for cancer. A cheap, plentiful, and safer radium substitute for use in the treatment of cancer is radioactive cobalt. Cobalt may be given lasting radioactivity by a relatively brief baking in a uranium pile.

Radioactivity is a term given to fast-moving streams of energy that come from the breaking up of matter. Stable atoms are bombarded with certain radiations in atomic reactors. Radioactivity cannot be seen or felt, but, because so much energy is involved, it is necessary to use sensible

safety measures in areas in which radioactive materials are known to be.

Radioactive isotopes have been used as a means of internal radiation of certain areas of the body where there is selective deposition of particular isotopes.

Application of principles

Physiology and chemistry. The human body possesses no sense organs for the detection of any of the wave energies of the electromagnetic spectrum except the heat waves and the visible section of the spectrum.

The effect of infrared radiation is entirely thermal. The depth of penetration depends on the nature of the underlying material, whether it is tendon, blood vessel, or muscle. Infrared rays vary in penetration from 0.05 to 10 mm. When heat is applied locally, blood vessels become dilated and the rate of blood flow is increased. As the warm blood is carried to other parts of the body, a generalized increase of temperature is produced. The temperature in the peripheral region is raised. As the blood supply in the area being treated is increased, the process of healing is hastened, since the healing elements come from the bloodstream. Local applications of heat increase phagocytosis and metabolism in the area.

The action of infrared is thermal and instantaneous, producing a burning sensation when the intensity is too great. Just sufficient heat should be applied to produce a faint blush on the skin.

Certain wavelengths of ultraviolet radiation have distinct physiologic effects. These effects are classified as photochemical in the skin and biologic in the blood and in the metabolism. Ultraviolet rays penetrate from 0.05 to 0.1 mm. Ultraviolet rays produce local redness, depending on the sensitiveness of the skin and the intensity of the radiation. Maximum erythema is produced by wavelengths from 2,500 to 3,200 Å. Ultraviolet radiation may cause pigmentation, which is produced in the epithelial and basal cells of the epidermis.

Radiation with ultraviolet rays in therapeutic doses increases the number of red blood cells and reticulocytes and the hemoglobin content. It may double the fat content in the blood. It coagulates and precipitates protein. It activates a substance called ergosterol in the skin in such a way that it becomes changed to vitamin D. Vitamin D in some way regulates the passage of calcium and phosphorus across the intestinal wall. The effect of ultraviolet irradiation on respiration is to make it easier, deeper, and less frequent.

Ultraviolet radiation may be prescribed by the physician to increase general body resistance against disease and to improve the healing of superficial wounds. It has been used in the treatment of rickets and tuberculosis and as a counterirritant in neuritis and fibrositis.

Ultraviolet lamps not enclosed in glass emit ozone, which is a very dangerous gas. Its presence is detected by its pungent, irritating odor, which causes coughing and headaches. To prevent these undesirable effects, good ventilation should be provided.

Diathermy produces increased temperature of the tissues. Hence vasodilation results. Greater heating effects are usually produced within the tissues than are produced on the body surface. Besides heat production, there are other physiologic effects of diathermy: a lowering of blood pressure, a general increase in oxidation and metabolism, and local analgesic effects.

Roentgen rays (or x-rays) and radium rays have physicochemical effects: contraction of tissues and molecular disintegration. The effects of x-rays result from energy actually being absorbed by the tissues. Radium destroys tissue cells, but its action is more intense on young, actively growing abnormal cells. Cells of malig-

nant tumors are poorly developed and therefore are destroyed by radiation doses that have little effect on normal cells. X-rays and radium not only damage the tumor cells but also induce dense fibrosis and contraction and strangulation of small vessels, which hamper the spread of the tumor and interfere with its nutrition. X-rays and radium produce necrosis in two ways: by direct effect on the cells and, indirectly, by causing vascular injury, thrombosis, and ischemia. Radioactive isotopes produce their physiologic effects through ionization of protoplasm. When cells undergo ionization, they die.

Microbiology. Almost all bacteria may be killed by sunlight or by radiant energy from 2,500 to 3,000 Å emitted by artificial sources of sufficient intensity and at sufficient exposure time. Ultraviolet rays kill bacteria within the depth of their penetration, which is about 1 mm. The shorter the wavelength, the greater the bactericidal power. The fundamental action that causes death is produced inside the bacterial cell by photochemical ionization induced in the protein body material of the bacterium. Ultraviolet radiation is used to sterilize air in operating rooms, pediatric departments, and communicable disease departments.

Within itself, electricity does not destroy bacteria, but it causes heat and changes in the tissues that may kill them. Tissues cannot tolerate temperatures that are required to kill most microorganisms.

Bacteria are practically as resistant to x-rays as normal tissue is. Radium retards the growth of bacteria.

Seeds, needles, and tubes of radium are sterilized by a chemical disinfectant or by boiling.

Pharmacology. The unit of measuring x-rays is known as r, the roentgen. The dosage can be suitably adjusted by varying the intensity of the rays by filters, by varying the distance between the apparatus and the patient, and by regulating the length of exposure. Usually the length of one treatment to a particular area is only a few minutes.

The dosage of radium or radon is determined by the amount of radium or radon used and by the length of time the preparation is applied. The dosage varies with the method of application and the disease to be treated. The standard dosage is expressed as milligram-hours and is obtained by multiplying the number of milligrams of radium by the number of hours it is applied. For example, 1 mg. of radium applied for 18 hours will give a dose of 18 mg.-hr. A millicurie is the radioactivity of 1 mg. of radium.

Units of measurement of radioactive substances are of two kinds: units of source strength and units of dosage. The common unit of source strength is the curie. The millicurie ($^1/_{1,000}$ of a curie) and the microcurie ($^1/_{1,000,000}$ of a curie) are used also. Source strength may be measured by an apparatus called a counter. The primary unit of dosage is the roentgen. Units of dosage are used chiefly for ensuring safety to personnel, while calculating dosage of radioactive materials to be administered to patients.

Radioactive iodine is used in the diagnosis and treatment of conditions of the thyroid gland. Given orally in a single dose, it has an affinity for the thyroid gland and seems to achieve an internal radiation. Other radioactive isotopes are phosphorus, used for chronic leukemia; gold, used in treating some forms of carcinoma; chromium, used to determine red blood cell survival rate; and cobalt, used for deep therapy similar to x-ray therapy. These isotopes are used in the diagnosis and treatment of disease. They may be given orally, intravenously, or as a radioactive implant. The dosage used in diagnosis is small and is not a source of danger, whereas the dosage used in therapy is greater. There are regulations concerning time and distance of the nurse from the patient and special handling of excretions, linens, trays, and so on.

Physics. Electromagnetic or wave radiation includes a wide range from radio waves to gamma rays. These waves represent a propagation of energy be means of waves traveling in all cases at the speed of visible light in a vacuum, which is 186,000 miles per second. The waves that produce heat are not hot in themselves, but they are converted into heat when they fall upon substances that absorb them. The amount of infrared radiation depends on the temperature of the generator of the heat.

Light rays or heat rays are most intense when the part to be irradiated is at right angles to the light source. A lamp can be arranged over a part or can be turned on its side. Ultraviolet rays, being absorbed at the point of contact, cannot penetrate clothing. The infrared rays have great penetrating powers and will go through any but the thickest clothing.

A mirror or a highly polished surface is a good heat reflector, yet it remains cold. Rough or black objects absorb radiant heat rapidly. Reflectors on the lamps should be highly polished so that the patient will receive maximum benefit from the radiation.

All conductors of electricity convert part or all of the electrical energy flowing through them into heat energy. The human body is a composite mass of tissues with varying electric conductivity. The relative conductivity of the various tissues is in proportion to their water content. Tissues that contain the most water are richest in ions and are therefore the best conductors. An electric current in diathermy moves against electric resistance in the body and thus produces heat.

X-rays, used in medicine, displace electrons in the atoms of the compounds of tissues and thereby produce chemical changes. X-rays differ from visible light by having extremely short wavelengths, 1.4

Å, whereas visible light is 4,000 to 8,000 Å. It would take 40,000 x-ray waves to equal the width of an average hair, or 40 μ. X-rays have the ability to penetrate objects that are opaque to ordinary light, such as body tissues, but they do not pass through substances such as lead. The rays vary in their penetrating ability. Those capable of deep penetration are "hard," whereas those capable of superficial penetration are "soft." The shorter the wavelength, the greater the penetration of the rays.

Radium undergoes continuous and spontaneous disintegration into helium and lead. As it breaks down, energy is released. This energy is used in treating disease. The rate of decay of radium is so slow that it would take 1,600 years for half of it to break up (called the half-life). Radium emits three distinct types of rays, called alpha, beta, and gamma rays. Alpha rays are not penetrating since their flight can be stopped by almost any obstacle. Beta particles travel ten times more rapidly than do alpha particles; consequently, they are more penetrating than alpha particles. Beta rays are divided into soft, medium, and hard rays, and they are used for the treatment of superficial tissues. Alpha and beta particles get together in due time to form the element helium. Gamma rays are the most penetrating and are used for treatment of deep structures. Radium is the most convenient element for a standard source of gamma rays because accurately measured quantities of radium are readily obtainable.

Radon is a radioactive gas that results when radium loses alpha particles or rays. It is used to produce radium action. However, it is not so effective as radium but is much cheaper. The half-life of radon is about 4 days. It is radium's first disintegration product.

Special detector instruments sensitive to radioactivity are used for locating radium when it is lost or discarded by mistake.

Nearly all the detection problems center on beta rays and gamma rays.

More than 375 radioactive isotopes of common chemical elements have been produced by nuclear bombardment. Isotopes are atoms of different masses but with identical chemical properties. Most of the artificially radioactive isotopes used in medical experiments emit beta rays. Some also emit gamma rays. Each radioactive isotope is characterized not only by type and energy of radiations emitted but also by a characteristic half-life. Radioactive atoms do not decay all at once. The time needed for them to lose half of their activity is called the half-life of the element, which is a very important number since it gives an indication of just how stable the nucleus of that element is (Table 25-2). The patient becomes deactivated in less time than the half-life because some of the drug is cast out in his eliminations.

In a few cases, artificially radioactive isotopes have proved useful as a means of administering a localized internal radiation therapy.

Radiation sickness

Of all the physical agents, ionizing radiation is potentially the most harmful to the human body. Exposure to excessive radiation injures not only organs and cells but also the molecules and atoms of protoplasm itself. When x-rays and the radiation given off by radioisotopes pass

Table 25-2 Half-life periods of the more common radioactive isotopes

Isotope	Half-life
Carbon 14	5,100 years
Cobalt 57	38.57 weeks
Cobalt 60	63.24 months
Gold 198	64.75 hours
Iodine 131	8.0 days
Iron 59	44.5 days
Phosphorus 32	14.3 days
Potassium 42	12.4 days

through matter, they cause a change in the matter, either a loss or gain in electrons, the negatively charged electric particles that are a part of the atoms composing the tissues. The original radiation energy is dispersed by collisions with atoms of the material through which it passes, which is termed *ionization.* This is an atom-splitting effect as the radiation traverses through the human body. Atoms within the body are split as a result of exposure to a radioactive source, causing alteration in the behavior of the affected molecules.

Ionizing radiation is the term applied to the effect responsible for the damage to body tissues. This phenomenon is used for the therapeutic destruction of cancer cells. Ionizing radiation is always harmful to living tissue. Even though tissue repair occurs following the injury, radiation is thought to leave some residual permanent radiation damage. Additive effects may be cumulative since man is continuously and unavoidably exposed to radiation over a lifetime.

The degree of damage from a dose of radiation is affected by time and the area of exposure. The greater the area of body exposed to a particular dose, the greater the effect. The dose over a longer time is less damaging than the same dose given in a shorter time.

Prolonged and continuous exposure to small doses of radiation produces both *physical* and *genetic* effects. The genetic effect is to increase the occurrence of *mutations,* which are a permanent part of the organism. Physical effects include leukemia, cancer of the skin, and bone cancer. Fetal exposure during the first trimester of pregnancy is associated with cancer in early childhood.

Radiation sickness follows exposure to large doses over a short period of time, the severity of the symptoms depending upon the dose absorbed. Mild symptoms may consist of slight fever, nausea, and perhaps diarrhea. Severe cases will manifest higher fever, nausea, abdominal pain, skin ulceration, purpura, leukopenia, hemorrhage, alopecia, and a variety of neurologic symptoms.

Some of the side effects of radiotherapy appear within a very short time (hours or days), while others are seen only after weeks, months, or years. The *prodromal* period with vague *malaise* lasts for a few hours to a couple of days, and it may be followed by a latent period of 2 to 3 weeks. The nausea, malaise, and anorexia are usually the first symptoms, with the skin changes, alopecia, scarring, and fibrosis following in the later phase if the radiation dose has been sufficiently large. Delayed effects that may occur years later are very serious, including malignant neoplastic change. Bone marrow and the gonads are more highly sensitive to radiation than other tissues; for this reason prolonged or repeated exposures at low dose rates can decrease fertility in both sexes.

Radiation harmful to man may result from high energy x-rays, used in diagnosis and therapy, and radium and related radioactive materials. Radioisotopes used in diagnosis are relatively low energy emitters, and the patient receiving them is not usually a radiation exposure hazard for the nurse.

Since avoidance of overexposure to ionizing radiation is the only way to prevent radiation injury, for which treatment is generally complex and unsatisfactory, it is extremely important that the nurse have understanding of the fundamentals regarding the nature of radiation, principles of radiation precautions, and the care of patients undergoing radiation therapeutic and diagnostic measures.

For the safety of everyone in the situation, the nurse should be informed about the radiation safety methods and rules in effect in the institution where employed and adhere to them meticulously (Fig. 25-

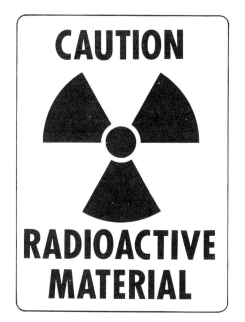

CAUTION

RADIOACTIVE
MATERIAL

Fig. 25-5. Warning cards of standard design are used to indicate the presence of radioactive material.

5). Personnel monitoring devices are worn by staff members whose responsibilities require exposure to radiation hazards. Radiation survey instruments, such as the Geiger survey meter, are used in area monitoring to detect contamination by radioactive materials. Emergency decontamination procedures should be instituted in the event spillage of radioactive materials or contaminated body fluids occurs. Cleanup should be followed by area monitoring.

Psychosocial aspects

The colors used for their emotional effect are in the visible section of the spectrum. Red is exciting—an angry, passionate color. Blue is soothing, but it can be depressing. Yellow is stimulating and hints of sunlight and joy. Violet is the least pleasant color; it has an emotional quality of depressed excitement or anger—slightly unhealthy. Orange contains sunlight, anger, and warning—the result being heat;

it has more personality than red. Green, halfway between stimulation and depression, is the most neutrally emotional color of all, thus restful Gray is also neutral, and the emotional qualities of the colors fade off as they are mixed with gray. For quiet, restful, or soothing effects, blues, greens, grays, and grayed violets (in fact, all the colors if mixed with sufficient gray) are used. Used for exciting or stimulating effects are reds, yellows, orange, pure violet, and greens when tending toward yellow.

Ultraviolet rays are stimulating and make the patient more cheerful. Infrared treatment is relaxing, warming, and healing. The mere mention of infrared creates in the minds of many persons a feeling of something mysterious. They do not realize that all warm objects emit infrared rays.

A calm and businesslike method of procedure is essential in order that the patient will not be frightened by the size of the apparatus used in radiation therapy. A patient should be told that diathermy treatments do not hurt and do not burn and that there is never more current administered than he can tolerate comfortably. The nurse never refers to radiation injury as "burns," since this term is associated with carelessness, but uses the terms "erythema," or "radiation reaction."

Patients receiving x-ray or cobalt treatments should be given special consideration, for it is necessary for them to return again and again. When the first treatment is given, they should be told what to expect and should be assured of the fact that they will be under constant observation during the treatment. The nurse should reassure the patient that the treatment is not painful. Patients may become distraught and panicky for fear of the x-rays and electricity used in running the machines. The fact that the patient must be left alone during the treatment is probably one of the great-

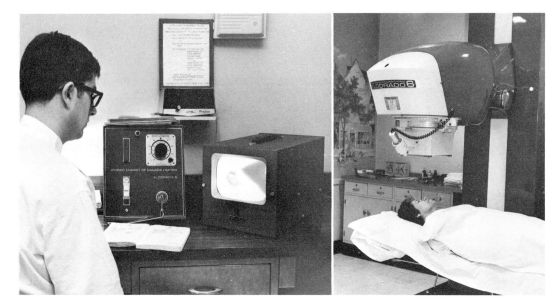

Fig. 25-6. During therapy, observation is maintained by closed-circuit television. (Courtesy Roanoke Memorial Hospitals, Roanoke, Va.)

est causes of fear. The nurse should explain that someone will always remain close by and will keep watch through the observation window or on closed-circuit television (Fig. 25-6). It should also be explained that there are automatic devices controlling the machinery that would come into effect in case of emergency.

Since x-rays are often indicated for the treatment of a malignant growth, an added problem of mental depression is usually present. There is a great difference between the outlook on life of the patient who knows he has cancer and that of the patient who does not have cancer. Most patients will benefit by having an opportunity to talk about their physical condition and the kind of therapy to be prescribed. The responsibility of informing the patient of the diagnosis rests with the physician.

A desirable mental attitude can be obtained through careful attention to the patient's surroundings, his room or unit being kept neat, attractive, and pleasant. Diversional activities should keep him busy and interested.

The nurse may apply infrared treatment. Other radiation treatments are applied by specially trained persons. The physician prescribes all the treatments. The nurse's part in the procedures is usually limited to the preparation of the patient, possibly accompanying him to the radiotherapy room, and aiding in positioning him for the treatment. The nurse cooperates with the physician and with the x-ray therapist for the proper treatment of the patient and is responsible for the before and after care of the patient. The nurse also observes the results of the treatment, especially any serious untoward effects, noting the time the patient goes to and returns from special departments, and communicates with the physician and therapists for the benefit of the patient.

It is important to win the patient's confidence and reassure him of the usual effectiveness of the treatment. Radium is applied and removed by the physician. It is cleaned and returned to its proper place so that it will be available for other treatments.

Techniques of care

In caring for the patient who is receiving radium or radioactive isotopes, it is sometimes necessary for the nurse to limit contact with the patient and radioactive equipment for self-protection. Shielding, distance, and time are the factors commonly combined to protect those exposed to radioactive substances.

Shielding. Shielding is the term used to describe the sealing off or barricading of radioactive material. Sealing off is best accomplished by use of lead in the form of sealed containers or heavy movable shields or sections.

Radioactive materials should be left in their original lead containers as long as possible and returned to them immediately after removal from the patient, only allowing time for checking and cleansing.

Lead shields in the form of screens or drapes may be used to separate the radioactive patient from hospital personnel and other patients. Lead gloves and aprons may be worn by those in direct contact with the radioactive materials.

Distance. A second factor used to reduce exposure is distance. Ideally patients under treatment should be placed in private rooms and preferably ones with outside walls. Exposure above and below the patient should also be considered, as well as adjacent exposure. If several patients must share a room, those patients of child-bearing age should be the farthest away from the source. All beds should be spaced at least 6 feet apart.

Proximity of the patient should also be considered during treatments and care. A minor detail, such as walking at the head of a stretcher while transporting a patient instead of alongside the patient, will greatly reduce exposure. The upper portion of the patient's body not only provides distance but also acts as a shield. In handling radioactive substances, long-handled forceps may add a distance of 12 to 18 inches. Under no circumstances should the material be picked up with the hands. Ordinary rubber surgical gloves offer little or no protection.

Time. The time factor (since radioactive results are cumulative) is of vital importance. Time may be utilized in the following ways.

Planning. The efficient nurse who prepares a plan of care so that activities in direct patient contact are limited during the high radioactive period can reduce the amount of exposure in relation to the time saved without sacrificing nursing care. As many nursing procedures as possible may be carried out on the day before the treatments are administered so that such steps will not be necessary while there is the greatest amount of exposure present. For example, a complete bed bath and change of linen before the treatment will probably be all that is necessary for at least 24 hours.

Staffing. Units that care for radioactive patients are usually heavily staffed so that it will not be necessary for the same nurse to answer the continuous calls of a patient who is emitting sufficient rays to be dangerous to others. Nurses are usually required to rotate shifts in order to avoid overexposure.

Swift movements. Swift movements may also shorten the time factor if quick disposal of contaminated articles and quick shielding of active materials is encouraged. This factor should also be considered when planning activities.

Half-life. The half-life or the time it takes for one half of the radioactivity to disappear may be effectively used in relation to unsealed isotopes. Many of them may appear in urine, vomitus, or perspiration. A quick cleanup and disposal or storage until the radioactivity is reduced offers increased protection. Limitation of contact during the early stages of even a few hours are highly effective in reducing exposure, especially in a short half-life, as of ^{198}Au, being less than 3 days. Routine monitoring and continu-

405

ous educational programs also add to the safety of personnel.

Care must be taken to explain to the patient such measures as are necessary so that he will not feel neglected or that the nurse is antisocial.

Consideration must also be given to protect personnel outside the hospital, so that contaminated linen is not released to public laundries until exposure levels are within safe limits and maintenance workers are kept accurately informed and instructed.

Basic rules for x-ray and radium protection have been issued by the International Commission on X-ray and Radium Protection. More detailed rules prepared in the United States are available from the Bureau of Standards. Every institution that uses radioactive drugs has regulations governing the use of the drugs.

Learning situations for the patient

Radium and x-ray therapy are used often in the treatment of cancer. Sometimes malignancy is not the reason for their use, and this fact should be explained to the patient. The patient may inquire about the nature of these treatments. The nurse should be able to answer the patient's questions in language he can understand. The patient may wonder why he may need to be hospitalized for x-ray and radium therapy. The nurse will explain that more careful observations can be made and results more quickly noted under controlled conditions in a hospital. Some people fear radiation even when having a chest x-ray film made, and they need to be reassured that the dose and frequency of use are safe.

The nurse should be well informed on the subject of radiation in order to answer questions that the patient may ask, but the answer should be given in terms the lay person can understand.

SUMMARY

Physical agents commonly used for their

therapeutic or diagnostic effects include heat, cold, light, and radiation.

Applications of heat and cold are universal and effective treatments. They are either moist or dry. Moist applications penetrate deeper than do dry ones. The effect of moderate heat is relaxation of blood vessels near the surface. Hence, more blood is brought to the area, which promotes healing. Cold contracts blood vessels and is used to prevent suppuration or discoloration. Heat is conveyed to the tissues by conduction, convection, and radiation. Because applications of heat and cold are common available treatments, patients need to be informed about their dangers. For greater effectiveness many heat treatments are administered by physical therapists using special equipment in the physical therapy department.

Radiation therapy includes the use of light rays, heat rays, electric rays, radium, x-rays, and radiation from radioactive cobalt and drugs. Infrared rays and diathermy are used as heat treatments. Ultraviolet light is used for its chemical effect on tissue. X-rays and radium are treatments often used for cancer. Because the equipment is large and is operated by electricity, the patient may fear the treatment. The nurse should have sufficient information to be able to answer the patient's questions and keep him from becoming unduly alarmed.

Effective communication and instruction of all personnel involved is necessary for the protection of personnel and other patients in radioactive units. The nurse utilizes the laws of physics involving distance, time, and half-life to reduce exposure levels of radioactive patients and materials.

QUESTIONS FOR DISCUSSION

1 Explain the expression "withdrawal of heat."
2 What treatments are included in hot dry applications? hot moist applications?

3 What is the purpose of applying local heat? cold?

4 How does a warm application on the skin relieve congestion in a deeper area?

5 What are the effects of heat on the tissues?

6 What are the effects of cold on the tissues?

7 How do you care for a hot-water bottle after use?

8 What factors influence the effect of heat?

9 Why may the patient having a sitz bath become faint?

10 Why does an ice bag filled with ice become wet on the outside?

11 In your physical therapy department, what methods of applying heat and cold have you observed patients receiving?

12 What is radiation?

13 Where is an infrared lamp placed in relation to the area under treatment?

14 What are radioactive isotopes? How do they produce physiologic effects?

15 How far do infrared rays penetrate?

16 What rays from the spectrum are bactericidal?

17 How is the dosage of radium measured?

18 What are the advantages of cobalt therapy over other types of radiation?

19 How would you gain the cooperation of a patient who feared to have an x-ray treatment?

20 How would you explain diathermy to a patient before he went to a physical therapy department to receive a treatment with diathermy?

21 What measures are used in your institution to protect personnel and patients from overexposure to radioactivity?

22 What symptoms might suggest to the nurse that the patient is experiencing radiation sickness?

23 Describe the effect of ionizing radiation on tissue.

LIFE SITUATION

You note that one of the female attendants on your unit is remaining longer than the designated safety time limit in the room of a patient having radium therapy. When you caution her she replies, "Oh, I did it on purpose. They say that radium will make you sterile and I don't want any babies when I get married." What will be your reaction?

SUGGESTED PERFORMANCE CHECKLIST
Applications of heat and cold
Comfort

1 Is the patient in a comfortable position during the entire treatment?

2 Is the material wrung as dry as possible?

3 Is the application as light as possible?

4 Is the hot-water bag covered?

5 Is the application renewed when it becomes cool?

6 Is the patient screened during the application?

7 Is the environment comfortable?

8 Is draping adequate?

9 Is drying thorough after removal of the application?

Therapeutic effectiveness

1 Is the liquid or the material at the prescribed temperature?

2 Is the application kept at the proper temperature to accomplish its purpose?

3 Is the application fastened securely in place?

4 Is the application renewed as often as necessary?

5 Is the treatment discontinued if unfavorable reactions occur?

6 Is the cooperation of the patient obtained?

7 Is adequate observation made during the treatment?

8 Is the charting pertinent and accurate?

Economy

1 Is all needed equipment at hand?

2 Is expensive equipment handled carefully?

3 Is equipment cleaned and put away properly?

4 Is heated material kept warm as it is carried to the patient?

5 Is the bedding protected from wetting?

6 If not sterile, is proper care taken of the materials so that they may be reused?

7 Is pinning avoided when using rubber or plastic materials?

8 Is the hot-water bottle or ice bag inflated with air when it is put away?

9 Are defects in materials reported at once?

10 Is the cover of the appliance changed often enough to keep it clean and dry?

407

Safety

1 Is the physician's order checked?
2 Is the equipment examined for defects before using?
3 Is a cover used if needed?
4 Is the skin area observed sufficiently?
5 Is moisture prevented when using electric devices?
6 Is the proper temperature maintained?
7 Is the patient kept warm during and after a heat treatment?
8 Is the heat treatment discontinued if the skin is too red?
9 Is the equipment sterile if need be?
10 Is sterility maintained during the treatment?
11 Is the application placed on the skin gradually?
12 Is the proper explanation given to the patient?

SUGGESTED READINGS

Early, Paul J., Razzak, Muhammad A., and Sodee, D. Bruce: Textbook of nuclear medicine technology, St. Louis, 1969, The C. V. Mosby Co.

Isler, Charlotte: Radiation therapy—the nurse and the patient, RN **34:**48, March, 1971.

Prosnitz, Leonard R.: Radiation therapy — treatment for malignant disease, RN **34:**52, March, 1971.

Rummerfield, Philip S., and Rummerfield, Marilyn J.: What you should know about radiation hazards, American Journal of Nursing **70:**780, April, 1970.

Principles related to therapeutic measures in common problems of illness

26 Pain

THE PROBLEM OF PAIN
Definition

Pain is a distressing sensation evoked by a wide variety of stimuli. Its perception is usually accompanied by reactions that are both emotional and physical in nature. Pain occurs on the physical and emotional levels when effective stimuli are relayed to the appropriate sensory area of the cerebral cortex, and the pain perception and interpretation are followed by the initiation of impulses that activate the physical and emotional responses to pain.

In considering pain, it is well to recognize that it is a complex phenomenon having two components: pain sensation, or perception, and pain reaction. Perception, which is the awareness or feeling of pain, depends to a greater extent upon its interpretation in the cerebral cortex than upon the exact nature of the causative stimulus, which may have been qualified by learned experiences. Because of these associations the individual's reaction to pain may be more intense than would be expected in relation to the apparent stimulus.

The term "pain" is generally used in reference to distressing experiences on either a physical or emotional level. For in-stance, if Mrs. Lewis burns her wrist on the oven door while removing a roast from the oven, she feels the unpleasant sensation in the burned area of her wrist. However, when she received word that her son had been killed in an automobile accident, she experienced nonspecific, generalized distressed or unpleasant feelings. Later, Mrs. Lewis might describe this emotional experience as "painful." Both the physical and psychologic components must be dealt with in the plan of nursing care if the patient's needs are to be met.

The patient's pain situation ought to be considered within the context of the total person for the purpose of assisting him with the pain experience. A number of current writers on the subject of pain have emphasized the idea that pain is the patient's own subjective, individual possession that cannot be verified by another. Therefore, if the patient says he has pain, his statement should be accepted. The fact that diagnostic measures are negative may simply mean that the cause of the pain is not known, but the patient's subjective report of pain should nevertheless be believed.

411

Anatomy and physiology of pain

The main structures necessary for the pain sensation, briefly summarized, include the following.

Receptors for pain. These are nerve endings found chiefly in the skin, muscles, joints, tendons, dura mater, periosteum, and arterial walls and to a lesser extent in the viscera. The lungs are said to be insensitive to pain because there are thought to be few pain receptors located in them. Pain perception is a protective mechanism when it warns of tissue damage or the presence of other harmful stimuli, such as excessive heat or cold or interference with the blood flow to a tissue. Common stimuli for visceral pain include muscle spasm of the digestive tract or distension of the intestine, common bile duct, or ureter.

Impulse pathways. Conducting nerves (sensory or afferent nerve fibers) transmit pain impulses to and within the central nervous system for perception, interpretation, and initiation of responses.

Cortical sensory areas. Pain impulses are relayed to the appropriate sensory area of the cerebral cortex, where awareness of pain and interpretation as to the site of the pain and its quality and intensity take place. Here, also, impulses are initiated that activate the physical and psychologic responses to pain.

Pathophysiology may be present that affects the receptors, impulse pathways, or cortical sensory areas, thus interfering with the individual's pain sensation or perception.

Pain stimuli

Effective pain stimuli include mechanical agents (force such as a blow, friction, cutting, distension), thermal agents (extremes of heat and cold), chemical agents (toxins produced by microorganisms), electric current, and, as indicated in the preceding paragraphs, ischemia and sustained muscle contraction.

Pain receptors differ from all the other sense organs in that they do not adapt, or accommodate, to continuous stimulation, such as occurs with the other sense organs. Most people have probably had the experience of no longer being aware of the presence of a particular sound until there is sudden silence. The sound stimulus continued over a period of time no longer excites the receptor. The nonadaptability of the pain receptors provides a very important aspect of the protective mechanism. It is protective in that the pain fibers are indefatigable in transmitting the stimulus warning that tissue damage, or potential damage, is in progress.

Pain threshold

The threshold for pain is the intensity at which awareness of pain is elicited by a stimulus. In the opinion of some authors, the presence of pain indicates the beginning of damage to the receptor nerve endings. According to this theory the pain threshold and the intensity causing tissue damage would be the same thing. The majority opinion also seems to indicate that the pain threshold may vary among different individuals and in the same individual under different circumstances.

Evidence also indicates that the pain threshold may be elevated by distractions, pain in another part of the body, and pathologic conditions affecting the pain receptors, impulse pathways, or cortical sensory areas. The threshold may also be raised by factors depressing the activity of the cerebral cortex, such as certin drugs, alcohol, shock, and general debilitation.

The pain threshold may be lowered in the presence of inflammation, injury to the involved or adjacent tissues, and reduction of other stimuli, which may account for the patient's apparent increase in awareness of pain during the night.

While there is some variation in the pain threshold level among individuals, there are wide variations in individual reactions to pain, depending upon such factors as ethnic and cultural backgrounds, childhood experiences, education, emotional status, previous experience with pain, or the presence of uncertainty, fear, and tension, that may exaggerate response to pain. Some people react strongly to the anticipation of pain. These points should be kept in mind by the nurse as a reminder of the patient's need for reassurance when facing a difficult or uncertain situation.

Types of pain

Pain is sometimes described as superficial or deep. *Superficial pain* occurs when the cutaneous receptors are stimulated. The pain has a sharp quality and is localized at the point of disturbance. *Deep pain* arises from deeper tissues (muscles, viscera, periosteum). It is usually dull and aching in character as compared to superficial pain, tends to be more persistent, and, since it is usually more diffuse, may be located less precisely.

Referred pain from a visceral lesion is felt in a part of the body distant from the actual lesion, usually in a surface area. A very commonly used example of referred pain is that which occurs as a result of ischemia of the heart muscle in angina pectoris. The pain originates in the ischemic heart muscle but the patient feels the pain in the substernal region, the base of the neck, and the inner aspect of the left arm.

Estimating the severity of pain

Evaluation of the intensity of the patient's pain should be based on a variety of factors:

Sensitivity to pain. One forms an impression of a particular patient's sensitivity and psychologic reaction to pain. This is affected by age, ethnic and cultural background, and emotional state.

Facial expression. Furrowed brow, drawn lips, clenched teeth, eyes fixed and

pupils dilated, and pallor may reflect the severity of pain.

Body position. The affected part is held rigid in a protected position; the position assumed is such as to afford the greatest comfort (for example, the knees are drawn up in severe, cramping abdominal pain).

Body movements. Some patients may be extremely restless and writhing in pain; others may respond by refusing to move or change position.

Blood pressure and pulse. Usually there is an increase as a result of reflex through the autonomic nervous system. Very severe and/or sudden pain may be so acute that peripheral vasoconstriction results in shock with falling blood pressure, sweating, and vomiting.

Psychologic (emotional) reactions. A variety of reactions may occur, such as fear, anxiety, anger, weeping, and depression, that contribute to the exhaustion of the individual. Consciously or unconsciously, the individual may either minimize or exaggerate his pain.

Nursing responsibilities

The nursing care of the patient manifesting pain can be summarized under the following broad areas.

Assessment of the problem. Assessment is based on observable factors, and using the five senses as described in Chapter 10. Through observation the nurse assesses such factors as:

1. The *presence of pain* and its characteristics in terms of location (body part and whether superficial or deep), severity, description (sharp, stabbing, gnawing, throbbing, dull, cramping, shooting, spasmodic, and so on), duration, recurrence, interference with activity, and other factors pertinent in an individual situation.

2. The patient's *behavioral responses* to the pain through body movements, facial expression, crying (or groaning, grunting, screaming, gasping), verbal expressions (that is, the significance of the pain to the

patient), and patterns of handling pain. Possible adverse psychologic effects of pain include fear, anxiety, depression, insomnia, irritability, anorexia, withdrawal, and similar behaviors.

3. The associated *physiologic factors* within the context of the total response of the patient. The so-called "fight or flight" reaction occurs in the first phase of brief, intense pain. This includes an increase in pulse and respiratory rates, increase in blood pressure, increase in muscle tension, dilated pupils, pallor, cold perspiration, and nausea. The specific levels and time lapse of the response vary with individual differences and other factors that may be present in the situation. These observable responses indicate a great deal of internal physiologic activity throughout the body that is necessary in order for these effects to occur. For example, the circulatory shift diminishes the blood supply in superficial vessels (thus contributing to the occurrence of pallor) and, in viscera where activity is decreased, in the structures essential for the "fight or flight" activity of the body. Following a brief, intense period of pain a rebound effect may be observed in which the physiologic reactions, such as the pulse and blood pressure, are lower than they were prior to the period of pain activation. Depending upon the subsequent course of the pain, other patterns of physiologic response may occur. They are described in detail in literature on the subject.

4. The *source of pain.* Sometimes factors contributing to pain are readily identifiable. For example, the observation of pressure from improperly fitting dressings, casts, binders, or other appliances, uncomfortable positioning, disturbing environmental conditions, distension resulting from either flatus or urinary retention, and need for oral hygiene or other physical discomforts indicate the need for supportive care. In other situations the pain may be intractable or associated with grave illness from which there will be no recovery. For some patients it may be possible only to diminish the pain, but not to obtain complete relief or to prevent recurrence. Therefore, the nurse will need to deal with personal frustration and anxiety in order to be able to offer support to the patient and his family.

Nursing intervention to provide relief of pain. On the basis of the information obtained through the process of observation and assessment, the nurse seeks to identify the real problems. A nursing judgment is then made that forms the basis for developing a plan of care devised to alleviate the pain. Through assessment the nurse tries to understand as much as possible the patient's experience of pain. This enables the nurse to recognize the need for nursing intervention and to devise intervention specific for the individual patient's needs. Nursing intervention includes management of both physiologic and psychologic factors.

Examples of specific nursing measures that may be effective in diminishing pain include provision for physical hygiene measures contributing to the general feeling of comfort; frequent changes of position to reduce pressure and tension on affected parts and to support the body parts in proper alignment; planning of activities so that the patient has time to rest; diversion, if it is acceptable, that may help the patient change his focus from the pain to something else, thus making the pain more bearable; quiet, well-organized environment with adjusted ventilation, temperature, and lighting; and limiting the number of visitors and personnel working with the patient. Recognition of the presence of anxiety, which frequently accompanies the experience of pain is, in itself, an important nursing responsibility. The anxiety may often be reduced by the presence of a nurse who understands the use of the communication skills of listening, reflecting, and open-ended questions, through which communication and reassurance of the patient is encouraged. Reassurance and comforting of the patient in pain may also be communicated through physical contact. It has been commonly observed that the individual experiencing pain will hold on to a trusted person and seem to derive courage and comfort from this contact. Therefore, it is appropriate for the nurse to place a reassuring hand on the patient's hand or arm. Some patients will respond to rubbing an area of the body, for example, rubbing the back.

Nursing intervention. Medical orders should be carried out in a manner that will bring the maximum therapeutic effect for the relief of pain. The administration of medications prescribed for the relief of pain, and particularly the exercise of judgment regarding the use of p.r.n. orders and evaluation of the patient's response to the medications, are important nursing responsibilities in the care of the patient.

Evaluation of the intervention. Through the process of evaluation, the nurse makes a judgment regarding the effect of the nursing care upon the patient.

1. Is the patient relaxed? apparently comfortable? sleeping? Why was the intervention successful or moderately successful?
2. Is the patient still restless? anxious? complaining of pain? If the intervention was unsuccessful, why did it not provide relief? What more can the nurse do to provide relief? to assist in the process of adaptation?

Problem-solving approach

The problem-solving approach facilitates the application of theories and principles related to pain in devising and administering patient care. Problem solving is related to the nursing process in carrying out the responsibilities just described, as demonstrated in Table 26-1.

It is helpful to recognize that one phase

Table 26-1

Nursing responsibilities	Steps in problem solving*
1. Assessment of the problem	1. Recognizing and defining the problem 2. Collecting the data from observation and experiment
2. Nursing intervention	3. Formulating and implementing a solution
3. Evaluation of the intervention	4. Evaluating the solution

*See Chapter 3.

of the process merges into another. For instance, referring back to the example of Mrs. Lewis, when she arrived for treatment of the deep and painful looking burn she was given immediate attention by the nurse, Miss Heston. As Miss Heston talked with Mrs. Lewis, gathering pertinent information about the patient and the burn, not only was she assessing the patient's problem and her reaction to it, she was also intervening through the reassurance of her presence with the patient and, through her listening and concern, was reducing Mrs. Lewis' anxiety and opening the way for further effective assessment, intervention, and evaluation in the patient's behalf.

SUMMARY

Pain is described as a distressing sensation accompanied by reactions that are both emotional and physical in nature. It is a complex phenomenon having two components: pain perception and pain reaction. Perception depends to a greater extent upon its interpretation in the cerebral cortex than upon the exact nature of the causative stimulus.

The term "pain" is used to refer to distressing experiences on either a physical or emotional level. Both the physical and psychologic components must be dealt with in the plan of nursing care if the patient's needs are to be met.

Essential structures necessary for the pain sensation include (1) receptors for pain, (2) impulse pathways, and (3) cortical sensory areas. A wide variety of stimuli are effective in evoking pain reactions.

The threshold for pain is the intensity at which awareness of pain is elicited by a stimulus. The threshold varies among individuals and may be raised or lowered by a variety of factors. Pain is described as superficial or deep and may be referred from a visceral lesion to a distant area of the body, usually the surface.

Nursing responsibilities in the care of the patient manifesting pain may be summarized under the following steps. However, it is helpful to recognize that one phase of the process merges into another.

1. Assessment of the problem, based on observable factors and using the five senses as described in Chapter 10. Through observation the nurse assesses such factors as:
   a. Presence and intensity of pain
   b. The patient's behavioral responses to the pain
   c. Associated physiologic factors within the context of the total response of the patient
   d. Source of pain
2. Nursing intervention to provide relief of pain
3. Carrying out medical orders
4. Evaluation of the nursing intervention

The problem-solving approach facilitates the application of theories and principles related to pain in devising and administering patient care.

QUESTIONS FOR DISCUSSION

1 How would you describe pain? How would you recognize its presence? How would you evaluate its intensity?
2 Why is the patient's subjective experience of pain significant to the nurse?
3 What physiologic manifestations are associated with pain?
4 What is the relationship of the general adaptation syndrome to pain?
5 What is the significance of physical contact with others in the individual's pain experience?
6 How may information be gained about the patient's ability to cope with pain? Why is this information significant to the nurse?
7 What is the effect of cultural influences on the patient's behavioral responses to pain?
8 Discuss possible ways that nursing action may alter factors that cause or increase the patient's pain.
9 Discuss appropriate nursing action when the patient's pain is unavoidable.
10 How may the nurse determine the effectiveness of her intervention in behalf of the patient's pain?

SUGGESTED READINGS

Barber, Janet M., Stokes, Lillian G., and Billings, Diane M.: Adult and child care—a client approach to nursing, St. Louis, 1973, The C. V. Mosby Co., pp. 119-123.

Belleville, J. W., and others: Age and postoperative pain, American Journal of Nursing 72:132, January, 1972.

Billars, Karen S.: You have pain? I think this will help, American Journal of Nursing 70:2143, October, 1970.

Chodil, Judith, and Williams, Barbara: The concept of sensory deprivation, Nursing Clinics of North America 5:453, September, 1970.

Rodman, Martin J.: Drugs for pain problems, RN 34:59, April, 1971.

Shafer, Kathleen N., and others: Medical-surgical nursing, ed. 5, St. Louis, 1971, The C. V. Mosby Co., chap. 7, p. 131.

27 Eye, ear, nose, and throat disorders

Man is very dependent upon sensory perceptions gained through the special senses of sight, hearing, and, to a lesser degree, smell. Much of the knowledge about his surroundings, so important in the ability to move about safely and to enjoy the beauty of color and form, is obtained through the senses. Yet sometimes these sensory abilities are taken for granted, when in reality prevention of impairment is of utmost importance.

The nursing role is concerned not only with prevention but also with the carrying out of the treatments when there are disorders; with the patient's anxieties when loss of vision or hearing is threatened; and with participating in the rehabilitation of the patient who has loss of sight or hearing.

Many patients with disorders of the eye or ear are successfully treated on an outpatient basis. Such patients are admitted to the hospital most frequently when major surgical or medical treatment is to be undertaken, or when there is a concurrent systemic condition that necessitates hospitalization.

Since the total care of patients with disorders of the eye, ear, nose, or throat will vary considerably, the focus in this chapter, therefore, is primarily on local treatments of these structures that the nurse may encounter in the care of patients, rather than on a total plan of care for individual patients.

SCIENTIFIC PRINCIPLES

Examples of principles have been included that are relevant to common treatments of the eye, ear, nose, and throat

417

and that seem helpful in understanding some of the practices that have been developed in carrying out common procedures. These statements provide some basis for determining their rationale and validity. Many others may be identified.

Principles relevant to the eye

Some visual disorders result in defective vision that, regardless of the cause, affects the individual's emotional, vocational, and social life, either temporarily or permanently. The following statements are relevant to the care of patients with visual problems.

1. Information received through the senses is essential for the individual's assessment and awareness of the environment.

2. The individual's ability to interact with the environment is dependent on the functioning of his sensory organs.

3. Disorders of the eye that prevent the reception of information about the environment immediately alter the individual's perception and interaction in the environment; therefore, much of the nursing care of such an individual should be directed toward the environmental adaptations made necessary by his altered perception.

4. Normally, a film of tears keeps the conjunctival surfaces of the eye moist and clean. Tears are:
   a. A slightly hypertonic, clear, watery secretion
   b. Secreted by the lacrimal glands
   c. Moved across the eye by blinking and gravity to drain into the nose via the nasolacrimal duct and removed as fast as formed

5. Fluids having a salt concentration varying much more than 0.6%, to 0.7% from physiologic saline solution are irritating to the conjunctiva.

6. The cornea is well supplied with pain fibers.

7. The structures of the eye have a large blood supply, except for the cornea.

8. Movements of the eyelids (blinking) are either voluntary or reflex and help to protect the eye from injury by foreign particles.

9. The conjunctiva and cornea are susceptible to inflammation caused by:
   a. Invading microorganisms
   b. Heat
   c. Trauma (for example, foreign particles, irritating solutions, rubbing)

10. The iris is an opaque tissue that regulates the amount of light allowed to enter the eye.
   a. Constriction of the pupil results from parasympathetic stimulation of the circular muscles of the iris.
   b. Dilation of the pupil results from sympathetic stimulation of the dilator muscle, increasing the size of the pupil.

Principles relevant to the ear

Sufficient knowledge is needed about the ear to be able to meet the patient's needs with understanding, to administer prescribed treatments safely, and to be alert to the presence of significant symptoms.

1. The structure of the ear provides for the reception of sound and for the sense of balance.

2. The external auditory canal is approximately $1\frac{1}{4}$ inches long in the adult.
   a. In the adult the external canal is somewhat S-shaped, passing inward, forward, and upward, then inward and slightly backward.
   b. In the child the canal is relatively straight.

3. The external canal is lined with extension of skin. It is relatively insensitive in the outer half and very sensitive in the inner half.

4. Ceruminous glands secrete cerumen (ear wax), which helps to protect the ear from the entrance of foreign substances.

5. The tympanic membrane, a thin layer of fibrous tissue separating the mid-

dle ear from the external canal, is set in motion by sound waves.

6. Vibrations of the tympanic membrane are transmitted by the three auditory ossicles stretched across the middle ear and transmitted as nerve impulses carried to the brain via the acoustic nerve.

7. Normally, the middle ear is filled with air; atmospheric pressure is maintained on both sides of the tympanic membrane by means of the eustachian tube connecting the middle ear with the nasopharynx.

8. Rapid warming or cooling of the fluid in the semicircular canals produces a change in the sensation of position, which may cause the individual to feel dizzy.

9. The middle ear is subject to attack by a number of pathogenic microorganisms.

10. An opening exists in the posterior wall of the middle ear and provides entrance into the mastoid cells. At this point the temporal bone is very porous, allowing easy access inward to the brain.

Principles relevant to the nose and throat

The nose and throat serve several different functions that need to be understood when administering treatments involving these structures or when answering the patient's questions.

1. The mucous membrane of the nasal cavity is continuous with the lining of the nasal sinuses.

2. The mucous membrane of the nasopharynx is continuous with that of the eustacian tube and extends to the middle ear.

3. Normally the sinuses are kept clean by the beating action of the cilia, which direct drainage into the nasal cavity.

4. The mucous membrane lining the nasal passages is extremely vascular. The vessels of these membranes may be readily dilated by irritants, with resultant swelling.

5. Inspired air is warmed, moistened,

and filtered as it passes over the highly vascular mucous membrane with its projecting cilia.

6. Nasal and sinus mucosa secrete approximately a quart of fluid daily.

7. Receptors of the olfactory nerve are located in the nasal mucosa above the superior turbinate.

8. In order for it to be smelled, a substance must be sufficiently volatile for its particles to come in contact with the end organs of the olfactory nerve.

9. A variety of bacteria, some pathogenic, are normally present in the mouth and nose. They may do no harm to an intact mucous membrane but may be harmful to other people.

10. The pharynx is a passageway for both food and air.

11. The gag reflex is stimulated by touching the uvula.

12. The mucous membrane of the mouth can tolerate temperatures higher than any other tissues in the body.

PRINCIPLES APPLIED TO TREATMENTS OF THE EYE
Structure and functions of the eye

Structures of the eye include the orbital cavity, the extrinsic muscles, the eyelids, the lacrimal glands, and the conjunctivas (Fig. 27-1).

The anterior fifth of the orbital cavity is occupied by the eyeball, which rests on a cushion of fat. The eyeball is nearly spherical in shape and is about 1 inch in diameter. Six extrinsic muscles move the eye in the orbit. The eyelids, loose folds of skin and connective tissue, serve to protect the eyes from external injury, foreign bodies, and drying. Lashes, which grow at the inside margin of the lids, serve to protect the eye from injury.

The meibomian glands are enlarged, modified sebaceous glands near the margins of the lids. They secrete a fatty substance that hinders the overflowing of tears.

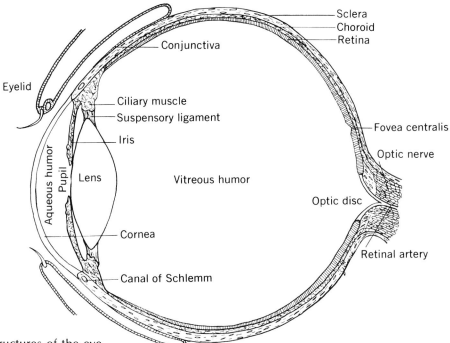

Fig. 27-1. Structures of the eye.

The eyeball has three coats. The sclera and the cornea make up the outer coat. The middle vascular coat is made up of the iris, the ciliary body, and the choroid extending backward. It furnishes the chief blood supply to the eye. The inner coat is the retina, which is a thin, transparent membrane that contains the visual receptors, extensions of the optic nerve. The interior of the eyeball is divided into two cavities, the anterior and the posterior. The posterior cavity is the larger and occupies the space between the lens and the retina. It contains a gelatinous substance called vitreous humor.

The anterior cavity is further subdivided into the anterior and posterior chambers. The anterior chamber lies between the iris and the cornea. The posterior chamber is the small space between the iris and the lens. Both chambers of the anterior cavity contain a clear, colorless, lymphlike fluid called aqueous humor.

The eyeball is covered with a sensitive mucous membrane called the conjunctiva, which is modified over the cornea. The same mucous membrane is continuous into the lacrimal sac, the nasolacrimal duct, and the nose. The part of the conjunctiva that covers the posterior surface of the lids is called the palpebral conjunctiva, that on the eyeball is called the bulbar conjunctiva.

The lacrimal apparatus consists of the lacrimal glands, located in a groove in the frontal bone, the lacrimal sac, and the lacrimal duct (Fig. 27-2). Tears are constantly being formed and are washed over the eyeball as the eye winks, which occurs normally about three to six times a minute. Tears keep the surface of the eye moist. Some of the tears are evaporated, while others find their way down the lacrimal sac and duct. The total secretion of tears is 0.5 to 0.76 ml. during the 16 waking hours.

Any type of stimulation of the cornea gives rise to pain. No sense of touch or temperature is present, but if the irrigating tip touches the cornea, pain will be experi-

420

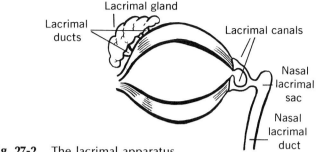

Fig. 27-2. The lacrimal apparatus.

enced. When the eyelids are separated for an irrigation, pressure is made on the bones of the cheek and brow to avoid injury to the cornea.

More than three fourths of all impressions come through the eye, so it is important to keep the eye in good condition. The health and nutrition of the entire body are reflected in the eyes. It has been estimated that one fourth of all physical energy is used in seeing.

The normal eye can become tired and strained from overuse by close work or by work done in artificial light. Prolonged close work should be balanced by rest or by looking at a distance occasionally. Eyestrain can cause irritability.

Constriction and dilation of the pupil are reflex acts stimulated by light or lack of it or by near or far vision. The pupil may contract or dilate by the action of certain drugs. If the cornea or the conjunctiva is touched, reflex winking occurs. Because of this fact, it is hard to hold the lids apart when eye treatments are carried out.

The optic nerve conveys sight impressions. The retina is supplied by a branch of the ophthalmic artery, which enters through the optic disk. Images falling on the retina stimulate the nerve cells contained in it to send appropriate messages to the brain. Seeing involves the interpretation by the brain of the image that is formed. Seeing is more than visual function. It is a normal activity of human beings and is intimately associated with efficiency, comfort, safety, and welfare.

Loss of accommodation that comes with advancing years is shown in Table 27-1. The greatest change is between 40 and 50 years of age.

Blood vessels dilate with the application of heat. The warm irrigating solution relaxes the eyes, brings more blood to the area, hastens healing, and gives comfort.

The eyelashes protect the eyes from dust. Tears contain a bactericidal substance called lysozyme, which protects the eyes from infection.

Common infections of the eye are caused by *Staphylococcus,* which is found in styes, *Gonococcus,* which causes conjunctivitis, and the Koch-Weeks bacillus, which is the cause of pinkeye. These infections are serious because there is a possibility that they may cause corneal ulcers, which impair sight.

In caring for patients with these conditions, the nurse keeps the hands away from the face and protects the eyes with

Table 27-1 Loss of accommodation

Age in years	Power of accommodation in diopters*
10	14.0
20	11.2
30	8.5
40	5.7
50	1.9
60	1.0
70	1.0

*A diopter is a unit used to measure lenses.

glasses or goggles if there is danger of splashing, such as during an irrigation. The nurse wears a gown to prevent cross-infection and washes the hands after caring for the patient.

In irrigation of an eye, further infection is prevented by turning the patient's head so that the solution flows from the inner to the outer canthus and hence does not go over the bridge of the nose to the other eye. The head is turned a little to the side of the affected eye to aid in drainage. Sometimes a transparent shield is put over an unaffected eye to protect it. Infection may be carried to the eyes by soiled handkerchiefs or towels. Eye drops are best administered by placing them inside the lower lid near the outer canthus, thus preventing injury to the cornea and loss of medication (Fig. 27-3).

The eyes may be affected by infections in the nose and throat because of continuity or proximity of structures.

Sterile drugs or solutions and sterile equipment are used in eye treatments and are kept sterile throughout treatment. Very low pressure is used in order not to injure the delicate conjunctiva.

Infected dressings or cotton used in irrigations should be wrapped well in paper and burned or discarded in containers provided for this purpose.

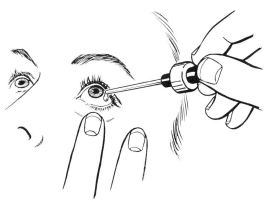

Fig. 27-3. A safe method for administering eye drops.

The pH of normal tears is 7 to 7.4. For comfort, irrigating solutions should be neutral in reaction. At pH 9 a slight feeling of irritation is produced, whereas a pH of 6.6 to 6.3 causes a slight feeling of dryness. A pH of 6 to 4.5 causes a severe burning irritation. However, boric acid in 5% solution with a pH of 4.2 produces only slight irritation since it is a weak acid (that is, weakly ionized).

Visual purple (rhodopsin) is an unstable chemical substance that is readily decomposed or altered by light and is dependent on an adequate supply of vitamin A in the retina, which comes from vitamin A present in food. Visual purple and visual yellow are substances that influence adjustment from light to darkness and from darkness to light, respectively.

Solutions used for eye irrigations are made from boric acid or sodium chloride. Weak solutions are used so that they will not be irritating. Boric acid is being used less frequently, since toxic side reactions and even death have been known to occur when it is taken internally by mistake.

Drugs used in the eye may be classed as antiseptic, astringent, mydriatic, miotic, or anesthetic. As antiseptics, the silver salts are used, commonly Argyrol and silver nitrate. Silver nitrate is used in the eyes of a newborn infant to prevent gonorrheal ophthalmia. Zinc sulfate drops (astringent) are put into the eye to reduce inflammation.

Mydriatic cycloplegic drugs frequently used to dilate the pupil for eye examinations and sometimes for other purposes are cyclopentolate and homatropine. An example of a miotic, or a drug to reduce the size of the pupil, is eserine, or physostigmine.

One of the first uses of cocaine was to anesthetize the eye. Antiseptic or soothing oils or ointments may be applied either in the conjunctival sac or on the lids.

Penicillin is used in treating some infectious conditions of the eye. Cortisone is the newest drug found useful in eye disorders. Fluorescein is a drug used in the diagnosis of lesions and foreign bodies in the eye.

Vitamins A, B, C, and D all affect the health of the eye. Vitamin A prevents night blindness. Vitamin B is useful in some conditions of the cornea, the retina, and the optic nerve. Vitamin C plays a part in the metabolism of the normal lens. Vitamin D has been used for some ocular conditions.

Weak beta rays have been used to treat the eyelids and the eyeballs, especially for conditions that involve new growths.

Light is the stimulus to the optic nerve. Intensity of light is measured by candle power. The term "1 foot-candle" means the amount of light cast by 100 candles at 10 feet. This is the minimum of light that should be used for reading. Close work needs 10 to 20 foot-candles on the work being done but not more than 20, because fatigue is produced by a pinpoint pupil. The pupil becomes smaller as more light is admitted. At least 2 to 5 foot-candles of general illumination should be maintained so that the eye will not have too much adjustment to make as it looks up from the work at hand. Factors influencing fatigue from close work are (1) size of print or object and color, (2) relative position of eyes and work, and (3) light. Good lighting prevents not only eyestrain but also the needless using up of untold amounts of nervous energy. The higher the intensity of light, the greater is the relaxation of the reader.

Glare is caused by light shining into the eyes or reflected into them. Glare is more tiring to the eyes than a dim light is. If images on the retina are not distinct because of impaired refractive power of the eye, glass lenses are used to refract rays of light and to aid in seeing.

Intraocular pressure averages 15 to 25 mm. Hg. Intraocular pressure displays hourly variations in normal individuals as well as in patients with glaucoma. It is lowest in the afternoon and highest in the early morning hours. The fluctuation in normal individuals is usually less than 5 mm. Hg, but in persons with glaucoma it may vary as much as 25 mm. or more.

Because the eyeball is a closed cavity, a pressure applied to its surface will be transmitted undiminished to the retina. Hence, in irrigations, pressure is kept as low as possible in order to secure a steady flow of solution yet not cause pain or injury to the delicate tissues. Pressure is controlled by hanging the reservoir low and using a tube of small diameter or by slowly pressing a bulb syringe.

The temperature of the solution for an eye irrigation is about 98° to 100° F. (36.6° to 37.3° C.) in order not to injure the conjunctiva, which is very sensitive to heat. The solution is carefully tested before it is used.

The surfaces of the eyelids are lubricated by tears, allowing them to move without friction. In trachoma the roughness of the eyelids breaks down the cornea into ulcers.

Friction is needed between the nurse's fingers and the eyelids in opening them for irrigation. If much solution wets the fingers, friction is reduced, and more effort is required to keep open the patient's eyelids, which are sensitive because of the condition that requires the irrigation.

Local treatments of the eye

The administration of treatments to the eye requires great accuracy, judgment, and gentleness of touch because of the high risk of irreparable damage that can result from improper instillation techniques or errors in medications and solutions used in the eye. A generally used guide in giving eye medications is that any preparation more than 1% in strength should be questioned.

Types of local eye treatments commonly administered by the nurse include (1) drugs applied as instillation of drops or ointments, (2) compresses, hot and cold, (3) irrigations, and (4) application of eye pads or dressings. Most hospitals have specific procedures for doing these treatments; therefore, details of techniques are not discussed here. However, the following practices should be observed regardless of the type of treatment.

1. The hands must be washed thoroughly before beginning any procedure in the care of the eyes.

2. All equipment and solutions used in or about the eye should be sterile.

3. Individual medicine bottles, droppers, tubes of ointment, and equipment should be used for the patient being treated for an eye infection.

4. A good light is essential when giving eye treatments.

5. Gentleness should always be used for any procedure involving the eye, such as opening the eyelid.

6. Pressure in opening the eye should be placed on the bony structures surrounding the eye rather than on the eye itself.

7. Eye pads are usually contraindicated in the presence of an eye infection.

8. Droppers, irrigating tips, and the like should not touch the eyelid or the conjunctiva.

9. Medications or irrigating solutions should be directed into the lower conjunctiva, not onto the corneal surface.

10. Cleansing strokes or solutions should be directed from the inner toward the outer canthus.

11. If infection is present, separate equipment should be used for each eye; solution should not be allowed to run from one eye to the other.

12. If the patient is helpless or unconscious, the cornea should not be allowed to become dry or irritated.

Examination of the eye

Visual acuity means sharpness of vision, and it is a measure of sight. The Snellen test card is commonly used to test visual acuity as a gross screening test. When vision is so poor that it cannot be tested with the card, an attempt may be made to have the patient count the examiner's fingers held in front of the eyes. If the patient cannot see the fingers, the examiner's hands may be moved in front of the eyes. If the patient cannot see the hand movement, he may be able to perceive light. If there is no light perception, the patient is blind. Blindness is defined in some states as visual acuity of 20/200 that cannot be corrected or peripheral field vision defect that limits vision to an angular distance no greater than 20 degrees.

An ophthalmoscope (Gr. *ophthalmos,* eye, + Gr. *skopein,* to examine) is used in examination of the eye. It lights and magnifies the view of the interior of the eye so that the retina, optic nerve, and blood vessels may be seen through the pupil. A flashlight may be used for testing the reflex to light. A tonometer is used for testing tension in the eyeball and thus is useful in detecting glaucoma.

Refraction is a procedure used to determine the degree to which the light-transmitting portions of the eye bring light rays into focus on the retina (Fig. 27-4). When the refractive error has been determined, corrective glasses or contact lenses can be prescribed. Perimetry is a method of determining limitation of the patient's visual field. Reduction in the field of vision is a common finding in the major disorders of glaucoma and retinal detachment.

Observation of the patient's eyes may reveal symptoms of a local eye disorder or manifestations of systemic diseases that may appear in the eye. A common example of the latter is the change that may occur in the retina when the individual has persistent systemic hypertension. Careful observation of the patient's eyes should be included in the process of assessing the patient's needs.

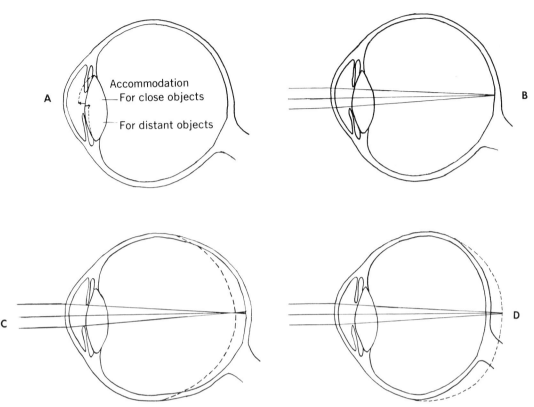

Fig. 27-4. Variations in structures of the eye causing abnormalities. **A,** Changes in the shape of the lens for focusing. **B,** Normal eye. **C,** Myopic eye. **D,** Hyperopic eye.

Psychosocial aspects

The eye is a very sensitive part of the body, and the patient fears that the simplest procedure may injure his eye or sight. Therefore he can be helped by careful explanations and modification of all procedures to meet his specific needs related to his visual problems. The patient who comes to the hospital to receive treatment for his eyes has many fears, such as (1) "Will this procedure cure me?" (2) "Will it be painful?" (3) "Will I be left totally blind?" (4) "How can I plan for my future and that of my family?" (5) "Will I become a dependent blind person?" (6) "Will my family be supported?" (7) "If things do not go right after the operation, how can I give my family proper care?"

The patient's emotional reaction to worry may cause him to be impatient and demanding or depressed and withdrawn. In either case it is important to establish communication with the patient, speaking frequently and reassuringly to him. One should always speak to him before touching him. If the patient cannot see, his unit should be arranged for his convenience and he should be well oriented to his surroundings. He will almost invariably feel very helpless and quite insecure, but the nurse can assist him to move toward independence by encouraging his efforts at self-care when he is permitted to begin such activities.

A patient who is wearing glasses for the first time may need encouragement in becoming adjusted to them or to the fact that a need for them indicates a changing vision. Sometimes the change of glasses to bifocals or to trifocals is a problem of ad-

425

justment not only to knowing where one is putting his feet when he is walking but also to the idea that he is growing older, which is revealed by the fact that he is wearing multiple lenses. He also may feel that the glasses are a sign of a physical defect and thus act as a barrier between himself and others. Man's desire to present a normal, unhandicapped appearance to the outside world is deeply rooted and intense. A knowledge of the community agencies that can help in rehabilitating the patient is essential.

Patients who are blind may be helped by the Office of Vocational Rehabilitation, the American Foundation for the Blind, and the Braille Institute of America. Schools or classes serve the blind. Talking books are stories in record form that are used by blind persons. Books in braille and talking books may be borrowed from many public libraries. The federal government recognizes the dependence of blind persons and allows two exemptions in income tax to a blind person. Persons with defective vision may be helped by the local chapter of the National Society for the Prevention of Blindness.

Special schools for children wherein sight is conserved are located in all large cities. To be admitted to classes for the partially seeing child, a child must have a visual acuity of not less than 20/70. The children use books with 18-point type, write with large crayons and chalk, and learn to type.

Many elementary schools require vision testing as part of the health program. Approximately 20% of children and 40% of adults of college age have defective vision. After the age of 60 years, the percentage increases to 95%.

Some diseases, side effects from medications, and accidents impair sight. The health program in industries includes methods of preventing eye injuries and strains.

Terminology

A vocabulary of commonly used terms makes the reading of literature dealing with the eye more understandable.

accommodation the focusing mechanism of the eye through which the shape of the lens is adjusted by action of the ciliary muscle.

amblyopia dimness of vision without a detectable organic lesion of the eye.

anterior chamber the space that lies between the cornea anteriorly and the iris posteriorly.

aqueous humor transparent fluid nourishing the lens and cornea.

astigmatism refractive error resulting from irregularity in the shape of the cornea.

blepharitis a chronic inflammatory process involving the margin of the eyelids.

canthus angle at either end of the eyelids.

cataract condition in which the lens of the eye becomes opaque.

chalazion infection of a meibomian gland.

conjunctiva membrane lining the eyelids and covering the front of the eyeball, except for the cornea.

cornea the clear, transparent anterior portion of the outer coat of eyeball.

cycloplegic medication producing paralysis of the ciliary muscle.

ectropion a turning-out of the eyelid because of spasm.

enucleation removal of the entire eyeball.

exophthalmos abnormal protrusion of the eyeball.

glaucoma disorder resulting from increased intraocular pressure caused by disturbance of the normal balance between the production and the drainage of the aqueous humor that fills the anterior chamber.

hordeolum an infection at the edge of the eyelid that orginates in a lash follicle (stye).

hyperopia farsightedness; condition in which the eyeball is shorter than normal and the image is formed behind the retina (Fig. 27-4, *D*).

iridectomy surgical procedure performed to relieve acute glaucoma by providing for unobstructed drainage of aqueous fluid.

keratitis inflammation of the cornea.

keratoplasty corneal transplant.

Koch-Weeks bacillus etiologic agent in epidemic pinkeye.

lens small, transparent structure that lies be-

426

hind the iris; one of the refractive media through which light passes.

meibomian gland sebaceous gland near the margin of the eyelids; the oily secretion prevents the tear film on the eyeball from evaporating.

miosis contraction of the pupil.

miotic a drug that contracts the pupil of the eye.

mydriasis abnormal dilation of the pupil.

mydriatic a drug that dilates the pupil.

myopia nearsightedness; a condition in which the eyeball is longer than normal and the image is formed in front of the retina (Fig. 27-4, *C*).

myosis *see* **miosis.**

ophthalmia severe inflammation of the eye, including the conjunctiva.

ophthalmologist (older term, **oculist**) medical doctor who has had special training in the diagnosis and treatment of eye diseases, including refraction and the prescription of glasses.

ophthalmoscope an instrument used to examine the interior of the eye.

optician fills prescriptions for glasses given by the ophthalmologist.

optometrist one who, though not a physician, has had special training in testing vision for refractive errors and prescribing and fitting glasses to correct such errors.

photophobia intolerance to light.

presbyopia the farsightedness of old age caused by loss of elasticity of the lens and leading to decreased ability to accommodate to near vision.

pterygium thickening of the conjunctiva on the cornea such that the growth tends to extend toward the center of the cornea.

ptosis drooping of the upper eyelid.

refraction ocular refraction is the process by which light rays are directed so that they will focus on the retina (Fig. 27-4).

retina inner coat of the eyeball that is a thin, transparent membrane containing the visual receptors, which are extensions of the optic nerve.

retinopexy treatment of detached retina with diathermy.

sclera outer coat of the eyeball.

scleral buckling surgical procedure for treating retinal detachment.

Snellen test visual screening device.

strabismus inability to direct both eyes to the same object, caused by lack of muscular coordination.

tonography method of measuring intraocular tension by using a tonometer.

uveitis inflammation of the uveal tract (iris, ciliary body, and choroid).

visual field the total area that the patient can see without turning his head.

PRINCIPLES APPLIED TO TREATMENTS OF THE EAR

Some understanding of problems relating to the ear are useful to the nurse in the care of many patients. Awareness of the serious complications that can follow minor infections of these areas leads the nurse to be concerned with reporting early symptoms and to instruction of the patient regarding preventive measures. Impairment of hearing may be slight, moderate, or so severe as to constitute deafness that in some cases might have been minimized or prevented by early therapy. Understanding of the handicapping effect of hearing loss contributes to the nurse's ability to be supportive of the patient who has already experienced hearing impairment and also leads to stressing preventive aspects in every way possible. Therefore, readings on more specialized care are listed at the end of this chapter.

Structure and functions of the ear

The ear has two physiologic functions: hearing and balance. Hearing depends on two factors, the sound conduction apparatus and the sound perception apparatus. The sound conduction structures are the eardrum, the ossicles, the eustachian tube, and the cochlea. The sound perception apparatus consists of the organ of Corti, nerve filaments of the eighth cranial or auditory nerve, and the hearing center within the brain. The funnel-shaped cartilaginous pinna or auricle serves to some extent to collect sound waves and to direct them into the bony unyielding ear canal. The acoustic meatus or auditory canal is a tubular passage about 2.5 cm. in length.

It is lined with skin, and modified sebaceous glands in the walls produce a waxlike secretion called cerumen. Normally this wax evaporates or dries and falls out. Sometimes it may become impacted and may impair the vibrations of the eardrum and diminish acuity of hearing.

The ear canal is not straight, and because it is not straight, the pinna is lifted upward and backward in order to straighten the external canal to provide for a more efficient irrigation and better drainage of the solution. In a child the ear canal is best straightened by drawing the pinna downward and backward.

The eardrum, or the tympanic membrane, consists of a cartilaginous ring across which is stretched a layer of fibrous tissue covered on its outer side with delicate skin and on its inner side with mucous membrane. It is elliptical, measuring about 10 mm. in height and 9 mm. in width. Its area is about 50 sq. mm. and is pearl gray in color. It receives sound waves entering the auditory canal, vibrates in harmony with them, and passes the vibration on to the middle ear.

The middle ear, or the tympanic cavity, is a chamber measuring about 15 by 5 by 2 mm. and is situated within the petrous bone. It is lined with a mucous membrane that is continuous with that of the pharynx through the eustachian tube, and it also communicates with the mastoid cells. The epithelium is ciliated except over the tympanic membrane and part of the inner wall.

A chain of three small bones, the malleus, incus, and stapes, joined together and loosely attached to the eardrum, serve to convey sound vibrations to the membrane of the oval window, which in turn conveys them to the inner ear. The eustachian tube is about $1\frac{1}{2}$ inches long and about $\frac{1}{8}$ inch in diameter at its narrowest part. It extends downward to the posterior wall of the pharynx. It is lined with cilia, which sweep both normal mucus secretions and sometimes pathologic discharges from the middle ear down into the throat. The eustachian tubes keep air pressure inside the eardrums the same as that on the outside. They are opened during swallowing and yawning and while blowing the nose (Fig. 27-5).

The stapes transmits the sound vibrations to the endolymph within the cochlea. Vibrations carried by the air change to fluid vibrations that are picked up by the receptors of hearing or hair cells of the organ of Corti. The sound vibration is conducted by the eighth cranial nerve to the auditory center in the temporal lobe of the brain.

The most important symptoms referring to hearing are deafening and ringing in the ears. The word "deaf" means complete loss of hearing. The word "deafened" means an impairment of hearing, or deafening. Deafness may be conductive, receptive, or cerebral. Anything that interferes with normal tension of the tympanic membrane, the three ossicles, and the footplate of the stapes may prove to be a cause of deafness in the conducting apparatus. With dysfunction of the organ of Corti, a receptive type of deafness occurs. Cerebral deafness involves conduction of the sound vibration to the brain and interpretation of the sensation.

If the difficulty is in air conduction, bone conduction may be substituted by using a hearing aid that magnifies sound to some extent, but bone conduction is not as effective as air conduction. Acuity of hearing may be measured by the audiometer.

The semicircular canals located in the internal ear are structures concerned with balance. The canals are innervated by a branch of the eighth cranial nerve. The semicircular canals may be affected if the temperature of an irrigating solution is too high or too low, and symptoms of imbalance, such as dizziness, staggering, or nystagmus, may appear.

Sound is a word used both for the sense impression with which the organ of hearing reacts and for the mechanical phe-

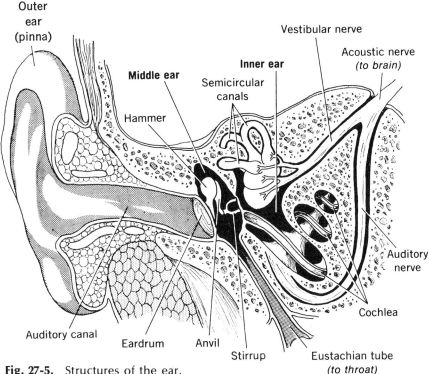

Fig. 27-5. Structures of the ear.

nomena, vibratory motions, that can produce that sensation. Sound waves are alternate condensation and rarefaction of air. Vibrations in the air cause the eardrum to vibrate. The vibration is then transferred through air to the stapes and beyond it through fluid, endolymph, to the auditory nerve. Thus the sensation of sound is produced. Sound may also be conducted through the bones of the skull.

Sound has three dimensions: loudness, related to the energy of the stimulus; pitch, which refers to lowness or highness of the sound on the scale; and timbre, a quality in overtones by which voices or instruments can be distinguished.

Intensity or loudness of sound is measured by the decibel. A decibel is just about the smallest change in the loudness of a sound that the human ear can detect. The decibel scale ranges from the threshold of audibility (where sound becomes barely audible) to the point at which sound be-

comes so intense that its vibrations can be felt as well as heard. Sound gains in loudness when vibrations increase in size. The voice in ordinary conversation produces 50 to 60 decibels. Sounds above 100 decibels can be felt. Sounds of 120 to 140 decibels cause discomfort in the ears. The ears become painful with sounds of 140 decibels, and the eardrums may rupture with sounds of 160 decibels.

Hearing losses of 40 decibels or more make it quite necessary for a person to use a hearing aid. With a loss of 60 to 90 decibels, a person is very hard of hearing. A loss of 90 decibels or more means practically no hearing. Much greater intensity is required for bone conduction than for air conduction.

Sound intensity can be increased by 10 or 15 decibels (1) by having the speaker talk louder or (2) by having the patient cup his ears. However, the most efficient and practical aid to hearing is the electric hearing aid, the main objective of which is to make speech intelligible. Two general types of receivers are the air-conduction type and the bone-conduction type. The newer types of hearing aids work by means of transistors and batteries. Three styles of hearing aids are the instrument worn on the body, the portable unit that can be placed on a table, and the group model. With the body instrument the battery can be worn on the chest, within the temple piece of eyeglasses, over the ear, or in the pinna of the ear, either monaurally or binaurally.

Pitch of sound is based on frequency of vibrations or on the number of air vibrations that reach the ear in 1 second. When the pitch is high, the vibrations are more rapidly produced. The normal ear can hear sound waves ranging from 20 to 20,000 vibrations in 1 second, a range of nearly ten octaves. The important hearing range is between 500 and 2,000 vibrations. Useful conversation lies between 256 and 2,048 cycles. Sounds whose frequencies are above 20,000, called supersonic or ultrasonic, have been used as a method of sterilizing some substances or treating some conditions.

Air in the middle ear cavity maintains air pressure equal to that outside, so that vibrations can take place. The eustachian tube keeps the air pressure against the inside surface of the eardrum equal to the air pressure against the outside surface of the drum. The faintest audible tone causes the eardrum to move less than 100 millionths of an inch.

The eardrum has an area twenty times that of the oval window (Fig. 27-6), so that the pressure of the sound wave is increased twentyfold when it acts on the base of the stapes. An increase of pressure is needed because the vibrations are transferred from a medium of low resistance or air to one of greater density, the fluid in the internal ear. The three ossicles can be regarded as a lever with two arms. Since fluids are incompressible, each vibration transferred through the endolymph is felt by the delicate hair cells of the organ of Corti, and the vibration causes movement of the round window.

The ears are delicate structures and must be guarded from infection or injury that might affect hearing. The tortuous external canal and the cerumen serve to protect the eardrum from infection. Sometimes boils occur in the canal, and they may be very painful because the canal is unyielding. Various forms of mold or fungi find ideal conditions for growth in the outer canal.

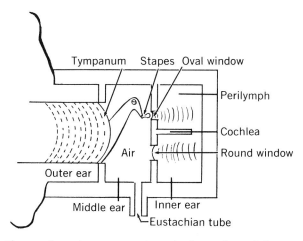

Fig. 27-6. The eardrum has an area twenty times that of the oval window.

Infection in the middle ear is called otitis media. The middle ear is subject to bacterial invasion by way of the eustachian tube from the nose and the throat. Infection may spread to the mastoid area because of continuity of the mucous membrane. It may spread to the meninges and cause fatal results. The middle ear provides a warm, moist, and dark environment for the development of microorganisms. *Treponema pallidum, pneumococcus,* and *Streptococcus* are destructive or virulent organisms that may attack the middle ear. The toxins of scarlet fever and other infectious diseases may produce complications in the ear.

Chronic otitis media is the commonest

ear disease and is the chief cause of progressive deafness. Extension of infection from diseased teeth, tonsils, and adenoids may affect the ear. The virus of the common cold may pass into the middle ear as a result of incorrect noseblowing, which forces organisms from the nasopharynx through the eustachian tube and into the middle ear.

Common diagnostic measures

The ear may be examined visually with an instrument known as an otoscope. It consists of a speculum and a magnifying lens. By means of a light reflected from a head mirror, the examiner can observe the condition of the external auditory canal

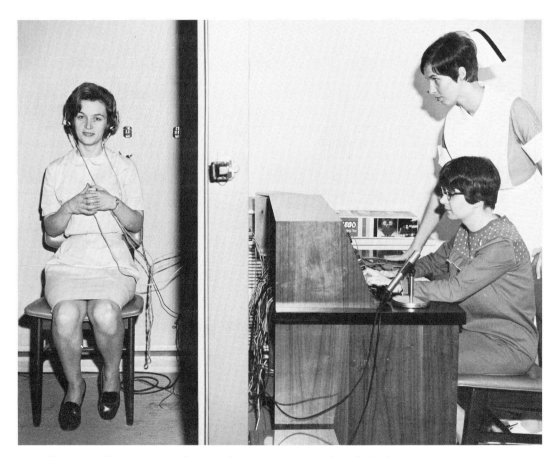

Fig. 27-7. The nurse works with the therapist in seeking help for the hard-of-hearing patient.

and the tympanic membrane. Minor treatments may also be administered through the speculum.

The ability to hear is tested with an electrical audiometer, and a chart of the hearing curve, which is referred to as an audiogram, is made (Fig. 27-7). An audiometer is an apparatus that produces sound waves of different pitch with variable intensity, and it is used for testing hearing acuity. Sometimes a tuning fork or a ticking watch is used. More often the vocal or the whispered word may be used for testing.

Local treatments of the ear

Treatments of the ear that a nurse performs include irrigation and the application of drugs in the form of liquid or ointment. An ear irrigation is the flushing of the external ear canal with a stream of solution. The irrigation may be accomplished by means of a rubber ear bulb or by means of a can suspended on a pole and small tubing, perhaps a catheter. A basin for the return flow and some protection for the bed will be needed. The metal Pomeroy syringe, which produces much pressure, is used for irrigation when the purpose is the removal of impacted wax. Liquid drugs may be instilled by means of a medicine dropper. Ointments are applied by means of an applicator. Drugs may be applied to the ear to soften the skin, to combat infections, or to soften wax.

Purposes of irrigation are to cleanse the external ear canal, to soften impacted wax, to dislodge a foreign body, or to supply heat.

The nurse may assist the physician in performing a myringotomy (L. *myringo-,* eardrum, + Gr. *tomé,* a cutting), which means an incision made in the eardrum. It is also called paracentesis of the ear. The technical term for eardrum is tympanum. Inflammation of the eardrum is called tympanitis (-*itis,* inflammation of). Otodynia (Gr. *ot-,* ear, + Gr. *odyné,* pain, +

-*ia,* condition) or otalgia (Gr. *algos,* pain) means pain in the ear. Otitis media is inflammation of the middle ear. Mastoiditis is inflammation of the air cells of the mastoid process.

Solutions used for ear irrigations are mild. They are usually made from boric acid or salt. If the purpose of the irrigation is to remove a foreign body such as beans or peas (which children sometimes put into their ears), alcohol may be used. It causes such foreign bodies to shrink, thus permitting them to be expelled easily. Oil may be used for other types of foreign bodies. It makes the foreign material slippery, permitting easy expulsion. Hydrogen peroxide is sometimes ordered to soften impacted wax and to aid in its removal. Some ear drops contain an anodyne, a drug that stops pain. Powders and ointments may be instilled in the outer canal to check the growth of fungous infections.

For general infections with complications in the ear the sulfonamides or penicillin may be ordered. Mild ointments or petrolatum may be applied to the skin of the auricle and neck to prevent irritation from ear discharges. Some drugs, such as quinine and the salicylates, cause dizziness, and this symptom should be reported. Vitamins A and B may be ordered as an adjunct in the treatment of some ear conditions to improve the patient's nutritional status in general.

Temperature changes affect the fluids in the internal ear. The eardrum is protected from drafts and changes in temperature by the length of the external canal. The temperature of irrigating solutions and liquid medication should be near body temperature, about 100° F. (37.7° C.), in order not to affect the fluids in the ear. Dizziness, a disturbance of the fluids of the semicircular canals, may occur from too high or too low temperature of irrigating fluid.

Pressure of flow in an irrigation is controlled by the height of the can or by the force applied to the bulb (Fig. 27-8). Pres-

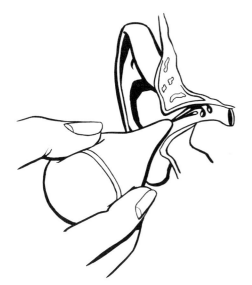

Fig. 27-8. Pressure in an ear irrigation is directed against the back wall of the ear canal.

sure should be low in order not to damage the eardrum. In order to remove impacted wax, pressure irigation may be used. However, irrigations and drops are usually not ordered when there is a perforation of the eardrum. When ointment is applied to the ear and neck to prevent irritation from drainage, the oily layer on the skin keeps the drainage from coming in contact with it.

Psychosocial aspects

Some patients have never had an ear irrigation. Patients who require irrigations may be suffering acute pain or may be in great discomfort. A careful explanation of the procedure will help to allay the patient's fears. The nurse's gentleness in touching the ear will encourage the patient's cooperation, and carefulness in performing the procedure will give the patient greater confidence. Irrigations of the ear can never be performed properly by the patient himself, so he is dependent on the nurse.

Anything unusual about an ear treatment should be reported immediately. The treatment and its results are recorded on the chart for the information of the physician and other nurses.

Every nurse should know how to communicate with a hard-of-hearing patient and should make certain that he understands what is being said, even if writing a note is required. A smile does much to buoy up the spirits of a patient with defective hearing or one who is deaf. The hard-of-hearing patient has some hearing, whereas the deaf person has no hearing. A person who is hard of hearing does not like to be called deaf.

Loss of hearing may be brought on by illness, occupation, or age. Almost everyone past the age of 50 years has lost some of his hearing power or clarity. About 10% of the population of the United States suffers from some degree of hearing loss. Loss of hearing may be temporary or permanent. Some people do not hear low tones well, while others do not hear high tones. Clear hearing can be an all-important factor in social acceptance by friends and family. All human beings need to be wanted and accepted by those near and dear to them and those with whom they come in contact each day. If a person feels he has to shout when he talks to one who is hard of hearing, he too is made to feel uncomfortable.

Many persons with a hearing loss prevent their own return to normal living because they avoid facing the fact, hoping against hope that their hearing may return. Even when they do recognize the problem, they may fail to realize that in many instances hearing can be restored. The first step is for the person to recognize that hearing loss exists and to have a desire to do something about it.

The hard-of-hearing person is usually sensitive about his condition. He tries to guess what people are saying. His hearing loss cuts him off from verbal communications. Frequently he is irritable and angry because he imagines people are

433

talking about him. He may be saddened by loss of contact with others, and he may suffer acute or deep depression as a result of the muffling or deadening of familiar sounds. Unless corrected, impairment of hearing leads to impairment of social and business contacts.

A hearing aid properly chosen and used makes communication with the world possible. It restores relationships with others, and social relationships become more enjoyable.

All hearing impairments are not alike, so hearing aids need to be fitted individually. It takes time, understanding, and determination to learn to wear an aid successfully. Many hearing aid companies keep in contact with their clients for several months and adjust the aids as necessary. With further developments in electronics, hearing aids are constantly improving.

When a person who wears a hearing aid is hospitalized, he should bring it with him and wear it in order to understand the nurses and doctors and to make his adjustment to the hospital easier.

About 3 million children of school age suffer with impairment of hearing, and very often a hearing loss is accompanied by a defect in speech. It not only is harder for deafened children to keep up with their classes, but it also sets them apart from other children. It may create, at an early age, personality problems that may last a lifetime. Some states require hearing tests as part of the school health program. About every 2 years children in each school are given a group audiometric test. The few children revealed to have a hearing deficiency are given individual acuity tests. These tests take from 5 to 15 minutes to administer. The degree of loudness for given tones are plotted on a chart called an audiogram. Any noticeable defect should be investigated promptly by an otologist so that the cause can be found and the condition treated before lasting damage occurs.

The nurse may be instrumental in promoting legislation favoring those with defective hearing and may aid in ear examinations of school children.

The American Society for the Hard of Hearing, founded in 1919 by Wendell C. Phillips, helps persons whose hearing is impaired. It has about 200 local chapters in large cities where persons who are hard of hearing and deaf may join together and promote their own cause.

The ancients considered deaf persons incapable of education, and it was not until the fifteenth century that any significant effort was made to teach deaf children. Now almost every state has a state school for the deaf. All large cities have classes for children who are deaf or hard of hearing. Gallaudet College in Washington, D. C., a national coeducational institution operated under the Department of Health, Education, and Welfare, is the only college for deaf persons in this country. Its students come from all fifty states. They return to their home states and help in educating others with hearing loss or impairment.

The nurse should know the location of local schools or classes for persons who are hard of hearing or deaf to be able to help such patients more effectively. Deaf persons tend to isolate themselves from social affairs because participation involves too great an effort. The nurse can encourage the patient to learn lipreading or to wear a hearing aid if a satisfactory one has been fitted. Many deaf persons use the sign language for communicating within the confines of their own homes. It is sometimes very difficult to reeducate children who have learned this form of communication in early infancy.

PRINCIPLES APPLIED TO TREATMENTS OF THE NOSE AND THROAT

The nose and throat are neighboring structures. Conditions of one very often affect the other. Treatments of the nose may be similar to treatments of the throat.

Structure and functions of the nose and throat

The external nose is composed of a triangular framework of bone and cartilage covered by skin and lined with mucous membrane. The anterior openings of the nose are called nostrils or anterior nares. The two nasal cavities are wedge shaped and separated vertically from one another by a partition or a septum formed by the vomer and adjoining cartilaginous septum. The septum is usually bent to one side so

that the cavities are not equally divided. This point should be remembered when giving nose irrigations. The floor of the nasal cavity is smooth and concave from side to side, $1/2$ inch or more wide, and nearly horizontal. It is shorter and wider than the roof. The roof of the nasal cavity has an anterior part, the slope of which corresponds to the slope of the nasal bridge; a middle portion formed by the cribriform plate of the ethmoid bone, which is perforated by the olfactory nerves; and a posterior part formed by the body of the sphenoid bone. Each chamber of the nose is divided into many spaces by the upper, middle, and lower turbinates,

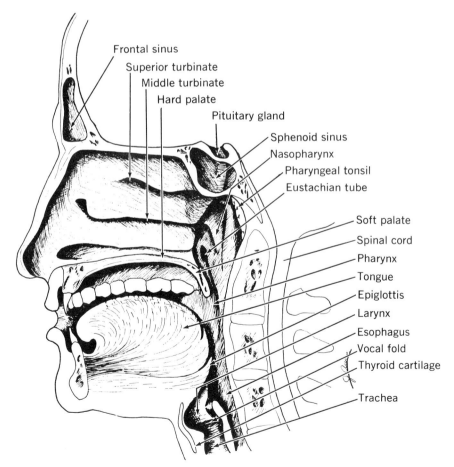

Fig. 27-9. Openings into the nasal canal.

which project diagonally into the lumen of the main cavity (Fig. 27-9).

The nasal cavity just within the external nares is lined with skin. The remaining parts are lined with mucous membrane covered by a layer of ciliated columnar epithelial cells. The mucous membrane is continuous with that lining the accessory nasal sinuses. This fact explains why an infection in the nose may extend into the sinuses. The sinuses are kept clear under normal conditions by the beating action of the cilia, which direct the drainage into the nasal cavity through small openings. The nasolacrimal ducts also empty into the nasal cavities. The mucous lining is extremely vascular, the blood supply being derived from the internal carotid artery. The blood vessels in the nose may be dilated by infections, irritants, allergies, and thermal states of the inspired air. In consequence, the mucosa may swell and narrow the air passage and interfere with the sense of smell.

End organs of the olfactory nerve have a limited distribution, an area about 2.5 sq. cm. in each nostril, in the superior part of the nasal cavity. Not all air that goes through the nose reaches this area. Sniffing will create currents that carry the chemicals in the air upward to the olfactory mucosa. During expiration, the air going from the pharynx does not traverse the olfactory area, and thus odors on expiration are not detected by the individual himself. By passing through the narrow meatuses, the inspired air is warmed, moistened, and filtered. Air is warmed as it passes over the highly vascular mucous membrane. The nasal and sinus mucosa secrete about a quart of fluid daily, a great part of which is used as water vapor to humidify the air passing through the nose. Small hairs in the nose act as an air filter.

The pharynx or throat cavity is a musculomembranous tube shaped somewhat like a cone. It communicates with the nose and the mouth. The part directly behind the nasal cavity is called the nasal pharynx, and that back of the mouth is called the oral pharynx. Mucous membrane lining the pharynx is continuous with that of the nose and mouth. The adenoids are located in the pharynx and sometimes are so large that they obstruct nasal breathing. The tonsils, which are the site of many throat infections, are located in the oral cavity.

A variety of bacteria, among which are the *Streptococcus, Staphylococcus, Meningococcus,* and influenza bacillus, are normally present in the mouth and nose. They do no harm to an intact mucous membrane. They are flushed out of the mouth during oral care or are swallowed into the stomach, where they are rendered harmless by the hydrochloric acid present. Many bacteria of the inspired air are caught in the mucus and are moved outward by the action of cilia in the respiratory passages. Microorganisms may invade the body, causing local or systemic symptoms.

Many communicable diseases begin in the nose and mouth: scarlet fever, diphtheria, pneumonia, tuberculosis, meningitis, septic sore throat, and the common cold. Because of continuity of the mucous lining, infection may spread to the ears or to the eyes. The most serious possibility is the extension of infection to the meninges by way of the olfactory nerve.

In caring for patients with communicable diseases and in handling their nose and mouth discharges, the nurse does so in such a way that the infection will not be spread. Medical aseptic technique is presented in Chapter 32. It includes such measures as use of an isolation gown, handwashing between patients, proper handling of linen and other equipment, and the provision of paper bags for disposing of wipes. The nurse avoids being in the direct line of spray from the nose or throat when the patient sneezes or coughs.

Common treatments of the nose and throat

Nose and throat irrigations are ordered, though infrequently. Drugs are sprayed into the nose and throat. Gargles and painting may be ordered for the throat. An irrigation is the flushing of a part by a stream of liquid. A nose irrigation may be called a nasal douche, and a throat irrigation may be called a pharyngeal douche.

The purposes of nose and throat irrigations are to soften and to remove discharges, to relieve pain and swelling, and to apply heat. Throat irrigations are more effective than gargling because the throat is more relaxed during an irrigation. The throat may be painted with an applicator in case of acute soreness. Liquid drugs are dropped in the nose to check bacterial growth or to shrink tissue.

The same equipment is needed for irrigation of both the nose and throat. Disposable equipment consists of a plastic bag and a plastic irrigating tip. A large basin for the return flow is also needed. Some kind of protector will be required for the bed and the patient, preferably a rubber apron, with a towel for the lap. An atomizer is used for spraying drugs into the nose or throat. Liquid drugs may be instilled into the nose by means of a medicine dropper.

Solutions used for nose and throat irrigations are made from mild nonirritating drugs: sodium chloride, sodium bicarbonate, or boric acid. The same solutions may be used for gargles. Sometimes syrupy solutions are used as gargles since they stick in the throat. Drugs used to paint the throat are stronger preparations than those used for irrigations or gargles. Such drugs may be silver nitrate, iodine, or merbromin (Mercurochrome). Ephedrine or phenylephrine hydrochloride, found in many nose drops, constrict the congested mucosa and makes breathing easier. Some nose drops contain antiseptics or anodynes. Some have an oil base that stays on the mucous membrane and softens crusts, and others have a water base. For general infections that begin in the nose or throat, the sulfonamides or oral antibiotics may be ordered. The antihistamines are used to ward off symptoms, and the analgesic antipyretic drugs are given to reduce fever and relieve general aches and pains. These drugs are usually administered systemically. Some drugs used for local effect are put up in the form of candy or chewing gum.

Pressure in a throat irrigation may be higher than in a nose irrigation, since in the latter case infectious material might be forced into the sinuses or the eustachian tube. Since the pressure depends on the height of the irrigating can, the can should be hung about 24 inches above the outlet in a throat irrigation and 12 inches above the outlet in a nose irrigation. Temperature of solution for a throat irrigation may be about 110° F., since the mouth can stand higher temperatures than any part of the body. The temperature of the solution for a nose irrigation may be 105° F.

The position of the patient for either throat or nose irrigation should be such that the solution will run freely in and out. The patient should be sitting with the head bent forward. When instilling drops in the nose, gravity will help if the head is hyperextended.

As the bulb of the atomizer is squeezed in a nose or throat spray, air is forced out of the bulb and moves along to the outlet, creating a low-pressure area on either side of the rapidly moving air. Atmospheric pressure on the solution in the bottle forces the solution into the low-pressure area,

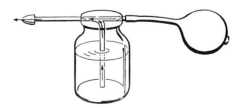

Fig. 27-10. The action of the atomizer is based on Bernoulli's effect.

and the solution is carried out with the next squeeze on the bulb in the form of a fine spray. This is known as Bernoulli's effect (Fig. 27-10).

Air reaches the olfactory area in the upper regions of the nasal chambers by diffusion. Since diffusion is hastened with increased motion of the air, sniffing, or drawing the air in forcibly, causes the air to reach the olfactory nerves quickly.

Psychosocial aspects

The patient who requires nose or throat treatments is very uncomfortable, if not in actual pain. He may be very irritable and does not wish to experience any more pain or discomfort than he already has. The nurse may explain that nose and throat treatments are comforting, that they bring easier breathing and relaxation, and that they may relieve pain caused by congestion. Use of the equipment is explained and the patient is allowed to hold the irrigator if it makes him feel more secure. Precautions are explained to him if he has an infectious condition. To elicit his cooperation if he is isolated because of a communicable disease, the nurse should explain why isolation techniques are carried out and find reasons to visit him often so that he will not feel cut off from the rest of the world.

A patient who is in bed suffering from a nose or throat infection is dependent on someone else to help him with his treatments. He may need to be reminded that he should not expose others to his condition, and he should think especially of his family. The reasons for isolation precautions need to be explained to visitors so that they will cooperate. The nurse reports to the physician any unusual symptoms or results of treatments and also records the treatment and its results on the chart.

Conditions of the nose and throat are important because many serious diseases have their beginnings with a cold. In the United States colds cost hundreds of millions of dollars each year and about 100 million working days, besides the cost of drugs and medical care. The common cold is continuously pandemic. More than one half the people in the United States have two colds a year. Colds are most frequent in March and October.

LEARNING SITUATIONS FOR THE PATIENT
Patients with therapeutic measures of the eye

The patient needs to be prepared for the effects that he will experience with some medications, such as temporary changes in vision or sensations that may be experienced following some eye drops. It is necessary to explain to the patient how he can assist by assuming the most helpful, comfortable, relaxed position, by fixing his gaze on some object, by closing (not squeezing) the eyelids gently after a treatment, and by keeping his hands away from his face.

The patient who is receiving eye treatments may have many questions. The nurse may explain the physician's directions to the patient and impress upon him the necessity of following them. It may be necessary to encourage the patient to continue treatments over a long period of time. If eye irrigations are to be continued at home, the patient and whoever will do the irrigating must understand the importance of using the prescribed method. An eye irrigation at home may require the cooperation of the entire family.

It may be appropriate to explain that eye health depends on the general health and nutrition of the entire body. Information about the importance of adequate lighting and correct body posture while reading and doing close work may be indicated for some patients. The nurse may have an opportunity to speak of measures to protect the eye from infections, such as keeping dirty fingers and soiled linen from the eyes, using individual towels and washcloths, not using the same eye covering on different children in blindfold games, and washing the hands before treating the eye.

The patient may be told of the danger of home remedies and be advised that an ophthalmologist should be consulted for any eye condition. The differences between an ophthalmologist, an optometrist, and an optician should be explained to the patient.

The nurse may remind the patient to have periodic eye examinations and may show the patient how to lay his glasses down so that the lenses will not be scratched.

The patient's family and· visitors may need to learn how they can aid in his recovery. Their conversations may be pleasant diversions for the patient who cannot use his eyes. They will need to learn not to jar the bed since the nerves of the eyes are very sensitive and to be told to identify themselves as they enter the unit of a patient whose eyes are bandaged.

Patients with therapeutic measures of the ear

It is usually best to observe the patient's level of understanding about his condition and health practices to avoid repeating what he already knows. It may be appropriate to discuss with individual patients the need for treatment of nose and throat infections by a physician, since microorganisms can be spread to the middle ear by way of the eustachian tube. The patient should obtain medical care for all forms of earache in order to keep the condition from becoming chronic and gradually endangering his hearing.

The patient should be warned against putting sharp or pointed instruments in the ear. If the external canal needs to be cleaned, a cotton-tipped toothpick may be used. Instruction should also be given against the indiscriminate use of drugs in the ear.

The proper method of blowing the nose may be explained to the patient—either to blow one side at a time or to keep the mouth open while blowing, thus preventing excessive pressure in the eustachian tube.

Ear infections may be prevented by proper diet, rest, and exercise. Many ear infections may seriously complicate some of the communicable diseases, and so the patient should be encouraged to obtain medical treatment for such diseases.

Since a child may be born with defective hearing as the result of syphilis, patients with syphilis must be made aware of the possible results of this disease and be encouraged to obtain and continue treatments.

The nurse can urge upon relatives the importance of treating a hard-of-hearing person as a normal individual. The necessity of talking in a normal voice directly to him should be pointed out. The relatives may be informed of local facilities for persons who are deaf or hard of hearing.

Although frowned upon by speech and hearing therapists, sign language is used quite commonly in the homes of the deaf. Some deaf children, because of other complications, may not be capable of learning to lipread. However, they may be able to learn sign language. It may also be quite easily learned by hearing parents of deaf children. Classes in sign language are sponsored by many local community churches and other organizations and are usually available at no cost.

The patient may be informed of the services of the Visiting Nurse Association when an ear irrigation is needed to be given at home. The visiting nurse may have an ear bulb in the equipment bag but will need a container for the solution and a pan for the return flow from household equipment. The nurse may instruct someone in the family how to make the solution, perhaps how to give an irrigation, and how to protect others in the family from an infectious condition.

Patients with therapeutic measures of the nose and throat

The administration of a nose or throat treatment provides an opportunity for the nurse to emphasize health habits to the patient. The purposes of the treatment and what he may do to cooperate in the treatment may be explained to the patient. Measures to assist in preventing reinfection may be suggested, together with discussion regarding the period of infectiousness and the mode of transmission of causative organisms. Specific instructions may include avoiding direct contact with others, using paper wipes that are destroyed properly, and guarding others from the spray of sneezing and coughing by placing a tissue over the nose or mouth.

A mother might receive suggestions about isolating her children at home and how to dispose of nose and throat discharges. A patient may be taught how to prepare a salt or soda solution at home for an irrigation or gargle.

The nurse should discourage the indiscriminate use of nose drops and other self-medication. When needed, nose drops should be prescribed by the physician. If they are needed by more than one member of the family, each should have his own medicine dropper and bottle of medicine.

SUMMARY

The nursing role in the care of patients receiving therapeutic measures of the eye, ear, nose, and throat is concerned with prevention, administering treatments, dealing with the patient's anxieties, and participating in the rehabilitation process, particularly for the patient with loss of a special sense.

Examples of principles relevant to such treatments are presented as being useful in meeting the patient's needs with understanding, administering prescribed treatments safely, and alerting the nurse to the presence of significant symptoms. These principles are applied to nursing responsibilities in common therapeutic measures of the eye, ear, nose, and throat.

QUESTIONS FOR DISCUSSION

1 What is the effect of a warm irrigation on the eye?
2 How may a nurse prevent eye infections among patients?
3 List several types of drugs that are used in the eye and give their purposes.
4 What should be the temperature of solution for an eye irrigation? Why?
5 Identify the specific nursing needs most apt to be encountered in the care of the patient with:
  a Cataract extraction
  b Retinal detachment
6 Identify the important points in technique for administering:
  a Eye drops
  b Eye ointment
  c Eye compresses
  d Eye irrigation
7 When giving on eye irrigation, why should the flow be directed from the inner canthus toward the outer canthus?
8 Give details of feeding a patient who has both eyes bandaged.
9 What social agencies are concerned with eye health?
10 What can you teach a mother about care of her children's eyes?
11 Describe the external ear, the middle ear, and the internal ear.
12 What are the purposes of ear irrigations?
13 What ear structures are concerned with sound conduction?
14 What structures are concerned with sound perception?
15 What is meant by deaf?
16 What bacteria cause most ear infections?
17 How is skin under the ear protected from drainage from the ear?
18 Of what significance is it to the nurse that the mucous membrane of the nasopharynx

is continuous with that of the eustachian tube?

19 What precautions should be observed when the patient has a perforated tympanic membrane?

20 Explain how a nurse may assist a hard-of-hearing patient to feel accepted.

21 What social agencies are interested in ear health?

22 What may you teach a mother in regard to ear health for her children?

23 How would you make a normal saline solution for a throat irrigation?

24 Why may more force be used in a throat irrigation than in a nose irrigation?

25 Describe the equipment used in irrigating a throat.

26 What passages open into the nose?

27 What bacteria normally inhabit the mouth?

28 Name several diseases that begin as a cold.

29 Explain the disadvantages of mouth breathing as compared with breathing through the nose.

LIFE SITUATION

1. Mrs. Jones, 79 years of age, is a patient in a four-bed ward in which there are three other patients who do much reading and insist on turning on the ceiling lights. Mrs. Jones complains that the ceiling lights bother her. How would you handle the situation?

2. Mr. Johnston, 69 years of age, has been hospitalized for a fractured femur. He is hard of hearing and wears a hearing aid. Because of his inability to move about, he sometimes misplaces his aid or fails to adjust it properly. When this happens, he becomes very upset and bangs on the furniture until the nurse arrives and fixes it for him. The other patients become frustrated with his noise and demand that the nurse teach Mr. Johnston to use his signal light to call the nurse instead of banging on the furniture. How should the nurse handle the situation?

3. The nurse instilled drops into Mr. Bond's nose. He said, "You put in only 3 drops. When I put them in, I put in a whole dropperful, blow my nose, cough some out, and then put in another dropperful. Why do you think your 3 drops will do any good?" How will you answer Mr. Bond?

SUGGESTED PERFORMANCE CHECKLIST

Comfort

1 Is the treatment explained beforehand?

2 Is the patient reassured during the treatment?

3 Is the patient told how he may hold the irrigating tip?

4 Is the patient comfortable in a sitting position?

5 Is the tube warmed before an irrigation by letting some solution run through it?

6 During an irrigation, is the solution introduced in a slow, steady flow?

7 Is the patient furnished with tissue wipes?

Therapeutic effect

1 Does the nurse speak as she approaches a blind patient or one whose eyes are bandaged?

2 Is the eye opened as wide as possible during an irrigation?

3 Is the treatment given on time?

4 Is the treatment given in the manner ordered?

5 Is gentleness shown?

6 Are pertinent observations made?

7 Are unusual symptoms reported?

8 Is charting pertinent and accurate?

9 Are the nurse's movements smooth and sure?

Economy

1 Is the equipment assembled quickly?

2 Is the equipment brought to the bedside in one trip?

3 Are the bed and the patient protected from wetting?

4 Is the basin for return flow of adequate size?

5 Is all equipment removed in one trip?

6 Is used equipment cared for at once?

Safety

1 Is sufficient light provided?

2 If solutions are used in the eye, is the percentage correct?

3 Is the temperature of the solution correct?

4 Is low pressure used in instilling the solution?

5 Are adherent eyelids moistened before opening?

6 Is pressure put against the forehead and the cheek in opening the eyelids?

7 Is the position the patient should assume explained before beginning the treatment?

8 Is care used not to let the irrigating tip or dropper touch the conjunctiva?

9 Is the dropper inspected before use?

10 If only one eye is treated, is the unaffected eye protected?

11 Is equipment sterile or clean as needed?

12 Is medical aseptic technique observed with infectious conditions?

13 Does the nurse wash hands before and after the treatment?

14 Are the nurse's nails short and well rounded?

15 Is the manner of breathing during a throat irrigation explained before beginning?

16 If a spray is used, is the pressure gentle?

17 Is the ear canal straightened before administering ear drops or irrigation?

18 Is the irrigating tip not inserted more than $1/4$ inch?

SUGGESTED READINGS

Condl, Emma D.: Ophthalmic nursing, Nursing Clinics of North America **5**:467, September, 1970.

Conover, Mary, and Cober, Joyce: Understanding and caring for the hearing-impaired, Nursing Clinics of North America **5**:497, September, 1970.

Cullin, Irene C.: Techniques for teaching patients with sensory defects, Nursing Clinics of North America **5**:527, September, 1970.

Hamilton, Mary Jo: What the nurse should know about eye banks, Nursing Clinics of North America **5**:483, September, 1970.

Havener, William H., and others: Nursing care in eye, ear, nose and throat disorders, St. Louis, 1974, The C. V. Mosby Co.

Linnell, Craig, and others: The hearing impaired infant, Nursing Clinics of North America **5**:507, September, 1970.

Ohno, Mary I.: The eye-patched patient, American Journal of Nursing **71**:271, February, 1971.

Parvulescu, Nina F.: Care of the surgically speechless patient, Nursing Clinics of North America **5**:517, September, 1970.

Payne, Peter D., and others: Behavior manifestations of children with hearing loss, American Journal of Nursing **70**:1718, August, 1970.

Rabb, Maurice F.: The present status of corneal transplantation, Nursing Clinics of North America **5**:477, September, 1970.

Seaman, Florence W.: Nursing care of glaucoma patients, Nursing Clinics of North America **5**:489, September, 1970.

28 Gastrointestinal disorders

GASTROINTESTINAL TRACT INTEGRITY AND BODILY NUTRITION

The physiologic needs of the individual for food, fluids, and electrolytes have been reviewed in previous chapters. Not only must the food materials be made available to the body, but they must first be processed into the form of usable substances suitable for cellular utilization. This implies that the foods ingested are dependent upon the functioning of the stomach and other portions of the gastrointestinal tract designed for food processing. The processing includes the chemical changes of digestion and the absorption of the processed nutrients into the bloodstream.

The passage of food through the gastrointestinal tract creates some mechanical stress on the structures, particularly in the stomach, where the lining is most apt to be traumatized by the undigested food particles and where the secretions are strongly acid.

It is not surprising that the stomach is subject to a rather high incidence of disorders, particularly in view of such contributing factors as faulty habits, for example, improper selection of food, rushing through meals, irregular meals, inadequate rest, stress, emotional conflicts, and psychic trauma. A variety of causative factors may lead to local irritation giving rise to malaise, nausea, vomiting, anorexia, hyperactivity of the gastrointestinal tract, abdominal cramps, and diarrhea.

Normally, the mucosa of the stomach is protected from the highly acid gastric juices by mucous secretions that coat the lining. In the event of either the increase in corrosive properties of the gastric juices as a result of hypersecretion or of local decrease in mucosal resistance, erosion and ulcer formation may occur.

When there is disturbance in the integrity of the food processing function, whether directly as a result of pathophysiology in the stomach itself or as indirectly

443

resulting from other disorders within the body, cellular nutrition will suffer. Nursing problems related to these disturbances include (1) carrying out various treatments of the stomach intended to maintain proper function, (2) maintaining adequate nutrition, and (3) participating in the administration of measures for the maintenance and/or restoration of fluid and electrolyte balance in the event of excessive vomiting or protracted diarrhea. The discussion in this chapter is concerned primarily with the common local treatments of the gastrointestinal tract.

COMMON DYSFUNCTIONS RELATED TO THE GASTROINTESTINAL TRACT

Common symptoms referable to the gastrointestinal tract, such as distension, flatulence, epigastric distress, complaint of nausea with or without vomiting, or pain, occur with many systemic conditions. These symptoms should be reported promptly so that the nature and severity of the problem may be evaluated.

Nausea and vomiting

Nausea and vomiting are symptoms seen in a great variety of medical and surgical conditions. Vomiting is a reflex response that is effective in removing potentially harmful ingested material from the stomach. To this extent it is a protective mechanism. However, severe vomiting results in dehydration, electrolyte depletion, and, if prolonged, interference with nutrition.

The physician will seek to determine the cause of vomiting and prescribe appropriate treatment for its control. His plan for treatment may include (1) antiemetic drugs such as sedatives, antihistamines, phenothiazines, and anticholinergics (the last causing delayed emptying time of the stomach through depressed gastric motility), (2) nasogastric intubation with continuous or intermittent suction to relieve

distension, and (3) parenteral therapy to replace fluids and electrolytes lost in vomitus.

Well-planned nursing care can accomplish a great deal toward decreasing the ill effects for the patient experiencing nausea and vomiting. The aims of nursing care would need to be adjusted according to the individual patient's problems but would include the following:

1. Minimizing factors contributing to vomiting or increasing its severity
2. Minimizing the problems that may occur as a result of vomiting, including:
   a. Aspiration of vomitus for the unconscious or semiconscious patient or for one who has defective reflexes for any reason
   b. Fluid and electrolyte depletion
   c. Interference with nutrition
3. Administering measures prescribed in the medical management for the patient in a manner so as to obtain the maximum desired effect of the therapy

To assist in minimizing the factors contributing to vomiting, the nurse may look for clues useful in determining its cause and progress. Information relating to the onset, frequency, duration, type, odor, color, amount, and character of emesis is significant. For example, the presence of red blood in the vomitus or coffee-ground appearance would be significant; the presence and odor of fecal material might indicate obstruction; observation of absence or presence of retching, or projectile type vomiting, or abdominal cramps and diarrhea would also be significant. Noting changes in symptoms is useful in evaluating the success of the medical therapy and the nursing plan for patient care.

Some of the problems associated with vomiting may sometimes be lessened in severity by such nursing measures as (1) changing the patient's position slowly to diminish vestibular nerve impulses; (2) administering prescribed medications at specified time intervals to maintain the effective blood level; (3) keeping the environment pleasant (for example, prompt cleansing of the emesis basin, providing mouthwash, clean linen, and ventilation as indicated after each emesis, eliminating disagreeable sounds and odors); (4) maintaining accurate intake and output records and noting symptoms of dehydration and electrolyte depletion; (5) maintaining drainage for the patient with nasogastric intubation; (6) encouraging oral fluids as soon as permitted, offering either hot or cold fluids, such as tea and carbonated beverages; and (7) identifying the patient's concerns early and providing emotional support.

Nursing action that may lessen the hazard of aspirating vomitus is directed toward maintaining an unobstructed airway. Artificial dentures should be removed, and unless contraindicated, the patient may be positioned on the side. When the head is supported over an emesis basin during episodes of vomiting, gravity will aid the outflow of vomitus. Use of suctioning equipment may be indicated to remove vomitus safely from the mouth and throat of some patients to prevent aspiration.

Accurate recording of observations, treatments, and nursing care and the patient's reaction to these is important in evaluating and adjusting the continuing plan of nursing care.

Diarrhea

Dysfunction of the lower intestinal tract may be manifested by accelerated or retarded movement of contents through the intestine. Accelerated movement of contents results in frequent unformed, or even liquid, stools. Like vomiting, diarrhea is a symptom of many different disorders that may be either systemic diseases or local conditions within the bowel.

An intrinsic disorder of the bowel resulting in diarrhea may be an organic disease with characteristic changes, or the bowel may be structurally normal, the hypermotility being functional. In other words, diarrhea is not in itself a disease but rather is a symptom with many possible different etiologic classifications.

The effects of diarrhea depend to some extent upon the cause. It may be temporary, subsiding as soon as the irritating causative factor is eliminated from the intestine, or it may tend to be persistent, as for example in diverticulitis. There may also be remissions and exacerbations. Whatever the cause, severe and prolonged diarrhea may result in depletion of body fluids, electrolytes, and nutrients lost in the frequent liquid stools, producing rapid loss of weight and strength. Serious and even irreversible fatal effects may develop rapidly, particularly when the diarrhea is accompanied by vomiting. This is especially true of infants and the elderly for whom prompt treatment is necessary at the onset.

The condition of diarrhea is usually quite disturbing to the patient because he is embarrassed by the frequency, urgency, and odor of the stools and because of the irritation that may develop in the anal region. However, anyone experiencing diarrhea for more than a day or two or who has repeated attacks should have medical attention.

During diagnostic procedures to determine the cause of the diarrhea, symptomatic and supportive measures are provided. In severe diarrhea these usually include the following:

1. Bed rest to help reduce peristalsis and conserve the patient's energy. Keeping a clean covered bedpan at the bedside may help the patient who is having great urgency to relax.

2. Record of fluid balance kept as accurately as possible.

3. Replacement of fluids and electrolytes, usually intravenously. When oral

445

fluids are tolerated, water, tea, fat-free broth, and cereal are allowed by most physicians, depending on the individual patient's total condition.

4. Local hygienic care of the anal region to control the irritation that usually develops. This includes cleansing with soap and water following each defecation and, after thorough drying, the application of medicated cream or powder as prescribed for the patient. Soiled linens should be changed promptly.

5. Application of the principles of medical aseptic technique usually indicated for the patient with a potentially infectious condition. It may be necessary to include disinfection of the feces before disposal. Even though the patient may not be isolated, it is still important to practice thorough handwashing between patients and after handling bedpans or linen.

6. Administration of medications that may be prescribed for a variety of effects in the treatment of diarrhea. The nurse needs to understand the purpose of each medication in order to properly observe and evaluate the effect of the medication on the individual patient. For example, camphorated tincture of opium (paregoric) may be given to reduce peristalsis; aluminum silicate (Kaopectate, kaolin) may be used to form a protective coating on the intestinal mucosa or as an adsorbent; or sulfonamide preparations, such as succinylsulfathiazole (Sulfasuxidine) when the diarrhea is a result of microbial infection. Sulfasuxidine is an example of a drug that is poorly absorbed and that therefore has a local effect in the intestine.

7. It may be appropriate for the nurse to discuss with the patient or family members the hazards of unrefrigerated foods, such as meats and creamed dishes, the importance of sanitary measures in the handling and preparation of foods, and the need for thorough handwashing after use of the toilet.

Constipation

Retarded movement of intestinal contents results in constipation, a dysfunction of the large intestine that interferes with the excretion of bowel waste. Constipation is characterized by hard, dry, infrequent stools because the prolonged retention of the fecal material permits the absorption of greater amounts of water, resulting in the unusual stool consistency.

As with diarrhea, there are a variety of causative factors that may be either functional or associated with organic disease. However, there is a wide range in patterns of defecation habits in apparently healthy persons that is considered normal for the individual. However, when changes occur in an individual's usual pattern of defecation, with delayed passage of hard dry stools, the problem of constipation may be said to have developed (Fig. 28-1).

Although many factors or combinations of factors may have caused the constipation, the prolonged distension of the rectum and the accompanying anxiety are usually associated with typical symptoms including flatulence, malaise, abdominal discomfort, anorexia, headache, and perhaps a coated tongue and unpleasant breath.

Management of the problem of constipation varies with the causative factors affecting a particular patient and the pathophysiology involved. Unless the problem proves to be temporary, diagnostic measures are instituted by the physician; these may include proctoscopic examination, x-ray studies, and examination of the stool. The finding of occult blood in the stool together with alternating constipation and diarrhea will suggest the presence of cancer. History of the patient's living habits, emotional problems, dietary and defecation patterns, and use of laxatives and enemas may reveal clues to some of the causative factors in chronic constipation.

Treatment measures initiated by the

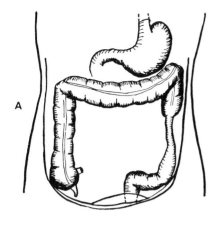

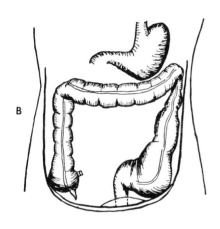

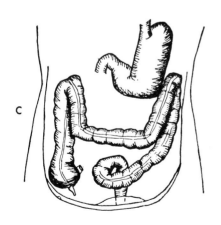

Fig. 28-1. Anatomic causes of constipation. **A,** Spastic; **B,** atony (loss of tone); and **C,** ptosis (sagging of transverse colon).

physician are directed toward correction of the causative factors, but palliative measures will usually be included: (1) dietary modifications as indicated for the particular individual (details are described in diet therapy texts); (2) adequate fluid intake; (3) exercises to increase strength of abdominal muscles; and (4) medications that may assist in restoring the defecation reflex (usually avoiding the individual's customary laxatives or enemas).

The problem of *fecal impaction,* which is an overloading of the bowel with a hardened fecal mass, is described in Chapter 19, Rehabilitation in Nursing, in conjunction with the abnormal functioning of body systems that tends to occur during the prolonged inactivity of bed rest.

The objectives of nursing care for the patient with retarded movement of intestinal contents must be adjusted according to the individual's total situation but usually will include participation in at least some or all of the following:

1. Identifying factors contributing to the patient's bowel problem

2. Administering prescribed treatments in a manner to obtain maximum effectiveness

3. Assisting in restoration and maintenance of a defecation pattern that is normal for the individual patient:

   a. Adjusting fluid and dietary patterns according to the individual patient's reactions

   b. Instructing the patient regarding diet, exercise, and normal ranges in patterns of defecation, clarifying any misinformation for him

   c. Providing uninterrupted time and privacy and adjusting routines to accommodate the patient's most opportune time for bowel movements

   d. Encouraging the patient to establish regular habits of dietary and fluid intake and exercise

COMMON TREATMENTS OF THE LOWER INTESTINAL TRACT

Treatments are given primarily to (1) aid elimination, (2) relieve intestinal flatus, and (3) administer medication for either local or systemic effect. Such treatments include the cleansing enema, the retention enema, the Harris flush, and suppositories. The suppository is a form of drug therapy and is discussed in more detail under medications.

The *cleansing enema,* or injection of fluid into the rectum, is an irrigation of the lower bowel. It may be administered for the purpose of promoting elimination of feces and flatus in constipation or to cleanse the lower bowel in preparation for examination, x-ray, or surgery. A cool solution may, on rare occasion, be injected to assist in reducing fever. The carminative enema is used to induce expulsion of flatus and the anthelmintic enema to aid in elimination of intestinal parasites. The type of irrigating fluid is selected according to the desired effect.

The *retention enema* is usually an oily preparation given for its lubricant action, that is, to make evacuation of feces easier in constipation or painful rectal conditions. Oils such as mineral oil, olive oil, or cottonseed oil are suitable to use for this purpose. Since the oil is to be retained for approximately 1 hour, a small amount is administered, about 150 ml. at room temperature, given slowly under low pressure.

Two other intestinal treatments that may still be seen occasionally in some parts of the country are the colonic irrigation and the proctoclysis. The colonic irrigation is a thorough flushing of the colon given to cleanse, to alter body temperature, or to help remove toxins from the large intestine. The proctoclysis is a slow injection of a large quantity of fluid into the rectum for absorption into the body. However, this treatment is seldom used because of the more effective results obtained by intravenous techniques.

The *Harris flush* is an irrigation of the lower bowel that is similar to the cleansing enema. It is given primarily to aid in the expulsion of intestinal flatus. It differs from the enema in that after the solution has been injected, the rectal tube is left in place and the solution is allowed to flow by gravity between the irrigating can and the intestine as the irrigating can is alternately raised and lowered above and below the level of the patient's hips. This process tends to stimulate peristalsis, which in turn encourages the onward movement of gas and its expulsion with the outflow of the irrigating fluid.

It may be necessary to give a cleansing enema prior to the Harris flush to avoid clogging the rectal tube with fecal material. Since the advent of early ambulation and the cholinergic drugs, which stimulate gastrointestinal motility postoperatively, the Harris flush is seldom used. When medications are used for this purpose, some physicians may order in addition such mechanical measures as application of heat to the abdomen and the insertion of a rectal tube to aid in removal of intestinal gases.

The *rectal tube,* intended to assist in expelling flatus, is inserted in the same manner as when giving an enema except that the distal end is placed in a container with a small amount of water rather than being connected to an irrigating can. Bubbles in the water indicate expulsion of flatus. The tube is left in place 20 to 30 minutes to provide for expulsion of flatus for the patient with depressed gastrointestinal tone and motility. Reinsertion of the tube at 2- to 3-hour intervals as needed will avoid fatigue of the anal sphincters.

Equipment used in intestinal treatments

Equipment for giving a nonretention enema will include a reservoir for the solution and the tubing. The reservoir may be an irrigating can, a rubber bag, or a pitcher. With a can or a bag, about 3 feet of tubing is needed, connecting the reservoir to the rectal tip or tube. With a pitcher, a funnel is attached to the rectal tube. Other materials needed are a lubricant, toilet tissue, a drape, a bedpan, and protection for the bed unless the patient can use the bathroom. The size of the colon tube depends on the size and the condition of the patient. Colon and rectal tubes vary in length from 20 to 30 inches and in diameter from 22 to 32 Fr. The French scale (one unit is 0.33 mm. in outside diameter) is used for measuring colon and rectal tubes as well as catheters and stomach tubes. Disposable enema equipment, consisting of a plastic container, tubing, clamp, and lubricant, is commercially available (Fig. 28-2). Some units also contain a small amount of concentrated liquid soap. Enema solutions also come in disposable plastic squeeze bottles with a prelubricated tip.

Equipment for giving a retention enema consists of a small colon tube or catheter, a funnel or Asepto syringe, and a container for the solution. No bedpan is necessary

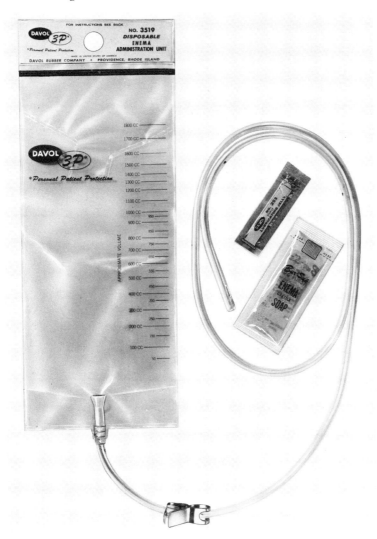

Fig. 28-2. Enema administration unit. (Courtesy Davol Rubber Co., Providence, R. I.)

but one should be available in case the enema is expelled prematurely. In most instances commercial preparations are used, in which case no special equipment is necessary.

Equipment for a colonic irrigation consists of an irrigating can, tubing with a Y connector, two spring cocks, a pail for overflow, a lubricant, toilet tissue, a drape, a pole, and a gallon pitcher for the solution.

For the patient who has a colostomy there are also available disposable colostomy irrigation sets.

Scientific principles

Some of the representative principles stated here appear in other contexts, which supports the premise that many principles useful in explaining the scientific basis for a nursing action are applicable in a variety of nursing situations.

1. Friction, which is the force opposing motion between two contacting surfaces, may be decreased by the presence of a lubricant smoothing and separating the two surfaces.

2. Fluids will flow only when there is a difference in pressure, the direction being to the area of lower pressure.

3. The rate of flow of a solution in a tube varies with the pressure, the caliber of the tube, and the density of the fluid.

4. The height of a column of fluid determines the amount of pressure exerted at the point of application.

5. Friction increases with the viscosity; hence, a thick solution flows more slowly than a thin solution.

6. Peristaltic action in the intestine may be stimulated by distension of the intestinal wall and by the action of cholinergic drugs.

The emphasis here is on *application of principles* from the various sciences rather than on procedural steps, since most agencies have established specific procedures. The discussion is intended to assist understanding of the essential principles guiding therapeutic effectiveness and safety in administering intestinal treatments in any situation, regardless of the equipment provided in the agency.

Application of principles

The terminal portion of the large intestine is the rectum and the anal canal. The rectum, from its origin at the third sacral vertebra, descends forward along the curve of the sacrum and coccyx and then turns sharply backward to form the anal canal. The anal canal is approximately 1 to $1^1/_2$ inches in length (2.5 to 3.8 cm.). It terminates with the external orifice, the anus, which is surrounded by strong fascia and muscles, the internal and external sphincters and the levator ani, which hold the anus closed except at defecation. The veins of the anal canal may become enlarged, resulting in the condition known as hemorrhoids.

These anatomic facts should be recalled when inserting a rectal tube. Relaxation of the sphincters guarding the anus facilitates passing the tube and is promoted by encouraging the patient to take deep breaths during the process of insertion. Very gentle, slow insertion of the tube, particularly when there are hemorrhoids, either external or internal, partially obstructing the anal orifice and canal, is necessary to avoid causing pain that will stimulate the sphincters to contract. If resistance is met, force should never be used in passing the rectal tube because it might injure the mucous membrane or any pathologic condition that may be present in the anus or rectum. A well-lubricated tube may usually be inserted smoothly past the anal sphincters if there is no obstruction.

Since the combined length of the anal canal and the rectum is about 6 to 7 inches in length, inserting the tube 3 or 4 inches should be sufficient for the enema solution to be carried up to the cecum by the force of gravity and the pressure of the inflowing solution. If the tube is inserted further, it probably will not negotiate the curve of the sigmoid flexure and may either be forced against the mucosa, causing injury, or kink back on itself.

It is usually recommended that the patient lie on his left side, since it is assumed that gravity will aid the inflow of fluid because of the position of the descending colon on the left side of the abdomen. If the patient cannot be positioned on his left side, it is still possible to give a successful enema. However, the patient should be lying down, not sitting up, in order to avoid the fluid collecting in the lower colon, thus creating the desire to evacuate before the solution can be effective. Sitting posture aids gravity during expulsion of the enema solution.

For the patient whose sphincter control is not sufficient to retain the enema solution while it is being given, it may be necessary to insert the rectal tube and then have the patient positioned on the bedpan while administering the solution. It may also be necessary for the nurse to hold the tube in place with a gloved hand during the procedure. Because of the direction of the colon, the head of the bed should not be elevated more than a few degrees. Otherwise, the pressure of the inflow must be increased in order for the fluid to ascend the colon against gravity, thus stimulating peristalsis, creating discomfort, and increasing the difficulty the patient will experience in retaining the fluid while it is being introduced.

Absorption of water through the intestinal wall is by osmosis. The speed of osmosis depends on the size of the area. Water is given for absorption by proctoclysis, and some drugs are given for absorption by retention enema. When drugs are given by rectum, they must be well dissolved to aid absorption.

Water combines directly with many substances, either with drugs in making solutions or with fecal material in the colon. Solutions commonly used for cleansing enemas are made from soap, sodium chloride, or sodium bicarbonate. Soap lowers surface tension of water and causes the water to combine more quickly with fecal material. Sometimes, however, soap solution is irritating to the mucous membrane. Sodium chloride solution, 0.9%, is isotonic with the blood and is not irritating. It is prepared by using ordinary table salt and tap water in the proportions of 1 teaspoon of salt to 1 pint of water. Sodium bicarbonate also softens water and is not irritating. When milk and molasses are mixed for a carminative enema, carbon dioxide gas is formed, irritating the intestinal muscles and causing contractions.

Tap water is hypotonic and may be undesirable to use in some cases since it may be absorbed and disturb the water balance in the body. It should not be used in large quantities or frequently.

Carminative enemas aid in expelling gas. The "1-2-3" enema may be used. This consists of 1 ounce of magnesium sulfate crystals (Epsom salt), 2 ounces of glycerin, and 3 ounces of hot water. If the proportions are doubled, the enema may be called a "2-4-6" enema. The magnesium sulfate is hypertonic, so that fluid is drawn out of the tissues and a liquid stool produced. Glycerin is adhesive to the mucous membrane and will be retained longer than water.

The chief ingredient in the commonly used commercially prepared Fleet enema is sodium biphosphate. This produces a rather mild salt reaction.

Soft, flexible tubes and hard tips used in treatments on the large intestine are usually lubricated with a commercially prepared water-soluble lubricating jelly rather than with a solid grease such as petrolatum. If the grease remains on the soft rubber a long time, it is absorbed by the rubber, causing it to become sticky and decomposed. Hence, grease, if used, should be removed from the rubber as soon as possible to prevent deterioration.

Cottonseed oil or mineral oil may be given by rectum to soothe the irritated mucosa or to lubricate hardened fecal material to make its passage easier. Usually 4 or 6 ounces (150 ml.) of oil are used. After a few hours, the oil injection may be followed by an enema of a cleansing solution.

The chief emollient drug used in enemas is cornstarch. The starch solution is boiled and prepared in a thin solution, the usual proportions being 1 dram of starch to 6 ounces of water. The solution is retained and coats the mucous membrane so that irritation is lessened.

Barium sulfate may be injected into the colon in order to outline the colon in x-ray examinations, since barium sulfate is opaque to x-rays. The barium, not being absorbable, is removed after the examination by a cleansing enema.

Sometimes drugs are given by rectum to be absorbed. Sedatives, chief among which are sodium bromide, chloral hydrate, and paraldehyde, are often administered by rectum to quiet the patient. These may be prepared in starch solution or in warm tap water. Sedative drugs may also be administered in suppository form. The dose of a drug given by rectum is larger than the dose given by mouth for the same effect because absorption is slower in the rectum.

The rate of flow of a solution in a rectal treatment varies with the pressure (gradient), the caliber of the tube, and the density of the fluid. Fluid will flow only when there is a difference in pressure between the solution in the container and the end of the outflow tube. Pressure depends on the height of the column of liquid. The pressure of aqueous solution in a container for irrigations has been established at about $1/2$ pound for every foot of elevation. In no irrigation should pressure exceed 1 pound. When increased pressure is desired in an enema, the container of solution may be raised. If pressure is too great, muscles

of the intestinal walls contract too quickly and cause so much pain that the patient will not be able to take sufficient fluid for the treatment to be effective. Too much pressure may cause injury to the mucous membrane.

Where low pressure is desired, the container may be lowered, a smaller tube may be used, or the caliber of the tube may be made smaller by a screw cock, thereby increasing the friction of the fluid against the walls of the tube and decreasing the speed of flow.

A thick fluid increases friction and flows slower than a thin solution, since specific gravity of a liquid influences pressure.

Pressure of gas against the walls of the intestines causes pain. Prolonged pressure against the small veins in the anal region may contribute to the development of hemorrhoids.

Fluid flows into the rectum and colon by the force of gravity. Gravity supposes a flow from a high level to a low one. A flow should start when the level of solution in the container is just higher than the rectum, but if there is internal resistance to the flow, the can must be held high enough to overcome this resistance. About 12 inches above the rectum is the usual height. Once the flow has started, the solution will keep flowing and the container may be lowered but with the level of the solution always higher than the rectum. Gravity aids the distribution of fluids. If the patient is in the left side-lying position, gravity will aid the inflow of solution. If it is possible to raise the backrest for expelling the solution, gravity will again help.

In a colonic irrigation, fluid flows out of the colon by the force of gravity. The end of the outflow tube is in a pail that should be the same distance below the rectum as the container of solution is above it in order not to have too much suction on the mucous membrane.

Sometimes when the solution of the

enema is not expelled, it is siphoned out with a colon tube. The free end of the colon tube is placed in the bedpan, which is placed on the bed and is lower than the level of the fluid in the rectum. The colon tube over the edge of the bedpan forms the siphon. The fluid runs out because the pressure in the colon is greater than the pressure at the free end of the tube.

Friction is caused by roughness, and it is reduced by smoothness and lubrication. Friction between the rubber tube and the fluid is reduced because of the smooth surface of the rubber. Friction between the rubber tube and the contracted anal sphincter muscles is reduced by lubricating the end of the tube before insertion. A solid grease such as petrolatum or a surgical lubricant is used for lubrication, since either adheres to the tube and is spread along the tube as it is being inserted. When pathology of the anal region exists, more lubricant than usual is needed.

Water is a good conductor of heat, and heat travels through the pelvic tissues by conduction. The solution is prepared at 105° F. (40.5° C.), which is comfortably warm to the mucous membrane.

Physics is also involved in the posture of the nurse. The patient and the materials should be placed within easy reaching distance. The nurse should stand with feet apart in giving a treatment in order to provide a wide base of support. Bending should be at the hips or at the knees. When carrying a bedpan, the nurse carries it close to the body (center of gravity) but without touching the uniform, to prevent strain in reaching.

Observations to be recorded include the approximate amount of fluid returned; the color, consistency, and amount of feces; presence of blood or mucus or other unusual material; the estimated amount of flatus expelled, small or large; and the general reaction of the patient to the treatment. The purpose for which the treatment is given will give clues as to pertinent ob-

servations. For example, following an anthelmintic enema, the presence or absence of visible parasites would be significant.

GASTRIC INTUBATION

Gastric intubation means the introduction of a tube into the stomach for therapeutic or diagnostic purposes. The tube is usually passed by way of the nose or throat, but it may be inserted through a surgical opening from the exterior, which procedure is referred to as a gastrostomy.

Intubation may be performed for the purpose of gavage, lavage, or gastric aspiration. Gastric gavage is a method of artificial feeding by means of intubation.

Gastric lavage means a washing out or irrigation of the stomach. It may be done to remove poisons or irritating matter from the stomach, to relieve nausea and vomiting, to cleanse the stomach in preparation for an operation on the stomach, or to remove cast-off epithelial cells for bacteriologic study.

Aspiration of the gastric contents—fluids, food, or gas—may be accomplished by introducing a tube into the stomach and applying suction to the end of it by means of a syringe or an electric suction machine. This procedure is carried out to keep the stomach empty, for example, following an operation in order to prevent nausea and distension, or for diagnostic testing.

For both gastric lavage and aspiration of the gastric contents the gastric tube and syringe are the essential pieces of equipment. For the stomach the Levin tube is used most frequently. Originally it was made of rubber, but more recently a plastic disposable material has been used. The Levin tube is narrow and can easily be passed through the nasal passages.

The duodenal tube most frequently used is the Miller-Abbot tube, which has a metal tip and a balloon on one end. The balloon is inflated after the tip has reached the duodenum. The tube is biluminal (that is,

453

there is a partition inside the tube), one passage for introducing air, water, or mercury to inflate the balloon and the other for drainage to flow out. The inflated balloon serves as a bolus of food does—to stimulate peristalsis. It passes into the intestines and may serve to locate or to break up an obstruction. Other tubes used are the Cantor tube and the Harris tube.

For a lavage, a solution basin and a return-flow basin will be needed. Also, some protection will be required for the bed and gown. A clamp may be needed for the tube in gastric suction.

Related scientific principles

Understanding of basic principles related to treatments of the stomach serves as an essential link between the biologic and physical sciences and patient care, thus enhancing the safety and effectiveness of the nursing ministrations received by the patient. Focusing on examples of relevant facts helps the nurse to move through a maze of information, to make use of that which is significant and which can promote useful understanding of patient care. Achievement in terms of behavioral objectives is a desired outcome of this approach.

The examples of principles cited here are helpful in identifying basic facts that should stimulate further study leading to deeper insight into the needs of patients having problems associated with the stomach.

1. Very little absorption occurs in the stomach.

2. Peristalsis is stimulated by a bolus of food.

3. Glands of the mucous membrane lining the esophagus and stomach normally produce mucus, but when irritated these glands secrete increased amounts.

4. Normally, the gastric mucosa acts as a protective lining for the stomach, preventing self-digestion through activity of hydrochloric acid and pepsin.

5. Specialized cells of the gastric mucosa

secrete hydochloric acid, which is responsible for the low pH of gastric juices.

6. The extreme acidity of the stomach is responsible for killing ingested bacteria; normally, this antiseptic action prevents putrefaction.

7. The chlorides used in the production of acids in the gastric juices are derived from chlorides of the blood.

8. Acid gastric secretions are inhibited by anticholinergic-antisecretory agents.

9. Gastric antacids counteract hydrochloric acid that has already been secreted in the stomach.

10. Certain metallic poisons, such as ingested mercury, will combine with protein to form harmless salt.

11. The siphon is a bent tube with unequal arms; the action depends on differences in atmospheric pressure (pressure gradient).

12. The negative pressure (vacuum) in hydraulic suction is produced by a column of water flowing from a higher level to a lower level.

13. Liquids exert pressure because of their weight.

Application of principles

The stomach is a hollow muscular organ whose function is to serve as a reservoir for retaining the bulk of food while the food undergoes certain chemical and mechanical changes. The mouth and the esophagus are lined with mucous membrane. When irritated by a foreign substance such as a tube, mucous glands produce more mucus. The additional amount acts to lubricate the tube, permitting it to be swallowed more easily. Swallowing of the tube is accomplished by muscular action. If the patient takes deep breaths it will help him to control gagging and vomiting.

Each time the patient swallows, the tube is advanced through the esophagus toward the stomach. Swallowing aids in ensuring that the tube will pass safely through the pharynx, which serves as a common passageway for both food and air. (Refer to Fig. 19-4). The tube should pass smoothly along the posterior wall of the pharynx and into the esophagus; otherwise, it may accidentally slip into the trachea and obstruct the patient's airway.

It is essential to be certain that the tube has reached the stomach before introducing fluid into the tube. A positive test for determining that the tip of the tube is in the stomach is aspiration of stomach contents. If the tube has slipped into the trachea the patient will experience difficulty in breathing and may become cyanotic. In this event the tube would be withdrawn and reinserted, directing it into the esophagus.

The mucous lining continues into the stomach where it is arranged in longitudinal folds or rugae that disappear when the stomach is distended with food. In irrigation of the stomach enough fluid (about 500 ml.) should be introduced to flatten out the rugae in order for the fluid to reach all parts of the mucous membrane.

The stomach is never entirely empty but always contains a little gastric juice that is secreted by numerous tubular glands in the wall of the stomach. In 24 hours the stomach secretes 1,000 to 1,500 ml. of gastric fluid.

Little absorption takes place in the stomach. Water leaves the stomach and enters the duodenum within 15 to 30 minutes after its ingestion. Absorption is a function of the small and large intestines. These facts are useful in the emergency treatment of poisons taken orally. After a poison is taken, immediate action should be initiated to remove it from the stomach before it enters the duodenum, in order to save the patient's life.

The opening from the stomach into the duodenum is guarded by a sphincter muscle called the pylorus or the pyloric sphincter. If the tube is to be passed into the duodenum, it is carried down from the stomach by peristalsis after several hours. Peristalsis consists of waves of motion in the stomach and intestines produced by successive contractions of the muscles in the walls, and it propels the contents onward.

A disposable tube is economical of time since it is discarded after use and does not need to be prepared for another patient. Reusable tubes are washed with soap and water and sterilized after each use to prevent transmission of bacteria, but tubes need not be sterile when used because the stomach is not a sterile cavity. Basins and pitchers for the solution need to be washed well. In handling them, even if they are not sterile, the nurse keeps the fingers on the outside. The nurse's hands should be clean when assisting with gastric lavage or gastric suction, and the drainage bottle used in gastric suction needs to be washed well to prevent odors as well as transfer of pathogenic organisms.

Gastric washings may be examined for tubercle bacillus or for cancer cells.

Gastric juice is clear, colorless, and acid in reaction. It is composed of water (97% to 99.5%), mucin, salts, hydrochloric acid (0.5%), and three enzymes: gastric protease, rennin, and gastric lipase. The hydrochloric acid is derived from the chlorides of the blood.

When the tube has been passed, litmus paper may be used to test the aspirated material. Fluid aspirated from the stomach will give an acid reaction and that from the intestines will give an alkaline reaction.

When there is excessive vomiting or when gastric suction is used for several days, the process removes much of the chlorides from the stomach. Since sodium chloride is necessary for the proper functioning of the body, it must be replaced by infusions of salt solution.

Sodium bicarbonate neutralizes the acidity in the stomach and makes a good irrigating solution. However, it is undesirable for routine use as an antacid in the

455

treatment of peptic ulcer or for relief of a feeling of fullness and burning sensation in the stomach, for at least two reasons. (1) The carbon dioxide gas that is released when sodium bicarbonate comes in contact with hydrochloric acid distends the stomach suddenly and, by putting pressure on the weakened base of an ulcer crater, may cause a perforation. (2) The alkalinity of the sodium bicarbonate hastens emptying of gastric contents into the duodenum where the sodium is rapidly absorbed systemically, which may result in sodium excess in the extracellular fluids.

Chemical antidotes of poisons are used to neutralize the effects of the poisons. An antidote for an acid poison is a mild alkali such as sodium bicarbonate. An antidote for an alkali poison is a mild acid such as vinegar.

Solutions used for lavage of the stomach are solutions of salt or soda or the antidote of a poison. Three types of antidotes are physical, chemical, and physiologic. A physical antidote is one that mixes with the poison and prevents its absorption or soothes and protects the mucous membrane. Milk and egg white are commonly used for metallic poisons. A chemical antidote reacts with the poison and neutralizes it. A physiologic antidote is one that produces an opposite systemic effect from that of the poison. Caffeine is the physiologic antidote for morphine poisoning. Household emetics (substances to produce vomiting) include warm solutions made with baking soda, salt, or soap. Apomorphine is given hypodermically to produce vomiting. Ointments for lubricating the tube may contain a local anesthetic.

Gastric lavage operates on the principle of the siphon. A siphon is a bent tube with unequal arms. The action of a siphon depends on differences in atmospheric pressure (pressure gradient). Liquids exert pressure because of their weight. After the proper amount of fluid is put into the stomach, the tube is reversed so that the funnel is below the stomach to form the long arm of the siphon. Fluid in the long arm of the siphon weighs more than fluid in the short arm. Hence, since more pressure is exerted, the fluid will flow from the stomach into the lower vessel. (See Fig. 28-3.)

Gastric suction depends on differences in presssure also. Although there are various methods by which suction may be created, a form of hydraulic suction is commonly used for the stomach. Hydraulic suction is based on the fact that negative pressure (vacuum) is produced by a column of water flowing from a higher level to a lower level. The apparatus used may make use of siphon suction or gravity suction. In siphon suction the top bottle is upright, and the bent tube connects it to the lower bottle (Fig. 28-4). In gravity suction the top bottle is upside down, and fluid flows out of it because of its weight (Fig. 28-5, A).

In either method of suction, as the water flows from the top bottle to the lower bottle, a partial vacuum is created in the upper bottle. In a, vacuum, pressure is below that of the atmosphere. Since the pressure in the stomach is at atmospheric pressure, the stomach contents will flow into the area of less pressure or into the upper bottle.

A three-bottle method has been devised (Fig. 28-5, B). The third bottle interrupts the tubing from the upper bottle to the patient's stomach. It is placed below the bed. The negative pressure is transferred to this third bottle, and as drainage comes out of the stomach it drops into the third bottle by gravity.

The force of suction depends on the distance of the fluid in the lower bottle from the stomach. It can be decreased by raising the lower bottle.

The electric suction pump (Fig. 28-5, C) operates on the principle that heat can be used to produce changes in air pressure. Air is heated in a compartment of the machine, and some of it is allowed to

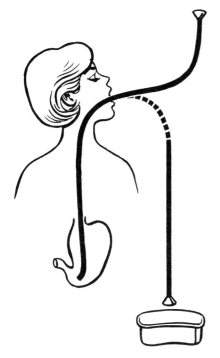

Fig. 28-3. The gastric tube acts as a siphon.

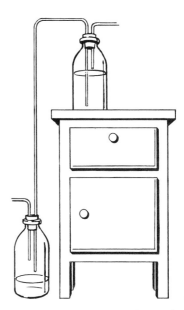

Fig. 28-4. Siphon suction. The siphon requires a bent arm.

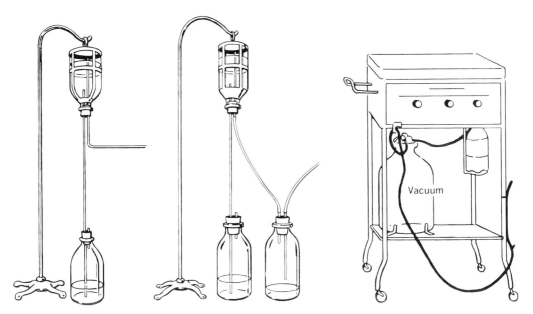

Fig. 28-5. **A,** Gravity suction. **B,** Gravity suction using a three-bottle method. **C,** Electric suction pump.

escape. The remaining air is cooled and so a vacuum is created. A flashing red light indicates the machine is operating efficiently.

Suction of $1/2$ to 4 pounds per square inch may be used in gastric treatments. Commercial automatic evacuators exert a maximum suction of $2^1/2$ pounds per square inch.

Since cold hardens the rubber tube and makes it easier to swallow, the tube is put on ice or in the refrigerator for some time before it is inserted.

Smoothness of the tube reduces the friction between it and the mucous membrane. The tube may be made smooth (lubricated) by dipping the end in water, by giving the patient water to drink while the tube is being passed, by applying a lubricating jelly, or simply by the excess mucus that is formed because of the irritation of the tube.

Before the tube is withdrawn, a clamp is applied to cut off air pressure on any fluid that remains in the tube and to prevent its dropping out as it passes the trachea.

PSYCHOSOCIAL ASPECTS

Patients fear pain. When a treatment is to be given, the nurse may explain how much pain is to be expected. Fright is aroused by some experience that is interpreted as dangerous, and the patient usually fears any treatment not experienced before. To overcome his fears, the nurse gives an explanation of the procedure and some suggestion of the result.

If a patient has been hurt by a treatment previously, he is not so likely to give the cooperation needed to provide relaxation in order to ensure good results.

Emotions may keep the patient so tense that the treatment is given with difficulty. Since tension may be caused by cold, the patient is kept covered with a warm drape. Tensing emotions may be decreased by ensuring privacy and as little exposure as possible and by distracting the attention of the patient through appropriate conversa-

tion. If the nurse wins the confidence of the patient, the treatment will usually be given with little difficulty.

The nurse-patient relationship needs to be therapeutic where necessary treatments are involved. The patient expects from the nurse knowledge of treatment details that make for safety and comfort, both physical and mental, expert skill in administering procedures, gentleness in touch, and poise and competence in work. Relaxation of the patient is needed in treatments on the large intestine for satisfactory inflow of the solution and for satisfactory outflow where indicated.

Having a tube inserted in the stomach is not a pleasant sensation. The treatment and its purpose need to be explained. The patient should be advised that the comfort obtained from the treatment will more than compensate for the discomfort involved. He also needs to be reassured and encouraged repeatedly during the passage of the tube. Sometimes a physician introduces the tube into the stomach, but in many instances the nurse may insert it. The nurse needs to obtain the confidence of the patient and to proceed slowly. Gagging causes fear and discomfort. If it occurs, the nurse should hold the tube where it is and have the patient close his mouth, take a deep breath, and rest a few seconds. When the patient is relaxed, the nurse may insert the tube farther. Passing the tube through the nose prevents gagging.

The chief discomfort from having a tube in the stomach for several days is irritation of the throat. The nurse may relieve some of this discomfort by giving good oral care and adequate amounts of fluids. After the treatment, the nurse may offer a mouthwash to remove the taste of rubber and to freshen the mouth.

When administering stomach treatments cooperation is needed between the patient and the physician or nurse who passes the tube and between the patient and the nurse who observes the treatment

458

in the physician's absence. Cooperation is needed between the nurse and laboratory workers if specimens are to be examined. If the physician is not present, the nurse reports to him any symptom or results that are unusual.

The treatment needs to be explained to relatives so that they may encourage the patient through an uncomfortable treatment.

The patient who has taken poison is dependent on quick thinking and acting of another in an effort to save his life. The patient may receive a gastric lavage in a hospital, in a clinic, in a physician's office, in his own home, or, in an emergency, wherever a tube is available.

SUMMARY

When the food-processing function of the gastrointestinal tract is impaired, bodily nutrition and well-being are affected. A variety of causative factors often lead to dysfunction in the stomach and intestinal tract, giving rise to symptoms that may require various nursing measures and treatments intended to assist in relieving symptoms and in maintaining or restoring proper function.

Nausea and vomiting are common symptoms seen in a great variety of medical and surgical conditions that the physician will seek to control through prescribed treatment. Well-planned nursing care can accomplish a great deal in decreasing or preventing ill effects for the patient experiencing these symptoms.

Diarrhea, constipation, and fecal impaction, which are dysfunctions of the lower intestinal tract manifested by accelerated or retarded movement of contents through the intestine, are like nausea and vomiting in that they occur as symptoms of many different disorders that may be either systemic diseases or local conditions within the bowel. These conditions are usually quite disturbing to the patient and, in the situation of severe diarrhea, may result in depletion of body fluids, electrolytes, and nutrients. The effects of fecal impaction, which is severe constipation, are discussed in context with the abnormal functioning of body systems that tends to occur during prolonged inactivity.

Objectives of nursing care for the patient with either retarded or accelerated movement of contents through the intestine are presented in relation to the individual patient's total situation.

Common treatments of the lower intestinal tract are the cleansing enema, the retention enema, the Harris flush, and the insertion of a rectal tube. Representative principles are stated that also appear in other contexts, which support the premise that many principles useful in explaining the scientific basis for a nursing action are applicable in a variety of nursing situations. The emphasis is on application of principles from the various sciences rather than on procedural steps in performing treatments. Accurate observation and recording are an important part of the nursing responsibility.

Common treatments of the stomach include gastric lavage, gavage, and gastric suction. Related scientific principles serve as a link between the basic sciences and patient care. Application of principles to patient care assists the nurse in gaining deeper insight into the needs of the patient with symptoms related to functioning of the stomach and in performing prescribed treatments effectively.

Cooperation of the patient is promoted by careful explanations given by the nurse to the patient and his family.

QUESTIONS FOR DISCUSSION

1 Define gastric lavage.
2 What is meant by aspiration of the gastric contents?
3 How is aspiration of the gastric contents accomplished?
4 Describe three kinds of tubes that may be put into the stomach.
5 Why are infusions of salt solution ordered for a patient who has continuous suction from the stomach?

6 Explain the physical principles regarding lavage.

7 Explain the physical principles of gastric suction.

8 Why would a relative worry about a patient who is receiving gastric suction?

9 How much pressure is used in administering a cleansing enema?

10 How far should a rectal tube be inserted? Why is it this distance?

11 What bacilli normally inhabit the colon? How may these bacilli get into other organs?

12 What nonirritating solutions may be used in enemas?

13 How does the Harris flush differ from a cleansing enema?

14 Explain the difference in amounts of solutions given for a retention enema and for the cleansing enema.

15 Discuss the serious effects of severe and prolonged diarrhea. Why is this apt to be more serious for an infant?

LIFE SITUATION

It is Mr. Smith's second postoperative day following a gastric resection. A Levin tube is in place in his stomach and is connected to a suction machine. The patient is very uncomfortable, states that he cannot tolerate the tube any longer, and threatens to remove it. The doctor refuses to give an order to discontinue the suction. What can you do to help make the treatment more bearable for Mr. Smith?

SUGGESTED PERFORMANCE CHECKLIST
Gastric intubation
Comfort

1 Is the tube chilled before use when this is indicated?

2 Is privacy provided during the passage of the tube?

3 Is the patient reassured while the tube is being passed?

4 Is water provided during the passage of the tube, if allowed?

5 Are mouth wipes provided?

6 Is mouthwash provided after the tube is removed?

Therapeutic effectiveness

1 Is the tube introduced slowly?

2 Has it been verified that the tip of the tube is in the patient's stomach?

3 If solution is used, is the amount sufficient?

4 Is the irrigation continued for a sufficient length of time?

5 If suction is used, is it maintained for the ordered time?

6 Does the nurse impart confidence to the patient and his family?

7 Is the charting pertinent and adequate?

Economy

1 Is the bed adequately protected?

2 Is equipment assembled before beginning treatment?

3 Is the apparatus? checked frequently for working efficiency

Safety

1 Are the nurse's hands clean?

2 Is the tube clean?

3 Are disposable tubes used?

4 Is the tube lubricated before insertion?

5 Is the tube clamped before removal?

6 If a solution is used, is the temperature correct?

7 Is the strength correct?

8 Is the entrance of air prevented while pouring the solution?

9 Is the pressure moderate?

10 Is the tube tested for placement?

11 If the tube is left in place for some time, is it fastened to the face?

12 Does the nurse give the patient adequate oral care while the tube is in place?

SUGGESTED READINGS

Barnes, Mauvine R.: Clean colons without enemas, American Journal of Nursing **69:**2128, October, 1969.

Dison, Norma G.: An atlas of nursing techniques, St. Louis, 1971, The C. V. Mosby Co.

Given, Barbara A., and Simmons, Sandra J.: Nursing care of the patient with gastrointestinal disorders, St. Louis, 1971, The C. V. Mosby Co.

Shafer, Kathleen N., and others: Medical-surgical nursing, St. Louis, 1971, The C. V. Mosby Co., chap. 24, p. 578.

Sill, Alice R.: Bulb-syringe technique for colonic stoma irrigation, American Journal of Nursing **70:**536, March, 1970.

29 Genitourinary disorders

PURPOSE OF THE CHAPTER

The focus of this chapter is on common manifestations of physiologic imbalance encountered by the nurse and on the related nursing care of the patient in either the hospital or community setting. These manifestations are not considered to be necessarily characteristic of specific diseases but rather to be responses in the presence of imbalance or needs that can occur when there is pathophysiology in various body systems. In Chapter 10 these manifestations were discussed as signs and symptoms that the nurse should recognize as indications of the patient's condition.

It is highly important that the nurse learn to understand and recognize normal ranges of well-being as a basis for perceiving significant changes in the patient's condition. Both the patient and the physician expect the nurse to recognize the presence of symptoms, discomforts, and problems that can be appropriately managed through nursing action and to recognize those manifestations of imbalance that should be promptly and accurately reported to the physician.

The purpose of this chapter is to provide a practical guide for general nursing action in some selected, commonly occurring patient-care problems.

DYSFUNCTIONS OF THE URINARY TRACT
Retention of urine

It is not unusual for a patient to experience difficulty in voiding. There are a variety of factors that may cause this distressing problem that predispose to further complications.

Inability to void may be associated with strong emotions, especially excitement, fear, or embarrassment, that greatly increase the tonicity of the muscles of the bladder resulting in retention (or frequency of urination in some persons). Retention may occur following surgery because of the effect of the anesthetic or when there has been injury to sensory or motor nerves involved in the act of urination, such as in spinal cord injury. Other causes include urethral strictures, pressure as in hypertrophy of the prostate gland, or edema following surgery or childbirth, which create obstruction.

461

Whatever the cause of the retention, the patient will experience a great deal of discomfort and anxiety. If the retention is allowed to continue, the resulting distension of the bladder and the stasis of urine predispose to infection. Back pressure is created on the ureters, and reflux of urine may lead to infection of the kidneys as well as of the bladder.

Retention of urine may be recognized by palpating the distended bladder above the symphysis pubis, but retention is to be suspected when the patient has not voided within an 8- to 10-hour period during which the fluid intake has been normal. The constant desire to void may be experienced by the patient but efforts to void are unsuccessful. Another common manifestation of a distended bladder is the passing of small amounts of urine, perhaps 25 to 50 ml., which the patient may or may not be able to control. *Retention with overflow* is a descriptive term for this occurrence.

Some nursing measures that may be helpful when the inability to void is associated with temporary causes include increasing fluid intake, providing privacy, or assisting the bed patient to assume as favorable a position as possible for use of the bedpan. The female patient may be assisted to use the commode if this permitted, or the male patient may be assisted to stand beside the bed. For the female patient, application of moist heat or pouring warm water over the perineum and, for some patients, the sound of running water may be effective in restoring the function of micturition. Every effort to induce normal voiding should be made before resorting to the procedure of urethral catheterization.

Residual urine

Even though there is the ability to void, the bladder may not be completely emptied at each voiding. The presence of residual urine is confirmed and the amount of residual determined by catheterizing the patient immediately after voiding. Residual urine is often associated with a partial obstruction of the bladder outlet, such as enlarged prostate. The resulting stasis of urine leads to bladder infection and calculus formation. Therefore, early detection and relief of residual urine is important. When catheterizing for residual urine, extreme precautions to avoid trauma of the mucosa and/or introduction of microorganisms should be employed.

Dysuria

Irritation and infection of the bladder and urethral mucosa usually produce such effects as an abnormally frequent desire to void, urgency, and painful urination. Voiding accompanied by a painful, burning, smarting sensation, intense desire to void immediately, or decreasing amounts of urine voided more frequently are symptoms that should be noted and reported at once.

Questions of concern to the nurse in evaluating the needs of a patient with any of these common problems related to functioning of the bladder or urethra include: Is the patient's fluid intake sufficient to maintain adequate fluid balance? Does he need assistance with fluid intake or diet? Is there difficulty or discomfort in voiding? Are there signs of urinary retention or residual? Is he incontinent? Are the laboratory reports normal, or do they show increased levels of nonprotein nitrogen in the blood or abnormal urinary constituents? Is the patient anxious or relaxed? Is he able to discuss his concerns with the nurse?

Whenever there is interference with the ability to empty the bladder, from whatever cause, nursing measures are appropriately directed toward (1) facilitating return of the normal pattern of voiding and (2) providing emotional support and comfort measures. When nursing measures are unsuccessful, the physician may order catheterization on the premise that the need for the patient to empty the bladder outweighs the possible hazards of catheterization skillfully performed.

REVIEW OF ANATOMY AND PHYSIOLOGY

The various structures of the urinary tract are illustrated in Fig. 29-1. Of particular interest in this context are the following facts.

1. Each kidney is abundantly supplied with blood by the renal artery, which is basic to the kidney performing its regulatory and excretory functions.

2. The ureter is a tube that conveys the formed urine from the kidney pelvis to the bladder.

3. The bladder is a hollow, muscular organ that serves as a reservoir for urine. The musculature is capable of great distension. The ability to distend is also increased by the fact that the mucous membrane is drawn into folds, or rugae, when the bladder is empty.

4. The mucous membrane lining the urinary tract is continuous throughout the urethra, bladder, ureters, and kidney pelvis.

5. Urine is retained in the bladder by an internal sphincter that is located at the opening of the bladder into the urethra.

6. The bladder is emptied by contraction of its muscles. The urge to urinate is caused by sensory stimulation in the bladder, which results from the pressure of the urine exerted against the detrusor muscle. This stimulation causes the muscle to contract and the internal sphincter to relax. The contraction is maintained until the bladder is empty. In a healthy adult urination is a voluntary act.

APPLICATION OF SCIENTIFIC PRINCIPLES

Attention is drawn to principles appearing in Chapters 17 and 19, some of which are applicable to catheterization and other treatments of both the urinary tract and of

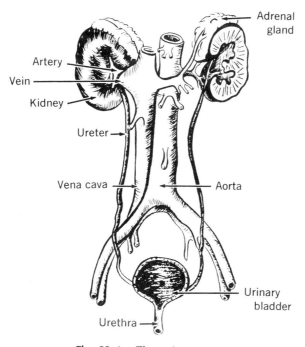

Fig. 29-1. The urinary system.

the large bowel. Review of these sections is suggested at this point.

The musculature of the bladder is capable of great distension to hold the urine that slowly and constantly accumulates in it. The capacity of the bladder varies greatly in health and in disease. The desire to empty the bladder occurs when about 300 ml. of urine have accumulated in it. Under disease conditions the bladder may be distended to hold 3,000 or 4,000 ml. of urine. The usual daily amount of urine excreted by a normal adult is from 1,200 to 1,500 ml. This amount varies with the weather, the fluid intake, and the action of food and drugs on the kidneys. In warm weather the volume of urine is low because of increased elimination of water through the skin (Fig. 29-2).

A healthy bladder is remarkably resistant to infection. However, if an infection is present in one part of the urinary tract, it may travel to another part because of the continuity of the mucous membrane.

The urinary tract offers a favorable location for the multiplication of microorganisms because it is dark, moist, and warm. The incidence of cystitis, or inflammation of the bladder, may be increased by highly concentrated urine, by irritating drugs used in irrigation and instillation, by introduction of bacteria, by overdistention of the bladder walls (causing the blood supply to be lessened), by injury, or by obstruction to the flow of urine.

The commonest organism causing urinary infections is the colon bacillus. Other bacteria responsible for bladder infections are the staphylococci and the streptococci, as well as the organisms that cause gonorrhea, typhoid, and tuberculosis. The cocci tend to cause a more acute condition than do the bacilli. About 30% of patients with typhoid fever excrete the bacilli in their urine. For this reason urine from these patients is disinfected before disposal where there is no adequate sewerage system.

Bacteria may be introduced into the bladder by an unsterile catheter. A catheter may also be a cause of injury because it may be too rough or too large, introduced with too much force, or manipulated carelessly. Trauma may also be caused by using a method that is too vigorous in disinfecting the urinary meatus. Another cause of trauma may be the nurse's long, pointed fingernails.

To keep pathogens from being carried into the bladder from the urinary meatus, different methods are used to cleanse the external area before introducing the catheter. The best method is to wash the glans penis or the perineal area with soap and warm water. An antiseptic solution may be applied to the area by means of soft

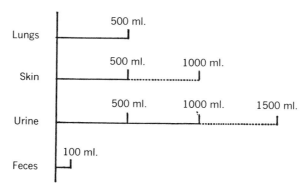

Fig. 29-2. The skin and the kidneys are complemental in regard to excretion of water —the more excreted by the one, the less by the other.

sponges or applicators. If stitches are present in the perineum, an antiseptic irrigation may also be used after voiding to prevent bacteria present in the urine from infecting injured tissue.

Bacteria are present in the air. Therefore, the sterile catheter is kept covered until ready to be used.

Rubber or plastic catheters are commonly used and are sterilized by autoclave. However, repeated exposures to high temperatures soften rubber. Silk woven catheters are usually sterilized by chemicals to avoid the destructive action of heat on them. The catheter should be smooth, sufficiently pliable to conform easily to the urethral passage, and lubricated to avoid trauma to the urethra.

Catheters are graded by the size of the lumen according to the French scale, varying from a small No. 8 to 10 Fr., commonly used for children; to No. 14 to 16 Fr., used for the adult female; to No. 20 to 22 Fr., which may be suitable for the adult male. It is important to select a suitable size catheter for the individual patient to avoid unnecessary discomfort and trauma to the urethra (Fig. 29-3).

Disposable retention catheters come in sterile packages ready for use. The lubricant added for use on the catheter must be sterile also. Disposable catheterization

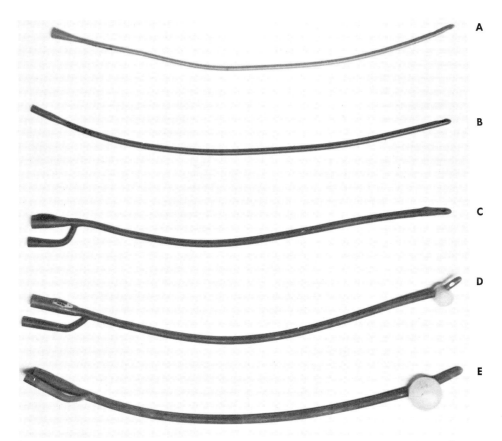

Fig. 29-3. Types of catheters. **A,** Plastic catheter. **B,** Rubber catheter. **C,** Foley catheter before inflation. **D,** Foley catheter, 5 cc. (ml.). **E,** Foley catheter, 30 cc. (ml.).

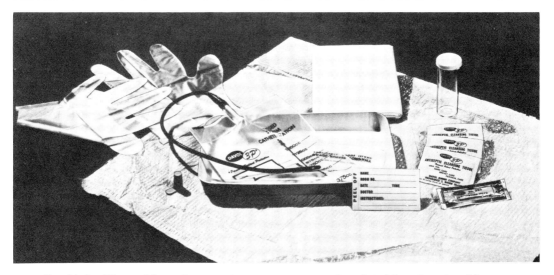

Fig. 29-4. Disposable catheterization set. (Courtesy Davol Rubber Co., Providence, R. I.)

sets containing all the materials needed for catheterization, even a graduated specimen container, are commercially available (Fig. 29-4).

Since the commonest method of transferring pathogenic bacteria is by contaminated hands and since the skin cannot be made absolutely sterile, the nurse wears sterile rubber gloves if it is necessary to touch a part of the catheter that will be introduced into the bladder. If gloves are not worn, the fingers with which the patient is touched are protected by rubber finger cots, by cotton, or by gauze. The nurse's hands are washed before and after a bladder treatment.

URINARY CATHETERIZATION

Catheterization is the introduction of a catheter through the urethra into the bladder for the purpose of removing urine.

Catheterization may be performed for several reasons, including (1) collection of a sterile urine specimen, (2) measurement of residual urine, (3) complete emptying of the bladder prior to surgery or delivery, (4) emptying of the bladder after surgery when the patient is unable to void, (5) removal of urine when it is not advisable for

the patient to void, such as when there is a radium implant in the vagina, and (6) gradual decompression of a greatly distended bladder in acute urinary retention.

This listing of reasons for catheterization might seem to imply that the procedure is used freely. However, the hazards of introducing a catheter into the bladder, including infection and trauma at a time when the patient's resistance is lowered, have resulted in decrease in the frequency of the procedure.

Normally, the sterility of the bladder is protected by such mechanisms as the emptying of the bladder at voiding and the slight acidity of the urine, which inhibits growth of invading microorganisms. The urinary meatus is never sterile, and because of its proximity to the vaginal orifice and the anus, microorganisms are readily introduced with the catheter. If the mucosa is irritated by the catheter or the urethra is injured by failing to introduce the catheter at the proper angle or by forcing it past a stricture, the predisposition to infection is greatly increased. For these reasons catheterization is rarely used unless it is absolutely necessary.

Other methods may sometimes be sub-

466

stituted to accomplish the purpose of catheterization. For instance, instead of catheterizing for a sterile specimen a "clean" specimen of urine may be collected for culture very simply by the following steps:

1. The external meatus is cleansed thoroughly but gently with soap and water or mild antiseptic solution such as aqueous benzalkonium (Zephiran).
2. The patient voids 50 to 100 ml., which is discarded.
3. Then the patient voids about 100 to 200 ml. into a sterile specimen bottle.
4. The remaining urine is voided and discarded.

Female

Most agencies have a specific procedure for performing catheterization that will usually incorporate the following suggestions.

Preparation of the patient includes both psychologic and physical factors.

The objective of psychologic preparation is to help the patient to achieve muscular relaxation through explanation that will reassure her as to the nature of the treatment, what to anticipate, and how she can participate in the procedure to make it more comfortable for herself. Privacy should be assured.

Physical preparation includes positioning the patient on a firm, smooth surface (the treatment table, preferably) in order for the patient's bladder to be at least level with the catheter outlet so that gravity will aid the outflow of urine from the bladder. Dorsal recumbent is the most favorable position for the patient to assume, with draping that will provide for warmth and avoid unnecessary exposure while providing for adequate visualization of the perineal area. Supporting the helpless patient's thighs with pillows will aid her in maintaining proper positioning of the legs during the procedure. An alternate position for catheterization is with the patient lying on her side and with knees flexed, the upper leg higher than the lower and supported with a pillow or blanket roll. Drapes are readily placed with the patient in this position.

Optimum visualization of the meatus can be provided by arranging artificial lighting. Adequate illumination is also important in avoiding contamination of the sterile field.

Placing equipment conveniently and arranging it in the order of use will promote efficiency and is consistent with aseptic techniques since it avoids the necessity of reaching over the sterile catheter while cleansing the perineum.

Thorough *handwashing* is important even when the procedure calls for the nurse to wear sterile gloves. Protecting the fingers with sterile cotton balls or gauze will help to keep them from slipping while exposing the meatus.

Exposure of the external meatus is accomplished by inserting the gloved thumb and first or second finger between the labia minora, pressing upward and backward with the thumb and finger to smoothe the tissues. The external meatus can usually be recognized as a small dimple located just above the vaginal orifice, although it may be difficult to locate because of an anomaly of the parts or the presence of edema.

Cleansing the perineal area is necesary, partly because of the proximity of the anus. (If indicated, the entire area may first be cleansed with soap and water using a washcloth.) The area immediately surrounding the meatus should be cleansed to avoid introducing microorganisms with the catheter. If soap is used it should be rinsed away before applying antiseptic solutions that may be inactivated by soap. Beginning above the labia, the nurse cleanses downward toward the anus, the direction of cleansing being from the cleanest to the more contaminated area. Each swab is used for only one cleansing stroke. Using a minimum of five swabs, the nurse cleanses the labia majora, the labia minora,

467

and then directly over the meatus. After cleansing the meatus the labia should not be allowed to touch either the meatus or the catheter in order to avoid introducing microorganisms into the bladder via a contaminated catheter (Fig. 29-9).

Insertion of the catheter is facilitated by using sterile lubricant on the tip of the catheter, which reduces friction of the catheter as it moves along the mucous membrane lining the urethra, making sure the lubricant has not plugged the eye of the catheter. Holding the catheter at least 3 inches from the lubricated tip with the gloved fingers of the free hand (or with sterile forceps), the nurse inserts the catheter through the external meatus, gently directing it obliquely inward in a slightly downward and backward direction (Fig. 29-5), avoiding the use of force. The catheter is inserted approximately 2 to 3 inches. The appearance of urine is evidence that the catheter is in the bladder.

The catheter should be held steady by resting the hand against the pubis. This will avoid the possibility of the catheter shifting outward and then inward again with possible contamination and irritation of the urethra. As the flow of urine decreases, the catheter is gradually withdrawn about $\frac{1}{2}$ inch at a time to remove any remaining urine.

Introduction of the catheter should not be painful, but it may produce sensations of pressure or desire to urinate. If the external meatus cannot be located, if the patient seems to be experiencing pain, or if the catheter cannot be passed for any reason, the procedure should be discontinued and the physician notified.

The purpose of the catheterization determines the steps to be taken following the procedure, such as the saving of a specimen or measuring the amount of urine collected for determining the quantity of residual urine. The procedure should always be recorded, including the amount of urine withdrawn, the color, clarity, or unusual odor of the urine, and any unusual discomfort or resistance encountered in passing the catheter.

Male

The principles, the equipment, and the measures for maintaining aseptic technique are similar for male and female catheterization. The differences in anatomy, however, must be understood in order for male catheterization to be performed without trauma to the urethra. Although

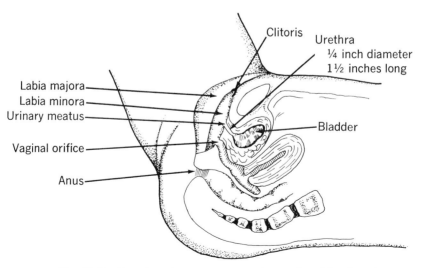

Fig. 29-5. Female urinary system and associated landmarks.

the procedure is usually carried out by the male nurse or the physician, there may be situations in which the female nurse will be expected to catheterize a male patient.

The male urethra is common to both the excretory and reproductive systems. It is approximately 7 to 8 inches long and consists of three parts: (1) the prostatic, surrounded by the prostate, (2) the membranous, and (3) the cavernous, extending from the external sphincter to the urethral meatus (Fig. 29-6). The cavernous portion of the urethra can be straightened by lifting the penis. The curvature of the remainder of the urethra is fixed because of the structures through which it passes. With the individual in the dorsal recumbent position the curvature is concave, first downward and then slightly upward.

The recommended position for the patient is dorsal recumbent, with knees flexed and legs slightly rotated externally. Careful draping, adequate explanation, and competent performance of the nurse will help to avoid embarrassment or fear on the part of the patient.

After cleansing of the external urinary meatus, the penis is grasped at the coronary sulcus and extended with slight traction to straighten the concave curvature at the mergence of the cavernous and membranous portions of the urethra.

Holding the catheter with the gloved fingers (or sterile forceps) the nurse inserts its lubricated tip into the urethral meatus and directs it about $1\frac{1}{2}$ inches, slowly and gently. Slight resistance may be felt as the catheter encounters Guerin's fold or the shallow depression of the fossa navicularis. Bypassing these structures is usually accomplished without discomfort to the patient by gently twisting the catheter while allowing it to find its own pathway. The catheter is advanced and the grasp changed at short distances, since it usually glides easily through the cavernous portion of the urethra.

Slight resistance may be again encountered at the bulbous pouch, where the catheter tip may push against the fold of the urethral mucosa as it traverses this portion of the urethra. A maneuver usually successful in guiding the catheter past this point is to apply more traction to the penis, withdrawing the catheter a bit, then lowering the penis and the catheter, directing the catheter forward by short, gentle movements. Passage of the catheter is facilitated by the patient taking deep breaths

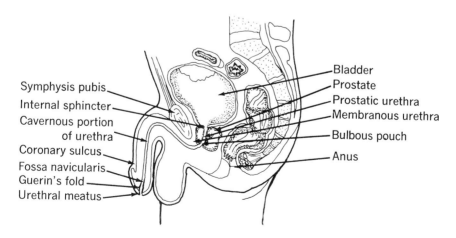

Fig. 29-6. Male urinary system and associated landmarks.

469

to avoid reflex muscular contractions. When the catheter passes through the internal sphincter and is in the bladder, urine will appear.

The indwelling catheter

An indwelling, or retention, catheter is one introduced into the bladder to remain for a period of time to keep the bladder empty. This may be necessary when pressure from a distended bladder is not desirable, for an incontinent or unconscious patient, for gradual decompression of an acutely distended bladder, or for intermittent bladder drainage and irrigation.

A typical indwelling catheter is the Foley catheter, which is constructed with a double lumen. The main channel is for drainage of urine and the other for inflation of the balloon through the sidepiece, using either sterile saline or water. The balloon is distended after the catheter has been inserted to keep the tip securely in the bladder (Fig. 29-7). Because the inflated balloon must be large enough so that it will not slip out through the internal sphincter, a range of sizes is available varying in capacity from 5 to 30 ml.

In most situations the method of inserting the indwelling catheter is the same as for the basic catheterization procedure, but equipment is added for inflating the balloon and for either straight or intermittent drainage and /or bladder irrigation. Equipment needed for inflating the balloon will vary. Some balloons must be inflated by a syringe fitted with an adapter and then the sidepiece clamped to keep the balloon distended. Another type of self-sealing balloon is filled with a syringe and a No. 20 needle. If the balloon is in the bladder, the patient should not experience discomfort or pain when the balloon is distended. However, if the balloon is still in the urethra the patient will experience considerable pain. In that event, the balloon is emptied, inserted a little farther, and inflated again. When the balloon is in the

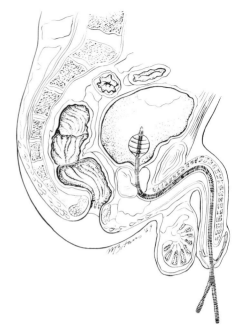

Fig. 29-7. Foley catheter in position with balloon inflated.

bladder it should inflate without any difficulty.

When the indwelling catheter is properly in place, the drainage channel of the catheter is connected with the collection unit using sterile connecting tubing. Usually the collection unit is a disposable plastic bag calibrated for convenience in measuring output. The straight drainage set generally used for this purpose is a closed system that decreases the danger of infection when used correctly. The connecting tube must be long enough for the patient to move about freely in bed but should not hang below the level of the collecting receptacle, which is attached to the bed frame as illustrated in Fig. 29-8. The tubing may be pinned or clipped to the bedding in order to hold it in place, and it may also be taped to the inner aspect of the patient's thigh to avoid tension on the catheter as he changes position. Tension on the tubing may cause it to separate from the catheter, allowing urine to drain onto the bed

470

and increasing the possibility of ascending infection.

Whether the connecting tube is placed over or under the patient's thigh often depends upon the opinion of the attending physician. If positioned over the thigh, urinary drainage from the bladder must be established and maintained against gravity. If positioned under the thigh the weight of the patient's leg resting on the tubing may compress it, again contributing to failure of efficient bladder drainage. Tubing that is too long or that is allowed to become kinked on itself will cause a similar problem. A plastic connector is generally used at the juncture of the catheter and drainage tubing for use in determining the patency

of the drainage system and for noting the character of the drainage.

In this drainage system the catheter acts as a siphon to empty the bladder of urine or of irrigating solution. Siphons depend on differences in pressure for their action. A fluid will flow in a siphon in the direction of the least pressure. The force that makes a siphon work is the weight of a column of water between two fluid surfaces (the gradient). A siphon is effective as long as the free surface of the liquid in one vessel is lower than the free surface of the liquid in the other vessel. The application of this principle is that the collection unit must be lower than the bladder or back flow into the bladder will occur; the greater the distance between the collection unit and the bladder, the greater will be the suction on the bladder.

The speed of flow of the urine will depend on the diameter of the catheter. A catheter with a large diameter, such as an 18 Fr., will produce a faster flow than one of small diameter, such as a 10 Fr. A unit in the French scale equals 0.33 mm. and measures the outside diameter of the tube.

The speed of flow of the urine will also depend on the specific gravity of the urine. Urine that is heavy with pus will flow more slowly than urine that is dilute because the weight of the urine offers more resistance to the tube.

Irrigation and care. Irrigation of the retention catheter is generally ordered when the patency of the drainage system requires it or if a bladder infection is present and the urine is cloudy from pus and cellular debris. The irrigating solution dilutes the sediment that tends to collect and aids in its removal from the bladder.

The solution used for bladder irrigation should be an aqueous preparation that will be nonirritating to the sensitive mucous membrane lining the bladder. Sterile normal saline is often used for this purpose. Equipment needed for open irrigation of the indwelling catheter is a basic irrigation

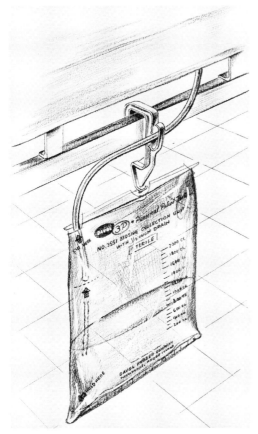

Fig. 29-8. Bedside collection unit. (Courtesy Davol Rubber Co., Providence, R. I.)

set (usually disposable) and the prescribed solution. Careful aseptic technique is absolutely necessary to minimize the possibility of bladder infection developing, if it is not already present. Unless otherwise prescribed, approximately 30 ml per each instillation in a bladder irrigation is used. The instillation is repeated three or more times, depending on the appearance of the return flow.

A deposit of urinary precipitates tends to form in the tubing and catheter and may necessitate changing them. However, the catheter is usually replaced only upon the physician's order because of the danger of infection. Sometimes an antiseptic solution may be added to the collecting unit to inhibit bacterial growth in the stagnant urine. When the catheter is disconnected —for example, to change the tubing, for the patient to ambulate, or for irrigation—it is essential that measures be taken to avoid contaminating either the catheter or tubing. In many situations small disposable sterile urinary catheter plugs are available for this purpose. They can be used as sterile covering for both catheter and tubing.

When the patient ambulates without the catheter being disconnected, the collecting unit must be removed from the bed frame and transported with the patient. However, it is essential that the patient understand the relationship between the level of the collecting unit and the bladder and the importance of avoiding backflow into the bladder. Otherwise he may inadvertently raise the collecting unit with resulting backflow. The patient needs to understand the working principle of bladder drainage and what he can do to help maintain its proper function, within the limits of his condition.

Open irrigation through the indwelling catheter may not be a suitable method of irrigation in some cases, either because of the infection hazard or because it is apt to be less efficient than a closed system of intermittent irrigation. In the closed method a container of sterile irrigating solution is hung on an intravenous pole and a tube from the container is connected by a Y connector to the catheter. The third arm of the Y is connected to the tube leading to the outflow container. The inflow and outflow are controlled by two clamps.

Bladder irrigation should always be performed gently to avoid injury to the mucous membrane of the bladder. The pressure of water in a container for irrigation has been established as approximately $1/_2$ pound for each foot of elevation. The pressure exerted by a column of water varies with its height—pressure can be lessened by shortening the column of fluid. Very low pressure is used for bladder treatments.

The nurse should maintain good posture during a bladder treatment. If the patient is brought to the near side of the bed, the nurse will find that there is less strain on arms and back and the treatment can therefore be carried out more efficiently.

PROBLEM OF INCONTINENCE

Incontinence is the involuntary voiding of urine, or the involuntary defecation of feces, or both occurring in the same patient. Incontinence may be either temporary, prolonged, or permanent, according to the contributing factors involved for any one patient.

Urinary incontinence. Involuntary voiding may be total, that is, constant dribbling because urine is not being stored in the bladder or because the bladder is not emptying normally. The dribbling occurs when the pressure in the bladder causes overflow but the pressure is not sufficient to empty the bladder. Incontinence may be temporary, for instance, during unconsciousness, or it may be a continuing problem such as that occurring in neurologic impairment, for example, in spinal cord injury.

Fecal incontinence. Involuntary defecation occurs when the anal sphincters fail to control the voluntary passage of feces and flatus.

Incontinence, urinary and/or fecal, is one of the most devastating of physical problems from the patient's viewpoint, and it causes him much embarrassment and emotional disturbance. It is a common problem for many geriatric patients who have suffered a cerebral vascular accident or those with atonic muscles. Depending on the cause of loss of control, the individual may be unaware of the need to void or defecate, or he may be aware of the need but unable to control the passing of urine or feces. The person with prolonged loss of control who remains incontinent because he has not had the benefit of a bowel or bladder management program is seriously handicapped in resuming his work and social life. Therefore, the situation should not be considered irremediable because the individual may benefit from a bowel and/or bladder training program, although some factors associated with incontinence may make management most difficult or only partially successful.

Nursing measures. The most immediate measures are concerned with cleanliness, skin care, and emotional support while participating in the efforts to help the patient regain functional control of bowels and bladder.

Constant diligence is required in order to keep the patient clean, dry, and free from unpleasant uriniferous and fecal odors and to prevent the development of skin problems. Decubitus ulcers develop very quickly when the patient's skin is irritated by contact with the ammonia of the urine, wet linen, and feces. Thorough washing and drying of the skin and use of clean linen promptly are essential each time soiling occurs. The problem of integrity of the skin is discussed further in Chapter 19.

Disposable incontinent pads may be used much like a diaper. However, for the mentally alert patient this may be very depressing unless it is managed with tact, understanding, and explanation to the patient. It is wise to avoid referring to the incontinent pad or protector as a diaper.

It is important psychologically for the patient to recognize that measures are being directed toward helping him to have restored normal function. Working with the patient to establish regular intervals for placing him on the toilet (or commode or bedpan) following meals and fluids, and perhaps at 2- to 3-hour intervals to give the patient an opportunity to attempt developing muscular control, would be appropriate in most cases. A regular schedule in which the patient learns to use a specific method to stimulate defecation and/or empty the bladder is essential for successful rehabilitation. *Bowel and bladder training programs* are developed essentially by such planning, worked out with the patient's participation, the goal being to achieve control on a regular basis (without enemas, laxatives, or catheters). Such a training program becomes an important part of the nursing plan of care through which consistency in assisting the patient is provided throughout the 24-hour period.

PROBLEMS RELATED TO THE REPRODUCTIVE TRACT

The system known as the *genitourinary system* consists of the urinary tract, male and female, and the male genital organs. Even though there is close relationship of the reproductive and urinary systems, some of the common problems encountered in the care of patients, while they may be related to the anatomy of both systems, particularly in the male, are most appropriately discussed in context with dysfunctions of the urinary tract, such as problems necessitating urinary catheterization.

Therefore, the focus at this point is primarily on problems related to the female genital tract. Problems of this nature assume different proportions because the reproductive system, unlike the urinary system, is not closely involved in the body's homeostatic mechanisms. On the other hand, its close relationship to the endocrine system and hormonal control means that there may be important psychic and somatic factors in pathophysiology of the reproductive system, regardless of the exact diagnosis. A review of gynecologic conditions, which may be found in most of the medical-surgical nursing texts, need not be repeated here, but it is suggested as a background for the following discussion of treatments of the vaginal canal.

Vaginal treatments

Treatments of the vaginal canal include douches, or irrigations, and the insertion of drugs in suppository, tablet, or powder form. The vaginal douche is an irrigation or flushing of the vaginal canal. It may be used simply to cleanse the vagina because of irritating discharges or as a preparation for surgery, to bring an antiseptic, disinfectant, or astringent solution in contact with infected or inflamed cervical and vaginal surfaces, or to apply heat to the pelvis to aid absorption of intrapelvic inflammations and exudates. Equipment used in giving a vaginal douche consists of a reservoir that is either a metal can or a plastic or rubber bag, some tubing, and a nozzle, which is usually of hard rubber or plastic. The entire equipment may be disposable. Solutions used are mild antiseptics or astringents made up in amounts of 1,000 to 2,000 ml. Drugs in suppository or tablet form are antiseptic and are inserted with a gloved finger.

Application of principles

The external genitals are made up of the mons veneris, the labia majora, the labia minora, the clitoris, the urinary meatus, the glands, and the vaginal orifice (Fig. 29-9). The mons veneris is a skin-covered pad of fat over the symphysis pubis. The labia majora are large structures composed

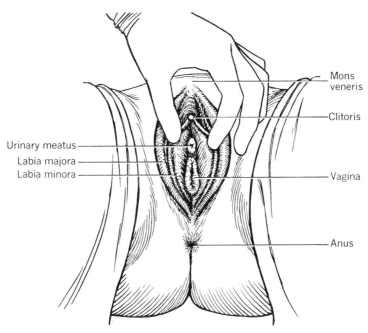

Fig. 29-9. External female genitals.

mainly of loose fat covered with skin. The outer surface is covered with hair, whereas the inner surface is smooth and free from hair. In the back-lying position with the knees flexed and apart, the labia majora separate. The labia minora are located inside the labia majora and are covered with modified skin resembling mucous membrane. They are freely supplied with blood. The labia minora come together in the midline and protect the vaginal and urethral orifices. They need to be separated before the vaginal orifice can be seen for introduction of the douche nozzle. The clitoris is a small organ composed of erectile tissue located under the junction of the labia minora. It contains many blood vessels and nerves. The urinary meatus is the small opening into the urethra situated between the labia minora below the clitoris and above the vaginal orifice. Bartholin's glands, two bean-shaped glands, one on either side of the vaginal opening, secrete a lubricating fluid. The vaginal orifice is the opening into the vagina. It is larger than the urinary meatus and may be partially or completely closed by the hymen. If it is completely closed, it is impossible to introduce the douche nozzle. If it is partially closed, a small nozzle or a catheter may be used. Since no sphincter muscle guards the vaginal tract, irrigating solutions return as they are being introduced.

The vaginal orifice opens into the vagina, which is a flattened but distensible muscular and membranous canal that extends upward from its orifice to the cervix of the uterus. Except during menstruation and late pregnancy, the opening into the cervix is closed. The vagina lies in front of the rectum and behind the bladder. In

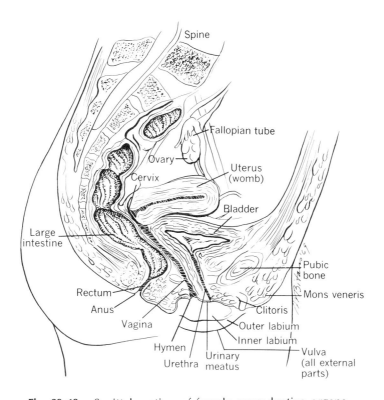

Fig. 29-10. Sagittal section of female reproductive organs.

475

the middle portion of its course, the anterior and posterior walls are in contact. The posterior wall is about 9 cm. long and the anterior wall is about 7.5 cm. long. The lining mucous membrane of the vaginal tract is a thick layer of stratified squamous epithelium. The mucous membrane is arranged in transverse folds called rugae, which makes a thorough cleansing of the area difficult. The mucous lining continues into the cervix, the uterus, and the fallopian tubes, which open into the peritoneum.

The direction of the vaginal tract is backward until the cul-de-sac is reached, and then it is slightly forward. This fact should be kept in mind in introducing the douche nozzle (Fig. 29-10). The walls of the vagina are made of strong muscle tissue. The blood supply to the vagina is from the vaginal branches of the uterine artery. The pelvic nerve, composed of parasympathetic autonomic fibers, arising from the second to the fourth sacral nerves, supplies vasodilator fibers to the external genitals. The nerves passing to the vagina are derived from the hypogastric plexus and from the fourth sacral and the pudic nerves.

The vagina is the habitat of a rod-shaped gram-positive bacillus described by Döderlein and known as Döderlein's bacillus. This bacillus is anaerobic and, by its effect upon the glycogen in the vaginal epithelium, gives an acid reaction to the normal vaginal secretion. The vaginal organisms are supposed to exert a bactericidal action upon any pathogenic organisms unless the latter are too numerous or too virulent. The normal protecting vaginal secretions are removed by frequent irrigations, and the vaginal tract thus is weakened in its resistance to pathogenic organisms.

The organisms most frequently responsible for pathogenic changes in the vaginal tract are the *Gonococcus, Streptococcus pyogenes, Staphylococcus albus, Staphylococcus aureus,* and *Escherichia (Bacillus)*

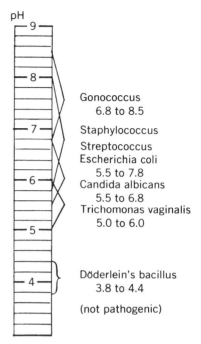

Fig. 29-11. Organisms found in the vaginal tract.

coli (Fig. 29-11). The gonococci grow best at body temperature and in oxygen but may grow without it. They thrive on delicate epithelium and do not invade tissue as a rule. Gonorrhea may spread upward to the fallopian tubes, or it may infect Bartholin's glands, Skene's glands, or the urethra. The gonococci do not attack the vaginal mucosa in an adult patient because the mucosa of the vaginal tract of adults is of resistant stratified squamous epithelium, unlike the softer epithelium of prepuberty girls. The gonococci may attack the conjunctivas and may cause blindness, so that precautions must be taken to prevent splashing when douches are given to patients who have gonorrhea. Hands may carry the gonococci from the vaginal area or from soiled perineal pads to the eyes. Patients are provided with facilities for handwashing after contact of the hands with the genital area. The nurse should wash the hands well before and after contact also. For inserting a tablet or a suppository, the nurse wears a glove to prevent infection.

The streptococci and the staphylococci may be introduced into the genital tract at the time of examinations or treatments. However, a break or an abrasion of the mucous membrane is necessary for their entrance into the tissues. Such an abrasion may be caused by using force in introducing a douche nozzle or by using too large a nozzle.

The colon bacillus *(Escherichia coli)* is the commonest type of bacterium normally inhabiting the intestinal tract. It may be found upon the skin surface of the vulva and the perineum. Drawing toliet tissue toward the back is a means of preventing contamination of the vaginal canal with organisms found in fecal material.

The upper part of the cervical canal and the endometrium are normally sterile. Near the external os the cervical mucus may be contaminated with bacteria of the vaginal vault.

Equipment used in giving douches usually is put up in sterile disposable packages (Fig. 29-12). In most instances, the sterility is not maintained. However, if stitches are present or if the tissues have been traumatized, the sterility of the douche equipment and solution is carefully observed. The nurse washes the hands before and after the treatment. Soiled perineal pads are wrapped in paper and burned. In case of a communicable disease, the nurse wears a gown. Sterile pads are used to prevent infection. It is best to secure them with a belt to prevent their slipping.

The vaginal epithelium contains much glycogen as a result of estrogenic activity. Through a series of changes the glycogen becomes lactic acid by the activity of Döderlein's bacillus. Before puberty and after the menopause, there is no glycogen, and Döderlein's bacilli are few because of insufficient nourishement. Therefore, normal lactic acid protection is lacking and susceptibility to infection is increased during these periods of life. The menstrual flow carries away the protective acidity, so that for a few days after menstruation the resistance of the vaginal mucous lining is low.

The normal reaction of the vaginal mucosa is acid, a pH range of 4 to 5. This is sufficient to be a protection against infection, since the pH range of most bacteria is from 4 to 7.5. The pH range of organisms that infect the vaginal tract has been well established. *Trichomonas vaginalis* needs a pH of 5 to 6. Loaded streptococci or staphylococci fields need a pH of 6 to 7. The gonococci need a pH of 8. Hyperactivity of the alkaline cervical secretion may increase the pH to as high as 6. Bacterial invasion may raise it to as high as 7. The acidity may be increased by douching with solutions made of acids whose pH is below 4 or 5, such as acetic acid, the pH of which is 3. Douche solutions may cause chemical irritation.

When the douche is ordered for its cleansing and thermic effect, a bland solution made with either sodium chloride, 0.9%, or sodium bicarbonate, 2%, may be ordered. When douches are used to allay inflammations, antiseptic or disinfecting agents may be added to the water. For deodorizing purposes, potassium permanganate solution, 1:5,000, may be ordered. Astringents sometimes ordered include acetic acid or vinegar solution, 1.5%, and borax or alum solutions, 3%.

Antiseptic suppositories are sometimes ordered. For skin irritation caused by the vaginal discharge, powders, soothing lotions, or ointments may be ordered to be applied to the skin. Petrolatum or mineral oil may be used to lubricate the skin to prevent burning when hot solutions are used.

Since pressure of the liquid from an irrigating tip is equal to the pressure of a vertical column of liquid extending from the level of solution in the can down to

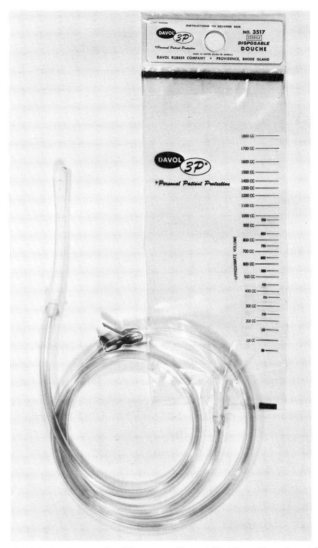

Fig. 29-12. Vaginal irrigation unit. (Courtesy Davol Rubber Co., Providence, R. I.)

the outlet of the tube, pressure of the solution in a vaginal douche varies with the height of the reservoir. Douches should be given or taken under low pressure. In no irrigation should pressure exceed 1 pound. Too much pressure in a vaginal irrigation may force infectious material into the cervical canal. Since great force is obtained by the bulb type of irrigator, it is seldom used for treatments.

Friction depends on the nature and the condition of surfaces. Friction is much di-

minished by proper lubrication. Wet surfaces give less friction than dry ones. The solution flowing through the nozzle as it is being introduced provides sufficient lubrication for it. Medication in suppository or tablet form needs to be lubricated to reduce friction between the drug preparation and the mucous membrane.

The vaginal mucosa will tolerate considerably higher temperatures than will the skin. Therefore it is important that a thermometer be used to regulate the temperature of solutions used rather than to rely on the patient's sensations or requests. Usually the temperature of the douche is about 105° F. Water is a good conductor of heat, and warmth is imparted to other pelvic organs by conduction. Where application of heat is the primary purpose, a sufficient quantity of solution is used to prolong the thermic effect.

Gravity will aid the inflow of solution if the hips are elevated and the head is low. Gravity also aids the outflow if the patient is raised to the sitting position at the completion of the treatment. The equipment should be arranged conveniently near the nurse to prevent strain and to save time during the treatment. The nurse should stand by the bed with feet separated to give balance and should bend slightly forward at the waistline.

Learning situations for the patient

The patient is cautioned against taking douches unless they are ordered, since the solution washes away protective secretions. If a douche is to be continued at home, the nurse may instruct the patient in regard to the proper method of making the solution and the proper way to take a douche. The person must be lying down in order for the solution to flush the entire vaginal tract. Equipment for the treatment may be purchased at a drugstore.

If applications of medications to the vaginal or the perineal area are to be continued, the nurse will make sure the patient understands how to carry out the treatment. It may be important to assist the patient in changing her attitude toward her own condition and to impress upon her that a gynecologic condition is not necessarily connected with venereal disease. Since the gonococci may affect the eye, emphasis is placed on the necessity of washing the hands after any contact with the genital area or with soiled perineal pads.

PSYCHOSOCIAL ASPECTS

Before receiving bladder treatment the patient should have some orientation to the procedure and its purpose. He should also have some idea as to the amount of discomfort to expect. Usually, bladder treatments promote comfort, particularly when the patient is relaxed. Relaxation is promoted by complete, warm draping of the body. Efficient draping also helps to decrease embarrassment.

Skillful manipulation of the catheter is important, for if the patient experiences unnecessary pain during a bladder treatment he does not cooperate so easily for subsequent treatments. Therefore, gentleness and consideration for the patient are indicated.

The patient requiring douches may feel embarrassed and have misconceived ideas about treatments of the genital tract. Some persons may have a feeling of guilt associated with conditions of the genital tract because venereal disease is feared.

Embarrassment may be caused by exposure of the genital area of the body. The embarrassment may be lessened by explanation of the procedure, by a matter-of-fact attitude on the part of the nurse, and by adequate draping to avoid unnecessary exposure of the patient. Explanation of how the treatment is to be given is especially helpful for the patient who has never experienced a douche before and fears it. The nurse may suggest that the warm solution will probably bring a feeling of comfort and that probably no pain will be noticed.

The patient requiring douches is often irritable and depressed. Through the cues given by the patient, verbal and nonverbal, the nurse is able to direct the communications into purposeful channels.

Accurate recording on the chart of the treatment given, solution used, character and amount of return flow and of any discharge (when present), and the reaction of the patient ensures availability of essential information to the other members of the health team, including the physician.

Although a well person may administer a douche to herself, illness brings dependence on others for many things, and the nurse gives the douche to the patient. If the patient desires a deviation from the usual procedure, this fact will be noted on the nursing care plan so that the patient's care will not be interrupted by change of personnel. The nurse may help the patient's relatives to understand her condition and to be more tolerant.

SUMMARY

The purpose of this chapter is to present common manifestations of physiologic imbalance that occur in response to pathophysiology in various body systems. The emphasis is on developing one's ability to recognize the presence of symptoms, discomforts, and problems that can be appropriately managed through nursing action and also to develop the ability to identify those manifestations of imbalance that should be promptly and accurately reported to the physician.

The central objective of the chapter is to briefly illustrate the steps of the nursing process in relation to the problem-solving approach in devising and administering patient care. Some selected, commonly occurring problems of illness are presented to illustrate the usefulness of principles as a foundation for devising and administering patient care.

The commonly occurring patient-care problems selected for discussion are urinary and reproductive disorders.

QUESTIONS FOR DISCUSSION

1 Give the meanings of the prefixes *a-* or *an-*, *olig-, poly-, py-,* and *dys-*. Define the term "micturition."
2 Describe three kinds of catheters.
3 How would you prepare 500 ml. of 0.9% saline solution for a douche?
4 How is an indwelling catheter secured?
5 What bacteria are most apt to cause bladder infections?

6 What are the common causes of urinary retention?
7 Identify nursing measures that may be employed to promote emptying the bladder without using a catheter.
8 For what purposes may the vaginal douche be prescribed?
9 What bacteria normally inhabit the vaginal tract?
10 What organisms may be pathogenic in the vaginal tract?
11 What methods are used to prevent pathogenic organisms from invading the vaginal tract?
12 What is the pH of the vaginal secretions?
13 What is the pH of organisms that cause infections in the vaginal tract?
14 What solutions are commonly ordered for vaginal douches?
15 How is pressure controlled in a vaginal douche?
16 How is friction reduced between the douche nozzle and the mucous membrane of the vaginal canal?
17 What is the danger in taking frequent douches?
18 Should a prescribed douche be administered during the menstrual period?

LIFE SITUATION

Mrs. Connor has had radium removed from the vaginal tract and has an order for a douche. While the treatment is being administered Mrs. Connor comments to the nurse, "Dr. Armstrong told me that I did not have cancer, but I have never heard of anyone who did not have cancer having a radium treatment. You know, doctors don't tell you everything. I am just wondering if he was telling me the truth." How would you reply to Mrs. Connor's statement?

SUGGESTED READINGS

Birum, Linda H., and Zimmerman, Donna S.: Catheter plugs as a source of infection, American Journal of Nursing 71:2150, 1971.

Dison, Norma G.: An atlas of nursing techniques, St. Louis, 1971, The C. V. Mosby Co.

Dobbins, Janet, and Gleit, Carol: Experience with the lateral position for catheterization, Nursing Clinics of North America 6:373, June, 1971.

Gibbs, Gertrude E.: Perineal care of the incapacitated patient, American Journal of Nursing 69:124, January, 1969.

Hassett, Marjorie: Teaching hemodialysis to the family unit, Nursing Clinics of North America **7:**349, June, 1972.

Shafer, Kathleen N., and others: Medical-surgical nursing, St. Louis, 1971, The C. V. Mosby Co., chap. 8, p. 131; chap. 19, p. 382; chap. 20, p. 433.

30 The surgical patient

THE PATIENT EXPERIENCING SURGERY

Regardless of its purpose, a surgical operation is always a stressful ordeal for the patient and his family. Uncertainty as to the outcome of the operation, dread of associated pain, fear of the anesthetic, and disquieting thoughts of altered personal plans are some of the factors adding to the physical stress of the patient.

Throughout the operative experience, the nurse, as a member of the health team, contributes to the care of the patient by constant, knowledgeable observation, assessment, and evaluation of his condition and needs; by skill in adapting and giving physical care according to his special needs as a surgical patient; and by sensitivity in supporting the patient psychologically in his efforts to cope with the apprehension he experiences upon entering the hospital and submitting himself to the surgical operation.

Scientific principles

Most of the principles presented in the preceding chapters may be applicable to the care of the surgical patient at some point in his hospitalization and should be reviewed in this connection. Some additional examples that are apt to apply generally in the event of surgical treatment are stated and possible applications are described.

Anatomy and physiology. Reflecting on the following pertinent biologic principles will stimulate analytic thought in planning effective nursing intervention for meeting specific patient needs in the process of maintaining or restoring optimal bodily function.

1. A relatively constant blood volume is necessary to provide for the changing demands of body organs.
   a. The volume of circulating blood varies with body weight and surface area, approximately 3 liters per square meter of body surface, or about 5 to 6 liters for the average-sized adult.
   b. Arterial bleeding is rapid and spurting.
   c. Venous bleeding is slow and regular.
   d. Capillary bleeding is slow and oozing.
   e. The rapid loss of more than 30% of

485

the total blood volume may result in death.

2. Adequate pressure is necessary in the vessels supplying the tissues in order to maintain the constancy of circulating blood volume.

    a. Overall vasoconstriction of the arterioles will lead to an increase in blood pressure.

    b. Overall vasodilation will lead to a fall in blood pressure.

    c. If the blood volume is reduced, as in hemorrhage, the blood pressure falls and the circulation becomes inadequate.

    d. A state of "surgical shock" occurs when there is marked interference with the circulation of the blood, which may be associated with dilation of the arteriolar beds and consequent lowering of arterial pressure; the decreased blood flow to vital tissues results in anoxia; blood flow may fall below the level essential to the welfare of the tissues.

    e. Dilation of the arterioles may result from a histamine-like substance formed in injured tissues.

    f. Vasodilation (or vasoconstriction) may be influenced by the relationship between the emotions and the autonomic nervous system; therefore, the emotional state of the individual may greatly affect the blood pressure. For example, psychic trauma may be a causative factor in the occurrence of shock.

3. The blood pressure in the arteries of the brain is less than at the heart level when a person is in the sitting or standing position. Since this difference disappears when a person is in the lying position, adequacy of the blood supply to the brain is promoted by the recumbent position with head at the level of the heart.

4. The inhalation of irritant gases (for example, an anesthetic) or too rapid administration of intravenous fluids may result in pulmonary edema. Edema occurs when congestion in the pulmonary blood vessels increases to the point that fluid oozes through the capillary walls into the air passages.

5. Any obstruction to breathing or to adequate drainage of respiratory secretions predisposes to respiratory tract infection. (See Chapter 19 for related principles.)

6. Venous stasis associated with obstruction of normal blood flow in the lower trunk and extremities may result in formation of a primary clot *(thrombus)*.

7. Obstruction of blood supply to the lungs by *emboli* or by mucous plugs results in impaired pulmonary function and possibly in tissue *necrosis.*

8. All the cells of the body require definite amounts of water and electrolytes for proper functioning.

Microbiology

1. The unbroken skin and mucous membranes offer natural barriers to invasion of the body by microorganisms. Infection results from the invasion of pathogenic *transient* microorganisms into the tissues. Members of the *normal flora* of the body may be pathogenic when introduced into the bloodstream or tissues through an unnatural route of entry, as in the case of a surgical or accidental wound.

2. The severity of an infection and the damage caused reflect the virulence of the pathogen and the host's capacity for defense against invasion and toxicity.

Chemistry. Solvents, such as alcohol, and bacteriostatic soap or detergent containing hexachlorophene remove skin oils and most of the superficial microorganisms.

Psychosocial aspects. An individual's personal sensitivity to pain is affected by his emotional attitude toward pain. His personal perception of pain may be affected by a variety of factors including state of consciousness, past experience, understanding of the origin and meaning of his pain, and the amount of fatigue and anxiety. (See Chapter 26 for related principles.)

PREOPERATIVE CARE

Surgical procedures are performed for the removal of diseased structures, for the restoration of normal functions, for palliative reasons, and for diagnostic purposes. To secure the best results for the patient, protective measures must be carried out before, during, and after the operation. Procedures performed and principles applied at this time may be divided into two groups, those occurring before the operation and those occurring after the operation, and they are usually referred to as preoperative and postoperative nursing care.

General preoperative care

Operations are of two types: those of an emergency nature and those for which a time may be chosen (called elective surgery). An emergency operation is one that must be performed within a certain period of time in order to save the patient's life. Some common examples of emergency operations are those dealing with the gastrointestinal tract, such as in acute appendicitis and ruptured peptic ulcers. Also, many lacerations and fractures resulting from accidents must be cared for immediately to prevent such complications as hemorrhage, shock, and infection.

An elective operation is one that the patient needs but that can be performed when it is convenient and more beneficial for the patient. Operations of an elective nature allow time to study the patient's condition thoroughly and to prepare him more adequately for the procedure.

All operations produce trauma and are a danger to the patient. Therefore, it is essential that the patient be in the best physical condition possible and that as many of the protective measures as feasible be carried out. With the aid of the newer drugs that control blood pressure and by the use of chemotherapy and the antibiotics, many operations that were quite impossible a decade ago can now be performed with safety.

Diagnostic and supportive measures. Upon admission of the surgical patient to the hospital, the attending physician, intern, or resident on the service usually takes a careful history, performs a complete physical examination, and orders blood and urine tests. Findings from these procedures help the surgeon to diagnose the presence of any other existing condition needing treatment before surgery and to determine how much risk will be involved in the operation and what precautions are to be observed. This diagnosis enables the surgical team to have such remedial measures as whole blood, blood constituents, oxygen, and other blood pressure stimulants in readiness.

Much postoperative discomfort and many complications result from improper preparation of the gastrointestinal tract. It is important that the patient be in a state of adequate nutrition, with proper fluid and electrolyte balance. The patient is usually allowed a full diet up to and including the evening meal before the day of the operation. Intravenous fluids and vitamins are usually given if indicated. They do much to prevent shock, dehydration, and electrolyte imbalance.

It is essential that the stomach be empty at the time of operation regardless of how minor the surgery, since vomiting can be produced by anesthetics, excitement, or slight tissue damage.

An enema may or may not be ordered, depending upon the preference of the surgeon. If the patient has regular bowel habits and the operation does not involve the gastrointestinal tract, it is now common practice to omit enemas, especially if early ambulation is expected. However, for operations on the gastrointestinal tract or pelvic or perineal areas, enemas are usually ordered until clear. Enemas should be effective so as to reduce the number, since repeated enemas, regardless of the solution, upset the electrolyte balance, irritate the mucosa, and tire the patient. If more than three are necessary, the nurse should consult the surgeon or resident. Sometimes the order will specify the number the patient is to have. A rested gastrointestinal tract will also do much to lessen postoperative nausea and other common disturbances often referred to by the patient as "gas pains."

Instruction of the patient. Although it is the surgeon's responsibility to discuss with the patient his condition and the nature of the impending surgical operation, the nurse has a responsibility for being informed about the patient's diagnosis, the physician's plan of treatment, and probable outcome for the patient and his family. When the patient or members of his family turn to the nurse for clarification of information they may not have understood, the nurse can reinforce and supplement the physician's explanation. The patient will thus find it easier to express his fears, giving the understanding nurse an opportunity to assist him to cope with these fears or to arrange assistance of the social worker, chaplain, or others when indicated. Meaningful communication with the patient may then open the way for the nurse to explain procedures he will experience and give him needed instruction in an unhurried manner that is conducive to understanding on the part of the patient as to what may happen and what may be expected of him.

Specific information that may be needed by a surgical patient could relate to various nursing procedures, treatments, fluids, diet, elimination, diagnostic tests, and preparation of the operative area. Instruction regarding experiences to be anticipated in the recovery room may also be indicated. Preoperative instruction usually should include explanation, demonstration, and practice of special exercises, such as deep breathing, coughing, turning, relaxing and contracting leg muscles, and early ambulation. As surgery becomes more intricate, so does preoperative instruction. For heart surgery it is sometimes necessary to have several teaching periods. Sometimes this is done in groups, thus enabling patients to share experiences. For children, it is now common practice to have them visit the hospital prior to surgery and play "doctor, nurse, and patient."

Legal data. A written permit required before surgery is usually obtained at the time of admission. However, in some hospitals it may be delayed until the day before the operation. The permit should be explained thoroughly to the patient, and he should not be under the influence of any sedative or narcotic drug during the explanation or at the time of the actual signing. If the patient is of legal age, he may sign his own permit. If not, a parent or legal guardian must sign it. In cases of removal of any of the reproductive organs, some states require the signature of both the husband and wife. For some gynecologic operations and special diagnostic tests, the patient may be requested to sign a special permit in addition to the general one. The nearest relative or otherwise legally designated person is requested to sign for a mentally ill, unconscious, or irresponsible patient. In emergencies a telegram or witnessed telephone call is accepted as legal permission.

Care of the skin. Cleansing of the skin is important in preventing postoperative infection from microorganisms on the skin. In addition to the general bath, special attention is given to the operative field. To minimize the danger of infection, the site of operation is shaved and thoroughly cleansed. Either a dry or wet shave may be done, depending on the area and time of operation. A sterilized razor and new blade should be used for each patient to aid in avoiding infection.

Scratching the skin is to be avoided since this increases the possibility of infection. Cuts and abrasions may be prevented by working up a good lather and by using a safety razor with a sharp blade. With some detergents, such as pHisoHex or G-11, more effective results are obtained by diluting the product with water rather than by adding more soap, since a concentrated solution will not give a good lather. Stretching the skin so that it is taut and shaving in the direction that the hair grows will produce both a closer and a more gentle shave. A dry shave is sometimes used for emergencies and on the extremities, and it can be made more effective by first drying the area and dusting with talcum.

Following either method of shaving, the area is thoroughly cleansed with soap and water. Most authorities believe that mechanical scrubbing of the skin is one of the best methods of preventing postoperative infections. By reducing the microbial flora, danger of autogenous infection through the surgical incision is minimized. Surgical preparation of the skin is often done in the operating room immediately prior to surgery.

Modern therapeutic drugs have now come to play a rather important part in the routine preparation of a preoperative patient. This preparation may include preventive therapy, with antibiotics given preoperatively to combat infection postoperatively.

Rest. Because it is essential that a preoperative patient secure a good night's rest preceding surgery, the surgeon usually orders a sedative such as one of the barbiturate preparations. This is usually administered at bedtime and is followed the next morning by a preoperative hypodermic injection. A calm and rested patient takes an anesthetic more easily, which in turn lessens the possibility of shock.

Psychologic preparation. Much of the physical preparation of the patient would be useless if it were not accompanied by the proper mental preparation. Doctors and nurses realize more than ever the close relationship between the physical and mental condition of a patient. Therefore, the surgical patient must be emotionally ready for the operation or the surgery should be delayed if possible.

Following are some of the common causes of worry and fear in the preoperative patient.

1. Fear regarding the outcome of the operation. Will it be a success? What about pain? Will I wake up? Will I be paralyzed by the anesthetic? How will the operation affect my future life?

2. Economic or home problems. If the patient is head of his household, his hospital stay may mean suffering for the whole family in terms of lack of food or clothing or the necessity of accepting help. If the patient is a mother, she may not be able to obtain the necessary rest because of worry over the care of young children left at home.

3. Worry of a personal nature. Examples include a delay in graduation for a college student, postponement of a business advancement for a young man, or the postponement of an engagement for a young woman.

The nurse can do much to aid the surgical patient. This aid can begin with his admission. Since first impressions usually are lasting ones, it is important that a surgical patient have nothing in his admission routine that will be unpleasant or make him feel unwanted. If the nurse appears hurried, the patient may get the impression that there will not be enough nurses to care for his needs while he is under the anesthetic and is not able to care for himself.

The surgeon usually explains the necessity of the operation to the patient. Most patients have faith in their doctors and trust the decisions they make. The nurse can do much to help the patient to keep this confidence.

The patient who is able to meet life's daily problems as they come usually will be able to withstand stress in time of emergencies. Sickness often brings about a renewal of one's faith in God, and for this reason some patients will desire or request a visit from their minister, priest, or rabbi before surgery. Most hospitals, as a courtesy, list the faith of each patient on admission, and this list is available to visiting ministers. For the out-of-town patient or the one with no particular faith, the hospital chaplain may be available. If the nurse feels that a patient might be in need of spiritual help, it is better to inform the chaplain so that he can approach the patient in a casual routine visit, avoiding the impression that the operation might not be a success.

Almost every patient comes from a community and belongs to a family, and for this reason others will also have an interest in his operation. More often the nearest relative is under a greater mental strain than the patient himself. Overanxious relatives often convey anxiety to the patient, or the patient may become worried about the relative. Courtesy to relatives at the time of admission can do much to lessen the patient's anxiety. If relatives have a feeling that the patient is in good hands, they can do much to transfer this feeling and assurance to the patient. Most patients desire a visit from some member of the family, clergy, or a close friend immediately before going to the operating room.

Flowers, get-well cards, and other tokens sent to the patient by members of his family, friends, co-workers, and church and club members also add to the patient's morale. A feeling of interest by others seems to instill in the patient a desire for a speedy recovery.

Immediate preoperative care

Some procedures are carried out at specific times in relation to the operation. Others may be done hours in advance of the operation, or, in case of an emergency, the majority may be done just preceding the surgery.

Whether the operation is elective or an emergency, certain procedures are performed immediately prior to surgery for the welfare of the patient and are generally referred to as immediate preoperative care. Most hospitals more or less adhere to the following routine.

Morning care. The patient should go to the operating room clean. Usually he has had a tub bath the evening before or rises early the morning of the operation and takes a shower. For a patient who has been heavily sedated or is unable to give self-care, a cleansing bed bath should be administered.

Good mouth care should be given to ensure both comfort and cleanliness. Many patients have fluids restricted after midnight and are in need of some fluid to cleanse and lubricate the oral tissues. An alkaline mouthwash or similar antiseptic is preferred to plain water to avoid tempting the patient to swallow it. Many surgeons order oral antiseptics routinely to avoid the postoperative complication known as surgical parotitis, which results from poor oral hygiene.

Dentures and partial plates may or may not be removed. Some anesthetists prefer that all artificial parts be removed since there is danger of their being broken or swallowed. Others claim that they help the patient maintain the normal contour of the face and facilitate breathing. If removed, they should be labeled and placed in a safe area. If left in place, a notation should be made in the nurse's notes on the chart.

The hair should be combed neatly and braided if long. All pins and combs should be removed to avoid injury to the patient.

A disposable cap or towel may be used to cover the head to protect the hair and help keep it in place.

Observation. The vital signs should be checked and recorded and any abnormalities reported to the charge nurse. The patient should also be observed for signs of a cold or other respiratory infections since these may mean a postponement of the operation.

Clothing and valuables. The patient is dressed in hospital apparel, which consists of a hospital gown that opens down the back. Surgical stockings or leggings are added for warmth if necessary.

All jewelry should be removed, placed in an envelope, labeled, and stored in the proper place until the patient asks for it. If jewelry is given to a relative, this should be done in the presence of another person, and a notation should be made on the chart. Wedding rings that are not removed should be tied to the wrist with a piece of string that has been looped through the ring. In many hospitals a piece of adhesive tape is placed around the ring, but the effectiveness of this is to be questioned since perspiration may cause it to come loose. Some hospitals permit the wearing of religious medals. If so, they should be taped to the body, preferably below the knee or fastened to the wrist tag that identifies the patient.

Artificial eyes and limbs, hearing aids, and other prostheses should also be removed, labeled, and placed in safekeeping. Other valuables, such as money, eyeglasses, and the like, may also be collected at this time in order to avoid a waste of time and the inconvenience of having several packages of valuables.

All personal articles should be removed from the top of the bedside table and placed in safekeeping until the patient again has need of them.

Elimination. The bladder should be emptied immediately before the patient leaves for the operating room. If emptied too soon, it may fill again if surgery is delayed after the patient reaches the operating room. There are two main reasons for an empty bladder: (1) to prevent accidental injury to the bladder during surgery and (2) to prevent early postoperative distension.

Many patients in whom fluids have been restricted may not have a desire to void but may be stimulated to do so when placed on the bedpan or given a urinal. Since most patients, although on nothing by mouth, receive intravenous fluids during surgery, many surgeons order retention catheters (Foley) as part of the immediate preoperative procedure. This is especially true of those patients having pelvic or extensive surgery. Failure to empty the bladder before surgery may lead to the necessity of catheterizing the patient during the operation.

Preoperative medication. Most patients are usually given some type of preliminary analgesic immediately prior to surgery. It usually consists of one of the narcotics, such as morphine, meperidine (Demerol), or a sedative of the barbiturate group. It is almost always combined with atropine or scopolamine, which helps to check the secretions, lessening the possibility of respiratory embarrassment and increasing the relaxation of the smooth muscles. The preliminary sedative helps to calm the patient, thereby lessening the tension that might increase as the time of operation draws near. The present trend is to include also a drug that has an antihistaminic action, such as promethazine (Phenergan).

The patient may become drowsy and may have only a vague memory of being transported from his room. Following the preoperative medication, he should be disturbed as little as possible in order to obtain the fullest benefit from the medication. Therefore, as many of the preoperative procedures as possible should be performed before its administration. The pa-

491

tient should be warned of the possibility of dizziness and should not be allowed out of bed after receiving the medication.

Visitors. Usually the patient will be visited by one or two relatives or close friends before going to surgery. If they arrive after the preliminary medication is given, they should be instructed to be as quiet as possible. In any case, they should try to keep calm and refrain from discussing any unpleasant subject with the patient.

Charting. Before surgery the chart should be completed, showing the latest temperature, pulse, and respiration, the time of voiding or catheterization and the amount of urine, and any treatment with drugs. The name, amount, and exact time of the administration of the preoperative medication should be clearly stated. Although laboratory reports are the responsibility of the medical or other departments, it is the duty of the nurse to see that such reports are in the chart before sending the patient to the operating room.

At the time the patient is transferred to the operating room, the chart is completed by adding the time of departure, and the chart is taken with the patient to the operating room.

Transfer of patient to operating room. If possible, the nurse who has cared for the patient during the preoperative period should accompany him to the operating room. Knowing that he has someone with him who knows and understands his condition gives him reassurance.

The patient may be transferred either in his bed or by stretcher. Both methods have advantages and disadvantages. During the transfer, there should be as little jarring and noise as possible, for a slightly sedated patient may be easily disturbed. The nurse accompanying the patient should remain until he has been received by the proper authorities in the operating room. The nurse then may return to the clinical area to prepare the patient's unit for postoperative care or may remain in the operating room during the entire operative procedure.

Consideration of relatives

A special waiting room should be provided for relatives. It should be located near the recovery room or near the unit to which the patient will be returned. If relatives are given an estimated time at which the patient will probably be returned to his room, they can more easily make plans to be occupied during the waiting period. If no information is given, they will wait restlessly, fearing to leave even for a coffee break. In prolonged surgery, information concerning the patient's progress is appreciated by the family. However, the nurse should never inform them of any direct findings by the surgeon or any unfavorable information unless ordered to do so. The surgeon usually visits the patient soon after his return to the unit and reports or discusses his condition with the family or responsible person.

POSTOPERATIVE CARE
Objectives

When the incision is closed, a major portion of the surgeon's task is accomplished, and the care of the patient again becomes the responsibility of the nurse. Recovery from the anesthetic and immediate trauma produced by the operation and a return to normal activity for the patient are the chief objectives in postoperative nursing care. Both of these objectives depend much upon the ability of the nurse to observe and make wise and sound decisions.

The postoperative care of the patient may be divided into two phases: (1) the care given immediately following the operation and (2) the general care given during the convalescent period. Both are designed to meet the two objectives previously mentioned. The responsibilities of the nurse will include observation, relief of postoperative discomforts, and prevention of complications. Effective nursing care given during the early postoperative period can do much to achieve the objectives of the surgery for the patient.

Environmental factors

As soon as the patient has left the clinical division, preparation for his postoperative care should begin. A main factor to consider is his environment.

Following surgery, the patient may be returned to his bed in his unit or may be

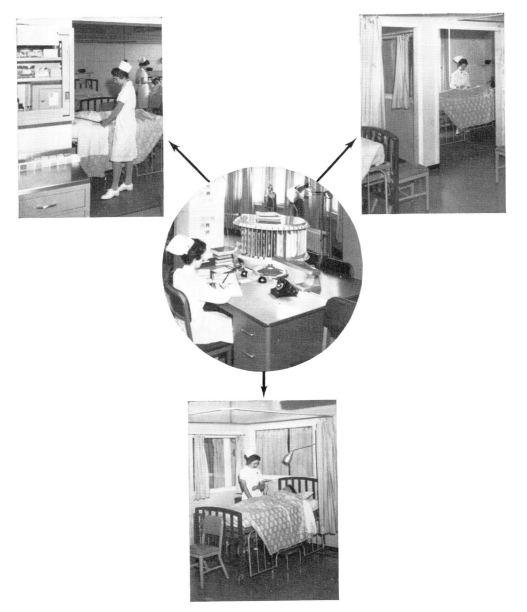

Fig. 30-1. Modern clinical facilities provide for close observation and communication between the charge nurse and patients at all times.

taken to a special room known as the recovery room or postanesthesia room.

If the patient must be returned immediately to a large clinical area, it is advisable to place his bed in an area that is under close supervision. The modern trend is to build clinical areas so that all critical patients will be within a short radius of the nurses' station, where they can be kept under constant observation (Fig. 30-1).

Personnel. All operations, regardless of their simplicity, subject the patient to some trauma and a slight degree of shock. Therefore, the first essential in the postoperative environment is a well-qualified nursing staff. Since the newly operated patient is completely dependent on nursing care, there should be a sufficient number of qualified nurses to care for his needs. Effective nursing care immediately following surgery hastens recovery and prevents many complications.

Since every human body is different from all others, no two patients will react the same. The nurse in charge should be a keen observer and should be well versed in postoperative dangers and complications.

Equipment. The postoperative bed, which is often called an anesthetic or ether bed, should be made as soon as the patient has been transferred to surgery (Fig. 30-2). Any waste or delay of time in preparing it may result in lack of a place to put the patient if he is returned sooner than the expected time.

If possible, a full set of clean linen should be used and other protection added if necessary so as to disturb the patient as little as possible later. In addition to the basic unit equipment, the modern recovery room contains special equipment that aids in the treatment of emergencies, such as a supply of oxygen, intravenous therapy carts, various types of suction machines, and cardiac and respiratory stimulants (Fig. 30-3).

Atmospheric conditions. The temperature of the room should be such that blankets will not be necessary. If placed on the bed routinely, they may do more harm than good by causing the patient to lose fluids through perspiration. If necessary, the blanket covering the patient on his return from the operating room may be left in place temporarily. The area should be free from drafts and undue exposure to any harmful object.

Immediate postoperative care

Immediately following the operation, the patient is transferred to the anesthetic bed or stretcher and is taken to the recovery room or intensive care unit or returned to his unit. Transportation should be done quickly and easily. By this time, however, the patient may be semiconscious or conscious. In every instance, care must be taken to prevent injury and exposure.

Position. The position of a newly operated patient will depend on the operation and type of anesthetic used. Unless contraindicated, the patient is placed in the lateral position with the back, abdomen, and extremities well supported. For the patient who must remain on his back, the head should be turned slightly to the side to ensure a free passage for breathing and avoid aspiration of vomitus.

Observation. A new postoperative patient should have constant watching and should never be left entirely alone. Upon his return, the nurse should check immediately for state of consciousness, color, respiration, pulse rate, and blood pressure. These are signals that tell the condition of the patient, and if watched closely, they may be used as warnings to prevent dangerous and serious complications.

Postoperative discomforts. The major portion of immediate postoperative care consists mainly of relieving the common postoperative discomforts. The chief ones are pain, anxiety, thirst, and restlessness. They are very closely related, and one may be the cause or result of another.

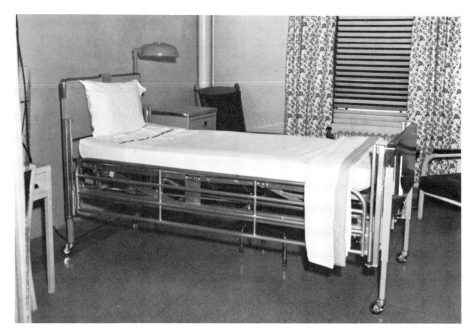

Fig. 30-2. A convenient method of opening a postoperative bed.

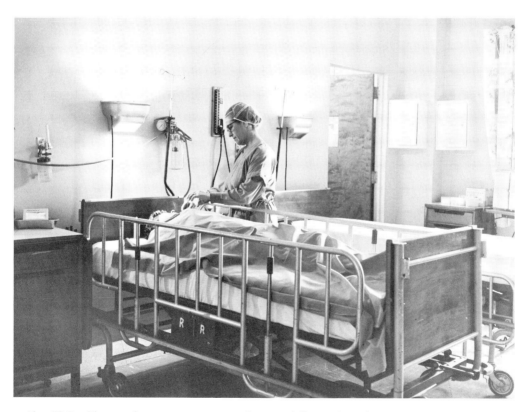

Fig. 30-3. The modern recovery room is especially equipped to meet emergencies in the postoperative patient.

Anxiety may be relieved by assurance from the nurse. Narcotics are usually ordered for the relief of pain and also help to relieve some of the tenseness. Thirst is prevented or treated by intravenous fluids.

If the patient is kept free from pain and other minor disturbances, he will be more likely to obtain the much-needed rest that is so important in the early stage of recovery. Effort should be made to find the cause of restlessness rather than to try to mask it with sedatives.

Restlessness may be caused by lying in one position too long, by the desire to urinate, by uncomfortable dressings, or by many other minor details, or it may be a symptom of one of the more severe complications such as shock or hemorrhage. For this reason, the nurse must base conclusions on not one but all observable symptoms.

Since most patients are unable to take food orally following surgery, nutrients are usually supplied by means of intravenous infusion. Physiologic saline and glucose solutions supplemented with vitamins and proteins are sufficient to keep up nutrition unless there is an imbalance in the electrolytes, in which case body salts are given.

Immediate postoperative complications

A list of principles relating to postoperative complications are included in those appearing on pp. 485 and 486 of this chapter. Reviewing them at this point will assist in identifying how they are related to the following discussion of postoperative care.

Shock. One of the most common and serious complications occurring during the early postoperative period is shock. It may be defined as a depression of all the vital centers, characterized by weak, thready pulse, shallow respiration, and cold, clammy skin. Shock is usually caused by pain, injury, hemorrhage, or exposure. One of the early characteristic signs of shock is a drop in blood pressure, and if blood pressure is taken frequently, shock may be detected soon enough to ward off any serious damage to the vital centers through the resulting anoxia.

The physician in charge should be notified immediately at the first signs of shock. The nurse should make other observations to determine the cause, if possible, and to report these findings to him upon his arrival. Treatment usually consists of the administration of fluids and whole blood or plasma for the purpose of restoring blood volume. Either vasoconstrictors or vasodilators may be administered, depending upon the condition of the patient. (See Suggested Readings.)

If pain is present, an analgesic is administered. The patient should be made as comfortable as possible, since pain and worry in themselves may increase the degree of shock. Care must be taken to observe the respirations when opiates are used frequently, since they usually depress the respiratory center. If conscious, the patient may appear anxious and restless and those in attendance should reassure him. Duties must be performed quickly but in a manner that will not excite the patient. If the patient complains of chilliness, blankets may be applied, but as a rule heat is not applied as a general therapeutic measure since it produces vasodilation, which is thought to decrease further the blood volume in the vital centers.

When shock results from hemorrhage, treatment is designed first to control the bleeding and then to institute other remedial measures.

Hemorrhage. Hemorrhage may be described as a sudden abnormal loss of blood. Its effect upon the patient will depend on his condition at the time of occurrence and on the amount of the blood loss.

Hemorrhages may be classified in several ways, the chief one being primary and secondary. A primary hemorrhage is one that occurs at the time of injury. A secondary hemorrhage is one that follows sometime later.

All patients, more or less, are subjected to primary hemorrhages. During the operation, this bleeding is controlled by the surgeon at that time by the use of sutures, ligatures, or cautery. If an extensive blood loss is expected, transfusions are instituted at the beginning of the surgery to compensate for any ill effects upon the patient.

Secondary hemorrhage following operation is usually caused by the slipping of a ligature, excessive pull or strain on a suture, or capillary oozing. Hemorrhage may occur from an artery, vein, or capillary. Arterial blood is bright red, occurs in spurts with each beat of the pulse, and must be controlled immediately. Fatal results may occur within a few minutes following hemorrhage from a large artery. Venous blood is darker in color and occurs in a steady flow, whereas capillary hemorrhage is a continual oozing.

Hemorrhage may be either concealed (internal) or evident (external). The external type can be detected immediately by frequent observation of the dressing, and it is most likely to occur in operations on the extremities. Since fluid has a tendency to flow downward, it is important that the nurse check the surrounding areas as well as the dressing itself.

Hemorrhage should never be confused with bloody drainage that often appears on dressings and in drainage bottles, since a small amount of blood may color a large area. The nurse should note the amount of fluid on the dressing or in the bottle, its consistency, and the rate of increase in volume. Actual hemorrhage will soon cause a variation in the vital signs.

Internal hemorrhage can be detected only by observation, and the alert nurse will note its symptoms early enough to prevent harm to the patient. Even the earliest symptoms of internal hemorrhage are grave danger signals, since sufficient blood has already been lost to produce changes in the vital signs. Early symptoms are a rapid pulse that increases gradually in rate and becomes more feeble, sighing respiration and air hunger, thirst, ringing in the ears, and a cold, pale skin. The patient usually becomes restless and very anxious.

Central venous pressure (CVP) and blood gas values (P_{H_2}, P_{O_2}, and P_{CO_2}) can be used to detect early indications of inadequate cardiac output, low blood volume, and electrolyte imbalance before these changes are otherwise apparent. Such determinations, evaluated in relation to each other and to the patient's clinical appearance, behavior, and other signs and symptoms, can provide useful guidelines in making medical and nursing judgments during the postoperative period as well as during other episodes of acute illness. As the amount of blood loss increases, the blood pressure drops and symptoms of shock appear. For this reason hemorrhage must be discovered early in order to differentiate it from shock, since the treatment is somewhat different. When shock is caused by hemorrhage, control of the hemorrhage itself is necessary for relief of the shock.

Treatment of hemorrhage usually consists of elevation of the part (if an extremity), reinforcement of dressings, and application of pressure bandages (if external). Sedatives and opiates are ordered to allay nervousness and to keep the patient quiet.

In the treatment of concealed hemorrhage, the patient is placed flat in bed or in shock position. Morphine is usually administered, and the patient is kept as quiet as possible. Whole blood or plasma is administered as both an emergency and a therapeutic measure. In some cases an emergency operation may be necessary to close off certain bleeding vessels, as in the case of ligatures or sutures that have slipped.

Vomiting. Vomiting may occur as the effects of the anesthetic wear off or because of a collection of food or fluid in the stomach. In nose and throat surgery it is often a result of the swallowing of blood and mucus. Care must be taken to prevent aspiration of the vomitus, which may present later complications. If vomiting persists, some type of gastric suction is usually ordered.

Delayed complications

Pulmonary disturbances. Pulmonary disturbances are probably the most serious of all the postoperative complications. Many of them can be prevented. It has been observed that patients who have some type of respiratory disease before the operation are more prone to develop complications, and for this reason every precaution should be taken.

Respiratory complications usually result from (1) the presence of preoperative infections of the mouth, nose, and throat that later spread to the lungs because of the patient's lowered resistance; (2) an irritating effect upon the mucous membranes by many of the inhaled anesthetics, causing an increase in the secretions that later may produce *atelectasis* (collapse of the lung because of blocking of one of the bronchi by a plug of mucus); (3) shallow respiration following surgery that may be caused by depression of the respiratory system by the anesthetic, sedatives, or opiates or by postoperative pain. Respiratory complications may predispose to bronchitis, pneumonia, or pleurisy.

Treatment of these conditions depends on the decision of the physician and usually consists of rest, fluids, and the administration of one or more of the antibiotics. As a preventive measure, many physicians order these routinely, along with deep-breathing exercises and early ambulation.

Intestinal and urinary complications. Intestinal and urinary complications sometimes occur. Intestinal obstruction, if severe, is treated by surgery. Otherwise it is treated by gastric suction.

Urinary complications are quite common and consist chiefly of cystitis or retention of urine. Postoperative therapeutic measures are the same as those for general treatment and have been discussed in Chapter 29 in relation to the urinary system.

Infection. A common complication following surgery is infection, not only of the wound itself but also elsewhere in the body, which may result from a break in surgical aseptic technique, from faulty sterilization, or from an endogenous source. Symptoms of infection in the surgical wound may appear about the third postoperative day and usually begin with fever. Treatment is directed toward mobilizing the body's defenses against microbial invasion. Special measures may be necessary for patients with organ transplants, who are susceptible to autogenic reaction. In organ transplants, potential complications of immunosuppressive therapy are infection and bone-marrow depression. Symptoms of rejection may duplicate those of infection but can be distinguished by electrocardiograph tracings.

Because of the possibility for cross-infection, surgical patients are sometimes segregated from other patients in a hospital. Most hospitals segregate patients to facilitate nursing care, but a more important reason is to protect certain types of patients from cross-infection, especially from those with upper respiratory and staphylococcal infections.

Because of slowed circulation resulting from sedation, the postoperative patient is predisposed to pneumonia. He is also more susceptible to many types of bacteria that the ordinary patient could resist. The patient should be kept free from drafts and from undue exposure to rapidly moving air to prevent chilling, since the patient may be perspiring profusely.

Circulatory complications. Postoperative patients should be observed for symptoms of clot formation in the veins of the pelvis and lower extremities. Venous stasis resulting from muscular inactivity and other contributing factors, such as obesity, debility, and old age, is thought to increase the occurrence of this potentially serious vascular complication. This clot formation is known as *thrombosis,* or *thrombophlebitis* when associated with inflammation of the veins. Since the *thrombus* is friable and easily detached, particles known as *emboli* may be carried via the bloodstream to the lungs, brain, or heart. The resulting *embolism* may be very serious, or even fatal, depending on the area of involvement. To avoid dislodging a possible clot, muscles of the patient's limbs should not be massaged without a specific order from the physician to carry out this measure, even though the patient may complain of pain in his limbs and request that they be massaged. Early ambulation and avoidance of pressure in the popliteal area are thought to be measures to aid in preventing pooling of venous blood in the lower extremities.

Psychosocial aspects

Most patients fear surgery even though they may not give evidence of doing so. The anesthetist usually tries to have the patient regain consciousness just about the time the operation is completed, and the surgeon may then inform the patient that the operation is over. Knowing that the operation was successful often puts the patient at ease and prevents much worry and restlessness. If nasal tubes, catheters, and other drainage tubes are in use, they should be explained to the patient so that he will not worry over their presence. If the patient has been prepared previously, he will expect to find certain equipment and will accept it as soon as he is aware of his surroundings.

Surgery brings dependence on others. Also, the patient may feel insecure and may want to seek help from others. For the first hours following major surgery, a patient must depend on others for his care, and this may be a hindrance later when the patient must again care for himself.

Early ambulation is necessary for the patient to regain his strength and to return to his normal activity. Explanation of the procedure before surgery will usually prevent the situation in which a patient desiring attention may resist or refuse to get out of bed. Many patients want to be up and out of bed because it shortens the recovery period and eliminates the use of the bedpan, thereby preventing constipation, retention, and many other postoperative discomforts. If the patient is given the proper instructions before surgery, he will look forward to early ambulation and will not fear it.

LEARNING SITUATIONS FOR THE PATIENT

For many patients who have had vital organs removed, a plan of rehabilitation must be initiated prior to discharge from the hospital. The nurse will share with other members of the health team the responsibility of teaching the patient or his family the care that he will need. Teaching should begin early in the recovery period so that the patient will have time to develop independence before discharge. A patient may obtain aid or nursing care following his return home through the liaison nurse working with the hospital and community organizations that provide these services.

SUMMARY

Surgery is always a stressful ordeal for the patient, and it necessitates expert nursing care both preoperatively and postoperatively. The nurse contributes to the care of the patient by informed observation, assessment, and evaluation of his condition and needs; by skill in adapting and giving physical care; by sensitivity in supporting the patient psychologically; and by maintaining effective channels of communication.

Biologic principles are presented as useful concepts in the planning of effective intervention for meeting the needs of the surgical patient. Emphasis is placed on psychosocial factors also as being important in the process of maintaining or restoring optimal bodily function.

Preoperative care is viewed as an important factor in reinforcing the patient's capacity to withstand the stress imposed by surgery. Recovery from surgery may be hastened by quality care following the operation. The alert nurse will recognize early symptoms of impending complications so that preventive measures can be applied.

The objective of surgical nursing is to assist the patient to return safely to independent functioning as quickly as possible and with the least amount of discomfort.

QUESTIONS FOR DISCUSSION

1 Outline a plan for instructing and assisting a preoperative patient with each of the following:
 a Relaxing and contracting leg muscles
 b Deep breathing and coughing to be done after abdominal surgery
 c Postural drainage
2 Describe the symptoms that the nurse should recognize as indicating these postoperative complications and problems:
 a Surgical shock
 b Internal hemorrhage
 c Thrombophlebitis if in a lower extremity
 d Pulmonary embolism
 e Infection of the surgical incision
 f Inability to void
 g Postoperative abdominal distention
3 Enumerate the ways in which respiratory ob-

struction or depression may occur during the immediate postoperative period. What measures should the nurse employ to maintain an open airway?
4 If your patient were to have skin preparation for abdominal surgery before going to the operating room, describe how you would proceed, using the following headings:
 a Explanation to the patient
 b Area to be included in the skin preparation
 c Equipment and solutions needed
 d Important points in the shaving process
 e Measures that can increase the effectiveness of the procedure
5 Identify the important points in moving an unconscious or semiconscious patient safely from the bed to a stretcher and then to the bed.
6 Following a general anesthetic, what fluid and foods should the nurse anticipate that the patient may be able to tolerate?

LIFE SITUATION

Mrs. Castro is a 60-year-old licensed practical nurse. She is married and has a 16-year-old daughter who lives at home. Her husband operates a local meat shop. Both Mr. and Mrs. Castro were born in Puerto Rico but speak English and Spanish equally fluently. They are practicing Catholics.

On admission Mrs. Castro appeared to be in mild distress. She walked with one hand over the upper epigastric region. She weighed 180 pounds and was 5 feet, 5 inches tall. Her obesity was noticeable and her appearance untidy. Her face appeared worn, she had a furrow on the forehead and dark circles under her eyes. She stated she had had some discomfort and pain in the upper epigastric region for several months. While working she had thought that it was caused by "gaseous foods" she ate or pulled muscles from moving heavy patients. She had very little illness previously. She gave birth to her only child in the hospital.

During hospitalization her major concern was her daughter. Both parents have shielded her considerably and are worried because no one will be at home when she gets in from school. She said her daughter still played with dolls.

Mrs. Castro's hospitalization was adequately covered by her husband's Blue Cross–Blue Shield policy.

She did well before and after surgery except during the period of preoperative instruction, when she appeared not to be aware of the need of postoperative coughing and deep breathings. Since her experience had been in a nursing home for the aged, she had not been able to keep up with techniques in other areas, but she was cooperative and very willing to do everything that was expected of her. In fact she stated that she wanted to work 1 or 2 days a week just to keep her "fingers in the pot."

When the liaison nurse made her call to Mrs. Castro's house 1 week after her discharge, she found Mrs. Castro quite upset because of a sharp pain in her incision. A call to her physician, who explained it was apparently a muscle spasm, settled the problem because it disappeared thereafter.

At the end of the study, Mrs. Castro was still under the care of her private physician.

Using the following data for Mrs. Castro, discuss or answer the following questions.

I. Identifying data, most of which was obtained from addressograph:
Name: Mrs. Castro
Doctor: Dr. W.
Age: 60
Occupation: L.P.N.
Marital status: Married
Diagnosis: Cholecystitis
Admitting date: 1/2/72
Religion: Catholic
Sacraments: 1/3/72
Principal language: English
Vision: Glasses
Hearing: Good
Dentures: Lower partial

II. Preoperative orders:

MEDICAL PLAN	MEDICAL PRINCIPLE
1. X-ray of abdomen	Stone formed by calcium carbonate will show up on flat x-ray
2. Blood for C.B.C. and clotting	Failure to absorb vitamin K will result in hypoprothrombinemia
3. Urinalysis	Urine from biliary tract obstruction will appear dark and frothy when shaken
4. Surgical scrub	
5. N.P.O. after midnight	
6. Teaching of deep breathing and coughing	

III. Postoperative orders:
1. I.V. fluids
   a. 1,000 ml. D5W and $\frac{1}{2}$ NaCl with 20 mEq. KCl run @ 125 ml./hour.
   b. 1,000 ml. D5W with 20 mEq. KCl @ 125 ml./hour.
   c. 250 ml. Albumisol @ 25 ml./hour.
2. Demerol, 50 mg., I.M. for pain q.4h.
3. N.P.O. except ice cubes
4. Nasogastric tube
5. Foley catheter
6. IPPB and chest physiotherapy q.4h.
7. Turn, cough, and deep breathe q.2h.

Questions:

1 What is the relationship between preoperative care and postoperative recovery?

2 What are the chief causes of anxiety in the surgical patient? (Chapters 7 and 30)*

3 How would a preoperative teaching plan for Mrs. Castro differ from that of the average lay person? (Chapter 5)

4 How does postoperative pain differ from other types of pain? (Chapter 26)

5 What is the importance of proper positioning during surgery?

6 What is the chief cause of postoperative dehydration? (Chapter 17)

7 What gastrointestinal and urinary problems might Mrs. Castro be expected to have had? (Chapters 28 and 29)

8 How could the nurse have aided in the prevention of the following infections in the above situation: pneumonia, urinary, wound? (Chapters 19, 29, and 31)

9 What are the effects of early ambulation or the lack of it in the surgical patient? (Chapter 19)

10 What are the chief causes of postoperative hemorrhage? How can they be prevented?

11 What are the advantages of a postanesthesia room (P.A.R.)? Disadvantages?

12 How do you account for the fact that Mrs. Castro's postdismissal pain disappeared so quickly following the physician's diagnosis of its cause? (Chapter 14)

SUGGESTED READINGS

Belleville, J. W., and others: Age and postoperative pain, American Journal of Nursing **72:**132, January, 1972.

*Chapters in parentheses indicate where related principles appear in this text.

Bosanko, Lydia A.: Immediate postoperative prosthesis, American Journal of Nursing **71**:280, February, 1971.

Chandler, James G.: The physiology and treatment of shock, RN **34**:42, June, 1971.

Collart, Marie, and Brenneman, Janice K.: Preventing postoperative atelectasis, American Journal of Nursing **71**:1982, October, 1971.

Connor, George, and others: Tracheostomy, American Journal of Nursing **72**:68, January, 1972.

Crawford, Christine F., and Palm, Mary L.: Can I take my teddy bear? American Journal of Nursing **73**:286, February, 1973.

Havens, Anita: Care of a depressed medical-surgical patient, American Journal of Nursing **70**:1070, May, 1970.

Harrell, Helen C.: To lose a breast, American Journal of Nursing **72**:676, April, 1972.

Klagsbrun, Samuel C.: Cancer, nurses, and emotions, RN **33**:46, January, 1970.

Levine, Dale C., and Fiedler, Jene P.: Fears, facts, and fantasies about pre and post operative care, Nursing Outlook **18**:26, February, 1970.

Merserko, Virginia: Preoperative classes for cardiac patient, American Journal of Nursing **73**:665, April, 1973.

Meyers, Billie L.: Patients in an OR corridor, American Journal of Nursing **72**:284, February, 1972.

Mezzanotte, Elizabeth J.: Group instruction in preparation for surgery, American Journal of Nursing **70**:89, January, 1970.

Myers, M. Bert: Sutures and wound healing, American Journal of Nursing **71**:1725, September, 1971.

Rodman, Morton J.: Drugs used in anesthesia, RN **33**:53, July, 1970.

Rodman, Morton J.: Vasopressors vs. vasodilators in treating shock, RN **31**:59, December, 1968.

Rodger, Bertha P.: Therapeutic conversation and post-hypnotic suggestion, American Journal of Nursing **72**:714, April, 1972.

Shafer, Kathleen N., and others: Medical-surgical nursing, ed. 5, St. Louis, 1971, The C. V. Mosby Co.

Smith, Brian R., and others: In a recovery room, American Journal of Nursing **73**:70, January, 1973.

Sun, Rhoda L.: Trendelenburg's position in hypovolemic shock, American Journal of Nursing **71**:1758, September, 1971.

Whitson, Betty J.: The puppet treatment in pediatrics, American Journal of Nursing **72**:1612, September, 1972.

31 Wounds

The verb form of the word "wound" means to injure or to damage. Therefore, any patient inflicted by a wound, whether accidental or intentional, as in surgery, will experience injury to a certain degree. In addition to the physical damage there is a degree of emotional injury. As was shown in earlier chapters there is a general bodily response to injury in addition to the local inflammatory or healing process. If the wound becomes infected, then the body's adaptive forces must be utilized in overcoming the invading organisms.

In many instances the physical wound may heal with little difficulty and the patient may experience little pain. However, the emotional injury may remain with the patient for the remainder of his life, as in the patient who has an ostomy or who has lost a vital organ such as an eye or limb.

One does not nurse a "wound" but the patient who has the wound; however, an understanding of wounds and the healing process, along with the therapeutic measures available for the care of wounds, will aid the nurse in giving care to the patient that will aid in the prevention of infection and promotion of healing with the least amount of permanent damage.

CLASSIFICATION OF WOUNDS

A wound is a break in the skin or mucous membrane, or other body structure, resulting from physical means. It may be superficial, affecting only the surface structures, or severe, involving blood vessels, muscles, nerves, fascia, tendons, ligaments, or bones. Even superficial wounds may be quite painful because of the sensitive nerve endings in the skin. Wounds occurring in tissues with abundant blood supply, such as scalp wounds, will bleed freely.

Wounds may be classified in a variety of ways, as in the following four groupings.

Classification according to continuity of surface covering

1. *Closed wounds* have no break in the continuity of the overlying skin or mucous membrane. Such injuries might be caused by a blow, by force exerted on the body part, or by an unusual or straining movement of the individual. This type of wound might involve a fracture as well as injury to other underlying tissues.

2. *Open wounds* are accompanied by disruption of the continuity of the skin or mucous membrane, with underlying tis-

sues exposed, and so providing the possibility of entry for microorganisms of all types, even though the break in the surface tissue may be minor.

Classification according to cause

1. A *surgical (incised) wound* is a clean, smooth cut made with a sharp cutting instrument, such as with a scalpel in surgery. *Stab wounds,* or those made with sharp objects, such as a knife or glass, are sometimes included in this category, even though they are accidentally produced.

2. *Accidental wounds* are those occurring under unexpected conditions and therefore more subject to infection.

Classification according to type of injury. The following descriptive terms are generally used:

1. An *abrasion* is a superficial wound produced by friction or scraping, such as the "floor burn" a basketball player receives when he slides along the floor with a skin surface in contact.

2. A *laceration* is similar to the incised wound except that the edges are jagged and torn. Examples might be wounds made by animal bites, machinery, or jagged objects; bleeding is apt to be profuse.

3. A *contusion* is a wound made by a blunt instrument. The surface tissues may or may not be broken. Bruising of the surrounding tissues results in extravasation of blood into the skin or mucous membrane, sometimes called an *ecchymosis.* The swelling resulting from hemorrhage into the tissues affected by the bruising is a *hematoma.*

4. A *puncture (stab)* is a wound made with a pointed object, such as a nail, wire, or bullet, that pierces to deeper tissues, leaving only a small opening on the surface. This type of wound, which tends to bleed very little and seals over quickly, is potentially dangerous because anaerobic pathogens such as *Clostridium tetani* or *Clostridium welchii* may have been carried into the depths of the wound by the punc-

turing instrument where conditions are favorable for their activity.

5. A *penetrating wound* occurs as a result of an instrument passing through skin or mucous membrane to deeper tissues and entering a body cavity or organ.

6. A *perforating wound* is caused by an instrument that both enters and emerges from a body cavity or organ. A gunshot wound may be perforating or penetrating.

Classification according to activity of invading microorganisms

Every wound will have some microorganisms present because surfaces of the skin and superficial membranes have a constant flora and because it is impossible to completely sterilize the skin or deeper tissues of a wound. Even an incision made in the operating room under strict surgical aseptic technique is subject to some airborne contamination. There is always an element of infectious risk in medical and surgical procedures.

1. A *clean wound* is one that has not been invaded by pathogenic microorganisms. The body defenses called into action have been successful in resisting any microbial invasion present, and therefore the "clean" wound heals without infection.

2. A *contaminated wound* is one in which the potential for microbial invasion is relatively great, such as in a wound occurring under accidental conditions without the benefit of aseptic technique. However, the body defenses may be able to resist the organisms present and the wound may still heal without clinical signs of infection.

3. An *infected (septic) wound* is one in which the invasion of pathogens is too great for the resistance of the first line of internal body defenses and clinical symptoms of infection develop.

BACTERIAL INVASION AND WOUND INFECTION

Pertinent concepts drawn from microbiology and physiology have been selected for their relevance to bacterial invasion of wounds.

Microbial properties

Regardless of the entry route, once the pathogen has entered the body, it may then induce damage in either one or both of two ways. (1) The pathogen may localize at the site of entry (most frequently in an accidental wound) and produce mechanical and physiologic effects in the surrounding tissues. (2) It, or its toxic products, or both, may be disseminated throughout the body. The damage produced may be either at the local entry site or in tissues far removed from the point of entry. Some organisms have invasive qualities through which they are disseminated in the body, or they may enter the lymphatics or the bloodstream and be widely distributed.

The production of infection in the body depends largely on (1) the pathogenicity of the invading organisms and its degree of *virulence*—virulence is displayed in terms of the two general qualities of *invasiveness* (ability to survive, multiply, and spread in the tissues) and *toxigenicity* (production of substances that are injurious to human cells and tissues and that are capable of causing imbalance in the body's homeostasis)—and (2) the body's defense mechanisms, which provide it with defenses against the invading pathogens.

Body defenses against microbial invasion

The human body is equipped with specific defenses, which are both external and internal, against invasion by pathogenic microorganisms.

External defenses include the natural barriers of unbroken skin and mucous membranes, which give mechanical protection to the deeper tissues. For the most part, the skin secretion has a distinctly acid reaction, with pH approximately 5.5, which is low enough to prevent growth of most transient organisms. Microorganisms usually present in the normal flora of the skin are nonpathogenic, except for staphylococci. Since organisms tend to penetrate the hair follicles and the glands of the skin where they cannot be removed by scrubbing with soap and water, they are always present, but the unbroken skin presents a more or less impassable barrier to invasion of underlying tissues by organisms.

The mucous membranes lining the respiratory tract and all other parts of the body that have external openings are impervious to microorganisms. The secretions of these membranes are mildly bacteriostatic. For example, lacrimal fluid (tears) tends to deter microbial growth and continuously bathe the conjunctival sac, washing away foreign material, including pathogens, from the eye. In the respiratory passages the secretions serve a similar purpose and, in addition, the hairlike cilia of the membranes have a wavelike motion that tends to move bacteria and irritating substances from the respiratory passages to the pharynx where they may be either swallowed or expectorated. If swallowed, they are destroyed by the gastric secretions. The nose and mouth ordinarily harbor many bacteria, including such pathogens as streptococci and pneumococci. These bacteria are usually not harmful because the ones in the mouth are swallowed with the saliva and destroyed by gastric secretions or by enzymes along the intestinal route. Normally, mucous membranes are moistened by protective secretions and are highly vascular, thus providing for the immediate operation of internal defense when organisms penetrate the natural barrier of intact mucous membrane. Reflex acts such as coughing and sneezing help to remove pathogens from the respiratory passages, and vomiting and diarrhea may eliminate transient bacteria and their toxic products from the gastrointestinal tract. Some pathogens may be eliminated from the body through the kidneys without harm unless there is an obstruction in the kidneys, ureters, bladder, or urethra or there is trauma such as may occur in catheterization. Normal flow of urine through the urinary tract, with complete emptying of the bladder, tends to prevent invasion of these tissues by washing out the organisms. Vaginal secretions are normally acid and inhibit entering pathogens, with some exceptions, such as the gonococci and spirochetes.

Internal defense mechanisms become operative when the external natural barriers to intrusion fail to control the invasion of the wound by pathogens. The host's internal defensive response to protect the body from entry by bacteria include the specific defenses of (1) *phagocytosis*—ingestion of microorganisms by white blood cells; (2) the *inflammatory response*—the process by which damaged cells release histamine into the surrounding intracellular fluid, thus causing local tissue reaction that is an attempt by the body to localize and overcome the damage of injury and bacterial invasion at the initial site; and (3) the *specific immune response*—the ability to resist a particular pathogen or its toxic products by the development of immune substances, or *antibodies,* which react specifically with the pathogen or its products.

The process of inflammation occurs whenever any agent (bacteria, chemical, foreign body, or severe blow) injures the tissues, resulting in the histamine response, with dilation and increased permeability of the surrounding capillaries, which then allows blood cells and serum to escape into the tissues. The swelling thus caused by the escaping fluid may result in painful pressure on nerve endings in the tissues. Thus the five cardinal symptoms of the inflammatory process are redness, heat, swelling, pain, and limitation of movement. The increased blood flow to the area allows a greater number of leukocytes (phagocytes) to migrate to the area of injury or invasion where they ingest bacteria and dead cells (process of *phagocytosis*).

During the process of phagocytosis in contaminated wounds, some leukocytes and bacteria are killed, some tissue is destroyed, and fluid accumulates at the site. When the invading pathogens are sufficiently great in number and in virulence to resist and destroy the leukocytes, phagocytosis then becomes a *purulent* exudate (pus), which is usually drained at the surface. The inflammatory process resolves when the leukocytes are able to remove the debris and, together with the blood, serum, and lymph, are reabsorbed into the capillaries and lymphatics.

When the local defenses lose the protective battle, the invading organisms will be carried by the lymphatics to the nearest filtering lymph node located along the course of the lymph channel, where they may be ingested and destroyed. The inflammatory process *(lymphadenitis)* continues in the node. If bacteria become bloodborne, they may be engulfed by *tissue macrophages* that are located along the course of blood vessels, spleen, liver, and other organs, which act similarly to lymph nodes. Pathogens and their toxic products are foreign proteins *(antigens)* against which the body has another line of defense known as the *antigen-antibody* response. Body cells become *sensitized* after contact with the antigen and tend to produce chemical substances to counteract the foreign protein. *Antibodies* are formed in response to pathogens; *antitoxins* are formed in response to toxins. The antitoxin or antibody is *specific* for each antigen. A thorough review of the antigen-antibody response at this point is suggested.

Other factors in the progress of wound infection

The outcome of the infection depends on the balance between the virulence of the organism and the internal defenses of the host *(susceptibility)*. Factors adversely affecting the internal defenses might include, for example, anything that causes *leukopenia* (decrease in the number of white blood cells) or else shock (because less circulating blood is available for the body's defense processes). Early therapy may be the supportive factor in enabling the body defenses to check an otherwise overwhelming infection.

The infection is called *septicemia* when pathogenic agents are present and are producing toxins in the bloodstream. These circulating bacteria may lodge in tissues far from the original site of infection, where a *secondary infection* may develop.

Symptoms of wound infection

Symptoms of wound infection do not appear until the *incubation period* is lapsing. This period is the time between entry of the bacteria into the body and sufficient cellular damage to produce the histamine response. It is relatively short in local wound infection, usually between 1 and 3 days.

The symptoms may be local in a very minor infection, or both local and systemic, depending on the severity of the infection and the resistance of the individual.

The characteristic local symptoms are the cardinal signs of redness, heat, swelling, pain, loss of function, and, depending on the nature of the causative organisms, the formation of pus. When the defensive reaction is successful in walling off the purulent material from the surrounding tissues, an *abscess* is formed. Bacteria most commonly causing suppuration are the *Staphylococcus, Streptococcus,* and *Pseudomonas.* When the pus formed is not walled off but spreads to surrounding tissues, the inflammatory process is called *cellulitis.* If the infection forms a channel from a normal body cavity or organ to the surface or to another organ or cavity, it is referred to as a *fistula.* A suppurating channel that ruptures onto the surface or into a body cavity is called a *sinus.*

General symptoms appear when toxic substances from the area of inflammation are absorbed by the bloodstream. They include elevation of body temperature, increase in rates of pulse and respiration, malaise, anorexia, nausea, headache, and possibly chills. It is believed that a rise in body temperature stimulates the production of white blood cells, and this is therefore considered to be an important indication of the mobilization of the body's defenses. The increase in *blood sedimentation rate* occurring in infection is thought to be caused by the increase in fibrinogen, a blood protein necessary for the healing process, and also is viewed as an indication that the body defense mechanism is operating.

WOUND HEALING

The healing process. As the debris is removed from the wound and the inflammatory process resolves, healing begins. New cells are formed in the base of the wound and from surrounding normal tissues to fill in the break in continuity of the tissues. Some types of body cells, such as those in the intestinal walls, tend to regenerate normal structural cells that function normally after the healing process. Other types of cells, for example, nerve cells, regenerate slowly or some not at all. In the latter, scar formation occurs with the growth of fibrotic tissue cells, which fill in the injured area but do not function as formerly.

Wound healing proceeds at a maximal rate if aseptic conditions prevail, if there is a good blood supply, and if no necrotic tissue or foreign bodies are present. Biologic factors that affect the rate of healing include age, nutrition, condition of the tissues, and efficiency of the circulation. Wounds heal faster in young individuals and more slowly in elderly persons. De-

507

hydration, hypoproteinemia, and insufficient intake of vitamin C definitely slow the rate of healing. Anemia and infection elsewhere retard healing. Other unfavorable factors are hemorrhage, bacterial invasion, presence of devitalized bodies or traumatized tissue, and lack of rest of the injured part. Both necrotic tissue and foreign bodies cause exudation and prolong the time required for regeneration of tissue.

Healing takes place in two ways: by primary union and by secondary union.

Healing by primary union. Healing by primary union occurs in a wound in which the surfaces have been approximated with-out tension by nonirritating sutures and the part kept at rest. In primary union a film of blood and lymph fills the narrow space in the wound, and fibrin and fibrils, precipitated by the process of clotting, glue the wound surfaces together. Serum and leukocytes pass through the endothelial wall, fibroblasts multiply and fill in the gap, and capillary buds penetrate and unite to provide a blood supply. Collagen fibrils form, and by about the fourth day the injured area is filled with a thin line of granulation, or scar tissue. Epithelium or mucous membrane will cover the scar, filling in from the edges.

Healing by secondary union. Healing by secondary union occurs when there has been tissue damage, when the edges of the wound have not been approximated, or when the wound has been infected. Healing will occur by a process similar to that in healing by primary union, but more slowly and with the formation of more granulation tissue since the wound defect to be filled is larger. Healing is complete when epithelium grows over the granulation tissue. Secondary healing generally causes a larger, uneven, relatively insensitive scar. Extensive scars tend to shrink, leading to contracture deformity and malfunction. In some people there may be excessive scar formation, known as a *keloid,* which may be disfiguring.

When wound tissues fail to heal, *necrosis,* or death of the tissues, may occur. Bacterial invasion results in decomposition, or *gangrene.* Such a wound must be debrided of the necrotic tissue before the healing process will occur.

SCIENTIFIC PRINCIPLES

Most of the concepts discussed in Chapter 30 regarding the care of the surgical patient can be applied to the care of the patient with a wound. Other essential science concepts relevant to understanding the nursing process in the care of wounds include the following.

1. Body cells require an internal environment with a pH of 7.4 for normal functioning; surface cells of skin and mucous membrane can resist a pH that is slightly acidic.

2. Most commonly encountered bacteria prefer a neutral or slightly alkaline environment. Therefore, the skin secretions having a pH of 5.5 and some mucous secretions containing acid, such as vaginal secretions, are bacteriostatic (Fig. 31-1).

3. The enzyme *lysozyme* in skin secretions, nasal mucus, and saliva is bacteriostatic because it has the ability to break down a polysaccharide found in the cell walls of many bacteria.

4. When the integrity of skin or mucous membrane is broken, either by injury or disease, routes of entry are opened for microbes.

5. Moisture of the skin and mucous membranes is an important factor in their integrity. Healthy skin is relatively dry; therefore, *maceration,* resulting from continuous, excessive moisture, and excessive *dryness,* resulting in cracking, decrease the surface structure's resistance to infection, while also providing an environment more favorable for multiplication of bacteria. Normally, mucous membranes are moist. Excessive dryness of mucosal surfaces, particularly of the respiratory pas-

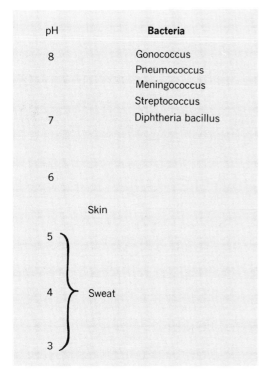

pH	Bacteria
8	Gonococcus
	Pneumococcus
	Meningococcus
	Streptococcus
7	Diphtheria bacillus
6	
	Skin
5	
4	Sweat
3	

Fig. 31-1. The acidity of the skin prevents the growth of bacteria.

sages, prevents the normal flow of protective mucus, which helps to keep the surfaces free of colonizing microorganisms through bacteriostatic and mechanical flushing actions.

6. Damage to vascular structures devitalizes the tissues because of decreased blood supply. Therefore the degree of trauma suffered by tissues is a determining factor in the development of wound infection.

7. The ability of a pathogen to cause infection in the human host is influenced by its degree of virulence.

8. The internal defenses of the human body against microbial invasion include phagocytosis, the inflammatory process, and the specific immune response.

9. The wound-healing process is an orderly and systematic formation of new tissue to replace that lost in the injury.

10. Microorganisms are always present on the surfaces of the body. Although the application of bacteriostatic agents decreases the number of organisms present, human body tissues will not tolerate sterilization processes. The use of friction and cleansing agents in handwashing decrease the transfer of contaminants.

11. Control of microorganisms is based on knowledge of the behavior of microorganisms, as in the following examples:

a. An absolutely dry field is necessary for maintenance of asepsis because fluids provide organisms with a transport system.

b. Control of air currents is a factor in decreasing the transmission of airborne bacteria.

c. Disinfection processes are based either on chemicals that interfere with the life processes of microorganisms or on length of exposure to moist heat at a degree sufficient to kill the microorganisms.

d. Maintenance of aseptic technique in care of wounds is facilitated by the knowledge that microorganisms are transferred from a contaminated surface to a "clean" or sterile surface by contact rather than by bacterial self-locomotion.

12. The absorption capabilities and wicking action of cotton material vary with the structure of the material. Therefore in planning care for a patient with a heavily draining wound, a nurse would select a dressing with maximum absorption quality and wicking action combined.

SUGGESTIONS FOR CARE OF WOUNDS

One of the objectives in caring for a wound is to prevent or reduce infection. This purpose is accomplished by maintaining aseptic technique during a dressing. Anything that touches a wound should be sterile—the dressing, instruments, sponges, solutions, and so on (Fig. 31-2).

509

Sterile dressings and sponges are individually packaged for use in the hospital and in the clinic, and disposable instruments may be used by a physician or nurse.

Bacteria are carried by capillary action from an unsterile surface into a dressing if the dressing is wet. Almost any bacteria may reproduce in a wound; examples of some common organisms that can produce severe infection are staphylococci, streptococci, and *Clostridium welchii,* which causes gas gangrene.

The nurse's hands should be washed before beginning a dressing. In order to avoid infection, the wound, the skin surrounding it, and the inner dressing should not be touched. Exposure time of the wound should be kept at a minimum. Sterile medications are applied to wounds by sterile tongue blades or sterile applicators. An irrigating tip is not touched to the wound.

Bacteria can enter a wound from the air, from a wet dressing or contaminated bedclothes, from mouths, noses, and fingers of the patients as well as nurses and physicians, and from instruments. Room air, if moving, may carry bacteria to sterile objects and wounds. Bacteria thrive in a warm moist environment. Bacteria cannot move by themselves. Sterile materials should be covered until time for use. Many dust particles are scattered by careless manipulation of bedclothing. Blankets and woolen articles, even when clean, harbor bacteria. Sheets on an occupied bed are invariably contaminated. Open wounds provide a ready culture medium for bacteria. Wound healing ceases when

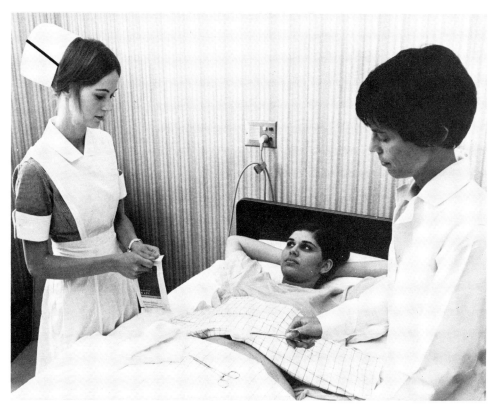

Fig. 31-2. Aseptic technique must be maintained until the wound is completely healed.

bacteria invade the tissues. Infection increases tissue damage and prolongs disability. The type of wound the nurse dresses is usually an infected one that has more or less drainage. Aseptic technique is used to avoid further damage to the wound, and the dressing should be changed often enough to keep the wound relatively dry.

No available antibacterial agent can completely sterilize an open wound. The skin around the wound is cleansed as well as possible with an antiseptic solution noninjurious to the tissues in order to prevent the bacteria on the skin from infecting the wound.

The foaming action of hydrogen peroxide may be employed to assist in cleansing and removal of foreign material from a punctured or lacerated wound.

Contaminated dressings are destroyed by burning. They are handled as little as possible and wrapped in plastic coverings before disposal in order to protect all workers.

A chemical solution used in the care of wounds is alcohol. It is most efficient in a 70% solution because its action is slow enough that it diffuses throughout the entire bacterium before its protein coagulates. When coagulation does occur, it is complete and the organism dies. Less than a 50% solution is not efficient as an antiseptic, whereas a solution greater than 80% hardens the surfaces of the bacteria and does not penetrate them, therefore not killing them.

Since most antiseptics combine with the proteins of the wound and within a short time become inactive, it becomes necessary to apply them to wounds frequently if their action is to be continuous. Wounds heal more quickly if protected from strong chemicals that destroy tissue cells as well as microorganisms.

Acetone is used as a solvent for adhesive that contains rubber and resins. It is also used to remove bits of adhesive that adhere to the skin when a dressing is removed. Other solvents may be pertoleum products such as benzine and naphtha and also carbon tetrachloride.

Besides alcohol, merbromin (Mercurochrome) in 1% to 2.5% solution may be used as a skin antiseptic. Silver nitrate is used occasionally as an astrigent and germicide to help in healing. Other skin antiseptics are benzalkonium chloride (Zephiran Chloride), nitromersol (Metaphen), and thimerosal (Merthiolate).

Protectives used on the skin include ointments, which may be applied directly to a wound or to sterile gauze that is laid on the wound. Zinc oxide ointment and petrolatum are widely used ointments. A powder such as zinc stearate powder keeps the drainage from irritating the skin. The antibiotics and cortisone are used to treat wounds locally. They are applied as solutions or ointments for treating or preventing infection. Systemic drug therapy is also used in the prevention and treatment of infections.

Ointments are used on the skin around wounds in order to prevect excoriation by drainage. Drainage, which contains much water, cannot penetrate through the oil because it is immiscible in oil. The molecules of oil or solid grease are adhesive toward the skin, but water is not adhesive to oil.

Fibers differ in their power to absorb. Gauze absorbs drainage by capillary attraction. The fluffier the gauze, the more absorbent it is. Ordinary cotton does not wet. When absorbent cotton is made, oil that interferes with wetting is removed. Cotton adheres to the edges of wounds, and therefore it should not be placed directly over them. When cotton is used in a dressing there is usually a gauze covering. A gauze drain conducts discharges out of a wound by capillary attraction (Fig. 31-3). A rubber drain conducts discharges out of a wound by gravity.

Pressure reduces the size of blood ves-

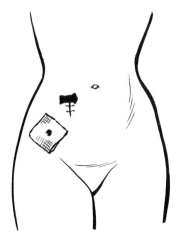

Fig. 31-3. A gauze drain conducts discharges out of a wound by capillary attraction.

sels. The tourniquet is a pressure bandage used to decrease the circulation in order to control bleeding. Pressure is also used around wounds to bring their edges together or to press out drainage. In applying a roller bandage, useless turns are avoided to keep the pressure as low as possible since each succeeding turn nearly

doubles the pressure. The distal part of an extremity that has been bandaged is observed for signs of pressure, swelling, coldness, and numbness. Friction between a bandage and the skin helps to hold it in place.

Tension of the sutures holds the edges of the wound together. However, tissues lose their capacity to hold sutures during the first 2 or 3 days after the wound is sutured, and, because the strength of the suture decreases, the wound is weakest on the third or fourth day after its repair. The capacity of tissues to hold sutures varies, and each has a characteristic capacity. This capacity is greatest in fascia and least in fat. Additional support is given by wide adhesive straps or by a binder.

Instruments used in dressing a wound include scissors, hemostats, and thumb forceps. Scissors and a hemostat are levers of the first class. The fulcrum is between the effort and the resistance. Thumb forceps is a lever of the third class, the effort being between the fulcrum and the resistance. (See Fig. 31-4.)

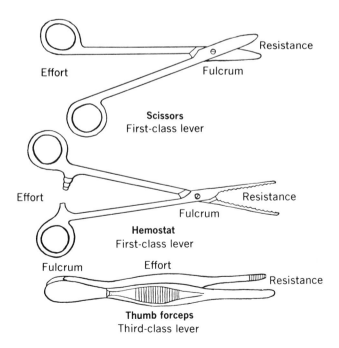

Fig. 31-4. Instruments as levers.

Friction between parts of instruments is prevented by lubricating the instruments with oil.

PSYCHOSOCIAL ASPECTS

Most wounds are painful. Patients fear treatments to their wounds lest more pain will be caused. A clear explanation of the treatment will help the patient to know what is to be done and whether pain may be involved.

Sometimes wounds are caused by accidents or other unpleasant situations, and scars remain as constant reminders. Sometimes the patient has lost a relative or close friend who was also involved in the accident and may have to cope with grief or feelings of guilt that may tend to retard his progress.

In contrast, a patient may have cosmetic surgery that may help him to forget his past and build a more promising future.

Patients' worry about having stitches removed may be relieved by the explanation that little pain will be experienced.

Some patients think their incisions will pull open if they turn about in bed. They may be reassured by the explanation that sufficient tension has been applied on the wound by the sutures and by the dressing to prevent its breaking open.

While a dressing is being done, the patient should be screened. Diversion may be provided by appropriate conversation. Soiled dressings should be removed as soon as possible. Ventilation should be provided to remove odors.

The physician often dresses a wound the first time, with the nurse assisting him and anticipating his needs. The nurse usually dresses a wound if the dressing is to be changed often and reports at once any observations that are unusual. The condition of the dressing and any observations for the information of the physician and other nurses are recorded on the chart.

SUGGESTIONS FOR BANDAGING
The roller bandage

Of all the types of bandages applied, the roller bandage requires the most skill. Typical roller bandage is made of gauze or woven elastic material (Ace bandage). The woven elastic material gives stronger support than gauze and is often used when support is the prime purpose of the bandage such as over varicose veins or for holding orthopedic appliances in place. The roller bandage in proper widths is used to cover the extremities, or parts of them, and the face and the head. The various widths of roller bandages are 1, $1^1/_2$, 2, $2^1/_2$, 3, 4, 5, and 6 inches.

Basic bandage patterns. The roller bandage is applied by using singly or in combination the five basic bandage patterns: circular, spiral, spiral-reverse, figure-eight, and recurrent.

Circular. In the application of the circular bandage pattern, each succeeding turn overlaps the entire width of the previous turn (Fig. 31-5, *A*).

Spiral. The spiral bandage pattern is used to cover an area of uniform circumference. Each turn overlaps one half to two thirds of the previous turn. (See Fig. 31-5, *B*.)

Spiral-reverse. The spiral-reverse bandage pattern is used on a cone-shaped part such as the forearm or leg. After the bandage is anchored, reverses (turning the bandage top to bottom) are made after each turn. Reverses prevent gaps and ensure a smooth bandage. (See Fig. 31-5, *C*.)

Figure-eight. The figure-eight bandage pattern is begun by forming two loops or turns, one above and one below a joint. Succeeding turns alternate above, where they descend, and below, where they ascend, until the joint is covered. This pattern is modified to form the spica bandage, where one circumference is much larger than the other. (See Fig. 31-6.)

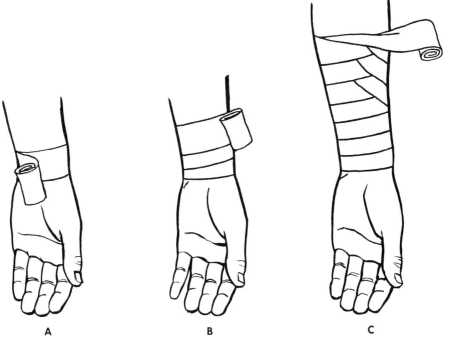

Fig. 31-5. A, The circular bandage pattern. **B,** The spiral bandage pattern. **C,** The spiral-reverse bandage pattern.

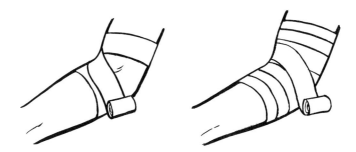

Fig. 31-6. The figure-eight bandage pattern.

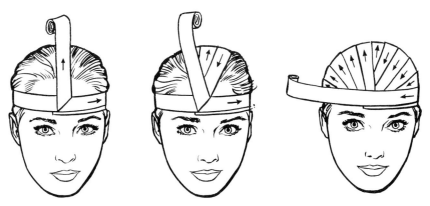

Fig. 31-7. The recurrent bandage pattern.

Recurrent. The recurrent bandage pattern is used to retain a dressing on the head, on a stump, or on the end of a finger. It is made by anchoring, or fixing, the bandage with two circular turns. The roll of bandage is then turned to cover the midline of the area. The following turns alternate on each side of the midline, passing back to front and front to back. Each turn overlaps one half the previous turn. When the entire area is covered, the bandage is ended with a circular turn directly over the first circular turn. (See Fig. 31-7.)

General instructions. General instructions for applying the roller bandage are as follows.

1. The patient should be placed in a comfortable position and the part to be bandaged should be in the position in which it is to be retained or used.

2. A bandage should accomplish its purpose. It may be used to hold dressings in place, to support a part, or to immobilize.

3. The bandage should be firmly anchored or fixed before starting the basic bandage pattern.

4. Two skin areas should not come in direct contact. They may be separated by either gauze or cotton. Special padding is used over bony prominences.

5. A bandage should be allowed to follow its natural course if possible. A bandage should not be pulled in order to make it fit.

6. Even pressure should be used insofar as possible, and the bandaging should be applied in the direction of the venous circulation. A portion of the distal area of an extremity should be exposed so that circulation may be observed.

7. All turns of a bandage are usually made clockwise. The roll is held in the right hand with the free end of the bandage in the left hand. The outer surface of the bandage is placed on the patient. As the roll is unwound, the bandage passes from the right hand to the left and back again.

8. When finished, the end of the bandage should be firmly secured, usually by adhesive. To hold wet dressings or dressings on the hand, the end of the bandage may be split and tied. Some modern bandages cling to bandage surfaces and do not need adhesive to hold them.

Special bandages for the hand

Finger bandage. The finger bandage is anchored by making one or two circular turns around the wrist. It is then carried by a wide spiral turn to the tip of the finger. If the tip is to be covered, sufficient recurrent turns are used to cover it. A circular turn is made to hold the recurrent turns in place or to start the bandage toward the hand. The finger is covered either by ascending spiral or spiral-reverse turns to the base. The bandage is then carried across the back of the hand to the wrist and secured by a final circular turn. (See Fig. 31-8, *A.*)

Thumb spica. The most common spica bandage applied by the nurse is the thumb spica. The hand should be placed in a semiprone position for working convenience. The bandage is anchored by making circular turns around the wrist. It is then carried to the tip of the thumb and anchored there. A turn around the thumb alternates with a turn around the hand, each turn covering one half the previous turn. When the thumb is covered, the bandage is anchored around the wrist. (See Fig. 31-8, *B.*)

Demigauntlet bandage. The chief use of the demigauntlet bandage is to cover the back of the hand. The bandage is anchored around the wrist. If the left hand is being bandaged, the bandage is carried from the wrist across the back of the hand and encircles the base of the thumb. It then is passed to the ulnar side of the wrist, forming a figure-eight. Then it is brought back across the hand, and the

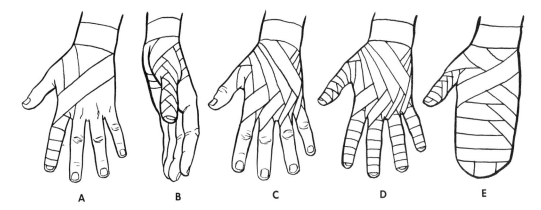

Fig. 31-8. Bandages for the hand. **A,** Finger bandage. **B,** Thumb spica. **C,** Demigaunt-let bandage, used to hold dressings on the back or palm of the hand. **D,** Full gauntlet bandage, used to cover the separated fingers. **E,** Mitten bandage.

second finger is enclosed in the same manner. The procedure continues until the back of the hand is covered. The right hand is begun in the same way with the sequence reversed, going from the little finger to the thumb. Additional strength may be added by making several turns over the palm before anchoring the bandage at the wrist. (See Fig. 31-8, *C.*)

Full gauntlet bandage. The full gauntlet bandage is used to cover the fingers separately or to cover one or more fingers and the back or palm of the hand. It is a combination of the finger bandage and the demigauntlet bandage. After the thumb or first finger is covered, the bandage is brought across the back of the hand to encircle the wrist and then across to the base of the next finger. A slow spiral turn takes it to the tip of the finger, and the procedure is repeated until each finger is covered. The bandage is anchored at the wrist. (See Fig. 31-8, *D.*)

Mitten bandage. The mitten bandage is used to cover the hand and fingers when it is essential to keep the fingers at rest. It is anchored at the wrist. If the thumb is to be bandaged, it is covered first with a finger bandage. The fingers are separated and protected by gauze or cotton and gauze. The bandage is brought over the

back of the hand, and several recurrent turns are made to cover the fingertips together. These are anchored by two or three circular turns around the fingers, and the bandage is continued with spiral or spiral-reverse turns over the hand. The bandage is ended by making figure-eight turns around the wrist and a final circular turn. (See Fig. 31-8, *E.*)

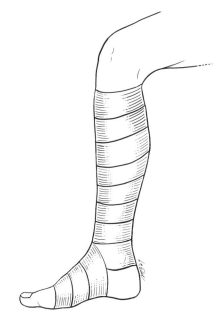

Fig. 31-9. Elastic bandage of the leg, or Ace bandage.

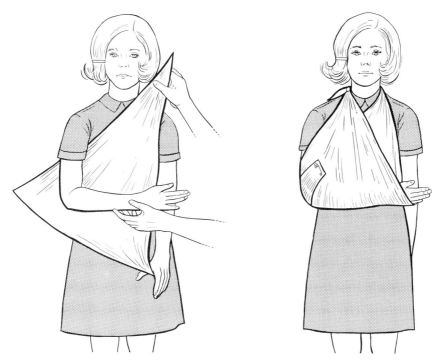

Fig. 31-10. Triangular bandage used as sling.

Miscellaneous bandages

Ace bandage. The Ace bandage, a commercially prepared bandage with an elastic weave, has several advantages over the conventional gauge bandage. It is used to give support, to apply pressure over varicose veins, and to help control hemorrhage. It is also available with adhesive backing. It is applied the same as the roller bandage. (See Fig. 31-9.)

Triangular bandage. A three-cornered bandage, often used as a first-aid bandage, is usually made of muslin and consists of a diagonal half of a square (1 yard in length and width). Its chief use is that of a sling to give support. (See Fig. 31-10.) It may also be folded to form the cravat bandage, which may be used for many other first-aid measures.

Binders. A binder is a special type of bandage used to apply pressure or hold dressings in place. Typical binders are those used for the breast, abdomen, and

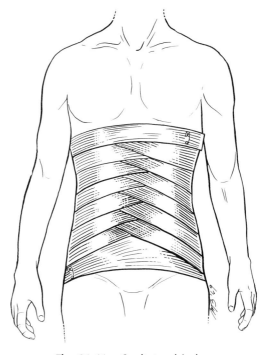

Fig. 31-11. Scultetus binder.

perineal areas. The one most commonly used is probably the Scultetus or many-tailed binder (Fig. 31-11). It is used for support and to hold dressings in place following an abdominal paracentesis.

The T binder is used for perineal dressing and may be one or two tailed and is referred to as a single T or a double T.

LEARNING SITUATIONS FOR THE PATIENT

The nurse may teach a patient how to dress a wound, what drugs are used on wounds, where to obtain dressings, how to handle materials, and why materials must be sterile.

A patient who has a long-term dressing, such as that on a colostomy, may need to learn how to do his own dressings. He will need to know where he may obtain dressings or how he may make them. Further, he will need instruction on safe methods of disposing of soiled dressings. He may also need to know how a bandage may be applied.

The patient should be instructed to keep his fingers away from the wound and off the part of the dressing that touches the wound.

SUMMARY

To function effectively in the care of a patient with a wound, the nurse must have basic concepts pertinent to understanding the various types of wounds, the factors influencing the speed and character of the healing process, the measures available for the care of wounds, and the ability to apply psychologic concepts in meeting the patient's needs. The nurse may have the responsibility for instructing the patient in continuing the application of his own dressings after discharge from the hospital.

QUESTIONS FOR DISCUSSION

1 What is a clean wound? an infected wound?
2 If a cut ¼ inch deep is made through the skin, what structures are involved?

3 Describe what happens in primary healing.
4 On the basis of science concepts stated in this chapter and in other references, how would you explain the physiologic effect of (a) moist, hot compresses applied to a wound? (b) cold compresses applied to a bruised wound immediately after the injury?
5 How do antibiotics and corticosteroids differ in their manner of action on the inflammatory response of body tissues to injury?
6 On the basis of scientific concepts presented throughout this text, list principles you would use in solving the problems you might encounter while at home in the event a member of the family receives a scalp laceration from broken glass.
7 How does gauze conduct drainage from a wound?
8 Why may a patient fear having a wound dressed?
9 List details of your explanation to a patient who would need to dress his own colostomy wound at home.
10 Define dressing, bandage, binder.
11 List three different materials used in making bandages.
12 What advantage does the elastic bandage have over a gauze bandage?

LIFE SITUATION

Mr. Jordan, a well-known local businessman, was admitted 2 days ago to the intensive care unit with gunshot wounds of the back and abdomen. He has refused to make any comments concerning the incident. Local newscasts indicate that he has been having trouble with his wife and that she is the suspect. If Mr. Jordan survives the initial trauma, he will be transferred to your unit to recuperate. What will be your attitude toward him? How will you communicate with him concerning his condition?

SUGGESTED PERFORMANCE CHECKLIST
Comfort

1 Is the procedure explained?
2 Is the patient relaxed during the dressing?
3 Is conversation used as a means of diversion?
4 Is the part supported during bandaging?

5 Is the bandage comfortable?

6 Is adhesive taken off with a minimum of trauma?

Therapeutic effectiveness

1 Is the ointment or solution of proper strength?

2 Is the patient's position adapted to the type of dressing?

3 Is infection prevented in the methods used?

4 Is the patient taught the value of asepsis?

5 Is the dressing neat, durable, and comfortable?

6 Is the wound observed carefully?

7 Does the nurse show skill?

8 Is an unusual condition reported?

9 Is charting pertinent and accurate?

Economy

1 Are sterile materials protected from contamination before use?

2 Is the bedding protected?

3 Is the proper size of dressing used?

4 Are no materials wasted?

5 Are materials all assembled before beginning?

6 If you are assisting a physician, are his needs anticipated?

7 Are useless turns of a bandage avoided?

8 Is the proper type of material used?

Safety

1 Are dressings and instruments sterile?

2 Is sterility maintained during the procedure?

3 Does the nurse wash the hands before beginning?

4 Is the cleansing away from the wound?

5 Is ointment used to protect the skin?

6 Are the soiled dressings disposed of in a safe manner?

7 Is the patient protected from chilling?

8 Is the bandage clean?

9 Is the bandage applied without too much pressure?

10 Is the nurse careful in using safety pins?

11 Is the safety pin or knot in a bandage on top of a part?

12 Is the dressing changed often enough to keep it dry?

13 Are skin surfaces separated in bandaging?

14 Are breaks in technique corrected at once?

SUGGESTED READINGS

Campbell, Emily B: Nursing problems associated with prolonged recovery following trauma, Nursing Clinics of North America **5:**551, December, 1970.

Lee, Jane M.: Emotional reactions to trauma, Nursing Clinics of North America **5:**577, December, 1970.

Myers, M. Bert: Sutures and wound healing, American Journal of Nursing **71:**1725, September, 1971.

32 Communicable disease

COMMUNICABLE DISEASE CONTROL

Communicable diseases have been known since the beginning of time, and certain measures have been instituted to prevent their spread. Moses received recognition as being the greatest sanitarian of biblical times because of the effort made by the ancient Hebrews to promote health and prevent disease. There is some evidence that these people had an authentic knowledge of some of the causes of disease and methods of controlling disease. Certain health measures practiced then that correlate with those of today are as follows: (1) rules and regulations controlling the preparation of food, (2) bathing, changing clothing, and washing the hands before eating, (3) putting out of the camp those suspected of having disease or thought to be unclean, and (4) showing certain skin lesions to the priest to ascertain an isolation or incubation period.

Hippocrates was probably the first to recognize a definite connection between disease and environment. He was greatly concerned with the effect of the weather on epidemics. He noted that pneumonia prevailed in the winter, whereas intestinal and malarial diseases were more prevalent during the summer months.

The Romans, influenced by the great Galen, followed with their contribution to environmental sanitation, and Venice forbade infected ships to enter her harbor.

With the coming of the Renaissance and the germ theory, modern concepts of medical asepsis were introduced, and in 1796 Edward Jenner vaccinated his first patient, thus winning the first battle with a communicable disease.

The prevention and control of infectious diseases advanced rapidly in the United States early in the twentieth century through organized public health efforts for immunization, efficient sewage systems, pure food and water supplies, and comprehensive programs to control insect, animal, and healthy human carriers of disease. A significant early contribution of the science of epidemiology was in relation to communicable disease control. Epidemiology is broadly considered to include the study of the various factors and conditions that determine the occurrence and distribution of health, disease, defect, disability, and death among groups of individuals. An early concern of epidemiology

520

for many years was the investigation of epidemics of communicable diseases, including tracing their sources, controlling spread, and developing measures to prevent recurrences. As infectious diseases have largely been brought under control through these efforts, the concern of contemporary epidemiology has focused on the noninfectious diseases that have gained increasing prominence.

A primary goal of modern public health is to update the application of control measures for sanitation, immunization, and quarantine to prevent the occurrence of communicable diseases. Although these control measures have largely freed the United States of major epidemics, for example, of typhoid, smallpox, and diphtheria, the potential threat of spread of communicable diseases is ever present. This threat is true for some of the more prevalent diseases such as salmonellosis and venereal diseases. Therefore specific programs for the prevention and control of acute communicable diseases are necessary, especially since this group of diseases, including smallpox, typhoid, schistosomiasis, and trachoma, are still the No. 1 health problem in some parts of the world.

PREVENTION

The most important factor in the modern control of communicable diseases is prevention. So much has been accomplished in this area during the last few decades that some diseases seldom occur. However, it is still important for the nurse to have knowledge in the prevention and control of communicable diseases. Natural disasters such as floods, earthquakes, and hurricanes may disrupt water supply and sewage disposal, which can result in conditions permitting the spread of these diseases. Changing cultural patterns and mores may also influence the spread of disease through social contact.

Although many different procedures have been used to prevent and control the spread of communicable diseases, all of them more or less are directed toward either increasing the patient's resistance or preventing the transfer of the causative organism. The majority of these measures are based on knowledge that has been accumulated since the discovery of the germ theory, and they vary from year to year as more advances are made in the sciences.

The modern trend is to divide preventive measures into two categories: public health and personal health.

Public health measures include (1) the destruction of breeding places of animals and insects that carry disease, (2) general disinfection of dishes and other materials used in public places, (3) the reduction of the bacterial count of air by ventilation, oil, and ultraviolet light, (4) a safe water supply, (5) proper disposal of sewage, and (6) aseptic care in the preparation and handling of food. Public health measures are usually effected by federal and community health laws.

Personal health measures include (1) the practice of hygienic living, (2) immunization, and (3) the use of proper techniques in the care of infected persons.

Communicable diseases, as well as other diseases, may be prevented by regular observance of simple, yet effective, measures of personal hygiene. If the body is kept in good physical condition, it can function to a greater capacity in resisting disease. Rest, sleep, exercise, a well-balanced diet, and emotional stability are just as vital in the prevention of a disease as they are in the treatment of it. Personal cleanliness, especially frequent handwashing and cleansing of the genital area, is essential in preventing spread of pathogens.

Infants are born with some natural immunity that they have received from their mothers. This suffices for a few months, after which time they must receive vaccines or toxoids in order to produce artificial immunity and escape the possiblity of contracting a communicable disease in the event of exposure. Natural immunity is uncertain, and the person may lose it.

The chief purpose of the vaccines and toxoids is to ensure immunity against the more virulent infections. Although no vaccine or toxoid is guaranteed, with the average practice of hygienic living artificial immunity does offer a high degree of protection. If cases occur, they are usually mild.

Vaccines and toxoids must be given early enough to enable the patient to build his own antibodies. Most pediatricians recommend that a normal, healthy child be started on the immunizations for childhood diseases at about the age of 6 months. Active, acquired immunity may last 1 year, several years, or a lifetime, but repeated immunizations at prescribed intervals for the specific diseases are recommended. This is usually explained to the mother when she takes her baby to the doctor for his first postnatal visit. Reimmunization of the adult is guided by occupation, travel, and military service.

In addition to vaccines, antibiotics and immune serums are used as prophylactic measures and also to treat the disease if it is contracted. Probably one of the most recent contributions of medical science is knowledge of the production of immunoglobulins. (For more information in this area, see Suggested Readings.)

The person who acquires a communicable disease should be separated from others. A very common procedure is to hospitalize the patient. If the patient is elsewhere, isolation may be more difficult. When physical separation is impossible, then general precautions would include the use of individual or disposable equipment for the sick, good housekeeping measures, the avoidance of contamination with nose and mouth secretion, excreta, or other body discharges, and frequent washing of the hands with soap and running water. Proper methods to use in the care of a communicable disease in the home may be learned in the Red Cross home nursing course.

DEFINITIONS AND TERMS

antibody an agent produced within the body that destroys or renders inactive certain foreign substances that gain access to the body, particularly bacteria and their toxins.

antigen a substance that, when introduced into the body, stimulates the body to produce antibodies.

antiseptic a substance that checks or inhibits the growth of bacteria.

antitoxin a substance found in the blood serum and other body fluids that neutralizes or prevents the action of a specific toxin. Antitoxins occur normally in the body in small amounts but may be increased greatly by the introduction of the corresponding toxin.

asepsis absence of septic matter, or freedom from infection.

carrier a person who harbors a pathogenic organism within his body and is capable of disseminating it to others. A carrier usually presents no symptoms and may or may not have had the disease.

channel of infection avenue by which pathogenic organisms enter the body.

clean when used in relation to communicable diseases, uncontaminated; not having come in contact either directly or indirectly with the contagious patient or his environment.

communicable disease a disease that can be transmitted either directly or indirectly from one person to another.

communicability period when the host is infectious.

contact a person or animal known or believed to have been exposed to a disease.

contagious capable of being transferred from one person to another either by direct or indirect contact.

contaminated soiled with infectious material or having come in contact directly or indirectly with an infected person.

disinfection the destruction of pathogenic microorganisms either by chemical or physical means directly applied.

disinfection, concurrent the immediate disinfection of objects that have been in contact with the patient or discharges from a patient.

disinfection, terminal the final disinfection of the unit and its contents after it has been vacated by the patient.

droplet infection infection conveyed by the spray from the mouth or nose while an individual is talking, coughing, or sneezing.

endemic a disease that is more or less present in an area or community continuously. The majority of the tropical diseases are endemic to locality.

epidemic a condition in which a disease attacks a large number of people in a community at the same time or during the same season. During an epidemic, the disease seems to spread rapidly.

etiology specific cause of a disease.

fomite any nonliving substance other than food that may harbor and transmit infectious organisms.

fumigation use of gas, smoke, or vapor for purposes of disinfection.

gamma globulin a protein formed in the blood. Ability to resist infection is related to concentration of such proteins.

host an animal or plant upon which a parasite lives.

immune protected against disease.

immune serum a serum taken from the blood of an immunized animal.

immunity a natural or acquired resistance to disease.

immunization process of rendering a person resistant to infection.

incubation period time intervening from initial infection to first appearance of signs and symptoms of the disease.

indigenous native to a particular locality.

infectious disease a disease caused by a microorganism.

infection the process by which a microbial organism invades and establishes a parasitic relationship with the host.

inoculation introduction of a disease agent into a healthy individual to produce a mild form of the disease followed by immunity.

isolation the separation of persons suffering from communicable diseases from other persons so that either direct or indirect transmission to susceptible persons is prevented.

lysin an antibody that causes disintegration of cells.

mode of transmission the manner of transfer of a microorganism from the source to a new host.

pandemic a very widespread or worldwide epidemic.

pathogenesis course of multiplication, further invasion, dissemination, and destruction of tissues by the etiologic agent following infection.

prophylaxis prevention.

quarantine the limitation of freedom of movement of persons or animals that have been exposed to a communicable disease for a period of time equal to the longest usual incubation period of the disease to which they have been exposed.

resistance condition of decreased susceptibility that can result from immunization and other factors.

sequelae deleterious effects, such as paralysis, resulting from an infectious disease.

specific pertaining to the special affinity of an antigen for the corresponding antibody.

sterile without living microorganisms.

susceptibility condition suitable for the establishment of an infection by invasion of an etiologic agent.

toxin the poisonous substance elaborated during the growth of pathogenic bacteria.

toxoid a toxin that has been treated in such a manner that its toxic properties are destroyed without affecting its antibody-producing properties.

vaccine a solution of dead or attenuated bacteria that, when introduced into the body, will produce the formation of antibodies without producing the disease itself.

virus a microscopic agent of disease that cannot be filtered by ordinary means and cannot be propagated on nonliving media.

SCIENTIFIC PRINCIPLES

Many of the biologic principles useful in the care of the patient with a communicable disease are related to characteristics of the causative agents. It is therefore suggested that pertinent portions of microbiology be reviewed, especially those presenting properties and activities of pathogenic microorganisms, defenses of the host against invasion, and factors in microbial control. Most of the principles stated in Chapter 30 in relation to wounds will be found useful in this context. Additional scientific concepts basic to understanding the nursing needs of a patient with a communicable disease appear in the following generalizations.

1. A human being spends his entire life in a never ending, constantly fluctuating microbial world.

2. The nature and variety of the *resident flora* is relatively constant in the various areas of the body. Members of the normal flora do not usually become parasitic, and as a rule their potential for inducing active disease is not great. *Transient flora* may establish a parasitic relationship with the host and, depending on their properties and on the resistance of the host, may establish active disease, parasitism implying some degree of harmful effect upon the host for the benefit of the parasite.

3. The behavior of microorganisms is closely related to their ability to estbalish a parasitic relationship with the host, with the following requirements:

a. Soluble nutrients, which they obtain from dead or decaying matter or from a living parasitized host

b. A narrow pH range, buffered to maintain approximate neutrality for most pathogens—this required pH is characteristic of the internal environment of the human body

c. Water, essential for keeping nutrients in a soluble form that can be absorbed through the cell wall of the organism

d. Oxygen—the aerobes require varying amounts of free oxygen, whereas the anaerobes obtain it chemically from the medium in which they are growing; oxygen is of significance in deep wounds that seal over so that anaerobic pathogens get their start in injured tissues in which the supply of blood and oxygen is limited

e. Temperature within relatively wide range for many kinds of microorganisms, but the range of temperature supported by the human body is most suitable for the physiologic activities of pathogens

f. Light—most bacteria do not require light or may be sensitive to ultraviolet rays in sunlight, a characteristic of importance in the control of communicable diseases

4. Bacteria are versatile in their ability to adjust to the changing demands of their environment. This characteristic is of practical importance in treatment with antibiotics or in the use of physical or chemical agents, including heat, disinfectant solutions, and the like, in the control of bacteria.

5. Bacterial mutations occur frequently, partly because of their rapid multiplication, producing antibiotic-resistant strains.

6. Toxins are products of bacterial growth and metabolism that are harmful to the host. *Exotoxins* diffuse out of the bacterial cell and may affect distant tissues, for example, toxins of diptheria, tetanus, and botulism. *Endotoxins* are a part of the bacterial cell's normal structure and are not liberated into the surrounding medium until the cell disintegrates, the endotoxic effect depending somewhat on the body tissues into which the bacterial cells themselves may be distributed.

7. The means of entry to the human body by microorganisms is accomplished through one or more of the four gateways: (a) via inhaled air into the respiratory tract, (b) ingestion with food taken via the mouth into the gastrointestinal tract, (c) penetration through the skin or mucous membrane via their own efforts, and (d) deposited directly into the deeper tissues, that is, via the parenteral route, as in the bite of an insect vector.

8. Essential to the communicability of a

disease are (a) availability to the invading pathogen of a portal or exit from the host body and (b) a route of transfer from one host to another host that has not been broked by the destruction of the microorganism.

9. Acidity of gastric secretions of the host kills many microorganisms swallowed with saliva. However, many organisms can survive at this pH level, including the tubercle bacillus and some other causative organisms such as the poliomyelitis virus and the bacteria of the *Salmonella* genus.

10. Pathogens differ in virulence according to their relative ability to display (a) *invasiveness* (ability to multiply and spread in the tissues of the host) and (b) *toxigenicity* (ability to produce substances that are toxic to the host tissues).

11. Establishment of parasitic relationship in the host by the invading organism is accomplished in one or both of two ways: (a) by localizing at the site of entry and spreading to surrounding tissues that are damaged through physiologic or mechanical means, or (b) by the organism itself, or its toxic products, or both, being disseminated from the portal of entry through the body. The organism and/or its toxigenic substances may be spread throughout the body via the bloodstream or lymphatic channels.

12. Nonspecific resistance factors of the host include those effective against microbes in general: (a) nonspecific constituents of plasma and leukocytes of the blood that are capable of phagocytosis, (b) phagocytes of the reticuloendothelial system, (c) phagocytes of the lymphatic system, (d) the inflammatory response, and (e) others associated with the resistance of the host, such as age, hormones, genetic and racial factors, nutritional status, stress, and climate.

13. Specific resistance of the host directed against a particular type of microorganism is the important characteristic of immunity, which may be either natural or acquired: (a) natural immunity, which includes species, racial, and individual immunity, and (b) immunity resulting from the production of antibodies in the host defending itself against the invasion by specific microorganisms or foreign substances.

14. Microorganisms can be destroyed by physical and chemical agents, depending on (a) the particular microbial group and its protective mechanisms, (b) the age of the bacterial cells, older ones being more resistant, and (c) the spore forms of some groups that are very resistant to destruction.

Through consideration of the background and implications of these generalizations the nurse may be assisted to a deeper insight into the battle of the patient versus the invading microbe and to more effectively maintain appropriate safeguards to prevent cross-infection of other patients and staff when caring for one with a communicable disease.

It is not possible to describe individual communicable diseases in a book of this type. However, suitable current literature on the subject is listed at the end of this chapter (Suggested Readings).

Although pathogenic organisms may contact the body in various ways, it does not always mean that disease will result. The human body is endowed with certain defense mechanisms that enable i to ward off or overcome invading organisms.

The body is protected with epithelial membrane that covers the outside as skin and lines the inside of the external cavities as mucous membrane. This membrane is said to be the body's first barrier against invasion. In addition, there are other mechanical structures that also aid. The hairs in the anterior nares protect the respiratory tract by serving as filters, the secretions of the open cavities wash away bacteria and other foreign material, and certain body fluids exert a high bactericidal action, such as the gastric juice that destroys many bacteria and their toxic products.

These anatomic and physiologic protectives are known as the body's first line of defense. When the first line of defense has been broken and bacteria do gain entrance into the body, the nonspecific defenses of phagocytosis and the inflammatory response attack the invaders. The purpose of the inflammatory process is to destroy the irritating and injurious agent and remove it from the body, or, if this is impossible, to limit its action throughout the body. If the organism perchance survives the inflammatory process, there is the next line of defense in the lymph nodes, which act as doors or filters at the vital passages to block the deadly enemy.

A second line of defense is that of specific immunity through the antigen-antibody response briefly described in Chapter 31.

There are two schools of thought in relation to immunity. The first is the humoral or chemical theory in which substances known as antibodies are produced in the bloodstream as a result of the introduction of an antigen. Antigens are usually of a protein nature, but some complex carbohydrates may be antigens. Each specific antigen produces its related antibody. Our most common antigens are found in bacteria, and their products are called toxins.

The second theory of immunity is the phagocytic or cellular theory. Certain body cells have the ability to ingest certain foreign materials in somewhat the same fashion as the feeding process of a unicellular organism such as the ameba.

It was once thought that these two theories were in opposition, but most modern immunologists now believe immunity to be a combination of the two, with one predominating as required by the nature of the invading organism.

Immunity may be classified in several

ways, the most common being natural and acquired. A natural immunity is one with which a person is born. This is evidenced by the action of phagocytes and other bactericidal powers of the blood. Natural immunity is more often associated with a race or species rather than with a certain individual. For example, Negroes and American Indians appear to have less resistance to tuberculosis than do Caucasians. An acquired immunity is one that an individual gains during a lifetime and is based on the chemical theory of the formation of antibodies in response to the introduction of a specific antigen.

Acquired immunity is classified as active or passive, depending on the part played by the body cells of the individual or animal. Active immunity is acquired either by a person's having the disease or by the introduction of bacterial or viral vaccine or toxoids into the body. In either case the individual builds his own antibodies in response to the antigen.

Passive immunity is obtained by injecting the individual with serum taken from the blood of a previously immunized animal. The animal is immunized by repeated injections of either the bacteria or their toxins. In this immunity the action is produced by the cells of the animal involved, and the recipient's cells remain passive. Hence, it is known as passive immunity. Passive immunity is produced at once and usually is of short duration. It is used as a preventive measure after exposure to a communicable disease.

Organisms may be transmitted either directly or indirectly. In direct transmission there is sufficient contact with the infected person so that the organism may pass directly from the host to the exposed person. Actual body contact is not necessary for the direct transmission of the organisms, for they may be spread by droplets, as in coughing or sneezing.

When a disease is transferred by direct contact, no time elapses from the moment the organism leaves the first host until it enters the second host, and no intermediate article is involved. A minute needle prick in a surgeon's glove may be sufficient to allow direct transfer of pathogenic organisms from the patient's bloodstream to the surgeon himself.

Organisms are transferred indirectly by way of articles handled by the infected person or by an intermediate host such as food, water, an animal, an insect, or a carrier.

The most common method of indirect transfer is by fomites. Fomites are articles to which organisms may cling. The term "fomites" is used to cover a large and varied list of articles such as clothing and bedding, money, dust, and so on.

Not all articles coming in contact with a patient having a communicable disease will contain pathogenic organisms. Contamination of the article will depend on whether it was in contact with the organism, and this contact will depend on the location of the organism in the patient and its portal of exit. Likewise, a person may contact contaminated articles and yet not receive the organism in question into his own body because that organism can enter the body of the host only through certain channels.

The various channels through which organisms may leave the body of the sick and enter that of another are (1) the nose and throat, (2) the gastrointestinal tract, (3) the genitourinary tract, (4) the mucous membrane of the eyes, and (5) a break in the skin. It is very rare that the organism in question will be present in more than one of these locations, so that the nurse can reasonably confine it to a specific area by the use of a good isolation technique.

Serums are used in the treatment of the disease itself and are also given after exposure to certain diseases when there is not sufficient time for the action of a vaccine or toxoid. Serums provide passive immunity in that they contain antibodies that have been produced by another animal or individual.

Whole blood and plasma are now among the preferred treatments for most diseases and are also beneficial in the treatment of communicable diseases. If the donor has recently had the disease in question, antibodies will be present in his blood, called immune or convalescent blood, but the usefulness of this type of treatment probably results more from the building up of the patient's entire system rather than providing immunity.

One of the greatest contributions to medical science during the last two decades has been the development of the use of anti-infective drugs, chiefly the antibiotics and the chemotherapeutic agents, which selectively inhibit the growth of or even kill pathogens. These medications should be administered only on the advice of a physician even though some of them may be purchased without a prescription. Their indiscriminate use may result in harm at a later date since certain chains of bacteria and viruses have a tendency to become resistant to various chemicals or the individual may become hypersensitive to them.

MEDICAL ASEPSIS

Meaning. Medical asepsis is the term used to describe the technique of preventing the transfer of the disease from its source or by reducing the number of pathogenic microorganisms.

One of the chief methods of confining an organism to a specific area is by isolation of the patient. Isolation means the separation of the patient and his unit from others to prevent the direct or indirect conveyance of the infectious agent to susceptible persons. Any article the patient uses or contacts should be destroyed or disinfected before being placed in general use again.

Methods. There are two main classifications of isolation techniques according to the physical setup—the unit type and the disease type. In the unit type a single patient is confined to an area. This area may be a private room, a cubicle, or a designated space in an open ward. In a ward screens should be used to mark the area, and at least 6 feet of space should be allowed between beds. In the disease type there is more than one patient, and the unit as a whole is set apart. This was once thought to be an adjunct to the care of the patient by having like patients grouped together. However, because of cross-infection and variance in organisms, its value is now questionable, and separation is advisable for all communicable disease patients.

Various methods of carrying out isolation have been designed. They are generally based on the route of entry and discharge of the organism. Some of the more common methods are respiratory isolation, intestinal isolation, and contact isolation.

Respiratory isolation. Respiratory isolation is used for diseases that are commonly spread by droplet infection and those in which the organism is present in the respiratory system. In this type of isolation the nurse usually wears a gown if close contact with the patient is expected (Figs. 32-1 and 32-2). All articles coming in contact with the patient, such as dishes, linen, trays, and the like, must be disinfected since there is a possibility of contamination. Many disposable materials (paper dishes, for example) are used in isolation, thus saving much disinfection. Urine and feces not contaminated may be emptied directly into the hopper or bedpan sterilizer. However, since the patient has come in contact with the outside of the bedpan and urinal, these articles are considered to be contaminated and must not be allowed to touch any clean article while being emptied.

In some hospitals it is customary for the

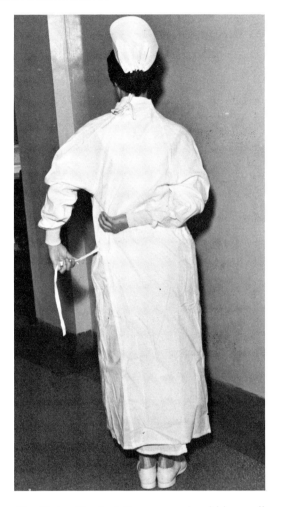

Fig. 32-1. The isolation gown should lap well in the back to afford complete protection for the uniform.

nurse to wear a mask while caring for a patient in respiratory isolation. This is advisable if the patient coughs frequently or is not aware of his behavior. However, masks in themselves may be a source of danger to the nurse unless properly handled. A fresh mask should be worn each time the unit is entered, and it should be changed every 20 minutes to provide adequate protection. It should be removed when the nurse leaves the unit and when it becomes soiled or damp. The warm, moist breathng of the nurse against the

528

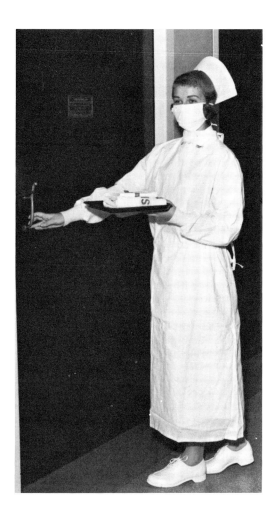

Fig. 32-2. The nurse wears a clean gown when entering the unit and removes the gown immediately prior to leaving the unit.

used with patients in whom the organism is present in the gastrointestinal tract. Feces are grossly contaminated and urine often is. In a hospital with modern plumbing facilities that empty into a sanitary sewage disposal system, it is permissible to dispose of excreta without previous disinfection if it is placed directly into hoppers or bedpan sterilizers, provided the procedure does not conflict with the policies of the community health department. In rural or small communities, excreta must be disinfected before disposal. In times of disaster, such as floods, earthquakes, hurricanes, and tornadoes, when the sewage system is not functioning, it is necessary to disinfect all excreta before disposing of it. For disinfection of excreta, most authorities recommend combining it with equal parts of a 0.5% to 1% chlorinated lime solution and allowing it to stand for at least 1 hour before emptying.

A patient on intestinal isolation is cared for much the same as a patient on respiratory isolation except that a mask is not necessary and any food left on the trays and bath water should be treated the same as excreta.

Contact isolation. Contact isolation is used when the organism is present in discharging wounds or in lesions of the skin. Care must be taken here to protect the hands of the nurse. Rubber or plastic disposable gloves are often used as a safety precaution. The nurse should avoid using harsh disinfectants, since they tend to make the hands rough, thereby creating a portal of entry. Wounds are kept covered, and soiled dressings are burned.

Care of linen. In almost all types of isolation, bed linen, towels, and other articles of clothing are considered contaminated and become a source of infection through indirect contact. Most institutions caring for contagious patients have devised methods suited to their needs, and this function may be delegated to the housekeeping department. However, it is

mask can provide a suitable environment for the growth of organisms.

Another technique is to have the patient wear a mask. This is of value when transporting the patient to and from the x-ray department and other areas where several people are involved. The greatest safety measure probably is teaching the patient to protect others by covering his mouth and nose with tissues and disposing of them immediately in a paper bag, which is burned.

Intestinal isolation. Intestinal isolation is

529

usually the responsibility of the nurse to see that the linen is prepared properly for transporting to the laundry and that both the nurse and the nonprofessional worker are protected. A satisfactory technique is to place the contaminated linen into a laundry bag within the unit and then to place this bag into a plastic or waterproof bag at the exit of the unit. The plastic bag is then closed with contaminated linen

sealed in and is now safe for removal to laundry. (See Fig. 32-3 and note position of nurses' hands.) Disposable linens are also now available at a reasonable cost.

Reverse isolation. Reverse isolation, as the name implies, is just the opposite of regular isolation in that it seeks to protect the patient from microorganisms in his environment. Reverse isolation is used mostly for patients who are critically ill or

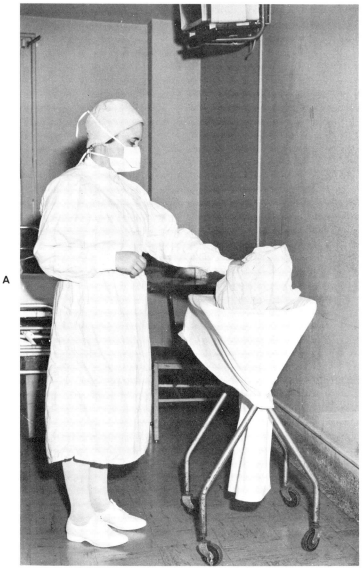

Fig. 32-3. A, Placing contaminated linen into bag within the unit. **B,** Transferring bag to plastic container at door of unit.

have a lowered resistance to disease. The procedure is somewhat similar to that of the technique used in the care of the newborn infant in the nursery. Effort is made in this case to protect the patient from invading microorganisms. In this type of isolation the nurse wears a mask and always washes the hands before contacting the patient. Unless the nurse is wearing a freshly laundered uniform, it may be necessary to cover it with a gown. In many instances, the nurse changes into "scrub dress" while on duty, thus reducing the possibility of outside contact with organisms in the commuting environment.

Patients placed on reverse isolation are usually seriously ill. The application of this technique is becoming common with patients receiving intensive chemotherapy, radiation, organ transplants, or extensive surgery.

Federal and community health laws. Regardless of how well an isolation technique is carried out, it alone will not prevent the spread of communicable diseases.

The greatest success probably lies in the community health laws and in the responsibility of each individual for assuming his share in the prevention of communicable diseases.

Many diseases are spread by food or water. Therefore, it is important that a community have a safe water supply and sewage disposal. Strict regulations must be observed in the handling of food. Food

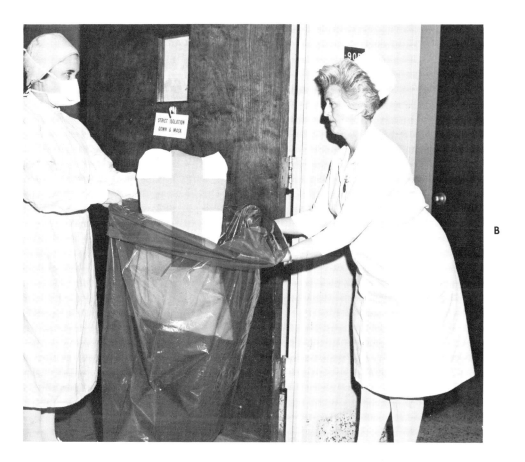

Fig. 32-3, cont'd. For legend see opposite page.

handlers usually have annual health examinations. Most firms require that employees wear special uniforms while on duty and that this apparel remain on the premises and not be taken to the home of the individual. Food handlers should not be allowed to work when ill, no matter how slight the symptoms, if it points to a possible communicable disease. Any person having symptoms of a cold or sore throat or an elevated temperature should be considered a suspect until ruled out. Most employers grant sick leave and provide for expenses through workman's compensation or sickness insurance. If this type of security is not provided, many may be forced to conceal certain symptoms for financial reasons.

The public health nurse from the board of health, from a visiting nurse association, or from the industry may visit the patient in his home to instruct and direct care.

Protective measures for the nurse. The health of the nurse caring for infectious patients must be guarded at all times. Various measures have been devised that include (1) an annual physical examination, including an x-ray film of the chest, (2) proper immunization, (3) routine nose and throat cultures, (4) a well-balanced diet and good elimination habits, (5) sufficient rest and sleep, (6) recreation, preferably outdoor, (7) good oral hygiene, (8) a daily bath with frequent shampooing of the hair, (9) well-cared-for hands, and (10) proper attire when entering the unit.

PSYCHOSOCIAL ASPECTS

The emotional reaction of the isolated patient may be one of tension and anxiety because of his need for additional care. He may feel resentment at being alone much of the time and may feel that he is different from other patients because his care is different. Since the No. 1 communicable disease of the present day is venereal disease, the patient may feel that his way of

life is not acceptable to the nurse. Also, the nurse may feel resentment toward the patient because of a difference in moral standards.

The patient should be told the reason for isolation (usually based on a written physician's order) and should be instructed in various ways in which he can cooperate. He should understand that the special methods are used to protect himself and others. The nurse will need tact and understanding to establish good rapport and to communicate with the patient and to teach him the importance of personal hygiene and disease prevention.

Diversions are important. Magazines and newspapers are usually available. However, they need to be burned after the patient has read them. Flowers, letters, and small gifts serve as welcome diversions.

Medical asepsis requires cooperation among all members of the health team. The isolation techniques practiced by the nurse should be observed by all others who come in contact with the patient.

Visitors are usually limited to members of the immediate family, and they must be properly instructed and gowned before being admitted to the patient's unit. A telephone in the unit helps him keep in touch with his family and friends.

The nurse should know the functions of official and nonofficial agencies concerned with communicable diseases such as the public health department in order to meet the health and social needs of the patient.

NURSING CARE

The communicable disease patient is most, often an acutely ill patient and, in some instances, also seriously or even critically ill, such as the patient who may have tetanus or smallpox. Even the so-called simple childhood diseases may produce permanent debilitating effects.

In the past so much effort has been spent on preventing the spread of the organisms

that little time was given to the actual care of the patient. In fact, in some instances, student nurses were assigned to care for these patients on the sole basis of acquiring skill in isolation techniques. (These techniques can be learned just as well in a "skills laboratory" without jeopardizing the comfort and welfare of the patient.) With the adjunct of the voluminous supply of disposable equipment now available and more hospital staff adequately trained in medical aseptic techniques, the nurse can now devote more time to the patient.

Objectives in the care of the patient should be:

1. To give the adequate care necessary for any acutely ill medical patient. This includes the administration of therapeutic measures and assisting with diagnostic tests. (These techniques are discussed elsewhere in this book under their relative headings.)

2. To prevent complications and secondary infections. This can best be accomplished by the effective use of the so-called general nursing measures of daily living, as covered in Chapters 15 and 16, and by having a knowledge of the specific disease conditions.

3. To prevent the spread of the disease to other members of the family and hospital personnel. A great majority of communicable disease patients are cared for in their homes. Here it will be necessary for the nurse to be skilled in effective teaching methods and home nursing procedures. The plan of care in the home must be adapted to the patient's family and the home setting. For principles applicable to this situation, one may refer to the nursing care plan in Chapter 14, which is adapted to a home setting.

In a hospital environment, the nurse usually follows the agency policy in the appropriate medical aseptic techniques, which are usually set up by an infection committee on which the nursing department should be well represented.

The National Communicable Disease Center has developed a manual of isolation techniques based on current concepts of the epidemiology of communicable diseases. The isolation categories are "strict," "respiratory," and "protective." Precautions are classified as "enteric," "wound and skin," "discharges," and "blood." Information concerning the manual may be obtained by writing the center.

It is also assumed that the future nurse practitioner will also be groomed in public health measures and have a fund of knowledge in the health sciences that will aid in devising the appropriate techniques needed. Agency techniques should be evaluated and revised routinely.

4. To give reassurance to the patient and his family. Illness is always a threat to a patient's security, and the added possibility of transmitting this illness to someone else brings more instability. Identification of the patient's individual needs will help to reduce feelings of anxiety and rejection. Fumbles by an inadequately trained aide may cause the patient to become embarrassed or feel he is imposing on the staff by requiring additional care.

Physical isolation does not necessarily mean mental isolation. Proper diversion following the acute stage can be planned with little or no added economic expense. Many children enjoy small toys such as miniature cars and trucks that can easily be replaced. In the home it is no longer necessary to deprive the patient of his familiar surroundings as many of the newer detergents are also antiseptic agents, so the patient may continue to use their regular clothing, pastel bed linens, and the like.

Acceptance of the patient regardless of the cause or source of his disease is always a priority in his care. Since most communicable diseases also involve the whole family, the nurse will use patience in teaching them the proper techniques, the need for protecting other members of the family, and the necessity of reporting certain diseases. No patient need be deprived of care and treatment because of a communicable disease, since public health departments are always ready to give assistance.

Since visitors in most hospitals are now limited to the immediate family, they need not be a problem of the communicable disease patient and may even aid in his care. For example, the parent or relative who is in the room and already gowned may assist in turning the patient or bringing a tray to the door, thus saving time for the staff. By the use of the proper protective measures the patient is thus able to remain in contact with the family, which will in turn lessen anxiety and aid in recovery.

LEARNING SITUATIONS FOR THE PATIENT

The nurse explains to the patient the benefits to be derived from cooperating in the techniques used. He is told how he can help. He learns the meaning of the words "clean" and "contaminated," if he is not already familiar with their use. He is also impressed with the importance of reporting a communicable disease and receiving treatment and, if of a social nature, the importance of reporting contacts and encouraging them to receive treatment.

The nurse also teaches the patient about the complications and other delayed effects of certain communicable diseases. Sometimes the experience itself becomes a learning experience for the patient.

SUMMARY

Communicable diseases are those that may be transmitted from one individual or animal to another. They are caused by microorganisms and are, therefore, infectious diseases. If there is knowledge of the causative organism, including how it enters and leaves the body, the elements necessary for its growth, and the means

of destroying it, a spread of communicable disease may be prevented.

The communicable disease patient is first of all an individual with an acute medical disorder who deserves the best nursing care possible, and unnecessary techniques should not take precedence over the patient's comfort and personal needs.

When an individual is known to have a communicable disease, the chief methods of preventing its spread are isolation of the individual and use of anti-infective therapy.

The health of a community depends largely on its health laws and on each individual's observance of them. A clean community is almost always a healthy community.

Effective immunizing agents are available for many communicable diseases and, if used early enough, help greatly in the reduction of the number of cases and their seriousness. The board of health is ready to give assistance at once in case of communicable disease.

QUESTIONS FOR DISCUSSION

1 Outline a program for immunizations that could be followed through a lifetime. Name specific diseases and specific agents against them.
2 Observe the isolation technique in use in your hospital. Identify scientific principles that justify each step. Are there practices that cannot be justified by scientific principles? If so, how might the practice be altered in order to be consistent with scientific principles?
3 Describe in detail an effective method of handwashing for use in carrying out isolation technique.

LIFE SITUATION

Lydia, a 5 year old, was admitted to the pediatric unit on a cold December day. Her mother stated that she had been lethargic, vomiting, at times delirious, and had had a high fever for the past 24 hours. This was Lydia's fourth hospitalization. She had a history of sickle cell anemia with embolic phenomenon that was diagnosed at age 2. She also had been hospitalized twice for acute respiratory infection.

Lydia lives in a well-kept middle income neighborhood. Her parents married at age 30. Lydia is their only child. Her mother is a public school teacher who expresses a great deal of anxiety about her recurrent hospitalization. Although she is educated, she has very little knowledge or understanding about sickle cell anemia. She stated that Lydia spends most of her time in the den on the couch. She usually has a great deal of pain in the lower legs and refuses to be active. It was necessary to hire a full-time housekeeper and baby-sitter since she is not able to go to kindergarten. Although she and her husband wanted a child, the confinement and limitation on their social activities have placed strain on the marriage. Lydia's father is a federal employee. It isn't difficult for him to get out of the house since the mother has assumed most of the evening care for Lydia.

Lydia's initial physical assessment revealed a red inflamed throat, marked nuchal rigidity, bluish spots on the lower extremities with edema of the dorsum of the feet and marked tenderness, equal and slightly dilated pupils, slight abdominal distension, rapid heart rate at 160 beats per minute, respirations 50, temperature 105° F.

A lumbar puncture was done that revealed a white cell count of 14,000 with a few red cells. The spinal fluid culture report revealed the presence of *Pneumococcus*. Complete blood count showed:

Hemoglobin: 8.9 Gm.
Red blood cell count: 3.54 million
White blood cell count: 63,200
Neutrophils: 74
Lymphocytes: 4
Bands: 14
100% polymorphonuclear leukocytes

A diagnosis of *Pneumococcus* meningitis was established.

Lydia was started on massive dosages of antibiotics. The tenderness in the lower extremities continued throughout the hospital period. She had two convulsions and experienced difficulty swallowing.

Physician's orders included:
Ampicillin, 300 mg. I.V. q.6h.
Penicillin, 1,000,000 units, I.V. q.12h.

5% Dextrose in water, 300 ml., q.6h.
Oxygen tent
Ice water to axillary and groin for temp. of 102° F.
Luminal gr. 1 (65 mg.) I.M. stat, then gr.ss q.6h. if restless
Packed cells, 250 ml., administer 50 ml./hour

Questions:

1 Lydia has many needs. To which will you give priority?
2 What is the significance of Lydia's high fever?
3 What is the action of ampicillin and penicillin against the invading organism?
4 What is the nurse's responsibility in the performance of a lumbar puncture?
5 How does the *Pneumococcus* enter the body? How does it leave the body?
6 What type of isolation technique will be used for Lydia? Why?
7 Why was Lydia placed in an oxygen tent?
8 What precautions should be taken when giving a temperature sponge bath?
9 How do you account for the fact that Lydia's mother knows so little about her daughter's chronic disease?
10 How will the presence of sickle cell anemia influence Lydia's acute medical prognosis?
11 What is the probable cause of Lydia's inactivity at home?
12 What information could be gained by doing a pediatric assessment of developmental tasks in this situation?
13 What needs other than those indicated above does Lydia have?
14 Outline a plan of care for Lydia to be used during her hospitalization and one to be followed after discharge.

SUGGESTED READINGS

Branchman, Philip S.: The new NCDC isolation manual—a brief review, Nursing Clinics of North America 5:175, March, 1970.

Brown, Mara A.: Adolescents and V.D., Nursing Outlook 21:99, February, 1973.

Francis, Byron John: Current concepts in immunization, American Journal of Nursing 73:646, April, 1973.

Garner, Julia S., and Kaiser, Allen B.: How often is isolation needed? American Journal of Nursing 72:733, April, 1972.

Hippie 'live in' cited in spread of pubic lice (notes and quotes), RN 31:23, September 23, 1968.

Hubbard, Charles William: Family planning education—parenthood and social disease control, St. Louis, 1973, The C. V. Mosby Co.

Is cervical cancer a venereal disease? RN **31**:23, December, 1968.

Jackson, Dolores E.: Sickle cell disease: meeting a need, Nursing Clinics of North America **7**:727, December, 1972.

Lentz, Josephine: The nurse's role in extending infection control to the community, Nursing Clinics of North America **5**:165, March, 1970.

Lenz, Philomene E.: Women, the unwitting carriers of gonorrhea, American Journal of Nursing **71**:716, April, 1971.

McDermott, Nancy King: The nursing role in a specialized infection control unit, Nursing Clinics of North America **5**:113, March, 1970.

Morrison, Shirley T., and Arnold, Carolyn R.: Patients with common communicable diseases— preventive measures, treatment and rehabilitation, Nursing Clinics of North America **4**:143, March, 1970.

Naismith, Grace: The plain truth about V.D., Reader's Digest **65**:19, September, 1972.

Sexual activity linked to cervical cancer, RN **31**:65, October, 1968.

Spicher, Charlotte: Nursing care of children hospitalized with infections, Nursing Clinics of North America **5**:123, March, 1970.

33 Long-term illness

INCIDENCE OF CHRONIC ILLNESS

In this chapter the expression "long-term illness" is used interchangeably with "chronic illness," which is defined by the Commission on Chronic Illness as "an illness of 3 or more months' duration." It usually refers to illness or disability that is permanent or recurrent and that requires a long period of care, hence the name "long-term." However, principles included here may also apply to any patient needing extended care, as for example, the leg amputee who may recover from surgery in a few days but who may require a very long period of rehabilitation.

There are at least fifty diseases that may be classified as chronic. The more common ones and those that result in permanent impairment are diseases of the heart and circulation, arthritis and rheumatism, diseases of the nervous system, cancer and other malignant growths, and a host of disabilities resulting from automobile accidents and military service.

The median age is rising as a result of medical discoveries that lead to longer life. The increase is not so much caused by the fact that people are living longer but by the decrease of the death rate in infancy, childhood, and youth. However, the prob-

lem of long-term illness not only affects elderly persons but also a number of young people. Results of a recent survey revealed approximately 30 million individuals with some type of mental or physical impairment. Only 8% were over 65 years of age, and more than one half were under 45 years of age. Accidents still involve a high percentage of young people, and a great majority of returning wounded veterans are under the age of 40. These facts show that age is not always a deciding factor in long-term illness.

Long-term patients have common needs. In addition to nursing care, the long-term patient may need financial assistance, rehabilitation services, and help with emotional problems. Many of the needs can be met, and the more specific ones are discussed in this chapter.

FACTORS INFLUENCING THE PATIENT'S NEEDS

Medical diagnosis. No set of standard rules can be laid down for nursing the long-term care patient. The term "long-term" is not a disease entity, such as cardiovascular or other similar classification. The long-term patient may be a diabetic who will need a special diet, and

537

maybe medication, for the rest of his life. He may be a physically handicapped cerebral vascular accident victim or a laryngectomee with a speech problem. The patient may be a rheumatic child who must fight life with conserved energies. He may be a mental patient with continuous personality problems, or a terminally ill cancer patient, or he may be an honored heroic veteran who at the height of his career must change his occupation. However, each long-term patient will automatically fall into a medical classification that will dictate some of his needs. The diagnosis will also probably determine where the patient will be cared for. As medicine becomes more specialized, so will nursing care. The nurse clinician in a coronary unit cannot be expected to give the same expert service in a cancer clinic or in a home for the aged.

Age. The patient's age should also be considered. If he is a child with an orthopedic disability, one would probably think of a Shriner's Hospital as a place of hope and recovery. Here the child would be with other children his own age, could attend school in his wheelchair, and be entertained by the most popular movie and television stars. For the elderly paralytic patient, the future is not quite so bright.

Prognosis. The prognosis becomes very important when setting goals for the long-term patient. Can the patient be expected to return to his normal daily routine, must he live with a physical handicap, must he remain under continuous medical therapy, or can he function within a scope of limited activities?

The condition may also be a terminal one. The patient with a metastatic breast cancer may fully recover from the surgical procedure but yet face imminent death.

One will note that each of the above factors will produce specific and varied needs in addition to the patient's own personal needs.

NURSING CARE

In Chapter 1, the focus of the nurse practitioner was on the patient and the process through which his health needs might be met. It was considered in relation to the five broad categories outlined by the World Health Organization Expert Committee on Nursing.

Much success will depend upon the stage in which the nurse first contacts the patient. The public health or school nurse will probably have most contacts during the health maintenance, increased risk, or early detection stages, but for the hospital or average nurse, the contact will be during the clinical stage, so most plans of care will be started at this time. The earlier the contact, the better the outcome.

Sometimes both physicians and nurses are so concerned over meeting the patient's needs during the clinical stage that little thought is given to the rehabilitation stage. When this stage is finally reached, irreparable damage may already be done. Sometimes it is a matter of life and death, and certain procedures must then be carried out regardless of later results. For example, in an emergency, a tracheotomy may have to be performed with unsterile equipment. This risk of infection must be considered or treated later.

Objectives in the plan of care for the long-term patient will be:

1. To endeavor to perceive the patient over a period of time and to think in long-term goals as well as immediate goals. This is especially important in the care of the stroke or cancer patient.

2. To continue or assist the patient in continuing his therapy. Failure to take medication or to return for treatment, whether it be physical or mental, can do much to interfere with a patient's progress. A patient may neglect his therapy because he "feels better," cannot afford it, denies his illness, or lacks knowledge about it.

3. To work with the health team in assisting the patient to accomplish the developmental task appropriate to his age—the child, to mature to adulthood; the mother, to manage her home; the father, to support his family; and the aged, to die with dignity.
4. To aid the patient in working through his grief process, since all long-term patients eventually lose to some degree a portion of their body functioning.
5. To work with the family in helping them to accept the patient and to aid in their adjustment of the problem or anticipated problems that might arise.

APPLICATION OF SCIENTIFIC PRINCIPLES

Depending upon the problems or patient's needs, the nurse can learn from the biologic or behavioral sciences principles that will form a basis for nursing intervention. Since many long-term patients come from the elderly group of citizens, the nurse should be well versed in problems pertinent to the aged. (See Suggested Readings.) Any good book on medical-surgical nursing will contribute to one's ability to observe and perform certain diagnostic tests and therapy.

Principles pertinent to hygenic care, problems of inactivity, and elimination have been presented in earlier chapters of this book.

All long-term patients require some rehabilitation. Principles pertaining to this process were presented in Chapter 19. Special effort has been made to give the nurse a psychologic and physiologic basis for understanding and caring for the dying patient in Chapter 20.

PSYCHOSOCIAL ASPECTS

It is usually a shock to a person when told that he has a condition that will last for a long period of time. Besides the ne-cessity of coping with his physical condition, he may be confronted with social and emotional displacement. A period of only 6 weeks may mean a complete change in the career and life of some patients. Many patients immediately have feelings of insecurity. If the person involved is the head of a household, he will be fearful of how it will affect the family financially. Some patients may be faced with finding a different occupation. If the mother is the patient, she will worry about her home and children. The full impact of the diagnosis may not come suddenly but may evolve over a period of days. The patient may become depressed, which adds to the stress and strain on the members of the family. Often he is moody, despondent, and apprehensive about his illness, the cost of treatment, and the prospects of recovery. Many patients have a feeling of guilt, and some consider chronic illness to be a form of punishment.

Loss is a common occurrence in long-term illness: loss of a part of the body or its function, loss of economic or personal independence, loss of a job, loss of a comfortable body image. Loss is usually followed by grief. The nurse who understands that grief follows loss is better prepared to help the patient.

The patient has many fears: fear of getting out of bed, fear of falling, fear of pain, fear of the unknown. Also helplessness, loneliness, and boredom are present with the long-term patient. Fear is lessened by knowledge and by a successful experience, even in a small way, and through motivation inspired by the nurse.

Often tension can be relieved if the patient is able to talk with someone about his condition, and in this instance the nurse can be a good listener. By a sincere interest in what he has to say, the nurse can add to his feelings of security and also obtain a greater understanding of the patient and what can be done for him. The long-term patient may admit himself to more social interest by wearing his glasses or hearing aid, if he has these appliances. The nurse should encourage him to waer them in order that he may be more aware of what is going on about him. The nurse may also increase awareness and sensitivity of attendants to problems, feeling, and needs of the patient. Indications that the patient needs to talk further to someone can be brought to the physician's attention so that he can make a referral or a social worker can be contacted, according to the policy of the institution. The chaplain can impart faith and encouragement.

One important question that is always faced is in what facilities to place the patient for care. Many persons seem to feel that their own home is the ideal place. However, with the trend in modern living, this may not always be an appropriate place. If the patient needs 24-hour surveillance or care, this may be much added expense or too demanding on other members of the family. If the patient has periods of regression or relapses of the disease itself, he may require immediate medical and nursing needs. For these patients the ideal situation is a type of nursing home or long-term service unit that offers custodial, rehabilitative, medical, and nursing care. Many of the better type homes for the aged now have both self-care and hospital units.

As was noted in Chapter 20 (Fig. 20-2), each family member shares in the patient's illness and loss. In the total plan of care, some priorities must be given to family members especially in the education of children, and sufficient time must be given for a mother to care for her family.

One of the biggest blocks in the care of the long-term patient is his lack of money. A patient's financial worries can compound his illness. Treating the financial ills may at times be as important as treating the physical illness. Two over-

whelming problems are maintenance of income and meeting the costs of illness. The responsibility of the nurse includes an awareness and understanding of the patient's financial problems, of the activity of referral, of the knowledge of sources of assistance, of the teaching of basic budget planning, and of savings possible through conservation of costly equipment and improvising materials in the home. A referral to a social worker for assistance with economic problems may hasten the patient's recovery. The nurse may be the only professional worker in the day-to-day contact with the patient and so should be aware of such agencies as Social Security Administration, Old-Age Assistance, Office of Vocational Rehabilitation, or the many private agencies. Since many patients are sensitive about receiving welfare aid, usually the matter of a patient's financial needs should be referred to a social worker.

Much cost of illness is covered by insurance. The most popular and reasonably priced health insurance is probably the Blue Cross and Blue Shield programs, both of which are community-sponsored nonprofit corporations organized to furnish specific types and amounts of hospital service and medical care in return for regular prepayments. The patient has free choice of both hospital and physician. Government-sponsored programs include Medicare and Medicaid.

Long-term patients may be cared for in several places. (1) They may enter a hospital for an acute stage of their illness and then return home. A few hospitals send personnel into the home for follow-up care on some patients. Also, patients may have care at home by the Visiting Nurse Association. (2) After an acute stage of illness has subsided, patients may remain in the hospital and be moved to a wing for chronic conditions. Since the already-established facilities of the hospital, such as administrative personnel, laboratories, and dietary departments, can be used in such a setup, general overall costs in the care of a chronically ill patient may be reduced. (3) Another facility for the care of long-term patients is the nursing home, which patients may enter following a hospital stay.

Medicare and Medicaid programs provide for hospital care, posthospital extended care services, including care in a nursing home or rehabilitation facility, and posthospital home health services.

Both governmental and voluntary agencies have developed some activities in the field of long-term illness. In 1963 the United States Public Health Service set up the Clinical Center of National Institutes of Health at Bethesda, Maryland, where inpatients are admitted for study in six research areas: arthritis and metabolic diseases, cancer, heart, allergy and infectious diseases, neurology and ophthalmology, and psychiatry. Besides this research, The United States Public Health Service develops methods for control of disease and

assists and advises states in their functions in the care of the long-term patient.

LEARNING SITUATIONS FOR THE PATIENT

Teaching by the nurse is of major importance in long-term illness. It is based on accurate information that the patient already has and is adapted to the patient's ability to learn. The patient with a long-term illness may need to accept more responsibility for treatments and medications after discharge from the hospital than the patient with a short-term illness. While nursing care is given, teaching may be focused on how the patient can adapt the treatment to his ability to perform it with the equipment he has at home. The nurse should give instructions slowly, allowing time for the patient to understand, especially if he is elderly. He may need assistance in changing his attitude toward himself and his family.

An understanding of the family's social, ethnic, and religious life is necessary if the

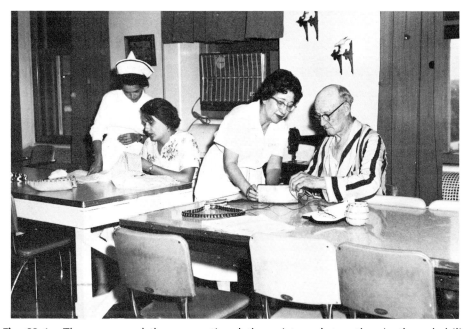

Fig. 33-1. The nurse and the occupational therapist work together in the rehabilitation of the patient.

nurse is to help plan the adaptation of treatments and living arrangements in the home. Adequate planning with the family provides for continuity of care as the patient moves from the hospital to his home. Plans for home care should begin just as soon as discharge is anticipated. If possible, plans should be made with the one who will actually give the home care. Things to consider are (1) the kind of equipment needed for home use, (2) where it can be obtained, (3) exercise and treatments, (4) diet and medications, (5) maintenance of role, and (6) a return for a visit to the physician's office or clinic. A written form or plan is most effective so that the person caring for the patient will not have to depend on memory. If special treatments or massage must be given, they could be demonstrated to the person assuming the care, or the patient might be referred to the local visiting nurse in order to start the home program functioning properly.

SUMMARY

Long-term illness is of great importance, since there is an increasing number of elderly persons in our population and many of them have long-term illnesses. The concern becomes not just a problem of the patient and his family but also of society in general. To be most effective, goals must be set in the early stages of illness. The nurse needs to keep abreast of changes in treatments and methods of dealing with specialized problems of chronically ill patients in order to give the best care medical science provides.

QUESTIONS FOR DISCUSSION

1 Why are posture and positioning often of more importance in the patient with a long-term illness than in one with a short-term illness?
2 Discuss the importance of occupational therapy in caring for the patient with a long-term illness.
3 What might be the reactions of a patient upon being told that his illness will last a long time?
4 Discuss the Medicare program.
5 What community agency provides bedside nursing care in homes?
6 Outline the broad topics covered in teaching a patient who has a long-term illness.
7 Name five community agencies whose concern is in the area of long-term illness.

LIFE SITUATION

Mr. Spurgeon, age 47, fell from a ladder while painting. He was not unconscious after the fall but immediately complained of pain in the back of the neck. He was unable to move his legs.

The initial medical assessment revealed:

Blood pressure: 80/0

Pulse: 56

Respirations: 26 and labored

Decreased chest excursions with entirely abdominal breathing

Neck resistant to passive motion and all motion was extremely painful

Tenderness at the cervicodorsal junction posteriorly

Some motor level between the biceps and triceps with absence of grip and dorsiflexion of the wrist

Biceps jerk bilaterally but no deep tendon reflexes below this level

Plantar response was flexor bilaterally

Complete sensory loss to just above the nipples bilaterally

Sensations present over the shoulders but absent in the hands

Bowel sounds absent

X-ray studies revealed compression of the sixth cervical vertebra with questionable chip fracture at the posterior inferior border of the body, but there was no dislocation. The lumbar puncture revealed an opening pressure of 170 with clear fluid. A diagnosis of compression of sixth cervical vertebra was established.

Initial medical orders included:

Cervical traction: 7 pounds

Oxygen therapy as indicated

Insert Foley catheter and irrigate with Neosporin I.V. solution

500 ml. 5% D.W.I.V. solution to run till noon tomorrow

Codeine 60 mg. q.3h. p.r.n. for pain

Soapsuds enema every other day

Ace bandage to groin and change each shift I.P.P.B. therapy with Isuprel and Dornavac for 10 minutes q.4h.

Decadron 4 mg. stat and q.6h.

As Mr. Spurgeon's condition improved, he was placed on diet as tolerated. His body position was changed frequently. He first had a poster brace, then he was given exercises, and finally he began ambulating.

Mr. Spurgeon is married and the father of six children ranging from ages 8 to 26. During his hospitalization his wife was admitted to the hospital with a respiratory infection. All of his children also had the flu. Therefore, there was a period of 2 weeks without visitors.

To supplement his income as a painter, he operates a small farm and often works for owners of larger farms. His wife does not work, but his oldest son, who still lives at home, helps with the painting and farming.

During the acute phase of hospitalization, Mr. Spurgeon was very depressed. He often stated, "I feel like a baby because I can't do anything for myself." As his condition improved, he became more cheerful and optimistic about his recovery. Two months after hospitalization, he could move his upper extremities but lacked ability to grasp with the hands. His legs responded with involuntary jerks. Use of Foley catheter with genitourinary irrigation continued and bowel training was started. However, Mr. Spurgeon was not doing well with coughing and deep breathing. He stated that he could not cough and appeared to experience periods of depression; however, he still expressed a desire to keep his farm and resume previous occupation if possible.

Questions:

1 Had you been Mr. Spurgeon's nurse at this time, what goals or objectives would you have included in your plan of care?

2 To be effective, at what stage of an illness should a program of rehabilitation begin?

3 Why do you suppose Mr. Spurgeon was still having difficulty in chest movements but seemed to be gaining activity in other involved muscles?

4 List at least three significant reasons for Mr. Spurgeon's depression. What could you do to help alleviate it?

5 What problems other than his illness do you suppose Mr. Spurgeon's family is experiencing?

6 Outline a postdismissal teaching plan for continued bowel and bladder training for Mr. Spurgeon in the event his physician decides to discharge him.

7 To what agencies could Mrs. Spurgeon go if she should have need for financial help?

SUGGESTED READINGS

Anderson, Helen C.: Newton's geriatric nursing, ed. 5, St. Louis, 1971, The C. V. Mosby Co.

Canady, Mary E.: SSPE—helping the family cope, American Journal of Nursing 72:94, January, 1972.

Carnes, G. D.: Understanding the cardiac patient's behavior, American Journal of Nursing 71:1187, June, 1971.

Conti, Mary L.: The loneliness of old age, Nursing Outlook 18:28, August, 1970.

Culbert, Pamela A., and Kos, Barbara A.: Aging: considerations for health teaching? Nursing Clinics of North America 6:605, December, 1971.

Dupuis, Pamela H.: Old is beautiful, Nursing Outlook 18:24, August, 1970.

Frenay, Sister Agnes C., and Pierce, Gloria L.: The climate of care for a geriatric patient, American Journal of Nursing 71:1747, September, 1971.

Gaspard, Nancy J.: The family of the patient with long-term illness, Nursing Clinics of North America 5:77, March, 1970.

Gress, Lucille D.: Sensitizing students to the aged, American Journal of Nursing 71:1968, October, 1971.

Hahn, Aloyse: It's tough to be old, American Journal of Nursing 70:1698, August, 1970.

Hutchins, Mary Helen: The geriatric patient: 'help me,' Nursing Clinics of North America 6:795, December, 1971.

Isler, Charlotte: New specialty: nursing in the extended-care facility, RN 31:30, June, 1968.

Larson, Laura G.: How to select a nursing home, American Journal of Nursing 69:1034, May, 1969.

Ornstein, Sheldon: Objective—a national policy on aging, American Journal of Nursing 71:960, May, 1971.

Roy, Sister Callista: Adaptation: a basis for nursing practice, Nursing Outlook 19:254, April, 1971.

Searcy, Laurel: Nursing care of the laryngectomy patient, RN 35:35, October, 1972.

Shepardson, Jan: A team approach to the patient with cancer, American Journal of Nursing 72:488, March, 1972.

Standards for geriatric nursing practice, American Journal of Nursing 70:1894, September, 1970.

Stone, Virginia: Give the older person time, American Journal of Nursing 69:2124, October, 1969.

Stuart, Sarah: Day-to-day living with diabetes, American Journal of Nursing **71**:1548, August, 1971.

Tyzenhouse, Phyllis: Care plans for nursing home patients, Nursing Outlook **20**:169, March, 1972.

Vincent, Pauline A.: Do we want patients to conform? Nursing Outlook **18**:54, January, 1970.

Walker, A. E.: Primex—the family nurse practitioner program, Nursing Outlook **20**:28, January, 1972.

Wang, Mamie, and Brayton, Robert: Health maintenance service for the high-risk chronically ill, Nursing Clinics of North America **5**:199, June, 1970.

Works, Roberta: Hints on lifting and pulling, American Journal of Nursing **72**:260, February, 1972.

Appendix

Common abbreviations

āā	of each (Greek, *ana*)
abd.	abdominal
A.B.R.	absolute bed rest
ac.	acid
a.c.	before meals
ad	to; up to
ad.	add
ad lib.	as desired
A-G	albumin-globulin (ratio)
A.H.A.	American Heart Association
alb.	albumin
alk.	alkaline
A.M., a.m.	antemeridian; ante meridiem; before noon
amp.	ampule
amt.	amount
A. & P.	auscultation and percussion; anterior and posterior
Aq., aq.	water
ax.	axillary
B.	bacillus
BCG	bacillus Calmette-Guérin
b.i.d.	twice a day
b.i.n.	twice a night
B.L.B.	Boothby, Lovelace, and Bulbulian
b.m.	bowel movement
B.M.R.	basal metabolism rate
B.P.	blood pressure
B.R.P.	bathroom privileges
B.T.	bedtime
BUN	blood urea nitrogen
C., c.	calorie; catheterized; gallon; 100; centigrade; colored
c,c̄,ċ,c̃	with (Latin, *cum*)
ca.	carcinoma
cap.	capsule
cath.	catheterized
C.B.C., c.b.c.	complete blood count
C.B.R.	complete bed rest
C.C.	chief complaint
c.c., cc.	cubic centimeter
Ck.	check
cm.	centimeter
C.N.S.	central nervous system
comp.	compound
C.S.	control station
C.S.R.	central supply room
C.T.	coated tablet
C.V.	cell volume
C.V.A.	cerebrovascular accident
d.	divorced; a dose

Common abbreviations, cont'd

D. & C.	dilation and curettage
dist.	distilled
diff.	differential count
dil.	dilute
disc.	discontinue
d.o.	right eye
D.O.A.	dead on arrival
dr.	dram
Dr.	doctor
D.W.	distilled water; dextrose in water
ECG	electrocardiogram
EEG	electroencephalogram
E.E.N.T.	eye, ear, nose, throat
EKG	electrocardiogram
elix.	elixir
1·2-3 en.	1 oz. Epsom salt, 2 oz. glycerin, 3 oz. hot-water enema
eos.	eosinophils, eosinophilic leukocyte
epith.	epithelial
E.R.	emergency room
et	and
etc.	and so on
ess.	essentially
exam.	examination
ext.	extract; external
F.	Fahrenheit; female
F. cath.	Foley catheter
fl., fld.	fluid
Ft.	make
ft.	foot
F.U.O.	fever of unknown origin
gal.	gallon
g.b.	gallbladder
GC.	*Gonococcus* (gonorrhea)
G.I.	gastrointestinal
Gm.	gram
gr.	grain
Gtt., gtt.	drop
g.u.	genitourinary
G. & W.	glycerin and water
G.W.	glucose in water
gyn.	gynecology
h.	hour
H. (H)	hypodermic
Hb., Hgb.	hemoglobin
HCT.	hematocrit
hr.	hour
h.s.	bedtime
H.T.	hypodermic tablet
ht.	height
h.w.b.	hot-water bottle
I.C.U.	intensive care unit
I.M.	intramuscularly
inf.	infusion
int.	internal
I.V.	intravenously
iss.	one and one-half
Kg., kg.	kilogram
kl.	kiloliter
K.U.B.	kidney, ureter, bladder
L.	liter; left
lab.	laboratory
lap.	laparotomy
lat.	lateral
lb.	pound
l'ft., L.	left
liq.	liquid
L.L.Q.	left lower quadrant
L.M.P.	last menstrual period
L.U.Q.	left upper quadrant
l. & w.	living and well
M.	male; meter; muscle; mix; one thousand
m.	married; in the morning (Latin, *mane*)
M., m.	meridian; noon
m., M., min.	minim
meg., μg.	microgram
mEq., meq.	milliequivalent
mg.	milligram
min.	minute
ml., mil.	milliliter
mm.	millimeter
m. & m.	milk and molasses
N.B.M.	nothing by mouth
neg.	negative
no.	number
N.P.N.	nonprotein nitrogen
N.P.O.	nothing by mouth
N.V.D.	nausea, vomiting, and diarrhea
O.	pint
O., o.	orally
OB.	obstetrics
occ.	occasional
o.d.	every day
O.D.	right eye

Common abbreviations, cont'd

oint.	ointment
Ol.	oil
o.m.	every morning
o.n.	every night
OPD	outpatient department
O.R.	operating room
os	mouth
O.S.	left eye
O.U.	both eyes together
oz.	ounce
palp.	palpable
P.B.I.	protein-bound iodine
p.c.	after meals
Ped.	pediatrics
P.E.G.	pneumoencephalogram
per	by
pH	potential of hydrogen, that is, hydrogen-ion concentration
P.H.	past history
P.I.	present illness
P.I.D.	pelvic inflammatory disease
Pil.	pill
P.M., p.m.	postmeridian; post meridiem; after noon
p.m.	post mortem; after death
P.O.	by mouth
p.o.	phone orders; postoperative
prep.	preparation
p.r.n.	whenever necessary
pt.	pint
pulv.	powder
q.	every
q.d	every day
q.h.	every hour
q.2h.	every 2 hours
q.3h.	every 3 hours
q.4h.	every 4 hours
q.i.d.	four times a day
q.n.	every night
q.o.d.	every other day
q.s.	sufficient quantity
qt.	quart
R.	roentgen; rate; rhythm
r.	rate; rectal; rhythm

R., r., rt.	right
R.B.C., r.b.c.	red blood count
Rh.	rhesus (monkey)
R.L.Q.	right lower quadrant
R.U.Q.	right upper quadrant
s, $\bar{s}$, $\dot{s}$, $\dot{\bar{s}}$	without (Latin, *sine*)
sat.	saturated
S.B.E.	subacute bacterial endocarditis
S.C.B.	strictly confined to bed
sed.	sedimentation
sep.	separated
Sig.	signify; write directions on medical package
S.O.B.	shortness of breath
Sol.	solution
solv.	dissolve
S.O.S.	if necessary, one dose only
sp.	spirits
spec.	specimen
sp. fl.	spinal fluid
sp. gr.	specific gravity
ss	one half
s.s.	soap solution
Stat., stat.	at once
Syr.	syrup
T. & A.	tonsillectomy and adenoidectomy
T.A.T.	tetanus antitoxin
tab.	tablet
T.b.	tubercule bacillus
Tbc.	tuberculosis
t.i.d.	three times a day
T.L.C.	tender loving care
T.P.R.	temperature, pulse, respiration
tr., tinct.	tincture
T.T.	triturate tablet
T.U.R.	transurethral resection
U.	unit
ung.	ointment
V., vol.	volume
vag.	vaginal
V.O.	verbal orders
w.	white
w.	widowed
W.B.C., w.b.c.	white blood count
w.d.	well developed
w.n.	well nourished
wt., W.	weight

Common drug abbreviations

ACTH	adrenocorticotropic hormone
A.S.	atropine sulfate
A.S.A.	acetylsalicylic acid (aspirin)
A.P.C.	aspirin, phenacetin, caffeine
B.S.P.	Bromsulphalein
D.D.T.	dichloro-diphenyl-tri-chloroethane
E.T.H.c. C.	elixir terpin hydrate with codeine
M.S.	morphine sulfate

N.P.H.	neutral protamine Hagedorn
N.S.	normal salt
N.S.S.	normal salt solution
PABA	para-aminobenzoic acid
PAS	para-aminosalicylic acid
Pot.	potassium
P.S.P.	phenolsulfonphthalein
P.Z.I.	protamine zinc insulin
Scop.	scopolamine
Sod. bicarb.	sodium bicarbonate
vit.	vitamin

Affixes

a-, an-	without, not
ab-	from
ad-	to, toward
adeno-	gland
adreno-	adrenal gland
-agogue	causes increased flow
-agra	seizure of pain
-algia	pain
ambi-	both
ambly-	dull, blunt
ambulo-	walk about
an-, a-	without, not
angio-	blood vessel
ante-	before
anti-	against
arthro-	joint
bacter-	bacteria
bi-	twice
bili-	bile
bio-	life
brady-	slow
cardio-	heart
cata-	down; destruction
-cele	protrusion, tumor; cavity
centi-	one one-hundredth
cephalo-	head
cerebro-	brain
chole-	gallbladder
chondro-	cartilage
-cide	kill
circum-	around
clin-	bed

col-	colon
colp-	vagina
con-, com-, co-	with, together
contra-, counter-	against
-cutaneous	skin
cysto-	urinary bladder
-cyte, cyto-	cell
de-	removal from
deci-	one tenth
deka-, deca-	ten
dent-, dento-	tooth
derma-, dermo-	skin
demi-	one half
di-	twice
dia-	through
diplo-	double
dolor-	pain
dorso-	back
dys-	difficult, bad
e-	from
ecto-	outside
-ectomy	removal of
-emia	blood condition
encephalo-	brain
endo-	interior
entero-	intestines
ento-	within, inner
ep-, epi-	upon
erythro-	red
eu-	normal, well
ex-	out
exo-	outside
extra-	in addition; outside

Affixes, cont'd

febri-	fever
fibro-	fibrous
gastro-	stomach
-genesis	origin
genu-	knee
gero-, geronto-	old age
glosso-	tongue
-gram	picture, mark
-graph	writing, instruments for writing
gravi-	pregnant
gust-	taste
hecto-	one hundred
helio-	sun
hem-, hema-, hem	blood
hemi-	half
hepato-, hepar-	liver
hetero-	other
histo-	tissue
homeo-	similar
homo-	same
hydra-, hydro-	water
hyper-	above
hypo-	beneath
hystero-	uterus
-iasis	morbid condition
-iatric	healing
-ic	pertaining to
idio-	self
il-	(see in-)
ileo-	ileum
ilio-	ilium, part of pelvis
im-	(see in-)
in-	in, into; not
infra-	below
inter-	between, among
intra-	within
ir-	(see in-)
ischio-	ischium, hip
ischo-, isch-	deficient, suppression
iso-	equal, same
-itis	inflammation of
juxta-	near
kilo-	thousand
klepto-	steal
labio-	lip
lacrim-	tears
laryngo-	layrnx
-lateral	side
leuko-	white
linguo-	tongue

lipo-	fat
litho-	stone
-logy	science of
lympho-	lymph
lyso-	dissovling
macro-	large; long
mal-	ill, bad
-mania	madness
manu-, mani-	hand
medio-	middle
medullo-	marrow; medulla
mega-, megal-	large
melano-	black; melanin
meningo-	meninges
meta-	change; beyond, abnormal
-meter, metr-	measure
-metra, metro-	uterus
micro-	microscope
milli-	one one-thousandth
mono-	single
multi-	many
my-	shut (*see also* myo-)
myco-, myceto-	condition caused by fungi
myo-, my-	muscle
myx-	mucus
naso-	nose
necro-	dead; corpse
neo-	new
nephro-	kidney
neur-	nerve
neutro-	neither
nevo-	birthmark
noct-	night
non-	not
noso-	disease
oculo-	eye
odyno-, odynia	pain
-oid	like, similar
-ol, oleo-	oil
oligo-	few, lack of
-ology	science of
-oma	tumor
oophoro-	ovary (egg-bearing)
ophthalmo-	eye
-opia	eye condition
oro-	oral
-orrh-	serum
ortho-	straight
-ose	sugar
-osis	disease, condition
osmo-	smell

Affixes, cont'd

osteo-	bone
-ostomy	artificial opening
oto-, ot-	ear
-otomy	incision
pan-	all
para-	beyond, beside, accessory to
par-, part-	give birth
-pathy	disease
-penia	lack, decrease of
peri-	around
-pexy	fixation
-phagia	eating condition
-phasia	speaking condition
-phil	love, affinity for
phlebo-	vein
-phobia	fear condition
-phone	instrument for transmitting sound
phono-	sound
photo-	light
phreno-	diaphragm; mind
phthisio-	wasting atrophy
physi-	nature
-plasty	shaping, repair
-plegia	stroke, paralysis
pleuro-	pleura
-pnea	breathing
pneumo-	lung; breath
-poiesis	making, formation
poly-	many, much
post-	after, following
pre-	before
presby-	old
primo-, primi-	first
pro-	forward, in front of
procto-	anus, rectum
pseudo-	false
-ptosis	dropping
pyelo-	pelvis
pyloro-	pylorus
pyo-	pus
pyreto-	fever
pyro-	fire, heat
quadr-	four
quinque-, quint-	five
re-	again, back
recto-	rectal

reni-	kidney
retro-	backward
-rhage, -orrhage	bursting forth (of bleeding)
-rhaphy, -orrhaphy	suturing
-rhea, -orrhea	discharge, flow
rhino-	nose
rubi-	redness
salpingo-	tube; fallopian tube
-sclerosis	hardening
-scope	instrument for viewing
-scopy	inspection
-section	cutting
semi-	one half
septi-, septic-	putrefying
septi-	seven
sphygmo-	pulse
spleno-	spleen
-stasis	standing still
stoma-	mouth
-stomy	artificial opening
sub-	inferior, below
super-	above, implying excess
supra-	above, over
sym-, syn-	with
tachy-	quick, fast
tacti-	touch
tensio-	stretch
tetra-	four
-therapy	treatment
thermo-	heat, hot
thrombo-	clot
-tomy	incision
torsi-	twist
tox-, toxico-	poison
trans-	across
tri-	three
ultra-	excess, beyond
un-	not
uni-	one
-uria	urine condition
vagino-	vagina
vago-, vagi-	wandering
verti-	turn
viru-	poison; virus
vit-	life
vox	voice
xero-	dryness

Chemical symbols and formulas

Carbon dioxide	CO_2	Potassium	K
Carbon monoxide	CO	Potassium iodide	KI
Hydrochloric acid	HCl	Potassium permanganate	$KMnO_4$
Magnesium sulfate	$MgSO_4$		
Mercury	Hg	Radioactive iodine	^{131}I
Nitrous oxide	N_2O	Sodium chloride	NaCl
Oxygen	O_2	Water	H_2O
Hydrogen peroxide	H_2O_2	Zinc oxide	ZnO

Symbols used in charting and laboratory reports

At	@	Number	#
Dram	ʒ	Male	♂
Female	♀	Ounce	℥
Large amount of	+ + + +	Recipe, take	℞
Moderate amounts	+ + +	Times	×
Small amount of	+	Micron	μ
		Microgram	μg

Apothecary-metric equivalents

Apothecary		Metric			Apothecary		Metric		
480 gr.	=	30 Gm.	=	30,000 mg.	$1/12$ gr.	=	0.005 Gm.	=	5 mg.
15 gr.	=	1 Gm.	=	1,000 mg.	$1/15$ gr.	=	0.004 Gm.	=	4 mg.
10 gr.	=	0.6 Gm.	=	600 mg.	$1/20$ gr.	=	0.003 Gm.	=	3 mg.
7 $1/2$ gr.	=	0.5 Gm.	=	500 mg.	$1/30$ gr.	=	0.002 Gm.	=	2 mg.
5 gr.	=	0.3 Gm.	=	300 mg.	$1/40$ gr.	=	0.0015 Gm.	=	1.5 mg.
3 gr.	=	0.2 Gm.	=	200 mg.	$1/50$ gr.	=	0.0012 Gm.	=	1.2 mg.
1 $1/2$ gr.	=	0.1 Gm.	=	100 mg.	$1/60$ gr.	=	0.001 Gm.	=	1.0 mg.
1 gr.	=	0.060 Gm.	=	60 mg.	$1/80$ gr.	=	0.0008 Gm.	=	0.8 mg.
$3/4$ gr.	=	0.05 Gm.	=	50 mg.	$1/100$ gr.	=	0.0006 Gm.	=	0.6 mg.
$2/3$ gr.	=	0.04 Gm.	=	40 mg.	$1/120$ gr.	=	0.0005 Gm.	=	0.5 mg.
$1/2$ gr.	=	0.03 Gm.	=	30 mg.	$1/150$ gr.	=	0.0004 Gm.	=	0.4 mg.
$3/8$ gr.	=	0.025 Gm.	=	25 mg.	$1/200$ gr.	=	0.00032 Gm.	=	0.3 mg.
$1/3$ gr.	=	0.02 Gm.	=	20 mg.	$1/250$ gr.	=	0.00025 Gm.	=	0.25 mg.
$1/4$ gr.	=	0.015 Gm.	=	15 mg.	$1/300$ gr.	=	0.0002 Gm.	=	0.2 mg.
		or		or	$1/400$ gr.	=	0.00015 Gm.	=	0.15 mg.
		0.016 Gm.	=	16 mg.			or		or
$1/5$ gr.	=	0.012 Gm.	=	12 mg.			0.00016 Gm.	=	0.16 mg.
$1/6$ gr.	=	0.01 Gm.	=	10 mg.	$1/500$ gr.	=	0.00012 Gm.	=	0.12 mg.
$1/8$ gr.	=	0.008 Gm.	=	8 mg.	$1/600$ gr.	=	0.0001 Gm.	=	0.1 mg.
$1/10$ gr.	=	0.006 Gm.	=	6 mg.					

gr. = grain; Gm. = gram; mg. = milligram.

Approximate equivalents for liquids

Household	Apothecary	Metric
1 drop	1 minim (♏)	0.060 ml.
1 teaspoonful	1 fluid dram (fl. dr.)	4 or 5 ml.
1 dessertspoonful	2 fluid drams	8 ml.
1 tablespoonful	4 fluid drams	15 ml.
1 ounce	480 minims	30 ml.
1 teacupful	6 fluid ounces (fl. oz.)	180 ml.
1 glassful	8 fluid ounces	240 ml.
2 glassfuls	1 pint	500 ml.
4 glassfuls	1 quart	1,000 ml.
16 glassfuls	1 gallon	4,000 ml.

Approximate equivalents for linear measures

English units	Metric equivalents
1 inch (in.)	2.5 centimeters (cm.); 25 millimeters (mm.); or 25,000 microns (μ)
1 foot (ft.)	30 centimeters or 3 decimeters (dm.)
1 yard (yd.)	0.9 meter (M.)
1 mile (mi.)	1.6 kilometers (km.)
0.6 mile	1 kilometer (1,000 M.)
39.4 inches or 1.1 yards	1 meter
4.0 inches	1 decimeter (10 cm.)
0.4 inch	1 centimeter (10 mm.)
0.04 or $1/25$ inch	1 millimeter
$1/25,000$ inch	1 micron (0.001 mm.)

Approximate equivalents for weights

Apothecary	Metric
1 grain (gr.)	0.060 Gm.
1 dram (dr.)	4 Gm.
1 ounce (oz.)	30 Gm.
1 pound (12 oz.)	360 Gm.

Note: 1 pound avoirdupois = 16 ounces; 1 kg. = 2.2 pounds avoirdupois.

Index

Italicized page numbers refer to illustrations.